Head and Neck Cancer Surgery: Advancements in Surgical Otolaryngology

Head and Neck Cancer Surgery: Advancements in Surgical Otolaryngology

Editor: Hugh Miller

MURPHY & MOORE
www.murphy-moorepublishing.com

www.murphy-moorepublishing.com

MURPHY & MOORE

Cataloging-in-Publication Data

Head and neck cancer surgery : advancements in surgical otolaryngology / edited by Hugh Miller.
p. cm.
Includes bibliographical references and index.
ISBN 978-1-63987-771-3
1. Head--Cancer--Diagnosis. 2. Head--Cancer--Treatment. 3. Neck--Cancer--Diagnosis.
4. Neck--Cancer--Treatment. I. Miller, Hugh.
RD661 .H43 2023
616.992 715--dc23

Murphy & Moore Publishing
1 Rockefeller Plaza,
New York City,
NY 10020, USA

ISBN 978-1-63987-771-3

Contents

Preface

The cancers which affect the throat, mouth, sinuses or nose are classified as head and neck cancers. There are various treatment options for this type of cancer such as surgery, radiation therapy, targeted therapy, immunotherapy and chemotherapy. Surgical treatment involves removing the cancerous tumor and some surrounding healthy tissue. One of the major advancements in head and neck cancer surgery is virtual surgical planning (VSP). It refers to a type of pre-operative planning technique that uses 3D imaging computer software to visualize a surgical procedure. 3D reconstruction of complex head and neck cancers can reveal crucial details like tumor location, range of invasion and blood supply. It also offers the possibility of preoperative simulation for complex defect repair. This book aims to shed light on some of the advancements in surgical otolaryngology related to head and neck cancer surgery. The readers would gain knowledge that would broaden their perspective in this area of medicine.

Significant researches are present in this book. Intensive efforts have been employed by authors to make this book an outstanding discourse. This book contains the enlightening chapters which have been written on the basis of significant researches done by the experts.

Finally, I would also like to thank all the members involved in this book for being a team and meeting all the deadlines for the submission of their respective works. I would also like to thank my friends and family for being supportive in my efforts.

Editor

1

Aesthetical and Accuracy Outcomes of Reconstruction of Maxillary Defect by 3D Virtual Surgical Planning

Yang Wang[1,2,3]*, Xingzhou Qu*[1,2,3]*, Junjian Jiang*[1,2,3]*, Jian Sun*[1,2,3]*, Chenping Zhang*[1,2,3] *and Yue He*[1,2,3]*

[1] *Department of Oral & Maxillofacial–Head & Neck Oncology, Shanghai Ninth People's Hospital, Shanghai Jiaotong University School of Medicine, Shanghai, China,* [2] *National Clinical Research Center for Oral Diseases, Shanghai Key Laboratory of Stomatology & Shanghai Research Institute of Stomatology, Shanghai, China,* [3] *Shanghai Key Laboratory of Stomatology, Shanghai Research Institute of Stomatology, Shanghai, China*

***Correspondence:**
Yue He
william5218@126.com

Background: Reconstruction of maxillary defect resulting from trauma or oncology surgery is of great importance for patients with physical and psychological complications. The virtual surgical planning (VSP) and 3D printing technics had been used in recent years which simplified the surgical procedure and promoted success and accuracy. To assess the accuracy and outcome of VSP surgery, here we report our experience in maxillary reconstruction retrospectively.

Method: Patients who received maxillary defect reconstruction from 2013 to 2020 were analyzed retrospectively. These patients were divided into two groups. Group 1 received VSP and 3D printed guiding plates in the surgery, while group 2 underwent free-hand surgery (FHS). Patients with different vertical and horizontal defects were classified according to Brown and Shaw classification. Clinical information and postoperative complications of all patients were collected. For patients with unilateral maxillary defect, orbit volume, orbit height, and the contour of the reconstructed side were compared with the normal side.

Result: Thirty-four patients who achieved the criteria were analyzed, of which 20 patients underwent VSP surgery. There were primary and secondary reconstruction cases in both two groups. Vascularized iliac crest flap was used in three cases, and fibula flap was performed in the other cases. One flap collapse occurred in FHS group. Seven patients in VSP group received dental implants, while the number in FHS group was 0. In vertical class III cases, the differences in orbit height (ΔD) and orbit volume (ΔV) between normal side and reconstructed side were measured and compared in the two groups. The mean ΔD is 1.78 ± 1.33 mm in VSP group and 4.25 ± 0.95 mm in FHS group, while the mean ΔV is 2.04 ± 0.85 cm^3 in VSP group and 3.25 ± 0.17 cm^3 in FHS group. The alterations of orbit height and volume in VSP group were much smaller than that in FHS group with statistical significance. From the perspective of aesthetics, the color-gradient map indicates a more symmetric and smoother curve of post-operation appearance in VSP group.

Conclusion: Compared with traditional free-hand surgical technics, VSP and 3D printing guiding plates can allow for a more accurate maxillary reconstruction with improved aesthetics.

Keywords: maxillary defect, virtual surgical planning (VSP), 3D printing, free flap, accuracy reconstruction

INTRODUCTION

The reconstruction of maxilla or midface with the rehabilitation of occlusion, speech, and normal vision was challenging in head and neck reconstructive surgery. Patients with maxillary defects usually suffered great psychological and physical trauma, compelling surgeons to try their best to achieve the ideal result of maxillary reconstruction. The optimal maxillary reconstruction includes separation of oral cavity and nasal cavity, rehabilitation of alveolar ridge and maxillary buttress, restoration of normal visual function, and satisfied soft tissue contour (1–3). With the development of microvascular surgery, several free flaps had been described for use in reconstruction of the maxillary defect, such as anterolateral thigh flap, scapular flap, fibula osteomyocutaneous flap, iliac crest flap, et al. (2–10).

In the past two decades, virtual surgical planning (VSP) had been developed to improve the surgical and anatomic accuracy, and consequently aesthetical appearance, vision function, and occlusion. Due to the high accuracy of VSP, surgical resections with good tumor margin control can be obtained during ablation (11–13), and the use of bone flap containing several segments can be possible and simplified. To assess the accuracy and outcome of VSP surgery, here we report our experience in maxillary reconstruction retrospectively, including traditional free-hand surgery (FHS) and VSP surgery. The facial appearance and reconstruction outcome of both groups were evaluated. The VSP surgery group exhibited better accuracy and improved satisfaction with appearance. Still there are some special considerations that need to be addressed.

TABLE 1 | Patient demography and clinical details.

Patient demography		VSP(N)	FHS(N)
Gender			
Male		14	9
Female		6	5
Age at surgery			
<20		3	0
20–40		11	8
40–60		6	6
Maxilla defect reason			
Malignant tumor		13	8
Benign tumor		6	5
Trauma		1	1
Stage			
Primary reconstruction		7	7
Secondary reconstruction		13	7
History of RT at surgery			
Yes		8	3
No		12	11
Brown's classification			
Vertical defect			
Class II		12	9
Class III		8	5
Horizontal defect			
Class b		12	9
Class c		2	2
Class d		6	3
Reconstructive technique			
Fibula free flap		17	14
Segments	1	0	1
	2	9	3
	3	7	9
	4	1	1
Vascularized iliac bone flap		3	0
Titanium mesh		4	3
PEEK		1	0
Recipient artery			
Superfacial temporal artery		16	7
Facial artery		3	6
Superior thyroid artery		1	1
Dental implant			
Yes		7 (35%)	0
No		13	14
Surgery complications			
Flap vascular crisis		3 (15%)	2 (14.3%)
Flap failure		0	1 (7.14%)
Inflammation		1 (5%)	2 (14.3%)
Exposure of titanium mesh or PEEK		3 (15%)	2 (14.3%)
Enophthalmos		3 (15%)	3 (21.4%)

PATIENT AND METHODS

Patients

From 2013 December to 2020 October, 34 patients undergoing maxillary reconstruction in Department of Oral & Maxillofacial–Head & Neck Oncology, Shanghai Ninth People's Hospital were incorporated, including 20 patients receiving operation with the use of VSP and three-dimension (3D) printing technics, and 14 patients received FHS. Clinical details are shown in **Table 1** and **Supplementary Table S1**. The maxillary vertical and horizontal defects were classified according to Brown's revised defect classification of maxilla and midface (14). Primary diagnosis result in the defect included malignant tumor, benign tumor, and trauma. Surgical techniques including donor site of flap, usage of titanium mesh or Polyetheretherketone (PEEK), and recipient artery were recorded. Complications and the treatment during follow-up were traced. Our study was approved by the Ethics Committee of Shanghai Ninth People's Hospital, Shanghai Jiao Tong University School of Medicine.

Virtual Surgical Planning and Surgical Techniques

All patients underwent preoperative computed tomography (CT) scans of craniofacial and lower extremities or pelvis. These CT images were converted into 3D virtual models, and surgical planning was performed using Mimics software

(Materialise, Leuven, Belgium). The 3D image of fibula or iliac crest free flap (ICFF) were superimposed onto the mirrored maxilla image reconstructed by the software, and osteotomies were performed in the digital fibula or ICFF so that the curve of the segments would match the contour of maxillary alveolar ridge and pterygomaxillary buttress (**Figure 1**).

Fibula flap was used in most cases for maxillary reconstruction. For Brown's class II vertical defects (**Figure 1D** and **Figure 2C**), the distal end of fibula bone graft was placed to the alveolar ridge according to the digital cutting plane, and the proximal end to pterygomaxillary cutting plane. So the vessel pedicle of fibula flap can traverse to anterior tragus area, and the anastomosis was accomplished with superficial temporal artery and vein. The reconstructed maxillary alveolar ridge was usually rehabilitated to the location of first molar, and another segment turned to form pterygomaxillary buttress in necessity.

For Brown's class III vertical defects, there were two strategies. One design strategy was just like what was used for class II defects (**Figures 1G, H**). Additionally, titanium mesh was used to form the floor of orbit and the infraorbital rim. Individualized titanium mesh was prebended according to the 3D model of reconstructed maxilla. Soft tissue like fat tissue of the skin paddle or part of flexor pollicis longus muscle should be placed around the titanium mesh to prevent its exposure. In terms of the other strategy (**Figures 1I, J**), the distal end of fibula bone graft was placed to form infraorbital margin, and the proximal part was shaped to form the alveolar

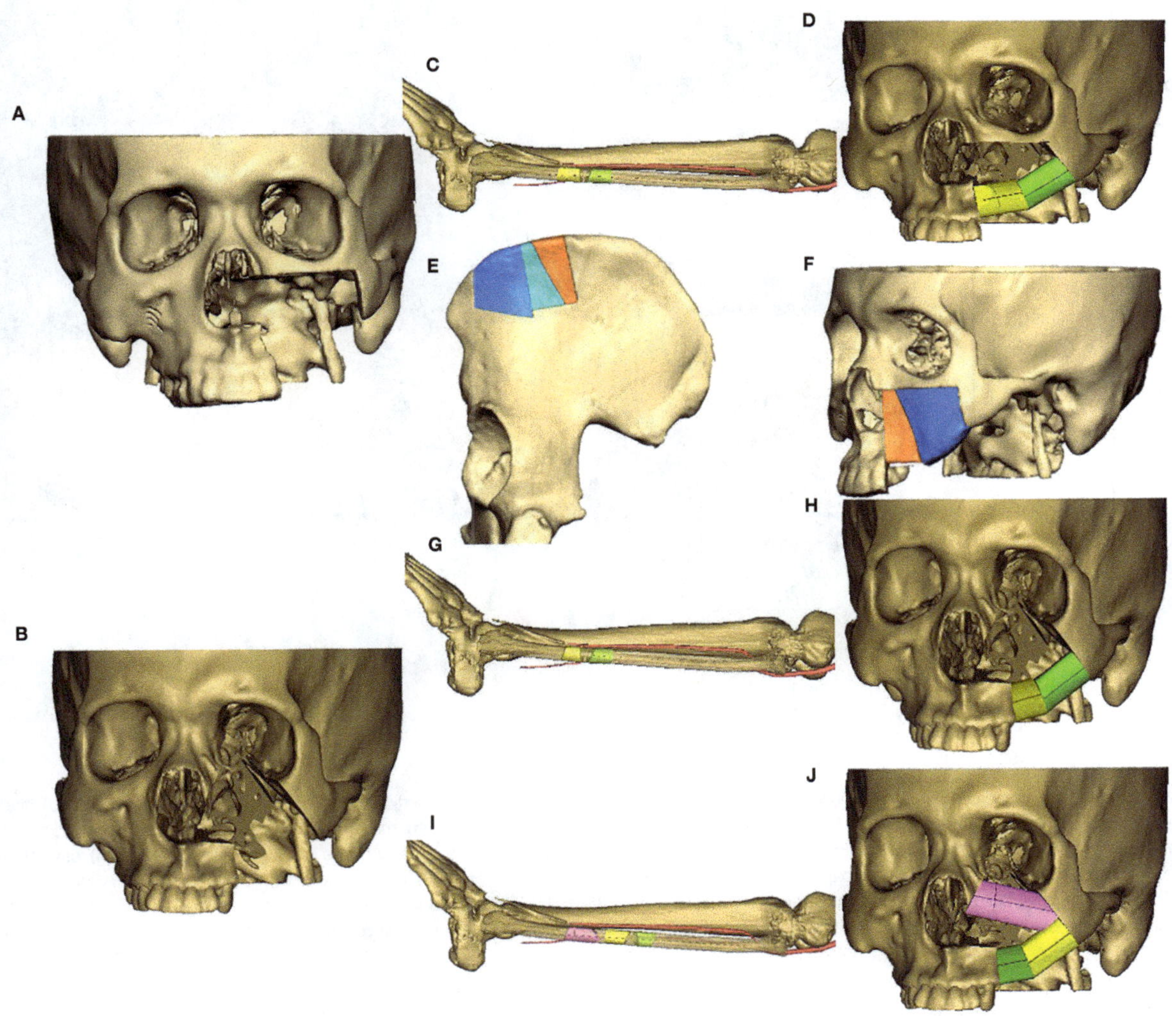

FIGURE 1 | Virtual surgical planning (VSP) strategy. **(A)** A virtual maxilla vertical defect of Class II; **(B)** a virtual maxilla vertical defect of Class III; **(C)** a virtual plan of osteotomy on fibula for defect in **(A)**, two segments were designed to render the curve of alveolar ridge and pterygomaxillary buttress; **(D)** virtual position of fibular segments according to defects in **(A, C)**; **(E)** a virtual plan of osteotomy on iliac crest for defect in **(A)**, osteotomies were performed to generate three segments, and the middle one was removed; **(F)** virtual position of ICFF segments according to defects in **(A, E)**; **(G)** a virtual plan of osteotomy on fibula for defect in **(B)**, two segments were designed to render the curve of alveolar ridge and pterygomaxillary buttress; **(H)** virtual position of fibular segments according to defects in **(B, G)**, titanium mesh was used to restore the infraorbital rim; **(I)** a virtual plan of osteotomy on fibula for defect in **(B)**, three segments were designed to render the curve of infraorbital rim, alveolar ridge and pterygomaxillary buttress; **(J)** virtual position of fibular segments according to defects in **(B, I)**.

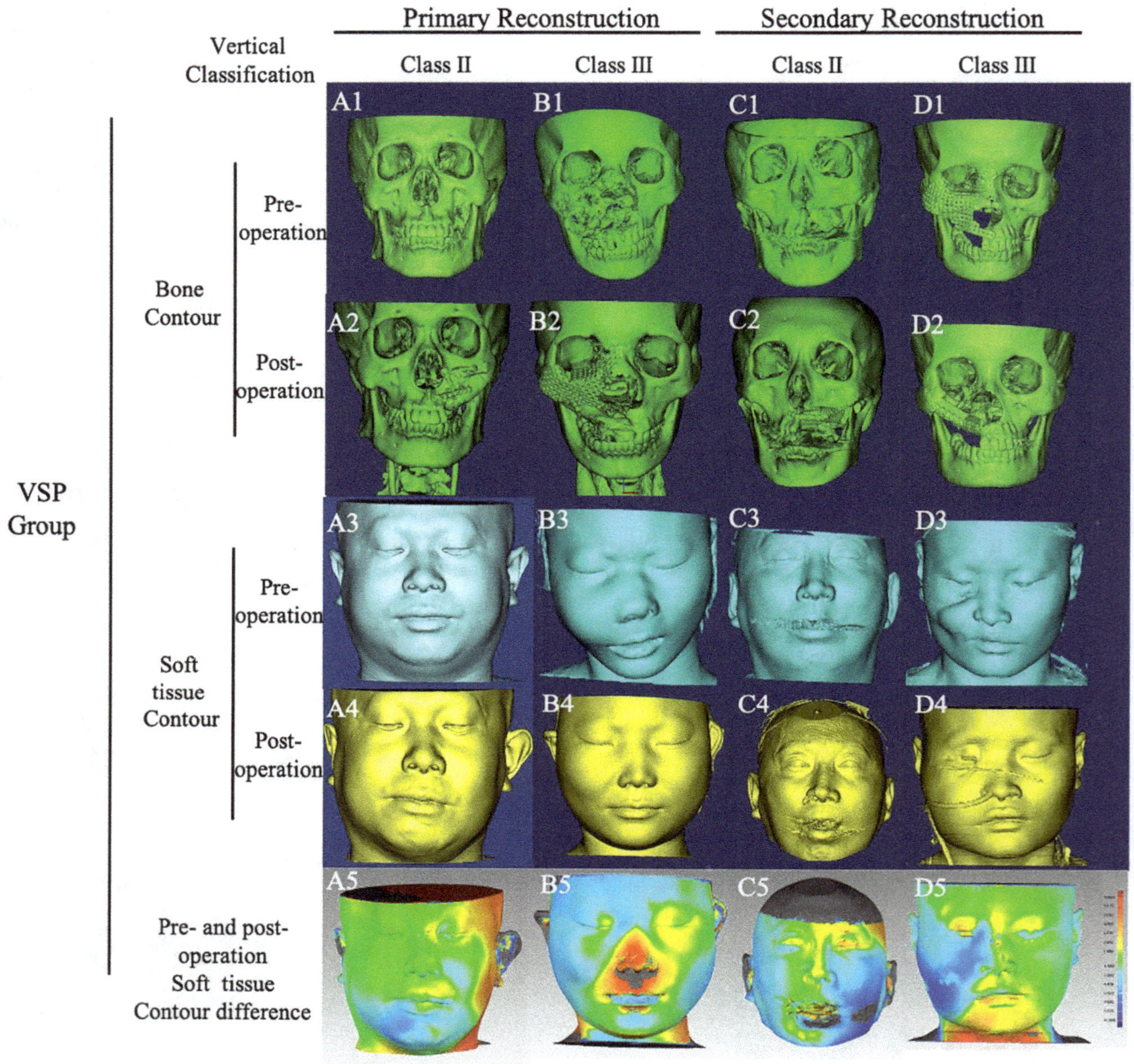

FIGURE 2 | Bone and soft tissue contour of cases in VSP group. Cases in VSP group were classified by vertical defect classification and surgery stage. CT images of all cases were converted into Mimics, and the bone and soft tissue contours were calculated. The color-gradient map indicating differences between mirrored symmetrical face and postoperative soft tissue contour was generated by Geomagic studio. Red color indicates ridge area, and blue indicates depressed area. **(A)**, case of primary reconstruction with vertical defect class II; **(B)**, case of primary reconstruction with vertical defect class III; **(C)**, case of secondary reconstruction with vertical defect class II; **(D)** case of secondary reconstruction with vertical defect class III. A1~A5, B1~B5, C1~C5, D1~D5 showed the pre-operation bone contour, post -operation bone contour, pre-operation soft tissue contour, post-operation soft tissue contour, pre-operation and post-operation soft tissue contour difference respectively.

ridge. In this case, the digital cutting plane of alveolar ridge was restricted posterior to canine; therefore, the vessel pedicle can traverse to submandibular area through a tunnel in buccal, and anastomosis was accomplished with facial artery and vein or others.

For cases using ICFF (**Figures 1E, F**), the surgical planning was performed as described before (15). Briefly, the contour of maxilla could be divided into two subunits of paranasal region and infraorbital region through a line segment from nasion to distal alveolar crest of maxillary second premolar. Osteotomies were performed in the bone graft of ICFF, and three segments were generated. The middle segment was removed, and the other two segments were spliced to match the curve of maxillary alveolar ridge and pterygomaxillary buttress. For Brown's class

III vertical defects, the floor of orbit and the infraorbital rim were established by bone graft of ICFF, too.

Special Surgical Technique

In FHS group, one case was graded class IIId (**Figure 3B**). To prevent enophthalmos, the anterior part of mandibular ramus including coracoid was cut off from sigmoid notch to retromolar area, with attachment of temporalis muscle. This pedicled bone graft was shaped and placed to form the floor of orbit (**Figure 3B2**). This technique was called coracoid-temporalis flap.

Reconstructive Accuracy Analysis

For cases classified as Brown's class III vertical defects, DICOM images of the postoperative CT scan were imported into Mimics software. Then a mask was established using bone tissue thresholds, and a 3D model was produced by calculation. In the frontier view, two lines were drawn as shown in **Figure 4A**.

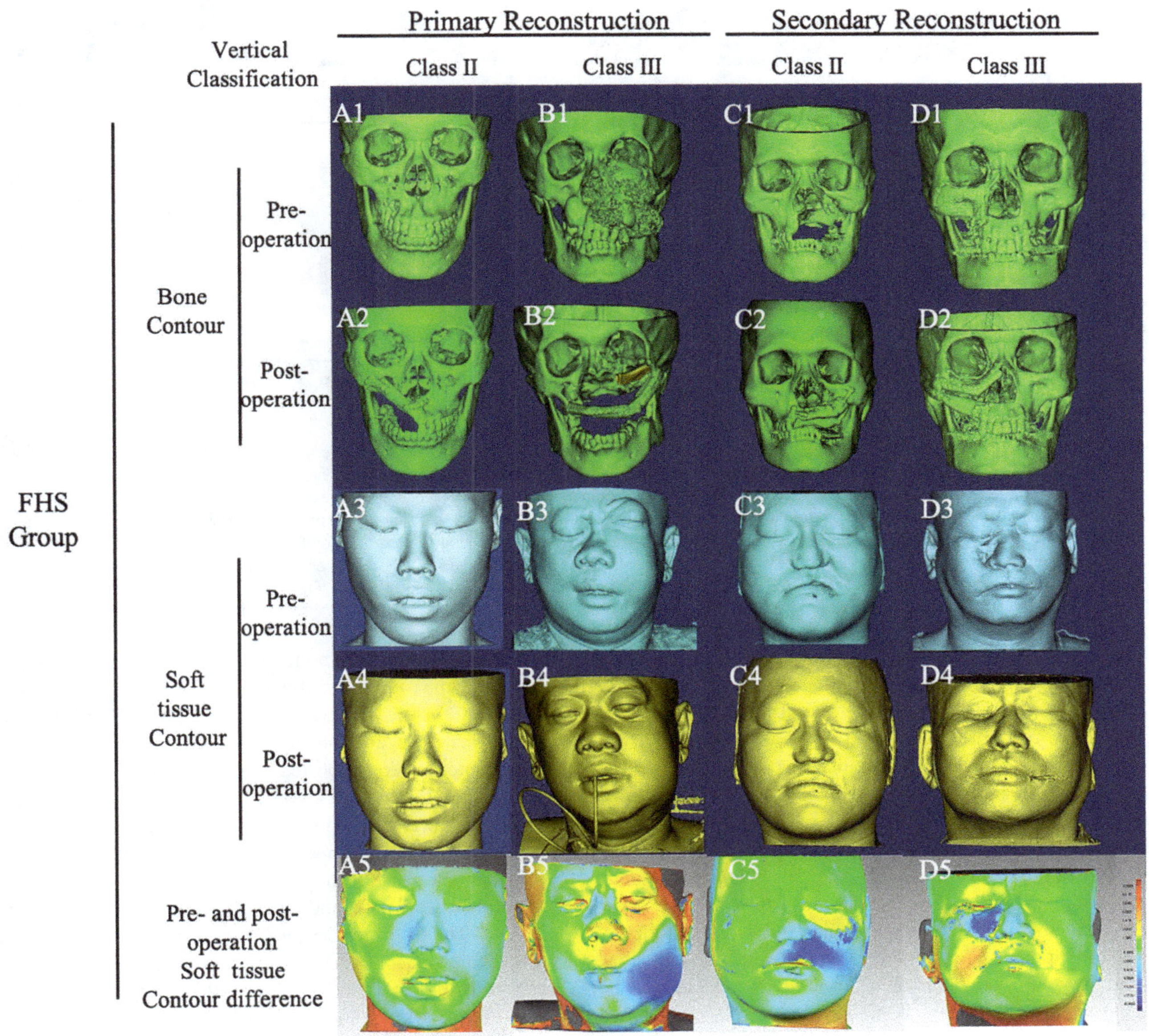

FIGURE 3 | Bone and soft tissue contour of cases in FHS group. Cases in FHS group were classified by vertical defect classification and surgery stage. CT images of all cases were converted into Mimics, and the bone and soft tissue contours were calculated. The color-gradient map indicating differences between mirrored symmetrical face and postoperative soft tissue contour was generated by Geomagic studio. Red color indicates ridge area, and blue indicates depressed area. **(A)**, case of primary reconstruction with vertical defect class II; **(B)**, case of primary reconstruction with vertical defect class III; **(C)**, case of secondary reconstruction with vertical defect class II; **(D)** case of secondary reconstruction with vertical defect class III. A1~A5, B1~B5, C1~C5, D1~D5 showed the pre-operation bone contour, post -operation bone contour, pre-operation soft tissue contour, post-operation soft tissue contour, pre-operation and post-operation soft tissue contour difference respectively.

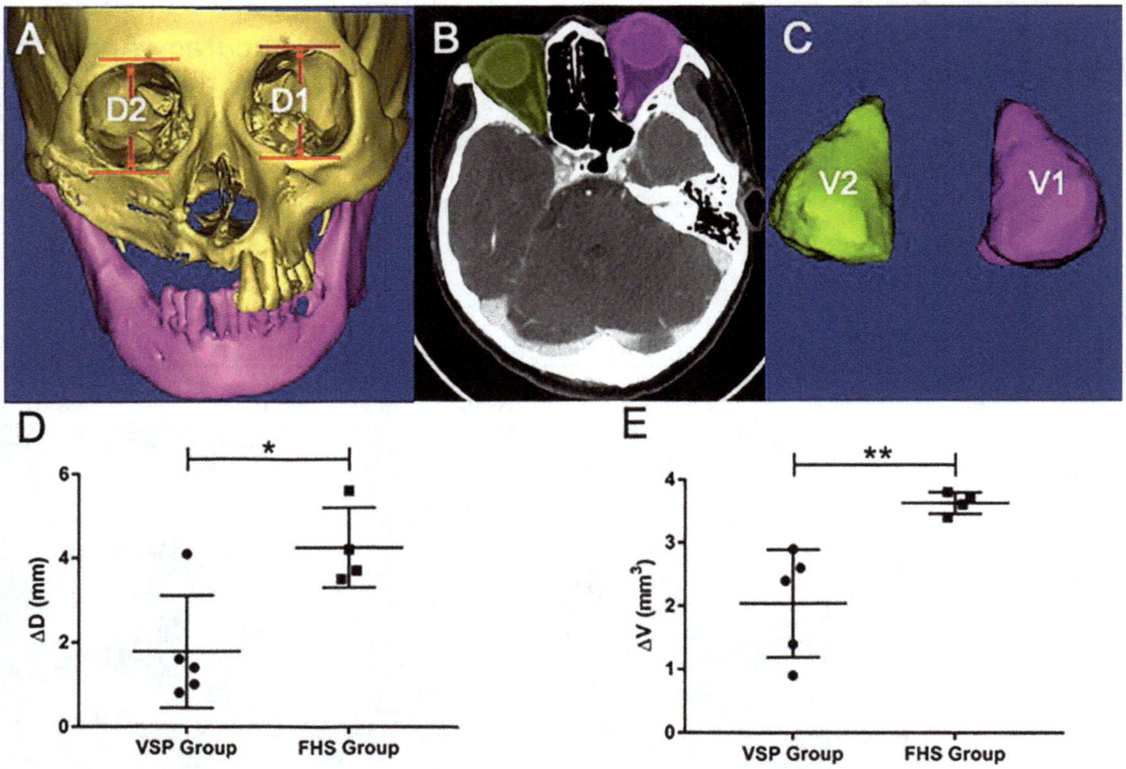

FIGURE 4 | Orbit height and orbital volume analysis in VSP and FHS group. **(A)** The definition of D1 and D2. In the frontier view, two lines were drawn. The upper line was horizontal to the lowest point of supraorbital margin, and the lower line was horizontal to the highest point of infraorbital margin. In the normal side, the vertical distance between these two lines was defined as D1. In the reconstructed side, the vertical distance was defined as D2; **(B)** the content of orbit was delineated in the normal side and reconstructed side; **(C)** the 3D model of orbital volume was established, the volume of normal orbit was defined as V1, and the volume of reconstructed orbit was defined as V2, which was calculated by Materialise Magics; **(D)** the absolute value of difference between (D1, D2) was defined as ΔD, which was analyzed in both VSP and FHS groups by two-tailed t test with statistical significance ($p<0.05$); **(E)** the absolute value of difference between V1 and V2 was defined as ΔV, which was analyzed in both VSP and FHS groups by two-tailed t test with statistical significance ($p<0.02$). *$p < 0.05$; **$p < 0.02$.

The upper line was horizontal to the lowest point of supraorbital margin, and the lower line was horizontal to the highest point of infraorbital margin. In the normal side, the vertical distance between these two lines was defined as D1. Accordingly, in the reconstructed side, the vertical distance was defined as D2. The absolute value of difference between D1 and D2 was defined as ΔD.

A new mask was established and the content of orbit was selected in all the slides (**Figure 4B**), then the 3D models of orbit were calculated (**Figure 4C**). The volume of the orbit 3D model was calculated using Materialise Magics software (Materialise, Leuven, Belgium). The volume of normal orbit was defined as V1, and the volume of reconstructed orbit was defined as V2. The absolute value of difference between V1 and V2 was defined as ΔV.

Both ΔD and ΔV were calculated in VSP group and FHS group. SPSS (Statistic Package for Social Sciences) 13.0 was used for data analysis. Two tailed t-test was used for statistical analysis.

Postoperative soft tissue contour of all case was analyzed using Geomagic studio software (Raindrop, USA) (**Figures 5, 6**). Subsequently, a mask was established using soft tissue thresholds, and a 3D model was generated by calculation. Using the mirror tool, a symmetrical face was obtained by mirroring to the normal hemiface. The.STL files of the symmetrical face and postoperative face exhibiting the soft tissue contour were imported into the software of Geomagic studio. The 3D models of symmetrical face and postoperative face were aligned with some anatomy landmarks, including nose, supraorbital and infraorbital line, zygoma, and midline. Then a color-gradient map showing differences in soft tissue contour of the reconstructed face and the contralateral normal side was obtained. The color-gradient maps were quantitatively analyzed using Geomagic control X (3D systems, USA). Four key points were set to analyze: Point1: midpoint of lower eyelid; Point 2: the cross point of ala nasi and nasofacial sulcus; Point 3: the point of philtrum; Point 4: point of mouth corner (**Figure 7**). The location of every point on the reconstructed face and the mirrored face was recorded as a three-dimensional coordinate, and the shift of every point was analyzed in X, Y, and Z axis, respectively. SPSS (Statistic Package for Social Sciences) 13.0 was used for data analysis. Two-tailed t-test was used for statistical analysis.

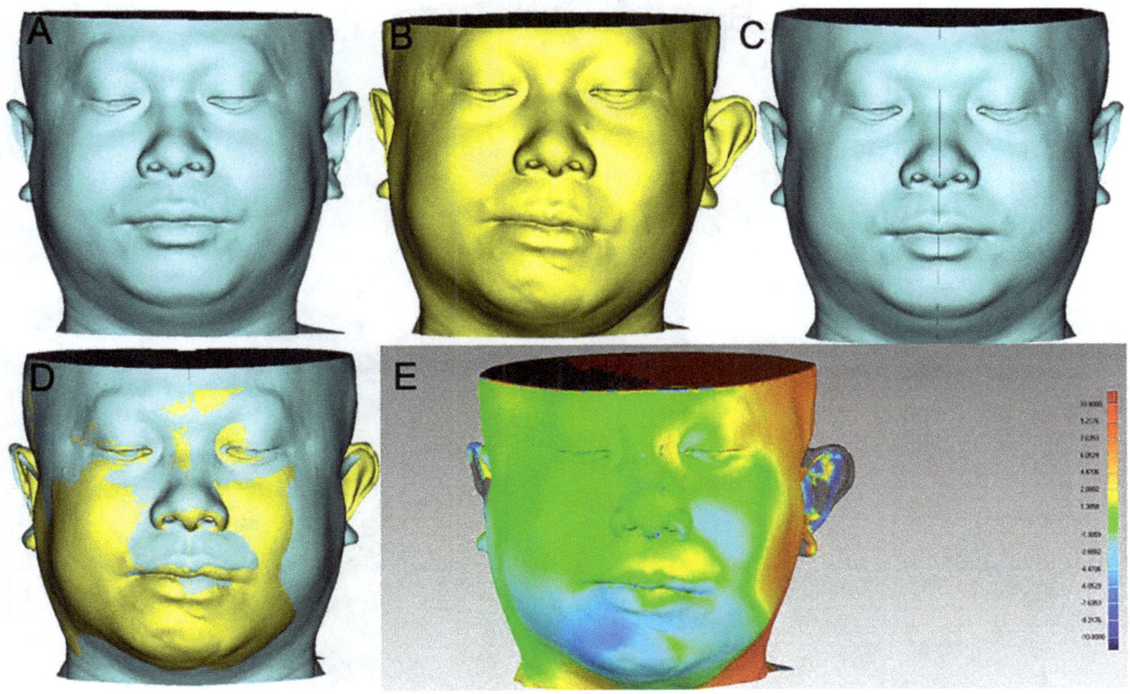

FIGURE 5 | Soft tissue contour of pre-operation and post-operation alignment in VSP group. **(A)** Pre-operation soft tissue contour; **(B)** post-operation soft tissue contour; **(C)** mirrored hemiface of normal side to form a symmetrical face; **(D)** post-operation soft tissue contour aligned with the symmetrical face in **(C)**; **(E)** the color-gradient map indicating the differences of soft tissue contour in **(D)**, red color indicates ridge area, and blue indicates depressed area.

RESULTS

Patient Demography

In the VSP group, there are 14 male and 6 female patients with the average age of 37.2 years (range from 12 to 52 years). Of the 20 subjects, 7 patients underwent primary reconstruction and 13 patients underwent secondary maxillary reconstruction. According to Brown's revised defect classification of maxilla and midface, cases in this study were classified upon vertical defect or horizontal defect. Eight cases had undergone radiation therapy at the time of reconstructive surgery. To reconstruct the defect, 17 cases were designed using fibula flap, and in the other cases, ICFF were carried out. During follow-up, seven patients got implant-anchored prosthesis.

In the FHS group, there are nine male and five female patients with the average age of 37.9 years (range from 25 to 58 years). Half of the patients underwent primary reconstruction, and the other half underwent secondary maxillary reconstruction. Among them, three patients had received radiotherapy at the time of reconstructive surgery. The vertical and horizontal defect was classified as described above. All cases of defect were repaired with fibula flap.

Comparison of perioperative characteristics including fibula segments, operation time, blood loss and transfusion, patient cost is shown in **Supplementary Table 1**. Two-tailed t-test was used for statistical analysis and showed no statistical significance between two groups.

Complications

In VSP group, titanium mesh was used in four cases to establish the floor of orbit and the infraorbital rim for class III vertical defect, while two cases, belonging to secondary maxillary reconstruction, exhibited exposure of the titanium mesh. Additional operation was performed to remove the mesh, and then enophthalmos developed. Temporalis muscle or free fat tissue transplantation was performed to improve the height of globe. The infraorbital rim was not settled up in only one case showing enophthalmos. In the VSP group, flap vascular crisis occurred in three cases, and all flaps were rescued.

In the FHS group, titanium mesh was used in three cases and exposed in two cases of class III vertical defect. In one case of class IIId (**Figure 3B**), the anterior part of mandibular ramus including coracoid was cut off from sigmoid notch to retromolar area, with attachment of temporalis muscle. This pedicled bone graft was shaped and placed to form the floor of orbit, and enophthalmos was prevented, while infraorbital rim was depressed yet. In the FHS group, flap vascular crisis occurred in two cases, and one of them was not rescued.

Reconstructive Accuracy Analysis

The bone and soft tissue contour of all patients were established and classified according to the vertical defect classification, and the corresponding primary or secondary reconstruction was shown in **Figures 2, 3**. For the aesthetical assessment, color-gradient map indicating the soft tissue contour difference was

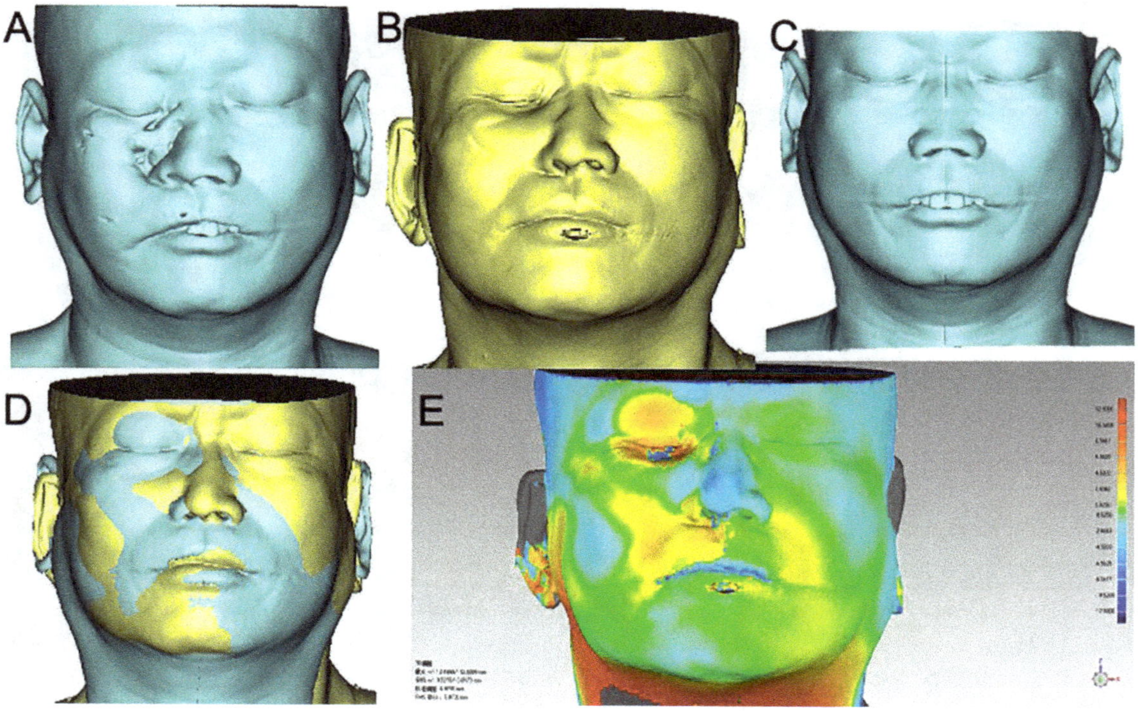

FIGURE 6 | Soft tissue contour of pre-operation and post-operation alignment in FHS group. **(A)** Pre-operation soft tissue contour; **(B)** post-operation soft tissue contour; **(C)** mirrored hemiface of normal side to form a symmetrical face; **(D)** post-operation soft tissue contour aligned with the symmetrical face in **(C)**; **(E)** the color-gradient map indicating the differences of soft tissue contour in **(D)**, red color indicates ridge area, and blue indicates depressed area.

performed in cases of both VSP and FHS group. The typical cases of two groups are exhibited in **Figures 5, 6**, respectively. In case of FHS group, the differences in area of infraorbital rim and the maxillary alveolar ridge were much bigger than that of case in VSP group, exhibiting larger area of orange and blue. In the VSP group, **Figure 2A** shows that a case of vertical class II reconstructed with ICFF exhibited a uniform change in the infraorbital region, and **Figure 2B** shows that a case of vertical class III reconstructed with fibula flap and titanium mesh exhibited better contour of infraorbital rim than the cases without titanium mesh as shown in **Figures 2D** and **3B**. For secondary reconstruction, cases in VSP group had smoother curve in the reconstructed region, whereas cases in FHS group showed some point with deep blue indicating obviously depressed surface. In vertical class III cases, the differences in orbit height (ΔD) and orbit volume (ΔV) between normal side and reconstructed side were measured and analyzed by t-test, the result of which is listed in **Table 2**. Mean ΔD is 1.78 ± 1.33 mm in VSP group and 4.25 ± 0.95 mm in FHS group, while mean ΔV is 2.04 ± 0.85 cm^3 in VSP group and 3.25 ± 0.17 cm^3 in FHS group. The differences in VSP group were significantly smaller than that in FHS group (**Figures 4D, E**).

The results of quantitative analysis of soft tissue appearance of reconstructed face are shown in **Table 3**. The distance shift in Z axis of Point 1 (midpoint of lower eyelid) and Point 4 (point of mouth corner) had statistical significance indicating more accurate of the reconstructed appearance.

DISCUSSION

The maxillectomy usually produces complex defect involving several structures, like tooth-bearing alveolar, nasal cavity, orbit cavity, palate, etc. Bone reconstruction was recommended for the defect higher than class II according to the Brown's vertical classification, while class I vertical defect was usually repaired by prosthesis (14). The complexity of maxillary reconstruction lends itself well to VSP surgery, which streamlines the shape of bone graft and improves the surgical and anatomical accuracy.

In VSP surgery, with the mirror function of the software, the images of contralateral normal maxilla were superimposed over the asymmetric flap side. The virtual plan and the bony framework were determined according to the mirrored normal maxilla to achieve a symmetric contour. With the introduction of 3D printing models and fabrication of surgical guides, complex resections can be planned preoperatively. In the reconstruction process, custom-made cutting guides helped to decide location and angulation of osteotomies, and the reposition guides determined precise position of the bone graft conducive for prosthesis rehabilitation. Studies analyzed vertical and horizontal changes between bone graft and normal side had demonstrated the better accuracy of VSP than FHS or traditional surgery (16–19). In our study, similar conclusion was obtained by comparing the orbit height and orbit volume in vertical defect Class III cases. More similar of orbit height and orbit volume in the reconstructed side indicated better sight function. And as

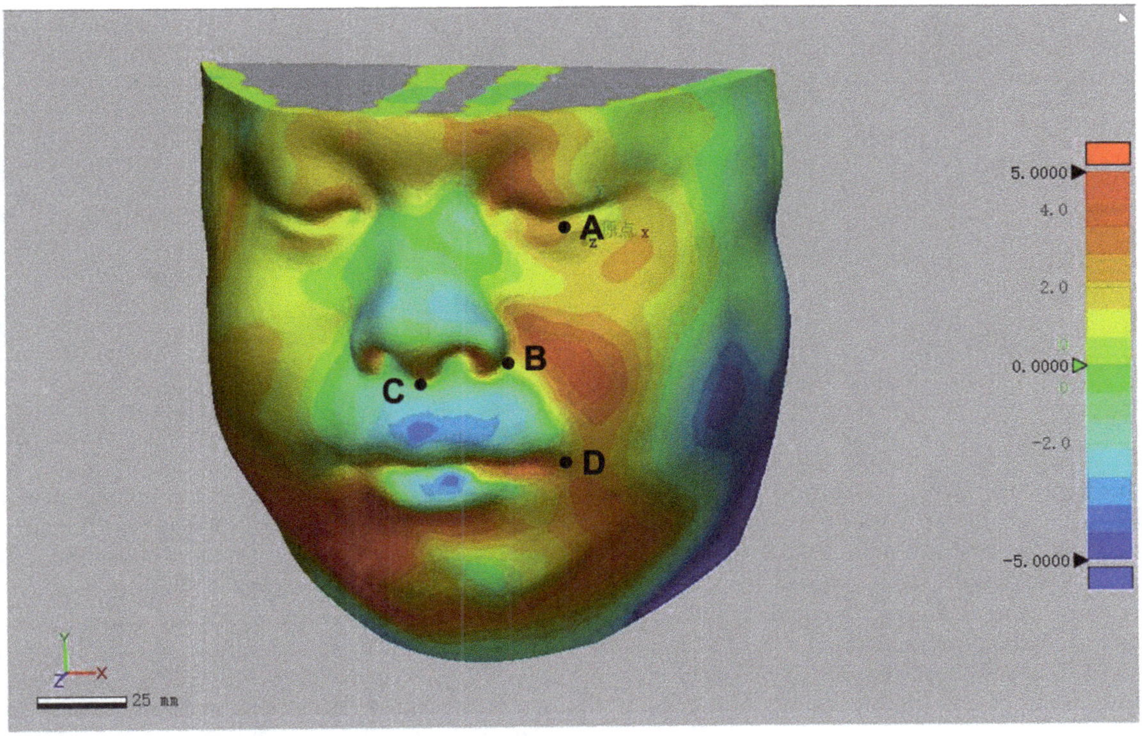

FIGURE 7 | Quantitative analysis of soft tissue appearance of reconstructed face. **(A)** Point 1: midpoint of lower eyelid; **(B)** point 2: the cross point of ala nasi and nasofacial sulcus; **(C)** point 3: the point of philtrum; **(D)** point 4: point of mouth corner.

shown in **Table 1**, seven cases in VSP group got implant denture, while no one in FHS group got prosthesis rehabilitation.

Complication comparation between two groups revealed a higher rate of complication in FHS groups (10/14). The other comparison of operation time, blood loss and transfusion, patient cost revealed no statistical difference in two groups, too, indicating that application of virtual surgical plan and 3D print in maxillary reconstruction was safe and economical and acceptable with better result.

To achieve the ideal goal of maxillary reconstruction, several variants of forearm flap, anterolateral thigh flap, fibula flap, scapular flap, and iliac crest free flap had been described. The fibular flap may be harvested as osseous flap, or chemical flap with muscle or muscle and skin paddle allowing to repair multi-kind of potential defects. And fibula flap usually provides a bone graft longer than 20 cm, which can be osteotomized into multiple segments (20, 21). Proper osteotomy makes the curve of fibula bone graft align well to the alveolar arch and maxillary buttress. The drawback of fibula flap was obvious that the width of the bone, 10 to 15 mm, was not enough for high maxillectomy defect. For class III vertical defects, titanium mesh or artificial-like specified PEEK should be installed combined with fibula bone graft. However, in secondary reconstruction, especially in cases with a history of radiation therapy, exposure of titanium mesh or artificial happened frequently. In our research, exposure of titanium mesh or PEEK occurred in three cases of VSP group and two cases of FHS group. In this situation, soft tissue like fat tissue of the skin paddle or flexor pollicis longus muscle is needed

TABLE 2 | Orbit height and orbital volume analysis in VSP and FHS group.

Group	D1(mm)	D2(mm)	ΔD=|D1−D2|(mm)	ΔD(mean ± SD)	V1(cm^3)	V2(cm^3)	ΔV=|V1−V2|(cm^3)	ΔV(mean ± SD)
VSP Group	35.9	40	4.1	1.78 ± 1.33	29.1	31.7	2.6	2.04 ± 0.85
	39.5	38.7	0.8		31.7	29.3	2.4	
	35.9	37.2	1		31.1	30.2	0.9	
	39.5	34	1.6		36.9	35.5	1.4	
	37.2	36.2	1.4		23.4	20.5	2.9	
FHS Group	39	43.2	4.2	4.25 ± 0.95	30.7	34.3	3.6	3.625 ± 0.17
	34.2	39.8	5.6		31.2	34.6	3.4	
	35.7	37.4	3.7		38	34.2	3.8	
	39.1	42.6	3.5		35.1	31.4	3.7	

TABLE 3 | Quantitative analysis of soft tissue appearance of reconstructed face.

Point	Point shift distance (mm, mean ± SD)			P-value
	Axis	VSP	FHS	
Point1	X	0.3232 ± 0.3474	0.6635 ± 0.3167	0.0577
	Y	0.2646 ± 0.3392	0.4176 ± 0.4272	0.4103
	Z	1.2363 ± 0.8999	3.5575 ± 1.7475	**0.0012**
Point2	X	0.7241 ± 0.6503	0.4945 ± 0.4507	0.4477
	Y	0.3079 ± 0.2923	0.1984 ± 0.2720	0.4491
	Z	1.3739 ± 0.5251	1.5446 ± 1.5356	0.7181
Point3	X	0.0966 ± 0.0841	0.1298 ± 0.1868	0.5933
	Y	0.4563 ± 0.5003	0.3025 ± 0.2453	0.4892
	Z	0.981 ± 0.8027	0.5656 ± 0.6026	0.2770
Point4	X	1.2703 ± 0.7117	1.6929 ± 2.4254	0.5613
	Y	1.2482 ± 0.7419	1.5368 ± 1.1510	0.5164
	Z	1.5765 ± 0.7210	3.0753 ± 2.5003	**0.0340**

Significant P values bolded.

to insert between the recipient skin and titanium mesh. Alternatively, double barrel of fibula bone graft can be taken into consideration. Just as shown in **Figure 3D**, the infraorbital rim and alveolar arch were both restored by bone tissue, exhibiting a good contour of bony framework. But the soft tissue contour showed a depressed area between this two-layer bone graft, which reduced aesthetics. The ICFF comes to be a better choice.

The ICFF, as described by Taylor, Sanders, and Mayou (22, 23), has demonstrated considerable utility in midface reconstruction when used as either an osseous, osteocutaneous, or osteomyocutaneous composition. ICFF provides a bulky bone graft of about 9 cm in length, which is enough for a hemimaxilla reconstruction, and 4 cm in height, which is enough for repairing a class III vertical defect. The iliac crest bone graft can be shaped to conform to the contour of infraorbital rim. Otherwise, the combination of ICFF with titanium mesh, if needed, prevents the exposure of titanium mesh. The iliac crest bone graft was a whole piece in vertical, which is another advantage of ICFF, preventing the depressed soft tissue contour as mentioned before in **Figure 3D**. In the situation of bulky soft tissue defect, ICFF can be raised with the internal oblique, assisting line oral cavity and nasal cavity wound. Furthermore, the caliber of the vessel pedicle of ICFF, the deep iliac circumflex artery (DCIA), is consistent with superficial temporal artery. Thus, adoption of ICFF for maxillary reconstruction should be considered and popularized in clinical practice.

Numerous researches before focused on the bone framework and the accuracy of bone graft position in VSP surgery, and the advantage of virtual surgery planning in modeling bone framework was obvious, but in terms of appearance or soft tissue contour, VSP was not always that useful. In our research we reported the soft tissue contour analysis and suggested that "Bone is bone, soft tissue is independent". To achieve aesthetical results, more attention should be given to soft tissue reconstruction, especially in some secondary reconstruction cases. For secondary reconstruction, the soft tissue defect is usually more complex than bone defects because of scar contracture deformities or stiffness caused by radiation therapy, limiting the applicability of VSP in real clinical practice. In our study, the exposure and inflammation of titanium mesh was not rare in VSP group. Titanium mesh was used in four cases, and two cases of secondary reconstruction exhibited titanium mesh exposure (**Table 1**). For secondary cases of class III vertical defect, soft tissue surrounding infraorbital region collapsed at varying degrees. When the contracture tissue was released completely with Weber-Fergusson incision, titanium mesh increased tension of the suture. The artificial infraorbital rim shaped by the titanium mesh overlapped with the incision, increasing the possibility of titanium mesh exposure greatly. Therefore, additional soft tissue was needed to cover the mesh, especially in cases after radiation therapy. In the case of complications of the exposed mesh, a secondary operation was performed to remove the mesh while transferring fat or pedicled muscle to prevent enophthalmos. The strategy that combines one-layer fibular bone graft and titanium mesh had been abandoned for reconstruction of class III vertical defect. Butterwort and Rogers reported a method of zygomatic implant perforated microvascular soft tissue flap (ZIP) to repair maxillary defect (24). For cases with bulky soft tissue deficit, using ZIP to fill the defect with soft tissue and rehabilitate occlusion by zygomatic implants, improved the quality of life, which could be taken into consideration.

Our research retrospectively analyzed 34 cases of maxillary reconstruction and proved the safety, accuracy, and functionality of virtual surgery *versus* traditional free-hand surgery. However, limitations remain in the application and the ultimate outcomes. For example, the application of virtual surgical plan and custom-made cutting guide simplified the bone framework modeling and positioned the bone graft precisely, but errors still occurred at the time of titanium plate shaping and fixation, for example. In this situation, introducing a navigation system that can discover the errors during surgery contributes to improve the outcomes. Also, we focused on the soft tissue appearance after surgery and revealed that soft tissue contour was an independent topic and should be taken into consideration. As the development of surgery planning software, we expect the utilization of soft tissue planning in software. Further study in maxillary reconstruction could focus on occlusion rehabilitation, combination of virtual surgical plan and navigation, aesthetical soft tissue reconstruction, etc., to resolve the limitation of this research.

CONCLUSION

VSP surgery and 3D printing techniques helped to improve accuracy and precise rehabilitation of normal contour, especially in bone framework. But soft tissue appearance was not always reflected by the bone contour, suggesting flexible treatment strategies to suit particular circumstance. In addition, the virtual planning of soft tissue reconstruction deserves further investigation.

ETHICS STATEMENT

The studies involving human participants were reviewed and approved by the Ethics Committee of Shanghai Ninth People's Hospital, Shanghai Jiao Tong University School of Medicine. Written informed consent from the participants' legal guardian/next of kin was not required to participate in this study in accordance with the national legislation and the institutional requirements. Written informed consent was obtained from the individual(s) for the publication of any potentially identifiable images or data included in this article.

AUTHOR CONTRIBUTIONS

YW drafted the manuscript. XQ and JJ analyzed data. JS and CZ revised the paper. YH conceived the study design. All authors contributed to the article and approved the submitted version.

SUPPLEMENTARY MATERIAL

Supplementary Table 1 | Comparison of perioperative characteristics.

REFERENCES

1. Triana RJ Jr, Uglesic V, Virag M, Varga SG, Knezevic P, Milenovic A, et al. Microvascular Free Flap Reconstructive Options in Patients With Partial and Total Maxillectomy Defects. *Arch Facial Plast Surg* (2000) 2(2):91–101. doi: 10.1001/archfaci.2.2.91
2. Sun J, Shen Y, Li J, Zhang ZY. Reconstruction of High Maxillectomy Defects With the Fibula Osteomyocutaneous Flap in Combination With Titanium Mesh or a Zygomatic Implant. *Plast Reconstr Surg* (2011) 127(1):150–60. doi: 10.1097/PRS.0b013e3181fad2d3
3. Futran ND, Wadsworth JT, Villaret D, Farwell DG. Midface Reconstruction With the Fibula Free Flap. *Arch Otolaryngol Head Neck Surg* (2002) 128 (2):161–6. doi: 10.1001/archotol.128.2.161
4. Kildal M, Wei FC, Chang YM. Free Vascularized Bone Grafts for Reconstruction of Traumatic Bony Defects of Mandible and Maxilla. *World J Surg* (2001) 25(8):1067–74. doi: 10.1007/s00268-001-0060-1
5. Ferri J, Caprioli F, Peuvrel G, Langlois JM. Use of the Fibula Free Flap in Maxillary Reconstruction: A Report of 3 Cases. *J Oral Maxillofac Surg* (2002) 60(5):567–74. doi: 10.1053/joms.2002.31857
6. Bianchi B, Ferri A, Ferrari S, Copelli C, Boni P, Sesenna E. Iliac Crest Free Flap for Maxillary Reconstruction. *J Oral Maxillofac Surg* (2010) 68(11):2706–13. doi: 10.1016/j.joms.2010.01.008
7. Swartz WM, Banis JC, Newton ED, Ramasastry SS, Jones NF, Acland R. The Osteocutaneous Scapular Flap for Mandibular and Maxillary Reconstruction. *Plast Reconstr Surg* (1986) 77(4):530–45. doi: 10.1097/00006534-198604000-00003
8. Bianchi B, Ferri A, Ferrari S, Copelli C, Sesenna E. Maxillary Reconstruction Using Anterolateral Thigh Flap and Bone Grafts. *Microsurgery* (2009) 29 (6):430–6. doi: 10.1002/micr.20619
9. Trosman SJ, Haffey TM, Couto RA, Fritz MA. Large Orbital Defect Reconstruction in the Setting of Globe-Sparing Maxillectomy: The Titanium Hammock and Layered Fibula Technique. *Microsurgery* (2018) 38(4):354–61. doi: 10.1002/micr.30199
10. Cordeiro PG, Chen CM. A 15-Year Review of Midface Reconstruction After Total and Subtotal Maxillectomy: Part II. Technical Modifications to Maximize Aesthetic and Functional Outcomes. *Plast Reconstr Surg* (2012) 129(1):139–47. doi: 10.1097/PRS.0b013e318221dc60
11. Kraeima J, Dorgelo B, Gulbitti HA, Steenbakkers RJHM, Schepman KP, Roodenburg JLN, et al. Multi-Modality 3D Mandibular Resection Planning in Head and Neck Cancer Using CT and MRI Data Fusion: A Clinical Series. *Oral Oncol* (2018) 81:22–8. doi: 10.1016/j.oraloncology.2018.03.013
12. Kraeima J, Schepers RH, van Ooijen PM, Steenbakkers RJ, Roodenburg JL, Witjes MJ. Integration of Oncologic Margins in Three-Dimensional Virtual Planning for Head and Neck Surgery, Including a Validation of the Software Pathway. *J Craniomaxillofac Surg* (2015) 43(8):1374–9. doi: 10.1016/j.jcms.2015.07.015
13. Witjes MJH, Schepers RH, Kraeima J. Impact of 3D Virtual Planning on Reconstruction of Mandibular and Maxillary Surgical Defects in Head and Neck Oncology. *Curr Opin Otolaryngol Head Neck Surg* (2018) 26(2):108–14. doi: 10.1097/MOO.0000000000000437
14. Brown JS, Shaw RJ. Reconstruction of the Maxilla and Midface: Introducing a New Classification. *Lancet Oncol* (2010) 11(10):1001–8. doi: 10.1016/S1470-2045(10)70113-3
15. Miao Yu, Huishan W, Jing H, Longwei Hu, Jiannan L, Yang W, et al. Two Subunit Osteotomy Approach of Vascularized Iliac-Internal Oblique Muscle Composite Flap in Total Maxillary Reconstruction. *China J Oral Maxillofac Surg* (2016) 14(5):430–4.
16. Zhang WB, Wang Y, Liu XJ, Mao C, Guo CB, Yu GY, et al. Reconstruction of Maxillary Defects With Free Fibula Flap Assisted by Computer Techniques. *J Craniomaxillofac Surg* (2015) 43(5):630–6. doi: 10.1016/j.jcms.2015.03.007
17. Zheng GS, Wang L, Su YX, Liao GQ, Zhang SE, Lao XM. Maxillary Reconstruction Assisted by Preoperative Planning and Accurate Surgical Templates. *Oral Surg Oral Med Oral Pathol Oral Radiol* (2016) 121(3):233–8. doi: 10.1016/j.oooo.2015.10.010
18. Swendseid BP, Roden DF, Vimawala S, Richa T, Sweeny L, Goldman RA, et al. Virtual Surgical Planning in Subscapular System Free Flap Reconstruction of Midface Defects. *Oral Oncol* (2020) 101:104508. doi: 10.1016/j.oraloncology.2019.104508
19. Navarro Cuéllar C, Martínez EB, Navarro Cuéllar I, López López AM, Rial MT, Pérez AS, et al. Primary Maxillary Reconstruction With Fibula Flap and Dental Implants: A Comparative Study Between Virtual Surgical Planning and Standard Surgery in Class IIC Defects. *J Oral Maxillofac Surg* (2021) 79 (1):237–48. doi: 10.1016/j.joms.2020.08.003
20. Wijbenga JG, Schepers RH, Werker PM, Witjes MJ, Dijkstra PU. A Systematic Review of Functional Outcome and Quality of Life Following Reconstruction of Maxillofacial Defects Using Vascularized Free Fibula Flaps and Dental Rehabilitation Reveals Poor Data Quality. *J Plast Reconstr Aesthet Surg* (2016)

69(8):1024–36. doi: 10.1016/j.bjps.2016.05.003

21. Lenox ND, Kim DD. Maxillary Reconstruction. *Oral Maxillofac Surg Clin North Am* (2013) 25(2):215–22. doi: 10.1016/j.coms.2013.01.004
22. Taylor GI, Townsend P, Corlett R. Superiority of the Deep Circumflex Iliac Vessels as the Supply for Free Groin Flaps. *Plast Reconstr Surg* (1979) 64 (5):595–604. doi: 10.1097/00006534-197964050-00001
23. Sanders R, Mayou BJ. A New Vascularized Bone Graft Transferred by Microvascular Anastomosis as a Free Flap. *Br J Surg* (1979) 66(11):787–8. doi: 10.1002/bjs.1800661111
24. Butterworth CJ, Rogers SN. The Zygomatic Implant Perforated (ZIP) Flap: A New Technique for Combined Surgical Reconstruction and Rapid Fixed Dental Rehabilitation Following Low-Level Maxillectomy. *Int J Implant Dent* (2017) 3(1):37. doi: 10.1186/s40729-017-0100-8

2

Augmented Reality and Intraoperative Navigation in Sinonasal Malignancies: A Preclinical Study

Axel Sahovaler[1,2†], Harley H. L. Chan[2†], Tommaso Gualtieri[1,2,3], Michael Daly[2], Marco Ferrari[1,2,3,4], Claire Vannelli[2], Donovan Eu[1,2], Mirko Manojlovic-Kolarski[1], Susannah Orzell[1], Stefano Taboni[1,2,3,4], John R. de Almeida[1], David P. Goldstein[1], Alberto Deganello[3], Piero Nicolai[4], Ralph W. Gilbert[1] and Jonathan C. Irish[1,2]*

[1] Department of Otolaryngology–Head and Neck Surgery/Surgical Oncology, Princess Margaret Cancer Centre/University Health Network, Toronto, ON, Canada, [2] Guided Therapeutics (GTx) Program, Techna Institute, University Health Network, Toronto, ON, Canada, [3] Unit of Otorhinolaryngology–Head and Neck Surgery, University of Brescia–ASST "Spedali Civili di Brescia, Brescia, Italy, [4] Section of Otorhinolaryngology–Head and Neck Surgery, University of Padua–Azienda Ospedaliera di Padova, Padua, Italy

***Correspondence:**
Jonathan C. Irish
jonathan.irish@uhn.ca

†These authors have contributed equally to this work

Objective: To report the first use of a novel projected augmented reality (AR) system in open sinonasal tumor resections in preclinical models and to compare the AR approach with an advanced intraoperative navigation (IN) system.

Methods: Four tumor models were created. Five head and neck surgeons participated in the study performing virtual osteotomies. Unguided, AR, IN, and AR + IN simulations were performed. Statistical comparisons between approaches were obtained. Intratumoral cut rate was the main outcome. The groups were also compared in terms of percentage of intratumoral, close, adequate, and excessive distances from the tumor. Information on a wearable gaze tracker headset and NASA Task Load Index questionnaire results were analyzed as well.

Results: A total of 335 cuts were simulated. Intratumoral cuts were observed in 20.7%, 9.4%, 1.2,% and 0% of the unguided, AR, IN, and AR + IN simulations, respectively ($p < 0.0001$). The AR was superior than the unguided approach in univariate and multivariate models. The percentage of time looking at the screen during the procedures was 55.5% for the unguided approaches and 0%, 78.5%, and 61.8% in AR, IN, and AR + IN, respectively ($p < 0.001$). The combined approach significantly reduced the screen time compared with the IN procedure alone.

Conclusion: We reported the use of a novel AR system for oncological resections in open sinonasal approaches, with improved margin delineation compared with unguided techniques. AR improved the gaze-toggling drawback of IN. Further refinements of the AR system are needed before translating our experience to clinical practice.

Keywords: augmented reality, intraoperative navigation, surgical margins, sinonasal tumors, surgical margin delineation

INTRODUCTION

The complex anatomy and close proximity of critical structures in the sinonasal region represent a major challenge for surgeons when treating advanced tumors in this location, and incomplete resections are not uncommon, both in open and endoscopic approaches (1, 2). Intraoperative navigation (IN) has been proposed as a potential strategy to improve surgical margins (3). IN enables co-registration of computed tomography (CT) and/or magnetic resonance imaging (MRI) studies with surgical instruments. As a result, real-time feedback of instrument location is provided in order to help the surgeon during the operation.

Our group has recently published an advanced IN system for open sinonasal approaches during the resection of locally aggressive cancers (4). This technology not only allows the surgeon to locate a registered instrument or pointer tool in two dimensions but also introduces planar cutting tool capabilities along with three-dimensional (3D) volume rendering. Therefore, the surgeon can anticipate the direction of the cutting instrument in 3D planes with respect to the tumor and improve accuracy of margin delineation. Still, one key drawback of all IN systems is that the information is displayed outside the surgical field, and therefore surgeons are forced to switch their gaze between the actual procedure and the navigation monitor, which can impact safety and efficiency.

Augmented reality (AR) uses visual inputs to enhance the user's natural vision and therefore can integrate navigation information onto the surgical field (5). This feature can potentially address the gaze-toggling drawback of IN and at the same time provide valuable information to the surgeon, for example, facilitating tumor localization and delineation. Reports of AR in otolaryngology–head and neck surgery are scarce, and most of them come from endoscopic sinus surgery (6), transoral robotic surgery (7), and otology (8, 9). Nevertheless, open sinonasal procedures also represent an adequate indication for AR. The rigid structure of the sinonasal region facilitates the co-registration processes required for AR, and the high rates of incomplete resections in advanced sinonasal tumors could be improved with the use of this technology.

The objective of this study was to report the first use of a novel AR system in open sinonasal tumor resections in preclinical models and to compare an AR approach with an advanced IN navigation system.

MATERIALS AND METHODS

Tumor Models

Two artificial skulls (Sawbones®) and a moldable material (Play-Doh®) mixed with acrylic glue were employed to build four locally advanced sinonasal tumor models (**Figure 1A**). Tumor surfaces were disguised with tape. Five different areas to be osteotomized were delineated: palatal osteotomy (Pa), fronto-maxillary junction (FMJ), latero-inferior orbital rim (LIOR), zygomatic arch (Zy), and pterygomaxillary junction (PMJ) (**Figure 1B**).

Image Acquisition and Tumor Contouring

Cone-beam computed tomography (CBCT) scans acquired 3D images of the skull models (9). Tumors showed higher x-ray attenuation than the artificial bone (**Figure 1C**). Tumor contouring was performed semiautomatically (10). First, a global threshold was applied to provide a quick, coarse segmentation, and then manual refinement was used to smooth the segmentation (**Figure 1D**).

Advanced Intraoperative Navigation System

An in-house navigation software package, GTx-Eyes, processed and displayed the CBCT images (11). This software has been proven useful in a breadth of surgical oncology subspecialties (12–15), and the technical aspects are described elsewhere (16). Tumor and margin segmentations were superimposed on triplanar views and also shown as 3D surface renderings (**Figure 2A**). Tool tracking was achieved by a stereoscopic infrared camera. Image-to-tracker registration was obtained by paired-point matching of predrilled divots in the skull by means of a tracked pointer. A four-sphere reference tool was drilled to the skull. A fiducial registration error of ≤1 mm was deemed acceptable. A three-sphere reference was attached to an osteotome and calibrated. This advanced IN system allows visualization of the entire trajectory of the cutting instrument with respect to the tumor in 3D views (**Figures 2B–D, Supplementary Video**).

Augmented Reality System

The AR system was composed of a portable high-definition projector (PicoPro, Celluon Inc., Federal Way, WA, USA), a stereoscopic infrared camera (Polaris Spectra, NDI, Waterloo, ON, Canada), a USB 2.0M pixel generic camera (ICAN Webcam 2MP, China), and a laptop computer (M4500, Precision laptop, Dell, Round Rock, TX, USA). A custom-made 3D printed case was fabricated to anchor a four-sphere reference tool and contain the other elements of the AR system (**Figure 3**). The technical details of this system including the kinematic transformation, reference system, and conventional image-to-tracker registration method have also been described elsewhere (17).

The AR system was registered into a single coordinate system by pairing correspondent landmarks using fiducial markers identifiable in both the images and projection surface (**Figure 4**). GTx-Eyes provided the 3D surface rendering of the tumors, which were projected by the AR system onto the skulls. The virtual tumor was delineated with CBCT imaging through ITK-SNAP software (ref below). The optical sensor mounted to the projector case facilitated real-time tracking of the AR device to allow the projector and/or skull to be repositioned during tasks without compromising projection accuracy (**Supplementary Video**), with a registration error <1 mm. This approach facilitated identification of the tumors and in consequence guided the virtual cuts of the participants (**Supplementary Figure S1**).

Gaze-Tracking System

A wearable gaze tracker headset was developed to continuously monitor and locate the user's gaze (e.g., surgical field *vs.* navigation monitor) during surgical tasks. This headset was used solely for gaze-tracking and did not project any

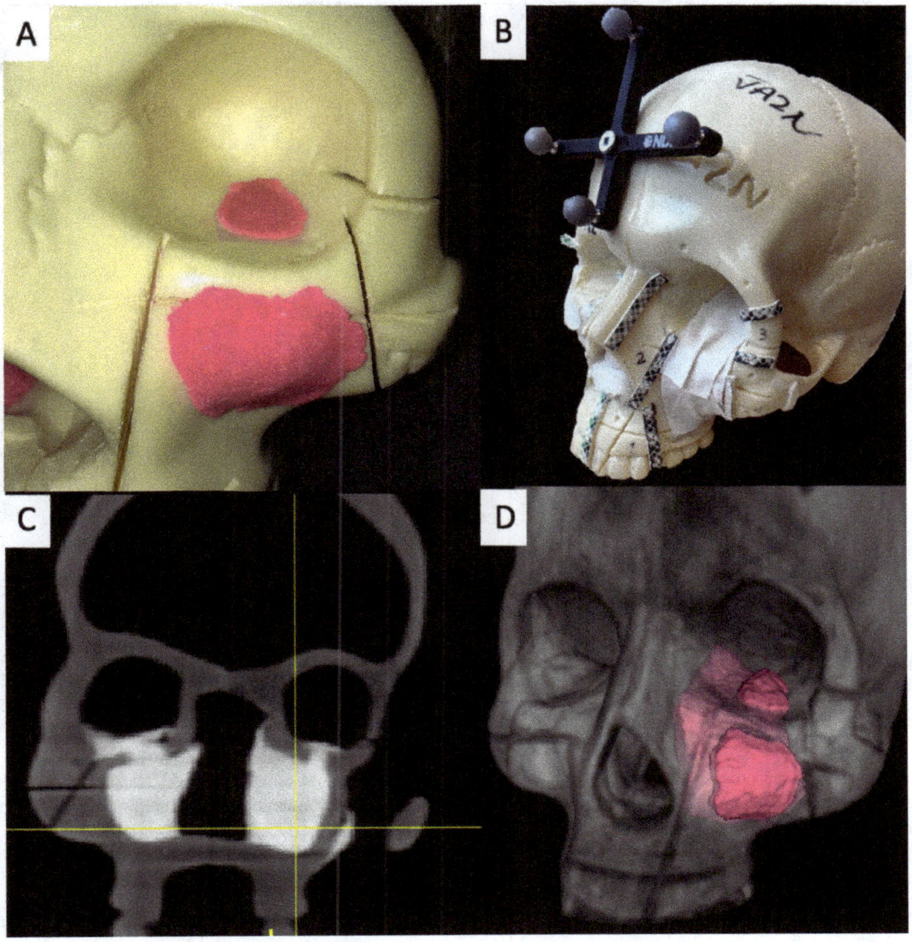

FIGURE 1 | Tumor models, image acquisition, and tumor contouring. **(A)** Artificial skulls with moldable material simulating advanced sinonasal tumors. **(B)** Final tumor model, with the tumors covered with white tape. The areas to be osteotomized are delineated with visible tape and marked with numbers. A four-sphere reference tool drilled to the skull to co-register the intraoperative navigation. **(C)** Higher attenuation of the artificial tumor models in the cone-beam computed tomography (CBCT) images. **(D)** Three-dimensional (3D) contouring of the left tumor.

information. The eye tracker (Pupil Labs, Berlin, Germany) consists of two cameras: one trained on the eye and the other, a "world camera", recording the individual's field of view. A series of computer vision algorithms are applied to the input from the eye camera to reliably detect the pupil throughout the eye's range of motion. A calibration step provides a triangulating mapping function between the pupil and world cameras, which enables the user's gaze to be precisely tracked (**Figures 5A–D**).

Simulations

Five head and neck fellowship-trained surgeons with 3–5 years of experience in oncologic ablations from the Department of Otolaryngology–Head and Neck Surgery of the University Health Network participated in the simulations.

Surgeons were instructed to position the osteotome between the delineated areas of the different osteotomy sites in a sequential order (Pa-FMJ-LIOR-Zy-PMJ) and to provide a 1-cm margin from the tumor along the plane trajectory. Instead of cutting the skulls, virtual cuts were performed in order to allow the reutilization of the models. This involved recording the osteotome position and orientation in the navigation software after the surgeon placed the osteotome in a certain direction and provided confirmation of obtaining the proposed cut. The analysis was performed on the virtual cutting trajectory after all the simulations were completed.

Four procedures were performed: 1) Unguided using axial, sagittal, coronal images; 2) Guided -AR-; 3) Guided -IN-; and 4) Guided -AR and IN-. This last group was possible, as both systems are contained in the same platform software and can be used simultaneously. Analysis of cutting planes was performed using MATLAB software. An area of 4 cm × 2 cm (1 cm on both sides with respect to the longitudinal axis) along the longitudinal axis of the cut was isolated from each plane. The minimal distance with respect to the tumor surface was calculated for each point making up the isolated area and reproduced as a distribution of distances shown as a 4 cm × 2 cm color scaled image. Distance from

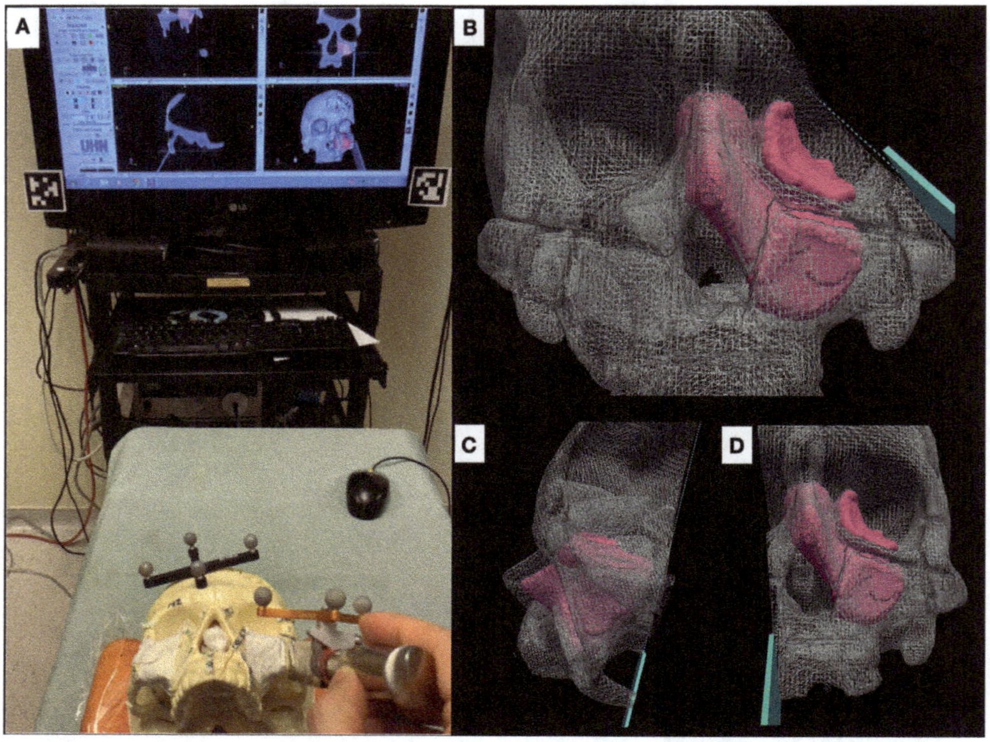

FIGURE 2 | Advanced intraoperative navigation system. **(A)** Setup of the system, depicting the triplanar cutting views and the three-dimensional (3D) rendering of the tumor on the screen. The skull and the cutting instrument (in this case an osteotome) are referenced to be tracked and co-registered. **(B–D)** The system allows users to visualize cutting trajectories of the instrument with respect to the tumor. **(B)** Cutting of the latero-inferior orbital rim, **(C)** pterygomaxillary junction, and **(D)** palate.

the tumor surface was classified as "intratumoral" when ≤0 mm, "close" when >0 mm and ≤5 mm, "adequate" when >5 mm and ≤15 mm, and "excessive" when >15 mm. The percentages of points at intratumoral, close, adequate, and excessive distances were calculated for each simulation plane.

The gaze-tracking system was calibrated to each participant, and it was used in all the simulations. The eye-tracking data were analyzed to identify each time point the participants switched their gaze between the navigation monitor and the surgical field. The metric reported is the percentage of total study time spent looking at the navigation monitor.

Finally, a NASA Task Load Index (NASA-TLX) questionnaire that measures the workload of a task was completed by the participants to evaluate the different approaches (18). This questionnaire is widely used and validated and rates the perceived workload to assess a task, system, or other aspects of performance (19–21). It has been employed to assess the workload of new technologies during surgical procedures (22). The total workload is divided into six subjective subscales, which assess mental, physical, and temporal demand, performance, effort, and frustration. Scores range between very low and very high.

Statistical Analysis

Statistical analysis was run through XLSTAT® (Addinsoft®, New York). Simulations were grouped into four categories: unguided, AR, IN, and AR + IN. Rate of intratumoral virtual cuts was the main outcome and was assessed with the Fisher's exact test. Multivariable analysis adjusting for surgeon and tumor was performed through logistic regression analysis. The groups were also compared in terms of percentage of intratumoral, close, adequate, and excessive distances from the tumor and duration of the simulations through the bilateral Kruskal-Wallis test and Steel-Dwass-Critchlow-Fligner *post-hoc* test. The Kruskal-Wallis test was also employed to analyze the gaze-tracking outcomes and the NASA-TLX scores. Level of significance was set at 0.05 for all statistical tests.

RESULTS

Intratumoral Cuts

A total of 335 cuts were simulated. Intratumoral cuts were observed in 20.7%, 9.4%, 1.2%, and 0% of the unguided, AR, IN, and AR + IN simulations, respectively ($p < 0.0001$). Univariate analysis comparing different procedures with AR showed that this technology improved margins with respect to unguided simulations. The advanced IN approach reduced the intratumoral cut rates compared with AR, and the combination of AR and IN did not significantly decrease the intratumoral cut rate compared with IN alone ($p = 0.51$). These differences were also seen in a multivariate model adjusted for tumor and surgeon (**Table 1**).

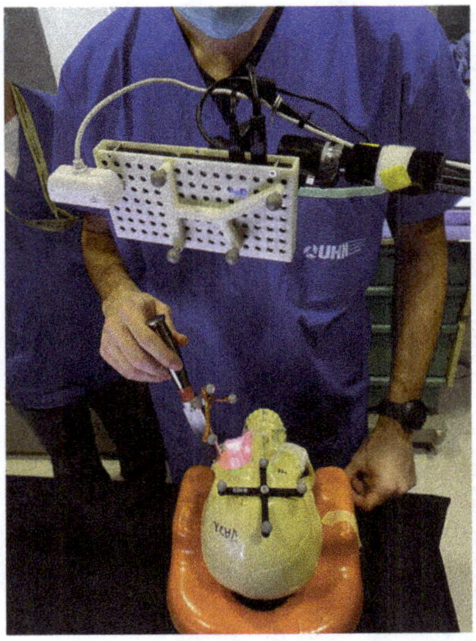

FIGURE 3 | Augmented reality system mounted and projecting.

TABLE 1 | Intratumoral cuts analysis.

INTRATUMORAL CUTS AND TYPE OF PROCEDURE				
Intratumoral cut/Guidance	**Unguided**	**AR**	**IN**	**AR+IN**
No	65	77	83	84
Yes	17	8	1	0
Total	82	85	84	84
Percentage	20.7%	9.4%	1.2%	0.0%
UNIVARIATE ANALYSIS OF INTRATUMORAL CUTS				
Guidance	**OR**	**95%-CI**	**p-value**	
AR	REF	REF	REF	
Unguided	2.44	1.00-5.02	0.049	
SN	0.16	0.03-0.97	0.046	
AR+SN	0.05	0.00-0.97	0.047	
MULTIVARIATE ANALYSIS OF INTRATUMORAL CUTS				
Guidance	**Adjusted* OR**	**95%-CI**	**p-value**	
AR	REF	REF	REF	
Unguided	2.54	1.05-6.17	0.039	
SN	0.16	0.03-0.88	0.035	
AR+SN	0.06	0.00-0.81	0.035	

*AR Augmented reality, IN intraoperative navigation, OR odds ratio, *Adjusted by tumor model and surgeon.*

Distribution of Points Forming Simulation Planes

The percentage of points forming the simulation planes was also registered. We observed that only the advanced IN system and the combined approach significantly decreased the percentage of intratumoral ($p < 0.0001$) and close margin points ($p = 0.008$) compared with the unguided resections (**Supplementary Table S1**).

Duration of Simulations and Gaze-Tracking Results

Mean total duration of the simulation was 215 s for unguided procedures and 117, 134, and 120 s in the AR, IN, and AR + IN, respectively. Participants required significantly more time to perform the unguided simulations compared to the AR- and IN-guided ones ($p = 0.004$). There were no differences between the AR-, IN-, and AR + IN-guided procedures. The percentage of time looking at the screen during the procedures was 55.5% for the unguided approaches and 0%, 78.5%, and 61.8% in AR, IN, and AR + IN, respectively ($p < 0.001$). Adding the AR technology to the combined approach significantly reduced the screen time compared with the advanced IN procedures alone (**Supplementary Table S2**).

NASA-TLX Scores

We found no differences in scores between the unguided and the AR procedures, and both of them exhibited a high degree of mental demand, effort, and frustration. Combining AR to IN showed a significant improvement on the previous scores (**Supplementary Graph 1** and **Supplementary Table S3**).

DISCUSSION

In this study, we observed that both advanced IN and AR technologies improved margin delineation compared with unguided procedures. Advanced IN was better for margin delineation than AR but required gaze-toggling between the surgical field and the navigation monitor, whereas AR allowed the surgeon to focus only on the surgical field. The combination of both technologies partially improved the flaws on margins and staring outside the surgical field of the AR and IN techniques, respectively. The integration of AR and IN also improved Mental Demand, Performance, Effort, and Frustration domains in the NASA-TLX questionnaires.

Margin control is among the most important prognostic factors and the only surgeon-controlled variable in head and neck cancer, and efforts have been centered around obtaining clear margins after tumor resections. Nevertheless, positive surgical margins represent a major issue, even in the hand of experienced surgeons. In a report from the largest tertiary referral head and neck cancer center in the Netherlands, 39% out of 69 resections of advanced maxillary tumors (>T3) were incomplete, being posterior and superior margins the most commonly involved (23). In a bi-institutional study from the Cleveland Clinic and the UC San Francisco (24), 24% out of 75 post-maxillectomy patients had positive margins in definitive pathology. Positive margins were associated with a 2-fold increase of risk of death, and in multivariate analysis after controlling for age, nodal stage, and surgical treatment, margins were independently associated with survival (25). Moreover, it has been reported that intraoperative frozen sections (which are probably the only intraoperative resource to evaluate adequacy of the resection) have only 40% sensitivity in open sinonasal approaches (26).

Currently, IN is employed in many centers in endoscopic sinonasal procedures (27–29). By point-tracking an instrument and locating it on two dimensions in triplanar views, IN has shown an increase in accuracy and a reduction in operative time, impacting favorably surgical outcomes and complications. Utilization of IN in open procedures to resect malignant tumors has been less reported, but promising results were obtained in margin status in small

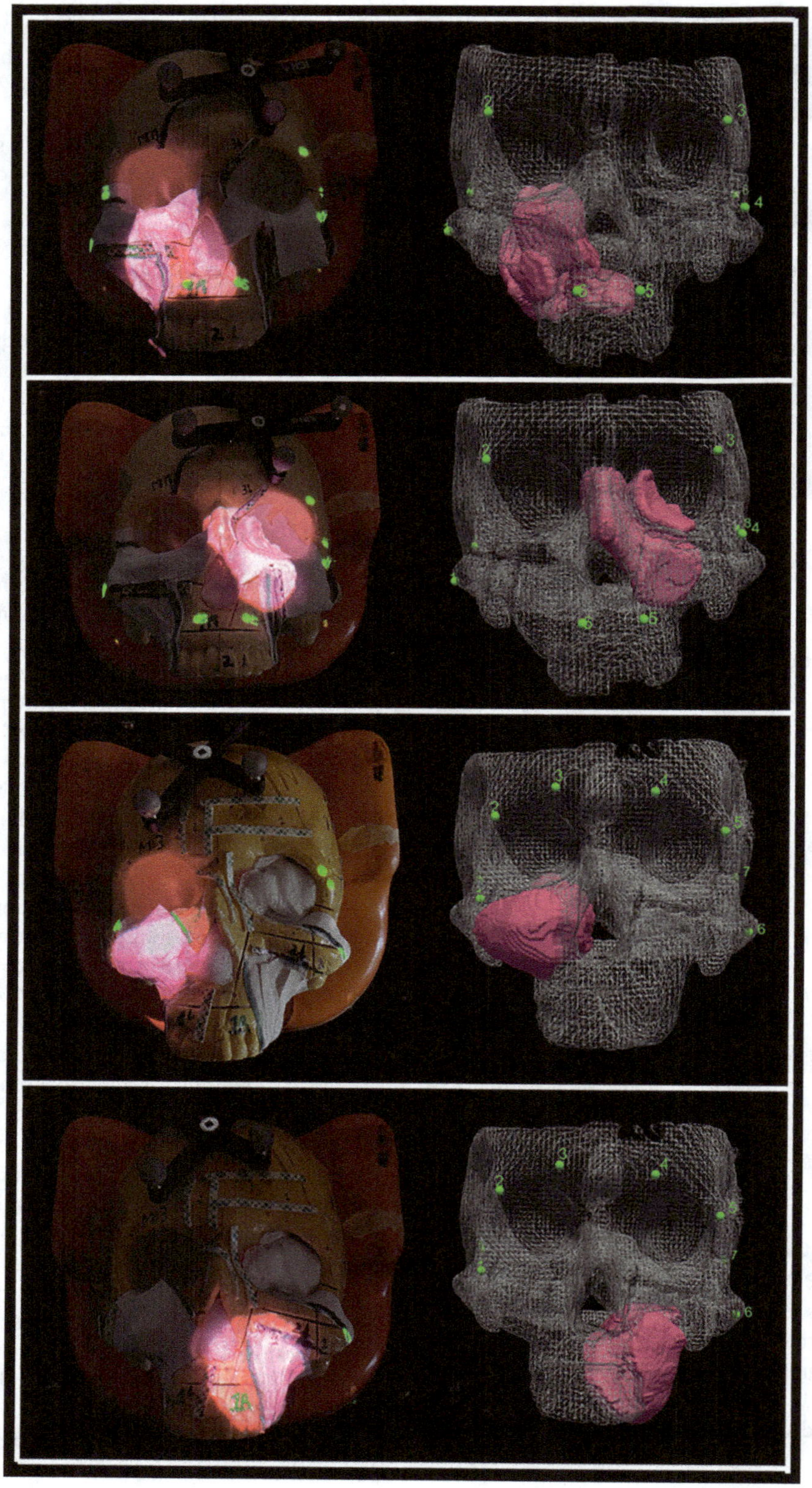

FIGURE 4 | Projection of the four sinonasal tumors using augmented reality, which enables tumor localization. The alignment points are depicted as well as the three-dimensional (3D) reconstruction of the tumors. Pictures were taken without light for demonstration purposes, but good visualization is obtained with light as well.

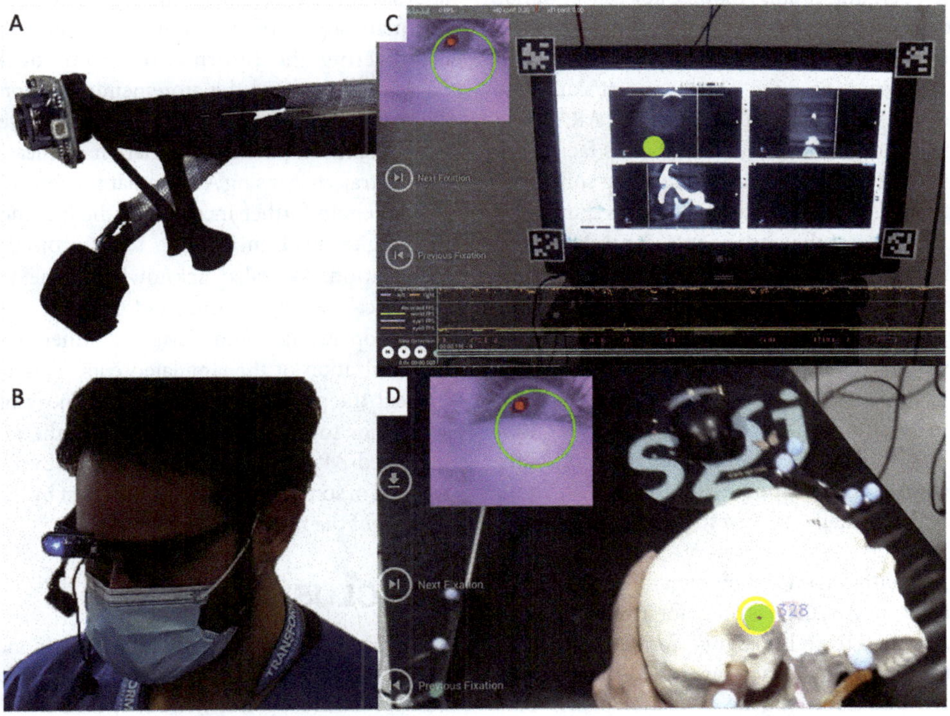

FIGURE 5 | **(A)** Gaze-tracking system with the two cameras that allow it to visualize the pupils and also the participant's view. **(B)** The device placed on one of the participants. **(C, D)** The "world camera" showing the participant's view, which could be either on the screen **(C)** or on the surgical field **(D)**. The green dot indicates the exact position of the gaze. A small picture-in-picture screen (upper left) shows the position of the pupil.

cohorts (3, 30, 31). Our group has recently published a preclinical experience utilizing the same advanced IN system used in the present study to assist in open sinonasal approaches (4). The main novelty is that our advanced IN system allows surgeons not only to track the desired instrument but also to visualize the entire cutting trajectory of a tracked cutting tool in 3D. In our previous experience using this technology, eight head and neck surgeons performed 381 simulated osteotomies for the resection of seven tumor models. The use of 3D navigation for margin delineation significantly improved control of margins: unguided cuts had 18.1% intratumoral cuts compared to 0% intratumoral cuts with 3D navigation ($p < 0.0001$). Furthermore, a clinical study using this advanced IN system for mandibulectomies demonstrated a <1.5-mm accuracy between the planned cuts and the actual bone resection in the post-resection imaging (15). One of the main criticisms to the system by the surgeons in this report was the multitasking challenge between the surgical field and the IN monitor, which can ultimately impact not only efficiency but also patient safety, as the surgeon has to look away from the surgical field.

AR enhances the surgeon's vision rather than replacing it: CT, PET-CT, or MRI scans can be visualized in 3D and in real time, granting "X-ray vision" to the physician (32, 33). It has recently gained interest by computer-assisted surgery researchers, as it integrates the imaging information onto the surgical field. This has the potential to overcome the main drawback of the IN technology, which stems from the frequent switching of focus from the navigation screens to the surgical field and the translation of 2D imaging data to a 3D anatomical structure (33). Despite having reports on AR application in the field of otolaryngology–head and neck surgery, the majority describe the use of AR using wearable computers (Microsoft HoloLens®, Microsoft Corporation, Redmond) and other head-mounted displays (HMDs), which might be cumbersome especially in long procedures, and preclude the use of loupes/headlights. There are literature reports about HMD limitations including heaviness of the devices, breaches in patient privacy/information, battery life, potential lag time secondary to preoperative image processing, and the potential of signal interferences of wireless Internet or Bluetooth connections that may cause intermittent data transmission of image (34). Moreover, most reports of HMD rely solely on the operator visual alignment between the projected images and the anatomical area of interest (35) without any co-registration steps between the projecting surface and the AR system, which can lead to errors. Lastly, there are descriptions of the use of AR in the operating room, but they are merely descriptive and not aimed to improve a surgical task (36) or for educational purposes only (37).

Our study reports several innovations. Tracking the AR projector as well as the projection surface with reflecting markers allowed us to be able to reposition the skull models and the projector without losing accuracy (17, 38), and this is something that was not described previously in head and neck surgery. This is paramount in computer-assisted surgery, as it allows precise projection even when movement occurs, as in real-time situations in the operating room. Another key aspect of our approach is the use of an external projector, which avoids the need for heavy wearable headsets. As a clarification, the headsets used in our study were for gaze-tracking only. The sinonasal/skull base region rigidity represents an excellent indication for AR, as the deformation of tissue is minimal and co-registration is facilitated. Deformation has to be taken into consideration during soft-tissue resections, as it is not possible to adjust the projections during AR (7, 39). By tracking the gaze of the participants, we were able to quantitatively measure the percentage of time that the surgeons had to look away from the surgical field. As our results suggest, there is significant improvement when AR is employed both alone or in combination with IN, addressing the main disadvantages of IN utility. Our AR system shares the same software platform as the advanced IN system, and both approaches can be used concurrently, allowing to evaluate the combination of both. Finally, there is a lack of user evaluation analysis with AR, so we utilized a validated questionnaire to investigate the differences between approaches.

Despite being significantly superior than unguided simulations in terms of intratumoral cut rates, there is room for improvement in our AR system. The advanced IN technology performed better than the AR in terms of intratumoral cut rates, as well as intratumoral and close distribution of points forming the simulation planes. This might be explained by the challenge in finding the correct angle between the projector and the projecting surface. We observed that if the angle differed greatly from 90 degrees, the image can be distorted and therefore lead to inaccuracies in surgical guidance to the operator. For example, when performing the PMJ cuts, by turning the skull 180 degrees, there were cases that the alignment was lost that might have impacted the positive margin cuts. Another important limitation is that the sense of depth can be lost in the projections, and the image can be interpreted in 2D on the surface rather than in 3D, especially with changes in ambient light. One last limitation of image projection is the parallax issue (40). This phenomenon occurs when there is a 3D space non-alignment between the viewer and the projection perspectives. Our system minimizes this issue by adjusting the perspective of the pico-projector close to the surgeon's sight. In addition, the AR system is fully integrated into our intraoperative navigation system with real-time tracking technology; therefore, the relocation/movement/displacement of the projector will not affect projection accuracy, with no need for further recalibration and registration procedure. These limitations were also reflected on the NASA-TLX scores, where mental demand, effort, and frustration rates for AR were higher than those for IN and similar to those of unguided approaches. Participants commented on the fact that when the adequate angle of projection was lost, they had difficulties interpreting the information from the AR system, which negatively impacted the aforementioned domains of the NASA-TLX questionnaire. A plausible way of improving these flaws, and in consequence improving the margin delineation, is to project the cutting trajectory using AR. Similar to the advanced IN capabilities, the AR could further incorporate the intended cut trajectories on the surgical field, in addition to its projection of the tumor for localization. We also acknowledge the limitations of using preclinical models that may not perfectly replicate the conditions of the operating room. Lastly, another limitation is the non-randomization of the simulated cuts. This was done in order to prevent the participant's retained memory of the guided views if seen prior to the unguided cuts. Still, the fact that the sequence unguided-AR-IN-AR + IN was followed by all surgeons could have resulted in some degree of learning effect by the participants toward the end of the tasks.

CONCLUSION

We reported the use of AR for open sinonasal approaches and improved margin delineation compared with unguided techniques. The advanced IN performed better in terms of margin delineation, but the AR improved the gaze-toggling drawback of IN. Further research within our group is currently underway before translating our experience to clinical practice.

AUTHOR CONTRIBUTIONS

All authors listed have made a substantial, direct, and intellectual contribution to the work and approved it for publication.

ACKNOWLEDGMENTS

The gaze-tracking system was developed by Dr. Kazuhiro Yasufuku's research laboratory.

SUPPLEMENTARY MATERIAL

Supplementary Video | Advanced Intraoperative Navigation system showing the entire cutting trajectory with respect to the tumor, and the Augmented Reality system providing the exact location of the tumor. The co-registration of the skull and the projector in the Augmented Reality system allows the image to be accurately projected and automatically adjusted despite movements.

REFERENCES

1. Deganello A, Ferrari M, Paderno A, Turri-Zanoni M, Schreiber A, Mattavelli D, et al. Endoscopic-Assisted Maxillectomy: Operative Technique and Control of Surgical Margins. *Oral Oncol* (2019) 93:29–38. doi: 10.1016/j.oraloncology.2019.04.002
2. Nishio N, Fujimoto Y, Fujii M, Saito K, Hiramatsu M, Maruo T, et al. Craniofacial Resection for T4 Maxillary Sinus Carcinoma. *Otolaryngol Neck Surg* (2015) 153(2):231–8. doi: 10.1177/0194599815586770
3. Catanzaro S, Copelli C, Manfuso A, Tewfik K, Pederneschi N, Cassano L, et al. Intraoperative Navigation in Complex Head and Neck Resections: Indications and Limits. *Int J Comput Assist Radiol Surg* (2017) 12(5):881–7. doi: 10.1007/s11548-016-1486-0
4. Ferrari M, Daly MJ, Douglas CM, Chan HHL, Qiu J, Deganello A, et al. Navigation-Guided Osteotomies Improve Margin Delineation in Tumors Involving the Sinonasal Area: A Preclinical Study. *Oral Oncol* (2019)

99:104463. doi: 10.1016/j.oraloncology.2019.104463

5. Moawad GN, Elkhalil J, Klebanoff JS, Rahman S, Habib N, Alkatout I. Augmented Realities, Artificial Intelligence, and Machine Learning: Clinical Implications and How Technology Is Shaping the Future of Medicine. *J Clin Med* (2020) 9(12):3811. doi: 10.3390/jcm9123811
6. Khanwalkar AR, Welch KC. Updates in Techniques for Improved Visualization in Sinus Surgery. *Curr Opin Otolaryngol Head Neck Surg* (2021) 29(1):9–20. doi: 10.1097/MOO.0000000000000693
7. Liu WP, Richmon JD, Sorger JM, Azizian M, Taylor RH. Augmented Reality and Cone Beam CT Guidance for Transoral Robotic Surgery. *J Robot Surg* (2015) 9(3):223–33. doi: 10.1007/s11701-015-0520-5
8. Creighton FX, Unberath M, Song T, Zhao Z, Armand M, Carey J. Early Feasibility Studies of Augmented Reality Navigation for Lateral Skull Base Surgery. *Otol Neurotol* (2020) 41(7):883–8. doi: 10.1097/MAO.0000000000002724
9. King E, Daly MJ, Chan H, Bachar G, Dixon BJ, Siewerdsen JH, et al. Intraoperative Cone-Beam CT for Head and Neck Surgery: Feasibility of Clinical Implementation Using a Prototype Mobile C-Arm. *Head Neck* (2013) 35(7):959–67. doi: 10.1002/hed.23060
10. Jermyn M, Ghadyani H, Mastanduno MA, Turner W, Davis SC, Dehghani H, et al. Fast Segmentation and High-Quality Three-Dimensional Volume Mesh Creation From Medical Images for Diffuse Optical Tomography. *J BioMed Opt* (2013) 18(8):86007. doi: 10.1117/1.JBO.18.8.086007
11. Daly MJ, Chan H, Nithiananthan S, Qiu J, Barker E, Bachar G, et al. *Clinical Implementation of Intraoperative Cone-Beam CT in Head and Neck Surgery*, Vol. 796426. KH Wong, DR Holmes III, editors. Lake Buena Vista, FL: SPIE (2011). doi: 10.1117/12.878976
12. Dixon BJ, Chan H, Daly MJ, Qiu d, Vescan A, Witterick IJ, et al. Three-Dimensional Virtual Navigation *Versus* Conventional Image Guidance: A Randomized Controlled Trial. *Laryngoscope* (2016) 126(7):1510–5. doi: 10.1002/lary.25882
13. Sternheim A, Daly M, Qiu J, Weersink R, Chan H, Jaffray D, et al. Navigated Pelvic Osteotomy and Tumor Resection: A Study Assessing the Accuracy and Reproducibility of Resection Planes in Sawbones and Cadavers. *J Bone Joint Surg Am* (2015) 97(1):40–6. doi: 10.2106/JBJS.N.00276
14. Lee CY, Chan H, Ujiie H, Fujino K, Kinoshita T, Irish JC, et al. Novel Thoracoscopic Navigation System With Augmented Real-Time Image Guidance for Chest Wall Tumors. *Ann Thorac Surg* (2018) 106(5):1468–75. doi: 10.1016/j.athoracsur.2018.06.062
15. Hasan W, Daly MJ, Chan HHL, Qiu J, Irish JC. Intraoperative Cone-Beam CT-Guided Osteotomy Navigation in Mandible and Maxilla Surgery. *Laryngoscope* (2020) 130(5):1166–72. doi: 10.1002/lary.28082
16. Daly MJ, Siewerdsen JH, Moseley DJ, Jaffray DA, Irish JC. Intraoperative Cone-Beam CT for Guidance of Head and Neck Surgery: Assessment of Dose and Image Quality Using a C-Arm Prototype. *Med Phys* (2006) 33(10):3767–80. doi: 10.1118/1.2349687
17. Chan HHL, Haerle SK, Daly MJ, Zheng J, Philp L, Ferrari M, et al. An Integrated Augmented Reality Surgical Navigation Platform Using Multi-Modality Imaging for Guidance. Máthé D, Ed. *PloS One* (2021) 16(4): e0250558. doi: 10.1371/journal.pone.0250558
18. Hancock PA , Meshkati N. Development of NASA-TLX (Task Load Index): Results of Empirical and Theoretical Research. *Adv Psychol* (1988) 52:139–83. doi: 10.1016/S0166-4115(08)62386-9
19. Rainieri G, Fraboni F, Russo G, Tul M, Pingitore A, Tessari A, et al. Visual Scanning Techniques and Mental Workload of Helicopter Pilots During Simulated Flight. *Aerosp Med Hum Perform* (2021) 92(1):11–9. doi: 10.3357/AMHP.5681.2021
20. Lebet RM, Hasbani NR, Sisko MT, Agus MSD, Nadkarni VM, Wypij D, et al. Nurses' Perceptions of Workload Burden in Pediatric Critical Care. *Am J Crit Care* (2021) 30(1):27–35. doi: 10.4037/ajcc2021725
21. Devos H, Gustafson K, Ahmadnezhad P, Liao K, Mahnken JD, Brooks WM, et al. Psychometric Properties of NASA-TLX and Index of Cognitive Activity as Measures of Cognitive Workload in Older Adults. *Brain Sci* (2020) 10 (12):994. doi: 10.3390/brainsci10120994
22. Lowndes BR, Forsyth KL, Blocker RC, Dean PG, Truty MJ, Heller SF, et al. NASA-TLX Assessment of Surgeon Workload Variation Across Specialties. *Ann Surg* (2020) 271(4):686–92. doi: 10.1097/SLA.0000000000003058
23. Kreeft AM, Smeele LE, Rasch CRN, Hauptmann M, Rietveld DHF, Leemans CR, et al. Preoperative Imaging and Surgical Margins in Maxillectomy Patients. *Head Neck* (2012) 34(11):1652–6. doi: 10.1002/hed.21987
24. Likhterov I, Fritz MA, El-Sayed IH, Rahul S, Rayess HM, Knott PD. Locoregional Recurrence Following Maxillectomy: Implications for Microvascular Reconstruction. *Laryngoscope* (2017) 127(11):2534–8. doi: 10.1002/lary.26620
25. Mücke T, Loeffelbein DJ, Hohlweg-Majert B, Kesting MR, Wolff KD, Hölzle F. Reconstruction of the Maxilla and Midface - Surgical Management, Outcome, and Prognostic Factors. *Oral Oncol* (2009) 45(12):1073–8. doi: 10.1016/j.oraloncology.2009.10.003
26. Murphy J, Isaiah A, Wolf JS, Lubek JE. The Influence of Intraoperative Frozen Section Analysis in Patients With Total or Extended Maxillectomy. *Oral Surg Oral Med Oral Pathol Oral Radiol* (2016) 121(1):17–21. doi: 10.1016/j.oooo.2015.07.014
27. Leong J-L, Batra PS, Citardi MJ. CT-MR Image Fusion for the Management of Skull Base Lesions. *Otolaryngol Neck Surg* (2006) 134(5):868–76. doi: 10.1016/j.otohns.2005.11.015
28. Kacker A, Tabaee A, Anand V. Computer-Assisted Surgical Navigation in Revision Endoscopic Sinus Surgery. *Otolaryngol Clin North Am* (2005) 38 (3):473–82. doi: 10.1016/j.otc.2004.10.021
29. Vicaut E, Bertrand B, Betton J-L, Bizon A, Briche D, Castillo L, et al. Use of a Navigation System in Endonasal Surgery: Impact on Surgical Strategy and Surgeon Satisfaction. A Prospective Multicenter Study. *Eur Ann Otorhinolaryngol Head Neck Dis* (2019) 136(6):461–4. doi: 10.1016/j.anorl.2019.08.002
30. Tarsitano A, Ricotta F, Baldino G, Badiali G, Pizzigallo A, Ramieri V, et al. Navigation-Guided Resection of Maxillary Tumours: The Accuracy of Computer-Assisted Surgery in Terms of Control of Resection Margins – A Feasibility Study. *J Cranio Maxillofacial Surg* (2017) 45(12):2109–14. doi: 10.1016/j.jcms.2017.09.023
31. Feichtinger M, Pau M, Zemann W, Aigner RM, Kärcher H. Intraoperative Control of Resection Margins in Advanced Head and Neck Cancer Using a 3D-Navigation System Based on PET/CT Image Fusion. *J Cranio Maxillofacial Surg* (2010) 38(8):589–94. doi: 10.1016/j.jcms.2010.02.004
32. Chen X, Xu L, Wang Y, Wang H, Wang F, Zeng X, et al. Development of a Surgical Navigation System Based on Augmented Reality Using an Optical See-Through Head-Mounted Display. *J BioMed Inform* (2015) 55:124–31. doi: 10.1016/j.jbi.2015.04.003
33. Gsaxner C, Pepe A, Li J, Ibrahimpasic U, Wallner J, Schmalstieg D, et al. Augmented Reality for Head and Neck Carcinoma Imaging: Description and Feasibility of an Instant Calibration, Markerless Approach. *Comput Methods Programs BioMed* (2020) 200:105854. doi: 10.1016/j.cmpb.2020.105854
34. Rahman R, Wood ME, Qian L, Price CL, Johnson AA, Osgood GM. Head-Mounted Display Use in Surgery: A Systematic Review. *Surg Innov* (2020) 27 (1):88–100. doi: 10.1177/1553350619871787
35. Battaglia S, Badiali G, Cercenelli L, Bortolani B, Marcelli E, Cipriani R, et al. Combination of CAD/CAM and Augmented Reality in Free Fibula Bone Harvest. *Plast Reconstr Surg - Glob Open* (2019) 7(11):e2510. doi: 10.1097/GOX.0000000000002510
36. Tepper OM, Rudy HL, Lefkowitz A, Weimer KA, Marks SM, Stern CS, et al. Mixed Reality With Hololens: Where Virtual Reality Meets Augmented Reality in the Operating Room. *Plast Reconstr Surg* (2017) 140(5):1066–70. doi: 10.1097/PRS.0000000000003802
37. Rose AS, Kim H, Fuchs H, Frahm JM. Development of Augmented-Reality Applications in Otolaryngology–Head and Neck Surgery. *Laryngoscope* (2019) 129(S3):S1–11. doi: 10.1002/lary.28098
38. Meulstee JW, Nijsink J, Schreurs R, Verhamme LM, Xi T, Delye HHK, et al. Toward Holographic-Guided Surgery. *Surg Innov* (2019) 26(1):86–94. doi: 10.1177/1553350618799552
39. Chan JYK, Holsinger FC, Liu S, Sorger JM, Azizian M, Tsang RKY. Augmented Reality for Image Guidance in Transoral Robotic Surgery. *J Robot Surg* (2020) 14(4):579–83. doi: 10.1007/s11701-019-01030-0
40. Mamone V, Ferrari V, Condino S, Cutolo F. Projected Augmented Reality to Drive Osteotomy Surgery: Implementation and Comparison With Video See-Through Technology. *IEEE Access* (2020) 8:169024–35. doi: 10.1109/ACCESS.2020.3021940

3

Surgical Navigation, Augmented Reality and 3D Printing for Hard Palate Adenoid Cystic Carcinoma En-Bloc Resection

Mónica García-Sevilla [1,2], Rafael Moreta-Martinez [1,2], David García-Mato [1,2], Gema Arenas de Frutos [2,3], Santiago Ochandiano [2,3], Carlos Navarro-Cuéllar [2,3], Guillermo Sanjuán de Moreta [2,4] and Javier Pascau [1,2]*

[1] Departamento de Bioingeniería e Ingeniería Aeroespacial, Universidad Carlos III de Madrid, Madrid, Spain, [2] Instituto de Investigación Sanitaria Gregorio Marañón, Madrid, Spain, [3] Servicio de Cirugía Oral y Maxilofacial, Hospital General Universitario Gregorio Marañón, Madrid, Spain, [4] Servicio de Otorrinolaringología, Hospital General Universitario Gregorio Marañón, Madrid, Spain

***Correspondence:**
Javier Pascau
jpascau@ing.uc3m.es

Adenoid Cystic Carcinoma is a rare and aggressive tumor representing less than 1% of head and neck cancers. This malignancy often arises from the minor salivary glands, being the palate its most common location. Surgical en-bloc resection with clear margins is the primary treatment. However, this location presents a limited line of sight and a high risk of injuries, making the surgical procedure challenging. In this context, technologies such as intraoperative navigation can become an effective tool, reducing morbidity and improving the safety and accuracy of the procedure. Although their use is extended in fields such as neurosurgery, their application in maxillofacial surgery has not been widely evidenced. One reason is the need to rigidly fixate a navigation reference to the patient, which often entails an invasive setup. In this work, we studied three alternative and less invasive setups using optical tracking, 3D printing and augmented reality. We evaluated their precision in a patient-specific phantom, obtaining errors below 1 mm. The optimum setup was finally applied in a clinical case, where the navigation software was used to guide the tumor resection. Points were collected along the surgical margins after resection and compared with the real ones identified in the postoperative CT. Distances of less than 2 mm were obtained in 90% of the samples. Moreover, the navigation provided confidence to the surgeons, who could then undertake a less invasive and more conservative approach. The postoperative CT scans showed adequate resection margins and confirmed that the patient is free of disease after two years of follow-up.

Keywords: surgical navigation, augmented reality, 3D printing, head and neck cancer, adenoid cystic carcinoma

INTRODUCTION

Salivary gland tumors account for approximately 5% of head and neck cancers (1) and are, in most cases, benign. Only 20% of these neoplasms are malignant, although this rate varies depending on the gland of origin (2, 3). Unlike most head and neck cancers, which are squamous cell carcinomas, salivary gland tumors comprise multiple histologic entities, each presenting a different clinical behavior (4). Mucoepidermoid carcinoma is the most frequent malignancy, followed by adenoid cystic carcinomas, representing less than 1% of all malignancies in head and neck cancers (5). These tumors can appear in both minor and major salivary glands. Most major salivary tumors occur in the parotid glands, while the palate is the most common location for minor salivary gland tumors (6).

Tumors located in the palate are often diagnosed in advanced stages of the disease due to indolent growth during early stages, with vague and unspecific symptoms (5, 7). In some cases, this phenomenon leads to extensive involvement of surrounding structures, such as the nose, paranasal sinuses, orbits, and even the middle cranial fossa, with the subsequent implication of vital structures such as the internal carotid artery, the jugular vein, and cranial nerves.

Regardless of whether it is followed by radiotherapy, surgery is the treatment of choice for midface tumors. To date, the surgical management of these tumors consists of radical maxillectomies combined with transfacial approaches, which are usually associated with significant functional and aesthetic sequelae. However, achieving safety margins is a therapeutic challenge. This is due to the complexity of the anatomical region, the reduced field of vision, the restrictive surgical field hindering the access and maneuverability of surgical instruments, and the risk of complications (bleeding, nerve injuries, or even cerebrospinal fluid leaks) (8). In addition, middle third tumors are frequently irregular in shape and invade neighboring structures. Consequently, it is not uncommon to set suboptimal cutting trajectories, which results in a high rate of positive margins.

An alternative approach for centrofacial tumors is the endoscopic-based resection, which considerably reduces the morbidity of surgery compared to open craniofacial resections. However, open surgery is still necessary for the most advanced stage cancers, often combined with endoscopic resection (9).

In these scenarios, tools facilitating local control during surgical resection and confirming adequate margins while minimizing morbidity are capital (10).

Computer-Assisted Surgery in Oral and Maxillofacial Surgery

In recent years, intraoperative navigation in craniofacial surgery has become an effective tool, improving results and safety while minimizing the risk of injuries (11, 12). Surgical navigation, also called image-guided surgery, was first described in the medical literature in the 70s when framed stereotaxy was introduced. This involved rigid fixation of the region to be treated, a situation that, on many occasions, entails significant mechanical limitations for the surgeon. Navigation was initially confined to neurosurgery as it provides a rigid and stable frame (13). However, technical advances in image processing and computed tomography allowed the development of frameless stereotaxy devices over the years, enabling the location of tools in 3D space intraoperatively without the need for rigid fixation. This 3D information, synchronized with preoperative computed tomography (CT) or magnetic resonance images (MRI), has given rise to 3D intraoperative navigation systems (14).

Surgical navigation enables the translation of the preoperative plan to the operating room, where anatomical structures can be identified in real-time. This technology allows intraoperative orientation regarding resection margins and surrounding vital structures, improving the safety and accuracy of the procedure. Also, recent advances have enabled navigation systems to be used not only as a simple localization device but also as a measurement tool that can provide other relevant information to the surgeons during different stages of the procedure.

There are currently several navigation solutions to track the positions of surgical instruments relative to patient anatomy. Usually, the selection of the tracking device depends on the specific surgical procedure. Optical tracking systems based on infrared cameras are the most common solution in interventions where a direct line of sight between the camera and the surgical instruments can be maintained. They are widely chosen, as they provide a large field of view and high accuracy (13, 15). In these interventions, retroreflective markers are fixed to the patient through a dynamic reference frame, allowing tracking of the patient's movements. The real-time position of these sensors is captured by the camera and translated to the navigation software. Other navigation solutions include mechanical or electromagnetic tracking systems (16).

Recent studies have also presented augmented reality as a tool for navigation. With this technique, virtual models can be superimposed onto the patient's anatomy instead of displaying them on an external screen. The virtual components can be represented in place either by following a manual alignment with the patient's anatomy (17, 18) or by using different tracking solutions such as electromagnetic or optical tracking systems (19, 20), features recognition (21), or optical markers (22–25). The information can be presented on an external screen, a smartphone, or a head-mounted display such as the HoloLens. Some examples include spine surgery (26, 27), craniosynostosis treatment (24), orthopedics (23, 28), or dental implant placement (29).

One of the most critical steps in surgical navigation is image-to-patient registration. This technique estimates the transform that aligns the preoperative images with the patient during the intervention. Registration can be either rigid or nonrigid. Nonrigid registrations are used as a secondary registration for pose refinement or to work with nonrigid surgical fields (30, 31). The most common algorithm is paired-points registration, where corresponding anatomical or artificial landmarks are located in the image and patient. Many systems include a secondary registration for refinement based on surface-points matching. In oral and maxillofacial surgery, the selected paired points are either anatomical landmarks or artificial fiducials, including skin stickers (32), dental splints (33), or bone-implanted screws (34). Surface-points matching is also widely applied by collecting points in the facial skin surface and aligning them with their corresponding landmarks in soft tissue models obtained from preoperative images (32, 35, 36).

The progressive evolution of intraoperative navigation systems has led to the use of this technology almost routinely in the field of neurosurgery (skull-base surgery, vascular lesions), otorhinolaryngology (endoscopic sinus surgery, lateral skull-base surgery, cerebrospinal fluid leaks), and, recently, orthopedic surgery (hip and knee arthroplasty, spinal procedures) (13). However, the extended application of this technology has not been widely evidenced in maxillofacial surgery (37, 38). In 2015, Dubois et al. (39, 40) presented the benefits of surgical navigation for accurate implant positioning secondary to orbital trauma by performing a cadaveric study. Four years later, Wu et al. (41) demonstrated the feasibility of using surgical navigation for zygomatic implant placement. Many other studies found in the literature have proved the benefits of surgical navigation, especially for complex procedures where a personalized approach is required.

Some applications of computer-assisted surgery (CAS) and intraoperative navigation have been described in this field, including orbital reconstruction (42, 43), implant surgery (44–46), or orthognathic surgery (47). Surgical navigation has also been used in tumor removal to delineate surgical margins and achieve safe and accurate resections (11, 48–50). The results are promising, but the clinical adoption is still reduced. The main limitations of this approach include complexity, technical support, cost, steep learning curve, or the rigid fixation of navigation references (14, 49), which are perceived as an entry barrier. Nevertheless, several commercial solutions exist in the market for oral and maxillofacial surgery. Some examples of navigation systems based on optical tracking are Columbia Scientific SIM/Plant software (Columbia scientific, USA) (51, 52), VISIT surgical navigation software (Vienna, Austria) (53, 54), and Vector Vision (Brainlab, Munich, Germany) (45) for dental implants placement, or Stryker Leibinger navigation system (Stryker, Leibinger, Freiburg, Germany) (50, 55, 56) for the removal of foreign bodies and tumors, or repairing orbital bone fractures. Although some studies have presented AR-based surgical navigation systems for oral and maxillofacial surgery applications (24, 57, 58), no commercial systems are available.

The application of CAS and intraoperative navigation in the midface, specifically in resections involving the maxilla and the middle cranial fossa, can become a valuable tool in complex procedures. Additionally, the presence of bone structures that do not modify their contours and volumes during the intraoperative process due to surgical maneuvers is an essential advantage for navigation (59). Therefore, these interventions provide an adequate scenario for navigation and can highly benefit from this technique.

In addition to intraoperative navigation, there are more resources that CAS procedures can provide in this field. Advances in preoperative planning with computer-aided design (CAD) and computer-aided manufacturing (CAM) have enabled the development of customized and prefabricated templates that facilitate both surgical resections and reconstruction (60–62). The recent introduction of intraoperative imaging, particularly computerized tomography (CT), has solved the limitations of morphological change, intraoperative edema, and soft tissue distortion that appear during the surgical resection and could not be considered in preoperative planning. Thus, the acquisition of intraoperative images once the resection surgery has been carried out provides additional information, allowing the verification and the achievement of adequate surgical margins (63, 64).

With the same objective of safety, accuracy, and minimization of sequelae in the treatment of tumors that involve the maxilla and midface, it is worth mentioning the endoscopically-assisted maxillectomy. The endoscopic transnasal approach provides advantages such as better control of the medial and posterior margins and the possibility of avoiding transfacial approaches when combined with intraoral procedures, minimizing the radicality of surgical resections (10).

Adenoid Cystic Carcinoma

Adenoid Cystic Carcinoma (ACC) is a rare malignant tumor accounting for 1% of head and neck cancers and 10% of salivary gland tumors (65). It is commonly found in palate small salivary glands, from where it spreads slowly but aggressively. These tumors settle in the upper palate and maxillary region and tend to local infiltration and perineural spread. Consequently, they may behave in an indolent and silent manner until late diagnosis, appearing as destructive masses that can even involve intracranial structures. In addition, this histologic type is characterized by a high predisposition to systemic dissemination, mainly hematogenous (lung, liver, brain, and bone) and lymph nodes. They present a high propensity to local recurrence and distant metastasis (5). The primary treatment consists of surgical removal with clear margins and complementary radiotherapy when needed. Data on the efficacy of systemic therapy or radiotherapy in recurrent or metastatic salivary gland tumors are limited, with some benefits described in proton-based radiotherapy (66–68) or the recent systemic use of Lenvatinib (69). Consequently, an effective primary surgical treatment with adequate margins is the best prognostic factor for these patients.

However, this intervention is highly challenging due to the occasional centrofacial tumor location, complex elective surgical approach, limited line of sight, and the need for immediate reconstruction. Additionally, the tumor boundaries are difficult to discriminate from the normal surrounding tissue.

In this type of intervention, where complex anatomy is present and high accuracy is needed, surgical navigation becomes a valuable tool to improve clinical outcomes. It can provide guidance that can help achieve accurate safety margins and protect vital structures. However, despite its great potential in these clinical applications, there are currently limited studies using CAS for midfacial tumor resection. Wei et al. (11) tested surgical navigation in patients who underwent surgery near the skull base, including five patients with adenoid cystic carcinoma at minor salivary glands of the palate. Their approach was limited by the invasive attachment of a reference frame to the patients' forehead and an image-to-patient registration based on non-precise anatomical landmarks, which can significantly reduce the navigation accuracy. Tarsitano et al. (49) followed a similar setup for maxillary tumors resection, screwing a dynamic reference frame to the patient's skull.

The aim of this study is to present and assess the accuracy of three different alternatives for surgical navigation in head and neck tumors based on 3D printing, optical tracking, and augmented reality visualization. These alternatives are less invasive than previous solutions (11, 49) and more convenient for these procedures than conventional registration solutions used in other disciplines such as neurosurgery as they do not involve fixation of the patient's head. A 3D printed patient-specific phantom was used for validation and assessment of the three navigation systems. One of the proposed solutions was then used to guide the tumor resection of a patient presenting a central palate carcinoma invading the nasal fossa floor and septum.

METHODS

Clinical Case

A 62-year-old woman was referred to the Oral and Maxillofacial Unit at our center for treatment. The patient presented an exophytic tumor of approximately 3x2 centimeters in the middle of the hard palate with normal oral mucosa (**Figure 1A**). Endoscopy showed a nasal extension of the lesion, and biopsy results confirmed an adenoid cystic carcinoma. A CT scan showed hard palate bony erosion, invasion for the nasal septum and floor of the right fossa, and an intact ipsilateral inferior turbinate (**Figures 1E, F**).

The chosen procedure consisted of an endoscopic nasal approach, a navigated transoral resection of the central palate with at least 2 cm margin (**Figures 1C, D**), and immediate reconstruction of the central hard and soft palate with a radial forearm free flap (**Figure 1B**). Alternative surgical approaches considered were a Le Fort I osteotomy (downfracture of the whole maxilla and resection of the central part) or a IIb maxillectomy (Brown classification, sacrificing the intact alveolar process and denture) reconstructed with a fibula free flap. Our purpose was to achieve functional rehabilitation, including a tight palate seal and maintaining the whole alveolar process of the maxilla. The proposed solution presented a more straightforward reconstruction involving only soft tissue, as bone reconstruction is not needed in horizontal class a defects.

The preoperative CT scan was used to extract the 3D anatomical models (bone and tumor) and perform the

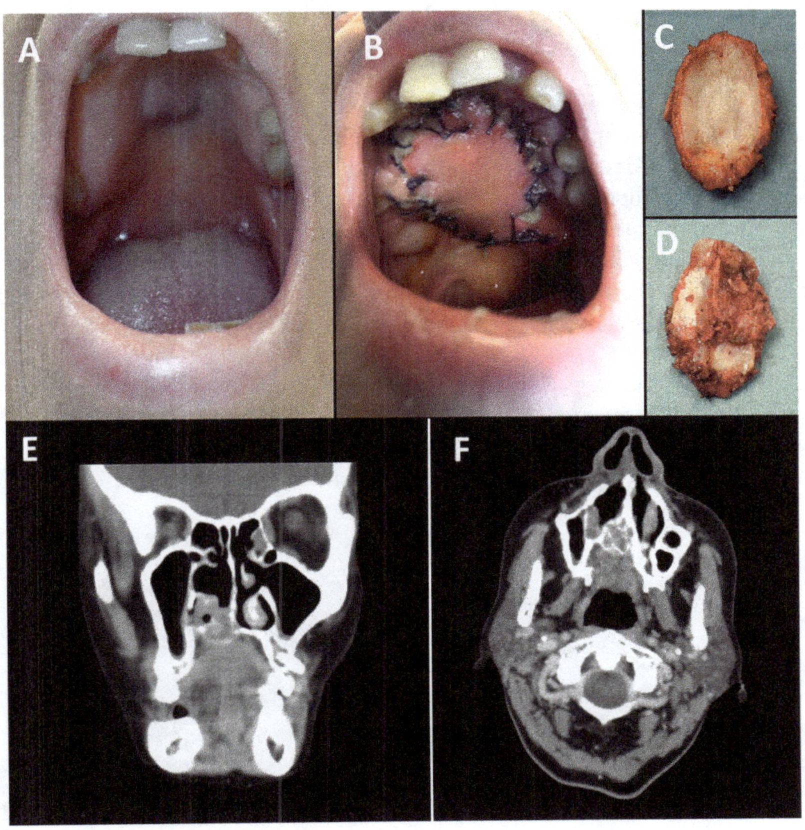

FIGURE 1 | Hard palate midline submucous bulging lesion **(A)** and palate reconstruction with radial forearm free flap (3 weeks after surgery) **(B)**. Resected specimen from **(C)** palate and **(D)** nasal view. **(E)** Coronal and **(F)** axial views of the CT image.

preoperative plan, defining the desired tumor margins for the resection. Using Autodesk Meshmixer software (Autodesk, Inc., USA), we increased the size of the tumor model 1 cm. The intersection of this model with the bone in the palate determined the surgical margins (1 cm margin with a thickness of 1 mm). Before image acquisition, five screws were attached to the maxilla above the upper teeth under local anesthesia as proposed by Zavattero et al. (70). This procedure provides unobtrusive, rigid, and exact landmarks that are clearly visible on virtual data sets (CT images) as well as during the navigation procedure. The position of these screws was identified in the scan for later use during intraoperative image-to-patient registration.

Surgical Navigation: Simulation

Based on the anatomical models of the patient, we designed and manufactured a phantom in polylactic acid using the desktop 3D printer Ultimaker 3 extended (Ultimaker B.V., NL). The phantom was used to simulate the intervention and to test the precision of three different solutions for surgical guidance (**Figure 2**).

The first solution consists in using an optical tracking system (NDI Polaris Spectra, CA) for computer-assisted navigation (**Figure 2A**). We attached a 3D printed dynamic reference frame to a silicone jig fabricated to fit on the patient's upper left teeth. The dynamic reference frame is used to compensate for head movements. This silicone jig consists of a mass given the shape of the patient's teeth during its malleable state. A picture of the fabrication procedure is provided as **Supplementary Material**. The image-to-patient registration is performed using the screws described in the previous section as artificial landmarks.

A second solution involves the same tracking device, but the reference frame is installed by means of a splint (**Figure 2B**) instead of using a silicone jig. This splint is designed from the 3D models of the teeth obtained from the preoperative images, and 3D printed in a biocompatible resin (Biomed Clear), using the Formlabs Form2 (Formlabs Inc., Somerville, MA, USA) 3D printer. In contrast to the first method, the registration in this case is computed with artificial landmarks added on the splint during the design process.

Finally, the third solution uses AR for surgical navigation (**Figure 2C**). We developed a specific smartphone app to visualize the patient's anatomy and the tumor margins. The application was implemented on the Unity platform (version 2019.3), using the Vuforia development kit (Parametric Technology Corporation Inc., Boston, MA, USA) for pattern recognition. The application displays the 3D models of the bone, tumor and surgical margins (obtained from the preoperative image and planning) and includes buttons to change the visibility of the models (modify opacity or hide). In order to display the virtual models in the correct position with respect to the patient's phantom, we attached a 3D-printed marker to the splint in a fixed and known position. This AR marker contains a unique black and white pattern printed using the double extruder functionality of the Ultimaker 3 extended 3D printer. The smartphone's camera detects this marker and displays the virtual models on the screen on top of the patient. **Figure 2C** and the video included as **Supplementary Material** show the appearance of the developed AR application.

The three configurations were tested on the phantom, where we performed the corresponding registration procedure for each configuration. After that, each navigation system displayed the position of the surgical margins defined preoperatively. Using the optical tracker and the pointer, we collected points (with distances of 1 mm between each other) following the indicated surgical margins. The process was repeated three times for each configuration, including the registration step. A similar number of points was recorded for each sample (around 100 points).

Inaccuracies in the registration step would generate errors in the displayed margins. Therefore, the collected points would present deviations from the position of the real surgical margins. In order to assess the accuracy for each configuration, we computed the distances between the collected points (following the margins indicated by each navigation system) and the real position of the tumor margins. For that, we obtained the closest point of the resection margins (a 3D model or pointcloud) to every recorded point and stored the distance. Then, we computed the median and quartiles for each solution. Finally, we conducted a statistical analysis to identify significant differences in accuracy between methods.

The surgical margins used as ground truth for evaluating the three methodologies were the ones defined during preoperative planning with the preoperative CT (1 cm margin). The real position of the tumor margins was obtained during assessment thanks to the rigid attachment of a reference frame to the phantom and a registration performed with artificial landmarks distributed all over the surface to ensure accurate

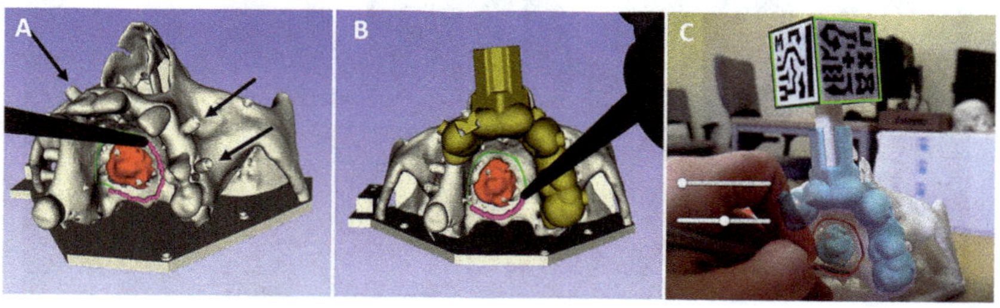

FIGURE 2 | Solutions for surgical navigation tested on the patient's anatomical model: **(A)** navigation with an optical tracking system and registration with screws (black arrows); **(B)** navigation with an optical tracking system and registration with a splint; **(C)** navigation with an AR application and registration with a cubic marker.

registration. These artificial landmarks were added as conical holes in the bone region and the base of the phantom and can be seen in **Figure 2**.

Surgical Navigation: Setup

Apart from tracking the patient with the 3D-printed dynamic reference frame (**Figure 3B**), two different instruments were tracked during surgery: a pointer tool to record points and a piezoelectric handpiece for tumor resection. We designed and 3D printed an adaptor with optical markers to fit in the handle (**Figure 3C**) for handpiece tracking. An additional tool was also designed and 3D-printed to fit the instrument at a specific position. This tool included six small conical holes for registration. The **Supplementary Material** shows a picture of the designed tool. Finally, as the handpiece is composed of an interchangeable saw with a non-fixed rotation around the longitudinal axis, we added an extra step in the registration procedure. This step consists in recording the position of the saw tip and automatically finding the rotation that corrects the orientation of the saw in the navigation scene. That is the rotation that minimizes the distance between the virtual tip point and the recorded point. The pointer and all 3D printed tools, including the dynamic reference frame, were sterilized before the intervention to maintain the asepsis of the surgical field.

We developed a custom module for surgical navigation in the 3D Slicer platform (71), a free and open-source software package for clinical and biomedical applications. We used the SlicerIGT kit (72) and the PLUS toolkit (73) to define the graphical user interface and manage the transforms sent by the optical tracker through the OpenIGTLink protocol. Intraoperative imaging was not used during the procedure. However, our software allowed the visualization of the CT preoperative image and the 3D models obtained of the patient (bone, tumor, and surgical margins) and the position of the instruments (**Figure 3A**). The three views of the CT (axial, sagittal, and coronal) could be updated in real-time to match the position of the instrument's tip for better guidance. The software also included other functionalities, such as modifying the point of view in the 3D view or recording points. The **Supplementary Material** includes a video showing the use of the software during the intervention.

Surgical Navigation: Intervention

Resection margins were controlled in real-time using the developed software through constant visual feedback displayed on a screen adjacent to the surgical field. During the intervention, we increased the surgical margin 1 cm from the preoperative segmentation to ensure adequate en-bloc resection with 2 cm of tissue free of disease. The final resection margins were recorded using the pointer. While not used for surgical guidance, AR was tested on the patient to validate the AR setup using the splint (**Figure 4**). The smartphone was introduced in a sterile case (CleanCase, Steridev Inc., Lansing, MI, USA) so that surgeons could hold it close to the patient.

After resection, a radial forearm free flap was harvested and placed to reconstruct the palate with an adequate seal. A postoperative CT scan was performed a week after surgery to assess the surgical outcome. Navigation accuracy was measured

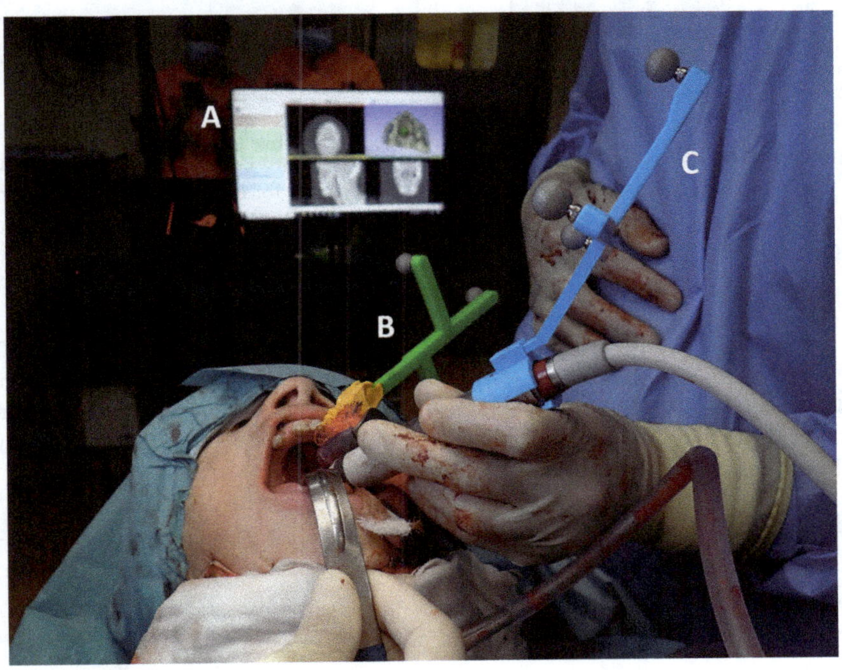

FIGURE 3 | Surgical navigation setup during the intervention: **(A)** surgical navigation software; **(B)** 3D-printed patient's dynamic reference frame; **(C)** 3D-printed adaptor for tracking of the piezoelectric handpiece.

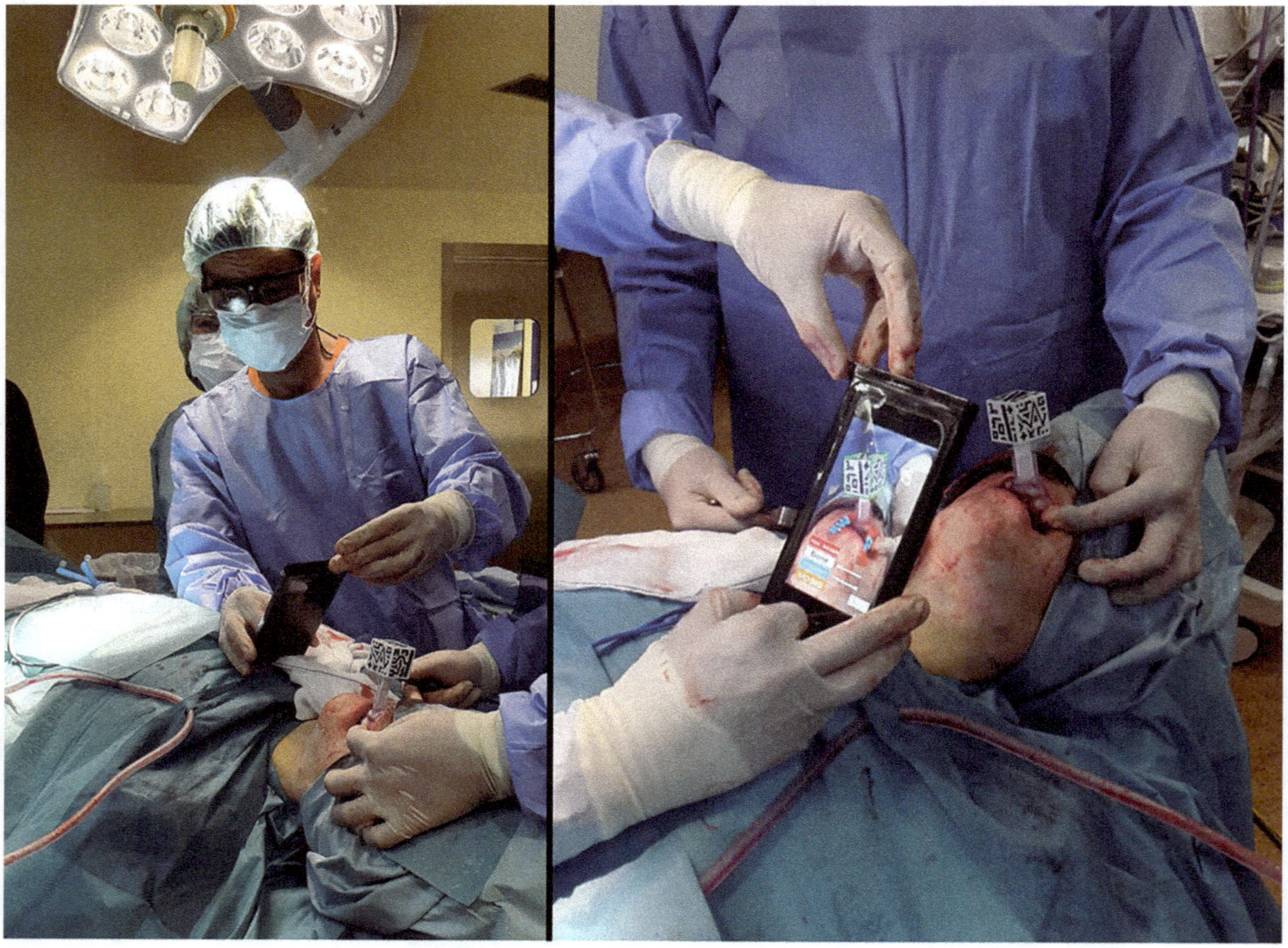

FIGURE 4 | Use of the augmented reality app during the intervention.

as the absolute distance between the points recorded intraoperatively and the real resection margins identified in the postoperative CT. A secondary CT scan was acquired 15 months after surgery for the patient's follow-up.

RESULTS

Surgical Navigation: Simulation

We analyzed the accuracy provided by each navigation solution on the 3D printed phantom by computing the distances between the collected points during guidance and the real resection margins. The results for each configuration are presented in **Table 1**.

All methods presented median values below 0.7 mm. Most of the points recorded using the optical tracking system for guidance presented deviations from the surgical margins below 1 mm. The results obtained when using AR for guidance presented the lowest median value (0.4 mm). However, they also presented the highest variation, with an interquartile range (IQR) of 0.89 mm compared to the ones obtained with optical tracking, where the IQRs for the screws and surgical guide configurations were 0.24 mm and 0.37 mm, respectively.

TABLE 1 | Mean and standard deviation of the distances between the tumor margins and the collected points with each navigation solution.

Navigation solution	Median	Q1	Q3
OTS (registration with screws)	0.57	0.34	0.81
OTS (registration with surgical guide)	0.61	0.30	0.98
AR	0.40	0.14	1.29

OTS, optical tracking system; AR, augmented reality; Q1, Q3, first and third quartiles (25th and 75th percentile).

A Kruskal-Wallis test was performed to explore the differences between each configuration proposed for this study. No statistically significant differences were obtained [$H(3) = 4.27$, $p = .12$]. Therefore, we can conclude that the three configurations present similar accuracy. The configuration using screws for registration was the one presenting lower error. Thus, it was the one chosen for the intervention.

Surgical Navigation: Intervention

The selected navigation system (optical tracker with screws for registration) was successfully used for guidance during the resection. Surgical instruments were accurately tracked with respect to the patient's anatomy, providing valuable feedback to the surgeons. The registration step was repeated three times during the intervention, obtaining a fiducial registration error of 0.77, 0.93, and 0.81 mm.

The points collected along the surgical margins with the navigation system were compared with the real surgical margins identified in the postoperative CT by measuring their absolute distance. We separated the analysis into four regions divided by left and right sides and posterior and anterior locations. **Figure 5** displays the results.

The mean distances were around 1 mm and below 2 mm in 90% of the samples. The posterior region presented higher errors compared to the anterior. The left side showed higher deviations than the right one. However, this deviation appears to be caused by the jig, which was still in place during the points collection and limited the pointer movements (**Figure 6**).

The AR app was also used inside the operating room, where surgeons visualized models of the patient's anatomy overlayed on the camera's image of an iPhone 6 (Apple Inc., Cupertino, CA, USA). The splint was inserted correctly and enabled AR display, where virtual models were represented aligned with the patient's anatomy.

DISCUSSION

The resections of head and neck tumors in deep and less accessible regions represent complex surgical scenarios requiring extreme dexterity, as the field of view and instruments maneuverability is limited. For middle third tumors such as palate ACCs, the preservation of normal bony tissue and surrounding soft tissues should be maximized. Tel et al. (67) advocate an open "box resection" where the tumor is resected within a three-dimensional volume of healthy tissue. In these scenarios, CAS represents a valuable tool to plan (74), guide (9) and verify (49) the resection margins.

Pu et al. (75) concluded in their study with 37 patients that surgical margins can be predetermined without compromising oncological safety, and that the difficulty in determining these margins lies more on soft than hard tissue. Thus, the use of CAS should be limited to cases with mainly bone involvement (76). Ricotta et al. (74) demonstrated how performing a volumetric virtual plan of the resection can improve accuracy and reduce the probability of finding positive margins.

Intraoperative navigation is highly indicated for resections in areas with restricted access (8), where the deep portion of the tumor is not clearly visible. Such is the case of deep maxilla cuts, where Hasan et al. (63) have reported resections errors below 2 mm when using intraoperative navigation. Surgical navigation systems also helps in achieving R0 (absence of disease) in deep sinonasal tumors (77).

Midfacial tumors usually present a small soft tissue involvement with a predominant three-dimensional bone infiltration, making them adequate for virtual planning. Tumors may be located in areas with limited access, making surgical navigation a valuable tool in these scenarios. In addition, the proximity to vital structures that cannot be damaged adds another advantage for guided resection of centrofacial tumors.

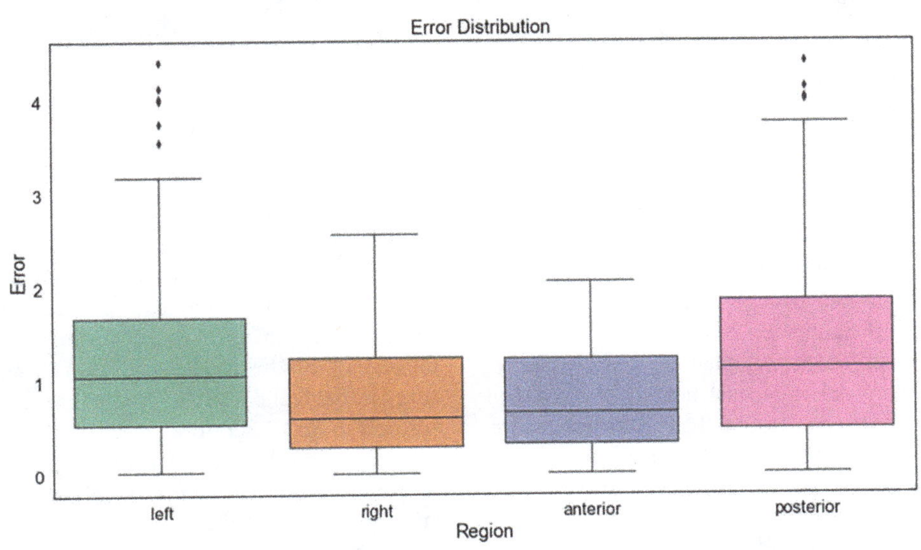

FIGURE 5 | Distances between the resection margins collected intraoperatively with the navigation system and those identified in the postoperative CT.

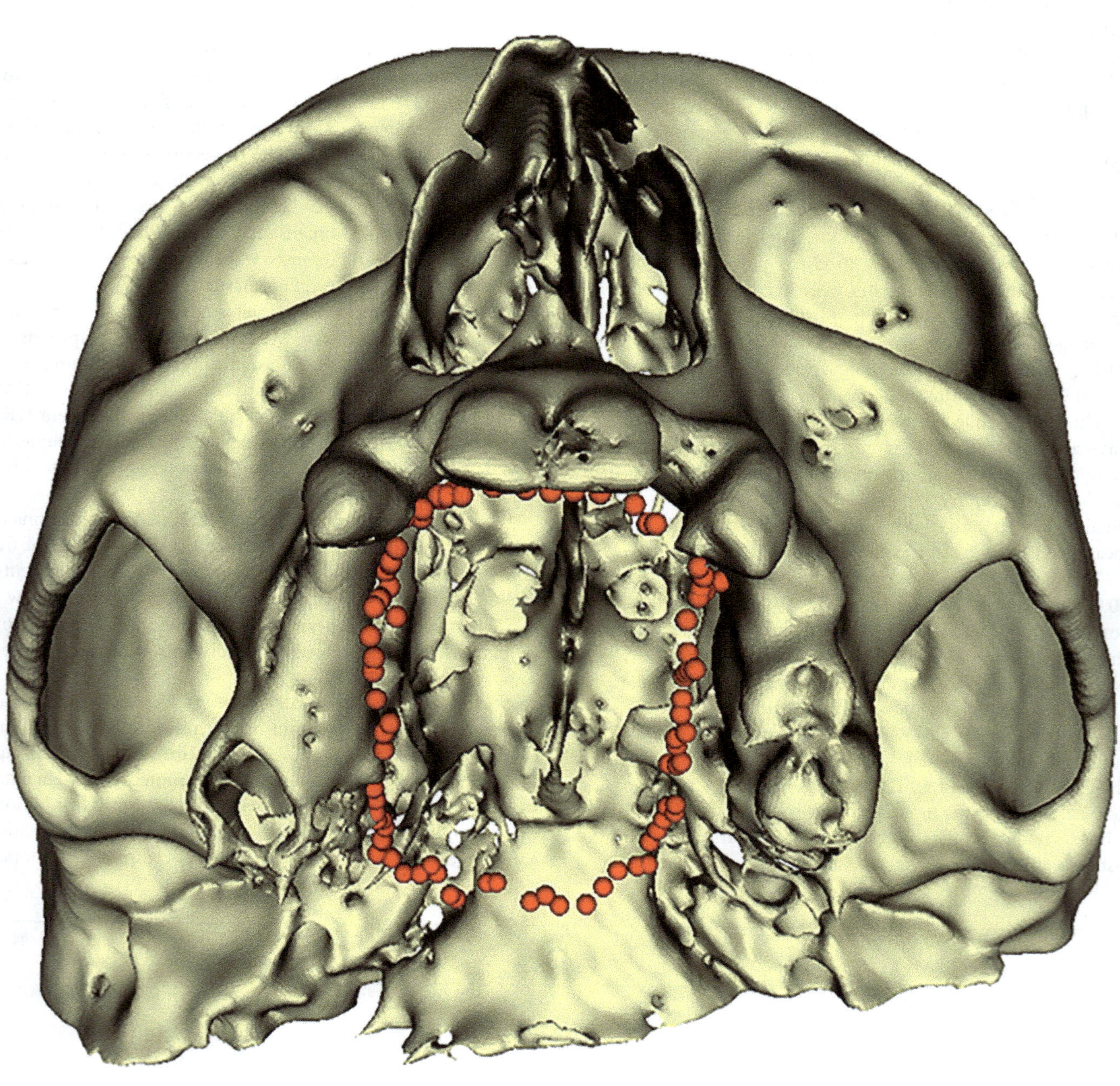

FIGURE 6 | Points collected intraoperatively along the resection margins.

Although the use of surgical guidance for tumor resections is a routine procedure in neurosurgery, the reports in the maxillofacial middle third tumors are scarce. The existing CAS applications mainly focus on virtual planning, intraoperative guidance for the free flap defect reconstruction, or validation of the reconstruction after trauma, not on the ablative procedure. Moreover, most existing commercial systems for surgical navigation use a three-point clamp (Mayfield clamp or similar) to fix the patient's skull and prevent head movements. Then, a dynamic reference frame is attached to the clamp to define a reference system for the patient and perform the image-to-patient registration. This setup is suitable for neurosurgery, and it can help achieve high accuracy. However, in the resection of middle third tumors, surgeons need free movement of the head to adjust the line of sight with the surgical field and enable proper angulation of the saw and surgical tools. Therefore, other solutions for tracking and registration need to be found for these procedures.

Some studies have presented alternative setups for tracking and registration. Malham et al. (78) use the SpineMask (Stryker, Leibinger, Freiburg, Germany) to track the patient's back and perform an automatic registration. This device is non-invasive, as it is an adhesive surgical tracker designed to be placed on the patient's back. The device contains markers for automatic registration, which are placed surrounding the surgical field. Other studies remove the dynamic reference frame from their setup and use conventional optical cameras to detect fiducial markers and constantly update the registration. These setups are usually based on computer vision algorithms for the detection of adhesive skin markers (79) or anatomical features in the bone (21). Other frameless systems use different devices such as hyperspectral cameras to detect skin features (80) or advanced methods such as 3D digital image correlation (also called stereo DIC). This last solution presents precise real-time tracking at a lower cost and based on small markers. Xue et al. (81) tested it for tracking the maxilla after a Lefort I osteotomy. However, it was not tested in a clinical setup where light conditions and external factors such as blood or saliva can condition the tracking and accuracy of the system.

Most of the existing alternatives focus on anatomical regions presenting deformations, where installing a dynamic reference frame and performing a rigid registration becomes inaccurate. Others are designed for specific applications, such as SpineMask, and are not applicable for reduced regions like the mouth. Also, we consider the systems based on skin markers not adequate for an open transfacial approach. Registration markers must be placed surrounding the surgical field to ensure an accurate registration, but in our scenario, the space is limited and a rigid position between markers is difficult to maintain.

Tarsitano et al. (49) presented a surgical navigation setup for the resection of maxillary tumors in a study with twenty patients, obtaining promising results with clear margins in 91% of cases. In their setup, a dynamic reference frame was screwed to the patient's skull. The registration was performed first with a point-to-point registration based on anatomical landmarks, obtaining a mean error of 2 mm, followed by surface matching for refinement. They computed the errors in preoperatively defined target points, finding values between 0.30 and 1 mm, and a mean error of 0.47 mm. Wei et al. (11) also used a similar setup in 15 patients with tumors involving the skull base, five of them presenting an ACC in the palate. In their case, they also installed the dynamic reference frame in the patient's skull but used bony skull landmarks and tooth cusps for registration. The registration errors and the resection accuracy in this study were not reported. Although these studies present a feasible setup for ACC resection, the installation of the dynamic reference frame is invasive. Moreover, the use of anatomical landmarks and surface matching with points in the face presents a suboptimal registration for ACC resection. Points used for registration should be close to the surgical area and surround it to provide accurate results. Anatomical landmarks and tooth cusps are not clearly defined and subject to intra- and inter-observer variability, leading to higher errors.

In our study, we have explored two different configurations for tracking and registration in ACC resection. They provide a non-invasive installation of the reference frame allowing for head movements and a registration based on artificial landmarks located close to the surgical field. The dynamic reference frame is fixed to the patient's teeth either through a silicone jig molded with the shape of the teeth or by means of a splint. The registration landmarks for the first solution (jig) consist of screws placed preoperatively. For the second solution, registration is performed through conical holes included in the splint. Both configurations were evaluated in an anatomical phantom providing equivalent accuracy results with no significant differences, and with deviations from the planned surgical margins of 0.57 and 0.61 mm respectively. These results are similar to the ones obtained by Tarsitano et al. (49). The jig and screws configuration was finally used in a surgical scenario of ACC resection, obtaining deviations from the surgical margin around 1 mm and below 2 mm in 90% of the collected points along the surgical margins. Errors were higher in deeper regions. This behavior was expected, since accuracy usually decreases in areas further from the registration landmarks (82, 83). The splint was also placed in the patient during the intervention for testing. Although the installation of screws in the maxilla has been previously described in other works as an unobtrusive and precise method for registration (68), we believe that using a splint could provide similar results while presenting a straightforward and less-invasive approach.

We have also proposed an alternative guiding method based on AR. A splint was again used for registration, to fix an AR marker in a known position and display virtual models of the patient. The precision of this system has been evaluated in a previous study, obtaining visualization errors below 3 mm (28). This solution was also evaluated in our phantom study, where we obtained a 0.4 mm (IQR = 0.89) median deviation from the planned surgical margins.

Previous studies have reported other registration methods for AR visualization. Gibby et al. (84) displayed the CT and virtual models indicating trajectories for pedicle screw placement in a lumbar spine phantom. They used the OpenSight software for the HoloLens to automatically register the data with the phantom. However, a manual adjustment was needed to correct the alignment. The pedicle screws were placed with deviations between 1.3 and 1.53 mm from their planned trajectory. Other studies rely only on manual alignment for registration (17) or use additional instruments like electromagnetic or optical tracking systems (19, 20).

Although all configurations are feasible, we found the AR app to be less convenient for this procedure, as the limited line of sight of the surgical field also restricts the movements and visibility with the smartphone. The sterilization of the smartphone was easily solved by introducing it in the sterile case. However, the need to hold the smartphone, leaving only one hand free, can present a limitation. The use of head-mounted displays such as HoloLens offers an alternative to the smartphone, although the possible points of view are as limited or more than with the phone. Therefore, AR can complement conventional navigation by allowing an inspection of the margins before or after surgery but is not adequate for resection guidance. The accuracy of the system depends on the quality with which the camera sees the AR marker. This factor is highly dependent on lighting conditions and the pose of the camera with respect to the marker. The detection is optimal when the camera is close to the marker and looks at it from the front. However, when the camera moves and detects the marker from a different angle, some inaccuracies can arise. This inherent holographic instability has already been noted by Gibby et al. (84) with the HoloLens.

CONCLUSIONS

The resection of an ACC in the palate is very challenging due to the limited visibility and the proximity to vital structures. Surgical navigation becomes a valuable tool to ensure adequate margins in such complex scenarios while performing a conservative approach. This study proposes and evaluates three different navigation setups for ACC resection. All configurations aim to provide accuracy with a non-invasive surgical procedure, improving the solutions proposed in previous studies (11, 49). Apart from providing a less invasive solution, the novelty of the proposed setups relies on the fact that all configurations, including AR guidance, are based on 3D printing to fabricate tools that enable navigation of the patient and surgical instruments. The splint, dynamic reference frame, AR marker, and adaptor for tracking the surgical instrument are all 3D printed with desktop 3D printers at a low cost. The three solutions were evaluated in an anatomical phantom, where they provided similar results, and tested in a surgical case. The configuration using an optical tracker and screws for registration was chosen for resection guidance during the procedure.

Surgeons combined the transoral navigated surgery with a nasal endoscopic approach, performing an optimal resection while preserving the whole alveolar process of the maxilla and upper teeth. The postoperative CT scans showed adequate resection margins. The pathological result was low-grade adenoid cystic carcinoma cribriform type, invading the mucosa, hard palate, nasal septum, and nasal floor with clear margins and perineural invasion. Head and neck tumor board established surveillance without adjuvant radiotherapy and a close follow-up. After two years, the patient is free of disease.

The results obtained from this surgery showing the accuracy and convenience of the proposed setups are promising. Navigation provided the confidence needed to undertake a more conservative approach and avoided the complete removal of the maxilla. The proposed navigation setup allowed a less invasive procedure compared to previous studies. We believe that image-guided surgery and 3D printing can provide a personalized, safe, and conservative en-bloc resection minimizing the need for reconstruction.

AUTHOR CONTRIBUTIONS

MG-S, RM-M, and DG-M designed the study and performed the data collection. MG-S wrote the manuscript and performed the analysis. GA contributed to the writing of the manuscript. SO and JP conceived the study. SO, CN-C and GS performed the surgery. All authors contributed to the article and approved the submitted version.

ACKNOWLEDGMENTS

The authors are grateful with the department of Oral and Maxillofacial surgery for their contribution to this study and for their interest in research.

REFERENCES

1. Boukheris H, Curtis RE, Land CE, Dores GM. Incidence of Carcinoma of the Major Salivary Glands According to the WHO Classification, 1992 to 2006: A Population-Based Study in the United States. *Cancer Epidemiol Biomarkers Prev* (2009) 18(11):2899–906. doi: 10.1158/1055-9965.EPI-09-0638
2. To VSH, Chan JYW, Tsang RKY, Wei WI. Review of Salivary Gland Neoplasms. *ISRN Otolaryngol* (2012) 2012:872982. doi: 10.5402/2012/872982
3. Shah GV. MR Imaging of Salivary Glands. *Magn Reson Imaging Clin* (2002) 10(4):631–62. doi: 10.1016/S1064-9689(02)00015-6
4. Son E, Panwar A, Mosher CH, Lydiatt D. Cancers of the Major Salivary Gland. *J Oncol Pract* (2018) 14(2):99–108. doi: 10.1200/JOP.2017.026856
5. Chundru NSV, Amudala R, Thankappan P, Nagaraju CD. Adenoid Cystic Carcinoma of Palate: A Case Report and Review of Literature. *Dental Res J* (2013) 10:274–8. doi: 10.4103/1735-3327.113372
6. Speight PM, Barrett AW. Salivary Gland Tumours. *Oral Dis* (2002) 8(5):229–40. doi: 10.1034/j.1601-0825.2002.02870.x
7. Mahajan A, Kulkarni M, Parekh M, Khan M, Shah A, Gabhane M. Adenoid Cystic Carcinoma of Hard Palate: A Case Report. *Oral Maxillofac Pathol J* (2011) 2(1):127–31.
8. Catanzaro S, Copelli C, Manfuso A, Tewfik K, Pederneschi N, Cassano L, et al. Intraoperative Navigation in Complex Head and Neck Resections: Indications and Limits. *Int J Comput Assist Radiol Surg* (2017) 12(5):881–7. doi: 10.1007/s11548-016-1486-0
9. Ferrari M, Daly MJ, Douglas CM, Chan HHL, Qiu J, Deganello A, et al. Navigation-Guided Osteotomies Improve Margin Delineation in Tumors Involving the Sinonasal Area: A Preclinical Study. *Oral Oncol* (2019) 99:104463. doi: 10.1016/j.oraloncology.2019.104463
10. Deganello A, Ferrari M, Paderno A, Turri-Zanoni M, Schreiber A, Mattavelli D, et al. Endoscopic-Assisted Maxillectomy: Operative Technique and Control of Surgical Margins. *Oral Oncol* (2019) 93:29–38. doi: 10.1016/j.oraloncology.2019.04.002
11. Wei B, Sun G, Hu Q, Tang E. The Safety and Accuracy of Surgical Navigation Technology in the Treatment of Lesions Involving the Skull Base. *J Craniofac Surg* (2017) 28(6):1431–4. doi: 10.1097/SCS.0000000000003624
12. Sukegawa S, Kanno T, Furuki Y. Application of Computer-Assisted Navigation Systems in Oral and Maxillofacial Surgery. *Jpn Dent Sci Rev* (2018) 54(3):139–49. doi: 10.1016/j.jdsr.2018.03.005
13. Cleary K, Peters TM. Image-Guided Interventions: Technology Review and Clinical Applications. *Annu Rev BioMed Eng* (2010) 12(1):119–42. doi: 10.1146/annurev-bioeng-070909-105249
14. Austin RE, Antonyshyn OM. Current Applications of 3-D Intraoperative Navigation in Craniomaxillofacial Surgery: A Retrospective Clinical Review. *Ann Plast Surg* (2012) 69(3):271–8. doi: 10.1097/SAP.0b013e31822a3ec3
15. García-Mato D, Ochandiano S, García-Sevilla M, Navarro-Cuéllar C, Darriba-Allés JV, García-Leal R, et al. Craniosynostosis Surgery: Workflow Based on

Virtual Surgical Planning, Intraoperative Navigation and 3D Printed Patient-Specific Guides and Templates. *Sci Rep* (2019) 9(1):17691. doi: 10.1038/s41598-019-54148-4
16. Berger M, Nova I, Kallus S, Ristow O, Eisenmann U, Dickhaus H, et al. Electromagnetic Navigated Condylar Positioning After High Oblique Sagittal Split Osteotomy of the Mandible: A Guided Method to Attain Pristine Temporomandibular Joint Conditions. *Oral Surg Oral Med Oral Pathol Oral Radiol* (2018) 125(5):407–14.e1. doi: 10.1016/j.oooo.2017.12.007
17. Pratt P, Ives M, Lawton G, Simmons J, Radev N, Spyropoulou L, et al. Through the Hololens™ Looking Glass: Augmented Reality for Extremity Reconstruction Surgery Using 3D Vascular Models With Perforating Vessels. *Eur Radiol Exp* (2018) 2(1):2. doi: 10.1186/s41747-017-0033-2
18. Mitsuno D, Ueda K, Hirota Y, Ogino M. Effective Application of Mixed Reality Device Hololens: Simple Manual Alignment of Surgical Field and Holograms. *Plast Reconstr Surg* (2019) 143(2):647–51. doi: 10.1097/PRS.0000000000005215
19. Meulstee JW, Nijsink J, Schreurs R, Verhamme LM, Xi T, Delye HHK, et al. Toward Holographic-Guided Surgery. *Surg Innov* (2018) 26(1):86–94. doi: 10.1177/1553350618799552
20. Kuhlemann I, Kleemann M, Jauer P, Schweikard A, Ernst F. Towards X-Ray Free Endovascular Interventions - Using Hololens for on-Line Holographic Visualisation. *Healthc Technol Lett* (2017) 4(5):184–7. doi: 10.1049/htl.2017.0061
21. Manni F, Elmi-Terander A, Burström G, Persson O, Edström E, Holthuizen R, et al. Towards Optical Imaging for Spine Tracking Without Markers in Navigated Spine Surgery. *Sensors* (2020) 20(13):3641. doi: 10.3390/s20133641
22. Moreta-Martinez R, García-Mato D, García-Sevilla M, Pérez-Mañanes R, Calvo-Haro J, Pascau J. *Augmented Reality in Computer-Assisted Interventions Based on Patient-Specific 3D Printed Reference.* Available at: http://digital-library.theiet.org/content/journals/10.1049/htl.2018.5072?crawler=true&mimetype=application/pdf&tags=noindex (Accessed 2018 Oct 8).
23. Moreta-Martinez R, García-Mato D, García-Sevilla M, Pérez-Mañanes R, Calvo-Haro J, Pascau J. Augmented Reality in Computer-Assisted Interventions Based on Patient-Specific 3D Printed Reference. *Healthc Technol Lett* (2018) 5(5):162–6. doi: 10.1049/htl.2018.5072
24. García-Mato D, Moreta-Martínez R, García-Sevilla M, Ochandiano S, García-Leal R, Pérez-Mañanes R, et al. Augmented Reality Visualization for Craniosynostosis Surgery. *Comput Methods Biomech BioMed Eng Imaging Vis* (2020) 9(4):392–9. doi: 10.1080/21681163.2020.1834876
25. Li L, Yang J, Chu Y, Wu W, Xue J, Liang P, et al. A Novel Augmented Reality Navigation System for Endoscopic Sinus and Skull Base Surgery: A Feasibility Study. *PloS One* (2016) 11(1):e0146996. doi: 10.1371/journal.pone.0146996
26. Edström E, Burström G, Nachabe R, Gerdhem P. Elmi Terander a. A Novel Augmented-Reality-Based Surgical Navigation System for Spine Surgery in a Hybrid Operating Room: Design, Workflow, and Clinical Applications. *Oper Neurosurg* (2020) 18(5):496–502. doi: 10.1093/ons/opz236
27. Ma L, Jiang W, Zhang B, Qu X, Ning G, Zhang X, et al. Augmented Reality Surgical Navigation With Accurate CBCT-Patient Registration for Dental Implant Placement. *Med Biol Eng Comput* (2019) 57:47–57. doi: 10.1007/s11517-018-1861-9
28. Moreta-Martinez R, Pose-Díez-de-la-Lastra A, Calvo-Haro JA, Mediavilla-Santos L, Pérez-Mañanes R, Pascau J. Combining Augmented Reality and 3D Printing to Improve Surgical Workflows in Orthopedic Oncology: Smartphone Application and Clinical Evaluation. *Sensors* (2021) 21(4):1370. doi: 10.3390/s21041370
29. Wang J, Suenaga H, Hoshi K, Yang L, Kobayashi E, Sakuma I, et al. Augmented Reality Navigation With Automatic Marker-Free Image Registration Using 3-D Image Overlay for Dental Surgery. *IEEE Trans BioMed Eng* (2014) 61(4):1295–304. doi: 10.1109/TBME.2014.2301191
30. Polfliet M, Hendriks MS, Guyader J-M, ten Hove I, Mast H, Vandemeulebroucke J, et al. Registration of Magnetic Resonance and Computed Tomography Images in Patients With Oral Squamous Cell Carcinoma for Three-Dimensional Virtual Planning of Mandibular Resection and Reconstruction. *Int J Oral Maxillofac Surg* (2021) 50 (10):1386–93. doi: 10.1016/j.ijom.2021.01.003
31. Manohar S, Alsadoon A, Prasa PWC, Salah RM, Maag A, Murugesan Y. A Novel Augmented Reality Approach in Oral and Maxillofacial Surgery: Super-Imposition Based on Modified Rigid and Non-Rigid Iterative Closest Point. *2020 5th Int Conf Innov Technol Intell Syst Ind Appl* (2020) 1–10. doi: 10.1109/CITISIA50690.2020.9371785
32. Hardy SM, Melroy C, White DR, Dubin M, Senior B. A Comparison of Computer-Aided Surgery Registration Methods for Endoscopic Sinus Surgery. *Am J Rhinol* (2006) 20(1):48–52. doi: 10.1177/194589240602000110
33. Bettschart C, Kruse A, Matthews F, Zemann W, Obwegeser JA, Grätz KW, et al. Point-to-Point Registration With Mandibulo-Maxillary Splint in Open and Closed Jaw Position. Evaluation of Registration Accuracy for Computer-Aided Surgery of the Mandible. *J Cranio-Maxillofacial Surg* (2012) 40(7):592–8. doi: 10.5167/uzh-60007
34. Šinikovič B, Kramer F-J, Swennen G, Lübbers H-T, Dempf R. Reconstruction of Orbital Wall Defects With Calcium Phosphate Cement: Clinical and Histological Findings in a Sheep Model. *Int J Oral Maxillofac Surg* (2007) 36(1):54–61. doi: 10.1016/j.ijom.2006.07.014
35. Hoffmann J, Westendorff C, Leitner C, Bartz D, Reinert S. Validation of 3D-Laser Surface Registration for Image-Guided Cranio-Maxillofacial Surgery. *J Cranio-Maxillofacial Surg* (2005) 33(1):13–8. doi: 10.1016/j.jcms.2004.10.001
36. Marmulla R, Eggers G, Mühling J. Laser Surface Registration for Lateral Skull Base Surgery. *Minim Invasive Neurosurg* (2005) 48(3):181–5. doi: 10.1055/s-2005-870906
37. Azarmehr I, Stokbro K, Bell RB, Thygesen T. Surgical Navigation: A Systematic Review of Indications, Treatments, and Outcomes in Oral and Maxillofacial Surgery. *J Oral Maxillofacial Surg WB Saunders* (2017) 75:1987–2005. doi: 10.1016/j.joms.2017.01.004
38. Anand M, Panwar S. Role of Navigation in Oral and Maxillofacial Surgery: A Surgeon's Perspectives. *Clin Cosmet Investig Dent* (2021) 13:127–39. doi: 10.2147/CCIDE.S299249
39. Dubois L, Schreurs R, Jansen J, Maal TJJ, Essig H, Gooris PJJ, et al. Predictability in Orbital Reconstruction: A Human Cadaver Study. Part II: Navigation-Assisted Orbital Reconstruction. *J Cranio-Maxillo-Facial Surg Off Publ Eur Assoc Cranio-Maxillo-Facial Surg* (2015) 43(10):2042–9. doi: 10.1016/j.jcms.2015.07.020
40. Dubois L, Essig H, Schreurs R, Jansen J, Maal TJJ, Gooris PJJ, et al. Predictability in Orbital Reconstruction. A Human Cadaver Study, Part III: Implant-Oriented Navigation for Optimized Reconstruction. *J Cranio-Maxillo-Facial Surg Off Publ Eur Assoc Cranio-Maxillo-Facial Surg* (2015) 43(10):2050–6. doi: 10.1016/j.jcms.2015.08.014
41. Wu Y, Wang F, Huang W, Fan S. Real-Time Navigation in Zygomatic Implant Placement: Workflow. *Oral Maxillofac Surg Clin North Am* (2019) 31(3):357–67. doi: 10.1016/j.coms.2019.03.001
42. Schmelzeisen R, Gellrich NC, Schoen R, Gutwald R, Zizelmann C, Schramm A. Navigation-Aided Reconstruction of Medial Orbital Wall and Floor Contour in Cranio-Maxillofacial Reconstruction. *Injury* (2004) 35(10):955–62. doi: 10.1016/j.injury.2004.06.005
43. Bell RB, Markiewicz MR. Computer-Assisted Planning, Stereolithographic Modeling, and Intraoperative Navigation for Complex Orbital Reconstruction: A Descriptive Study in a Preliminary Cohort. *J Oral Maxillofac Surg* (2009) 67(12):2559–70. doi: 10.1016/j.joms.2009.07.098
44. Casap N, Wexler A, Persky N, Schneider A, Lustmann J. Navigation Surgery for Dental Implants: Assessment of Accuracy of the Image Guided Implantology System. *J Oral Maxillofac Surg* (2004) 62(SUPPL. 2):116–9. doi: 10.1016/j.joms.2004.06.028
45. Sießegger M, Schneider BT, Mischkowski RA, Lazar F, Krug B, Klesper B, et al. Use of an Image-Guided Navigation System in Dental Implant Surgery in Anatomically Complex Operation Sites. *J Cranio-Maxillofacial Surg* (2001) 29 (5):276–81. doi: 10.1054/jcms.2001.0242
46. Watzinger F, Birkfellner W, Wanschitz F, Millesi W, Schopper C, Sinko K, et al. Positioning of Dental Implants Using Computer-Aided Navigation and an Optical Tracking System: Case Report and Presentation of a New Method. *J Cranio-Maxillo-Facial Surg* (1999) 27(2):77–81. doi: 10.1016/S1010-5182 (99)80017-1
47. Li B, Zhang L, Sun H, Shen SGF, Wang X. A New Method of Surgical Navigation for Orthognathic Surgery: Optical Tracking Guided Free-Hand Repositioning of the Maxillomandibular Complex. *J Craniofac Surg* (2014) 25 (2):406–11. doi: 10.1097/SCS.0000000000000673
48. Sure U, Alberti O, Petermeyer M, Becker R, Bertalanffy H. Advanced Image-

Guided Skull Base Surgery. *Surg Neurol* (2000) 53(6):563–72. doi: 10.1016/S0090-3019(00)00243-3

49. Tarsitano A, Ricotta F, Baldino G, Badiali G, Pizzigallo A, Ramieri V, et al. Navigation-Guided Resection of Maxillary Tumours: The Accuracy of Computer-Assisted Surgery in Terms of Control of Resection Margins – A Feasibility Study. *J Cranio-Maxillofacial Surg* (2017) 45(12):2109–14. doi: 10.1016/j.jcms.2017.09.023
50. Schramm A, Gellrich N-C, Gutwald R, Schipper J, Bloss H, Hustedt H, et al. Indications for Computer-Assisted Treatment of Cranio-Maxillofacial Tumors. *Comput Aided Surg* (2000) 5(5):343–52. doi: 10.3109/10929080009149852
51. Hagiwara Y, Koizumi M, Igarashi T. Application of CT Imaging for Dental Implant Simulation. *J Oral Sci* (1999) 41(4):157–61. doi: 10.2334/josnusd.41.157
52. Stockham CD. Using CT. And SIM/Plant to Plan Implant Therapy. *Alpha Omegan* (1996) 89(4):35–8.
53. Wagner A, Wanschitz F, Birkfellner W, Zauza K, Klug C, Schicho K, et al. Computer-Aided Placement of Endosseous Oral Implants in Patients After Ablative Tumour Surgery: Assessment of Accuracy. *Clin Oral Implants Res* (2003) 14(3):340–8. doi: 10.1034/j.1600-0501.2003.110812.x
54. Wanschitz F, Birkfellner W, Watzinger F, Schopper C, Patruta S, Kainberger F, et al. Evaluation of Accuracy of Computer-Aided Intraoperative Positioning of Endosseous Oral Implants in the Edentulous Mandible. *Clin Oral Implants Res* (2002) 13(1):59–64. doi: 10.1034/j.1600-0501.2002.130107.x
55. Gui H, Yang H, Shen SGF, Xu B, Zhang S, Bautista JS. Image-Guided Surgical Navigation for Removal of Foreign Bodies in the Deep Maxillofacial Region. *J Oral Maxillofac Surg Off J Am Assoc Oral Maxillofac Surg* (2013) 71(9):1563–71. doi: 10.1016/j.joms.2013.04.001
56. Kim Y-H, Jung D-W, Kim TG, Lee JH, Kim I-K. Correction of Orbital Wall Fracture Close to the Optic Canal Using Computer-Assisted Navigation Surgery. *J Craniofac Surg* (2013) 24(4):1118–22. doi: 10.1097/SCS.0b013e318290266a
57. Wagner A, Rasse M, Millesi W, Ewers R. Virtual Reality for Orthognathic Surgery: The Augmented Reality Environment Concept. *J Oral Maxillofac Surg Off J Am Assoc Oral Maxillofac Surg* (1997) 55(5):453–6. doi: 10.1016/S0278-2391(97)90689-3
58. Wanschitz F, Birkfellner W, Figl M, Patruta S, Wagner A, Watzinger F, et al. Computer-Enhanced Stereoscopic Vision in a Head-Mounted Display for Oral Implant Surgery. *Clin Oral Implants Res* (2002) 13(6):610–6. doi: 10.1034/j.1600-0501.2002.130606.x
59. Guo R, Guo YX, Feng Z, Guo CB. Application of a Computer-Aided Navigation Technique in Surgery for Recurrent Malignant Infratemporal Fossa Tumors. *J Craniofac Surg* (2015) 26(2):e126–32. doi: 10.1097/SCS.0000000000001350
60. Bernstein JM, Daly MJ, Chan H, Qiu J, Goldstein D, Muhanna N, et al. Accuracy and Reproducibility of Virtual Cutting Guides and 3D-Navigation for Osteotomies of the Mandible and Maxilla. *PloS One* (2017) 12(3): e0173111. doi: 10.1371/journal.pone.0173111
61. Liu B-Y, Cao G, Dong Z, Chen W, Xu J-K, Guo T. The Application of 3D-Printed Titanium Mesh in Maxillary Tumor Patients Undergoing Total Maxillectomy. *J Mater Sci Mater Med* (2019) 30(11):125. doi: 10.1007/s10856-019-6326-7
62. Metzger MC, Hohlweg-Majert B, Schwarz U, Teschner M, Hammer B, Schmelzeisen R. Manufacturing Splints for Orthognathic Surgery Using a Three-Dimensional Printer. *Oral Surg Oral Med Oral Pathol Oral Radiol Endod* (2008) 105(2):e1–7. doi: 10.1016/j.tripleo.2007.07.040
63. Hasan W, Daly MJ, Chan HHL, Qiu J, Irish JC. Intraoperative Cone-Beam CT-Guided Osteotomy Navigation in Mandible and Maxilla Surgery. *Laryngoscope* (2020) 130(5):1166–72. doi: 10.1002/lary.28082
64. Ivashchenko O, Pouw B, de Witt JK, Koudounarakis E, Nijkamp J, van Veen RLP, et al. Intraoperative Verification of Resection Margins of Maxillary Malignancies by Cone-Beam Computed Tomography. *Br J Oral Maxillofac Surg* (2019) 57(2):174–81. doi: 10.1016/j.bjoms.2019.01.007
65. Hassmann-Poznańska E, Skotnicka B, Musiatowicz B, Hubert E. Adenoid Cystic Carcinoma in the Head and Neck: Clinical and Pathologic Review. *Otolaryngol Pol = Polish Otolaryngol* (1993) 47(5):399–405.
66. Cozzi L, Fogliata A, Lomax A, Bolsi A. A Treatment Planning Comparison of 3D Conformal Therapy, Intensity Modulated Photon Therapy and Proton Therapy for Treatment of Advanced Head and Neck Tumours. *Radiother Oncol J Eur Soc Ther Radiol Oncol* (2001) 61(3):287–97. doi: 10.1016/S0167-8140(01)00403-0
67. Steneker M, Lomax A, Schneider U. Intensity Modulated Photon and Proton Therapy for the Treatment of Head and Neck Tumors. *Radiother Oncol J Eur Soc Ther Radiol Oncol* (2006) 80(2):263–7. doi: 10.1016/j.radonc.2006.07.025
68. Kandula S, Zhu X, Garden AS, Gillin M, Rosenthal DI, Ang K-K, et al. Spot-Scanning Beam Proton Therapy vs Intensity-Modulated Radiation Therapy for Ipsilateral Head and Neck Malignancies: A Treatment Planning Comparison. *Med Dosim Off J Am Assoc Med Dosim* (2013) 38(4):390–4. doi: 10.1016/j.meddos.2013.05.001
69. Locati LD, Galbiati D, Calareso G, Alfieri S, Singer S, Cavalieri S, et al. Patients With Adenoid Cystic Carcinomas of the Salivary Glands Treated With Lenvatinib: Activity and Quality of Life. *Cancer* (2020) 126(9):1888–94. doi: 10.1002/cncr.32754
70. Zavattero E, Ramieri G, Volpe F, Borbon C. Navigation-Assisted Resection and Fibula Free-Flap Reconstruction of an Extensive Maxillary Tumor. *J Craniofac Surg* (2021) 32(5):e450–2. doi: 10.1097/SCS.0000000000007304
71. Fedorov A, Beichel R, Kalpathy-Cramer J, Finet J, Fillion-Robin JC, Pujol S, et al. 3D Slicer as an Image Computing Platform for the Quantitative Imaging Network. *Magn Reson Imaging* (2012) 30(9):1323–41. doi: 10.1016/j.mri.2012.05.001
72. Ungi T, Lasso A, Fichtinger G. Open-Source Platforms for Navigated Image-Guided Interventions. *Med Image Anal* (2016) 33:181–6. doi: 10.1016/j.media.2016.06.011
73. Lasso A, Heffter T, Rankin A, Pinter C, Ungi T, Fichtinger G. PLUS: Open-Source Toolkit for Ultrasound-Guided Intervention Systems. *IEEE Trans BioMed Eng* (2014) 61(10):2527–37. doi: 10.1109/TBME.2014.2322864
74. Ricotta F, Cercenelli L, Battaglia S, Bortolani B, Savastio G, Marcelli E, et al. Navigation-Guided Resection of Maxillary Tumors: Can a New Volumetric Virtual Planning Method Improve Outcomes in Terms of Control of Resection Margins? *J Cranio-Maxillo-Facial Surg Off Publ Eur Assoc Cranio-Maxillo-Facial Surg* (2018) 46(12):2240–7. doi: 10.1016/j.jcms.2018.09.034
75. Pu JJ, Choi WS, Yu P, Wong MCM, Lo AWI, Su Y-X. Do Predetermined Surgical Margins Compromise Oncological Safety in Computer-Assisted Head and Neck Reconstruction? *Oral Oncol* (2020) 111:104914. doi: 10.1016/j.oraloncology.2020.104914
76. Ren W, Gao L, Li S, Chen C, Li F, Wang Q, et al. Virtual Planning and 3D Printing Modeling for Mandibular Reconstruction With Fibula Free Flap. *Med Oral Patol Oral Cir Bucal* (2018) 23(3):e359–66. doi: 10.4317/medoral.22295
77. Tel A, Bagatto D, Tuniz F, Sembronio S, Costa F, D'Agostini S, et al. The Evolution of Craniofacial Resection: A New Workflow for Virtual Planning in Complex Craniofacial Procedures. *J Cranio-Maxillo-Facial Surg Off Publ Eur Assoc Cranio-Maxillo-Facial Surg* (2019) 47(9):1475–83. doi: 10.1016/j.jcms.2019.06.016
78. Malham GM, Parker RM. Early Experience of Placing Image-Guided Minimally Invasive Pedicle Screws Without K-Wires or Bone-Anchored Trackers. *J Neurosurg Spine* (2018) 28(4):357–63. doi: 10.3171/2017.7.SPINE17528
79. Burström G, Nachabe R, Homan R, Hoppenbrouwers J, Holthuizen R, Persson O, et al. Frameless Patient Tracking With Adhesive Optical Skin Markers for Augmented Reality Surgical Navigation in Spine Surgery. *Spine (Phila Pa 1976)* (2020) 45(22):1598–604. doi: 10.1097/BRS.0000000000003628
80. Manni F, van der Sommen F, Zinger S, Shan C, Holthuizen R, Lai M, et al. Hyperspectral Imaging for Skin Feature Detection: Advances in Markerless Tracking for Spine Surgery. *Appl Sci* (2020) 10(12):4078. doi: 10.3390/app10124078
81. Xue Y, Cheng T, Xu X, Gao Z, Li Q, Liu X, et al. High-Accuracy and Real-Time 3D Positioning, Tracking System for Medical Imaging Applications Based on 3D Digital Image Correlation. *Opt Lasers Eng* (2017) 88:82–90. doi: 10.1016/j.optlaseng.2016.07.002
82. West JB, Fitzpatrick JM, Toms SA, Maurer CR, Maciunas RJ. Fiducial Point Placement and the Accuracy of Point-Based, Rigid Body Registration. *Neurosurg* (2001) 48(4):810–7. doi: 10.1097/00006123-200104000-00023
83. Fitzpatrick JM, West JB, Maurer CR. Predicting Error in Rigid-Body Point-Based Registration. *IEEE Trans Med Imaging* (1998) 17(5):694–702. doi: 10.1109/42.736021
84. Gibby JT, Swenson SA, Cvetko S, Rao R, Javan R. Head-Mounted Display Augmented Reality to Guide Pedicle Screw Placement Utilizing Computed Tomography. *Int J Comput Assist Radiol Surg* (2019) 14(3):525–35. doi: 10.1007/s11548-018-1814-7

4

Computer-Assisted Dental Implant Placement Following Free Flap Reconstruction: Virtual Planning, CAD/CAM Templates, Dynamic Navigation and Augmented Reality

Santiago Ochandiano [1,2], David García-Mato [2,3], Alba Gonzalez-Alvarez [2,3], Rafael Moreta-Martinez [2,3], Manuel Tousidonis [1,2], Carlos Navarro-Cuellar [1,2], Ignacio Navarro-Cuellar [1,2], José Ignacio Salmerón [1,2] and Javier Pascau [2,3]*

[1] Servicio de Cirugía Oral y Maxilofacial, Hospital General Universitario Gregorio Marañón, Madrid, Spain, [2] Instituto de Investigación Sanitaria Gregorio Marañón, Madrid, Spain, [3] Departamento de Bioingeniería e Ingeniería Aeroespacial, Universidad Carlos III de Madrid, Madrid, Spain

***Correspondence:**
Santiago Ochandiano
sochandiano@hotmail.com*

Image-guided surgery, prosthetic-based virtual planning, 3D printing, and CAD/CAM technology are changing head and neck ablative and reconstructive surgical oncology. Due to quality-of-life improvement, dental implant rehabilitation could be considered in every patient treated with curative intent. Accurate implant placement is mandatory for prosthesis long-term stability and success in oncologic patients. We present a prospective study, with a novel workflow, comprising 11 patients reconstructed with free flaps and 56 osseointegrated implants placed in bone flaps or remnant jaws (iliac crest, fibula, radial forearm, anterolateral thigh). Starting from CT data and jaw plaster model scanning, virtual dental prosthesis was designed. Then prosthetically driven dental implacement was also virtually planned and transferred to the patient by means of intraoperative infrared optical navigation (first four patients), and a combination of conventional static teeth supported 3D-printed acrylic guide stent, intraoperative dynamic navigation, and augmented reality for final intraoperative verification (last 7 patients). Coronal, apical, and angular deviation between virtual surgical planning and final guided intraoperative position was measured on each implant. There is a clear learning curve for surgeons when applying guided methods. Initial only-navigated cases achieved low accuracy but were comparable to non-guided freehand positioning due to jig registration instability. Subsequent dynamic navigation cases combining highly stable acrylic static guides as reference and registration markers result in the highest accuracy with a 1–1.5-mm deviation at the insertion point. Smartphone-based augmented reality visualization is a valuable tool for intraoperative visualization and final verification, although it is still a difficult technique for guiding surgery. A fixed screw-retained ideal dental prosthesis was achieved in every case as virtually planned. Implant placement, the final step in free flap oncological reconstruction, could be accurately planned and placed with image-guided surgery, 3D printing, and CAD/CAM technology. The learning curve could be overcome with preclinical laboratory training, but virtually designed and 3D-printed tracer registration stability is crucial for accurate and predictable results. Applying these concepts to our difficult oncologic patient subgroup with deep anatomic alterations ended in comparable results as those reported in non-oncologic patients.

Keywords: virtual surgical planning, 3D printing, computer-aided surgery, free flaps, dental implants, dynamic navigation, augmented reality, static navigation

INTRODUCTION

Head and neck tumor treatment entails an irreversible anatomical distortion and a loss of essential functions such as chewing, swallowing, or phonation. Facial contour disfigurement is also common, especially when adjuvant radiotherapy is required. Therefore, functional restoration of the oral cavity is one of the main challenges for head and neck surgeons. In this context, microsurgical free flaps enable the three-dimensional (3D) repair of orofacial defects on an individual basis to restore lost tissue.

In 1991, Urken (1) stated the main functional objectives for the reconstruction of the oral cavity (1): primary restoration of bone continuity with rigid fixed vascularized bone (2), immediate positioning of osseointegrated implants to ensure rapid rehabilitation of occlusion (3), placement of thin and pliable tissue for reconstruction of the floor of the mouth and tongue, and (4) restoration of soft tissue sensitivity: labial competence and restoration of sensation in intraoral tissue.

In 1988, Riediger (2) was the first author that fitted delayed implants in an iliac crest microsurgical flap. One year later, Urken et al. (3) were the pioneer in fitting implants immediately during the hard tissue reconstructive procedure with DCIA flap (deep circumflex iliac artery, the iliac crest flap). Since then, shape reconstruction using flaps and function restoration with implant-supported prostheses have become well-established methods.

As stated by Schoen et al. (4), in any curative cancer treatment, the placement of dental implants should be evaluated. Roumanas et al. (5) studied chew impairment after tumor resection. They concluded that microsurgical reconstruction and conventional dental restoration contribute to chewing function recovery. However, this study showed a statistically significant improvement when dental rehabilitation was based on osseointegrated implants. It is well reported that quality of life improves after dental implant-supported rehabilitation in oncologic patients in terms of self-assessed masticatory ability, social and psychological disability (6), or good to excellent speech intelligibility and aesthetics (7).

Prosthetic-based implant placement in oncologic patients poses major challenges for the surgeon because these patients have small mouth openings, flat reconstructed ridges, reduced tongue mobility and lip seal, thickened and retracted mucosa, xerostomia, skin scars, etc. (8). An ideal prosthetic rehabilitation should provide appropriate support, retention, and stability, preventing soft tissue injuries; this is why we consider that implant-based dental restoration is the only alternative to reestablish cosmesis and function in oncologic patients.

Smolka et al. (9) reported a significant difference between successful osseointegration and the ability of implants to provide valuable and functional restoration. A 92% osseointegration success rate fell to 42% in the functional evaluation owing to factors such as lack of patient cooperation or implant malpositioning. In our department, Cuesta-Gil et al. (10) found that 4.4% of malpositioned implants are due to a critical lack of parallelism, excessive angulation, or else lingual or vestibular deviation, demonstrating that adequate implant placement is crucial for long-term prosthetic success. More recently, we reported less than 2% of malpositioned, non-load-bearing, osseointegrated implants in oncologic patients (11). Clark et al. (12) estimated that about 7% of complications might be related to implant malposition. Nowadays, the goal is not only to load all the osseointegrated implants but also to place the fixtures so that they are guided by the prosthesis in an accurate and biomechanically ideal position. Poor implant positioning would lead to biological complications due to the inability to maintain proper hygiene, peri-implantitis, unfavorable mechanical load, and, finally, loss of implant at an early stage (13).

In head and neck oncology, virtual surgical planning (VSP) and image-guided surgery (IGS) have become widely accepted methods to improve resection and reconstruction reproducibility, speed, and accuracy (14). Based on CT or MRI data, this concept could also be applied to implant surgery in cancer patients to overcome the aforementioned challenges. Our dental implant placement philosophy has changed in numerous ways. From placing freehand implants in maximum bone volume and density, we moved to prosthetically driven surgery, guided surgery, and finally, computer-assisted surgery.

Computer-assisted implant surgery (CAIS) was introduced in 1995 by Fortin et al. (15), seeking an increased precision and accuracy with a particular interest in complex oncologic reconstructed patients. Several authors have demonstrated the CAIS concept in treating oncologic patients reconstructed with free flaps (8, 16, 17).

The prosthetically driven implant placement method is based on 3D image reconstruction and planning of virtual implant placement in the optimal position. Gargallo-Albiol et al. (18) classified implant navigation surgery as dynamic and static. The ideal plan is transferred to the actual surgical site through a custom-made template in the case of static CAIS (sCAIS) or through real-time tracking and guidance of the surgical drill in dynamic CAIS systems (dCAIS) (19).

Regarding the type of drilling and implant placement, static navigation can also be divided into fully guided (FG) and half-guided (HG) implant surgery. During FG navigation, drilling and insertion of the implants are performed through the rigid guide, whereas during HG navigation the drilling procedure is guided while the implants are inserted freehand without the guide in place. Furthermore, depending on the type of surgical visibility and guide support, we can differentiate between open and closed guided (flapless) or mucosa, bone, and tooth-crown-supported guided navigation. Both approaches, static and dynamic, rely on how the presurgical information is translated into the surgical procedure, offering different advantages and limitations.

When comparing dynamic and static guidance versus freehand placement, the literature shows consistently improved accuracy for the guided procedure (20). When studying guided techniques, Kaewsiri et al. (21) and Mischkowski et al. (22) concluded that dynamic navigation provided higher accuracy than the static guide system. Therefore, any guided method yielded better results than freehand implant placement techniques (17). Dynamic navigation is accurate, is useful in edentulous and mouth-restricted opening patients, and allows intraoperative updates. Static-guided surgery is simple, is cheaper, allows flapless surgery, and produces excellent results in dentate patients.

Another cutting-edge technology used in computer-aided surgery is augmented reality (AR). AR enables the surgeon to visualize virtual information from the patient (e.g., virtual surgical plan or medical images) overlaid on the surgical field (23). Clinical application reports of AR in implantology are scarce. Pellegrino et al. (24) presented the feasibility of adopting AR to facilitate the use of dynamic navigation for dental implantology and evaluated AR's accuracy compared to dynamic navigation in two cases.

To the best of our knowledge, this is the first time where the advantages of combining both guided techniques, static and dynamic navigation, are presented through a workflow that comprises virtual surgical planning, patient-specific 3D-printed tools, dynamic guidance based on real-time optical tracking, and augmented reality visualization. We have already applied these technologies to improve the surgical management of craniosynostosis (25–27). Our research has demonstrated that integrating these solutions into the surgical workflow has a positive impact on surgical outcomes, increasing the reproducibility and efficiency of the interventions (28). Therefore, we hypothesize that virtual prosthetically driven implant placement planning could be accurately translated to our oncologic reconstructed patients by combining static navigation, dynamic navigation, and AR visualization.

MATERIALS AND METHODS

Population

Eleven head and neck reconstructed oncologic patients (5 epidermoid carcinomas, 1 mucoepidermoid carcinoma, 1 adenoid cystic carcinoma, and 4 ameloblastomas), 9 males and 2 females, ages ranging from 18 to 84 years, with different bone and soft tissue defects, were treated with virtually planned and fully guided dental implant placement to restore form and function. Surgical reconstructions included free and regional flaps, 2 iliac crest free flaps, 2 double-barrel fibula flaps, 4 conventional osteocutaneous fibula flaps, 1 ALT with vastus lateralis flap, 1 radial forearm flap, and 1 pectoralis major after a failed fibula flap. Two patients received adjuvant radiotherapy. **Table 1** summarizes the characteristics of each patient included in this study.

All patients signed an informed consent for study participation. The study was performed in accordance with the principles of the 1964 Declaration of Helsinki as revised in 2013 and was approved by the Research Ethics Committee at Hospital General Universitario Gregorio Marañón in Madrid.

Treatment Protocol for Computer-Assisted Implant Surgery

Our treatment protocol follows these fundamental steps:

- Cone-beam computed tomography (CBCT) and patient plaster model scanning.
- Virtual planning: virtual dental prosthesis design, definition of prosthesis-guided implant location, and surgical guide design, including a modification for dynamic navigation (holes and sleeves for registration markers).
- Fabrication of surgical drilling guides on biocompatible resin with a 3D printer.
- Surgical-guided procedure. Static, dynamic, or mixed technique. Intraoperative verification with augmented reality
- Postoperative CBCT and analysis of position differences between planned and final results.

A bimaxillary CBCT scan was acquired for each patient (**Figure 1A**). Then, impressions of both arches were taken with either silicone or alginate materials, and the plaster was scanned to obtain 3D digital models with a D700 3Shape® scanner. These 3D models were manually aligned with the CBCT scan using anatomical landmarks. Then, VSP was performed on a computer workstation for optimal prosthetically guided dental implant placement using either Nobel Clinician-DTX® studio implant licensed software or Blue Sky Bio® open software (**Figure 1B**). VSP started with the virtual screw-retained prosthesis design. Once teeth are in the ideal occlusal position, implant locations were defined, focusing on achieving an appropriate angulation and depth while avoiding any interference with osteosynthesis screws. Finally, we ended with a virtual objective of treatment (**Figures 1C–F**). In all patients we placed Ticare®Osseous (Mozo-Grau, SA, Valladolid, Spain) and Ticare®Osseous Quattro (Mozo-Grau, SA, Valladolid, Spain).

Regarding virtual surgical planning translation to the surgical field, in our initial four patients (**Figure 2**) we followed a silicone jig tooth-supported dynamic navigated procedure. We built the virtual plan in the NobelClinician-DTX® studio implant software (Nobel Biocare®, Zurich, Switzerland) and manually created a silicone tooth-retained jig to hold the 3D-printed dynamic reference frame by articulating upper and lower jaw

TABLE 1 | Characteristics of the patients participating in this study.

Localization and tumor	Surgery	Reconstruction	Guided method	Implants	Prosthesis	Results
Mandibular right body and ramus ameloblastoma	Segmental mandibulectomy	Fibula flap	sCAIS	2 flap, 1 failed	Fixed screw retained	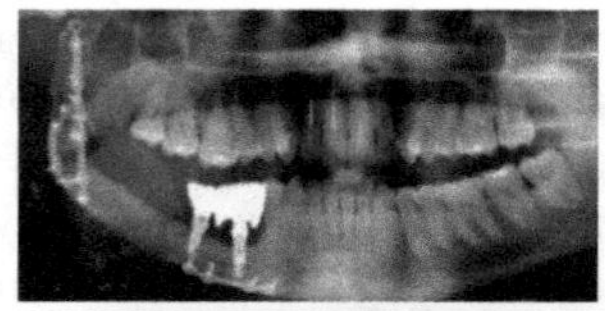
Right mandibular body epidermoid carcinoma	Segmental mandibulectomy and neck dissection	Double-barrel fibula flap	dCAIS	3 flap	Fixed screw retained	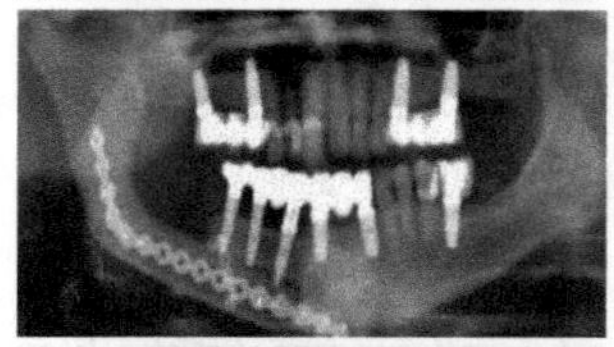
Left mandibular body epidermoid carcinoma	Segmental mandibulectomy and Neck dissection	Iliac crest free flap	dCAIS	2 flap 2 Mdb	Fixed screw retained	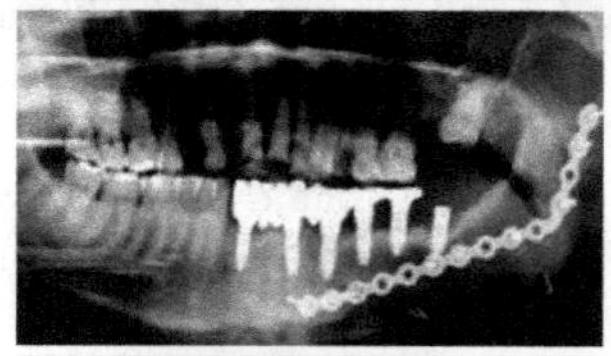
Left mandibular body ameloblastoma	Segmental mandibulectomy	Fibula flap	dCAIS	4 flap	Fixed screw retained	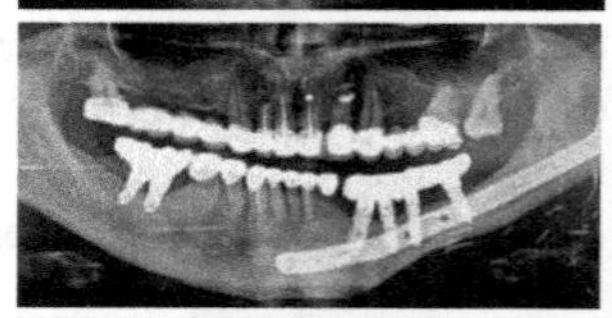
Right mandibular body ameloblastoma	Segmental mandibulectomy	Fibula flap	dCAIS and freehand	3 flap	Fixed screw retained	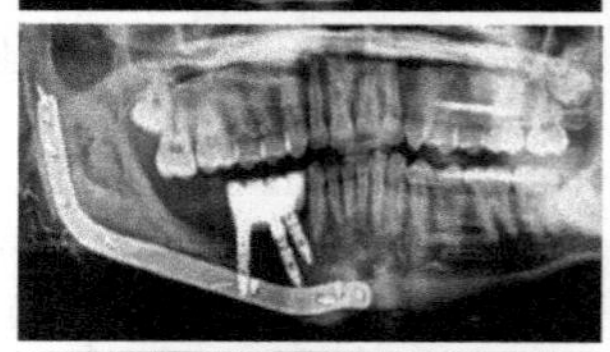
Hard palate adenoid cystic carcinoma	Central maxillectomy	Radial forearm flap	dCAIS and sCAIS	5 Mx 4 Mdb	Fixed screw retained	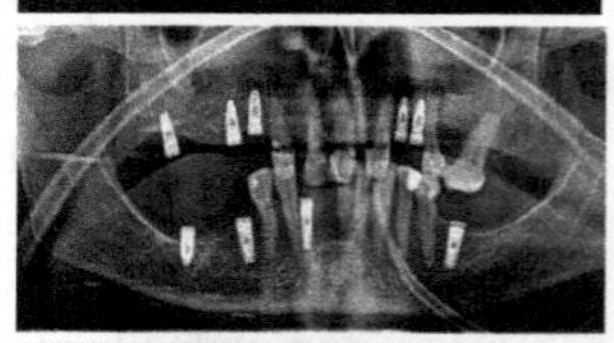
Left maxilla tuberosity adenocarcinoma	IIb Brown maxillectomy	Iliac crest free flap	dCAIS and sCAIS	3 flap	Fixed screw retained	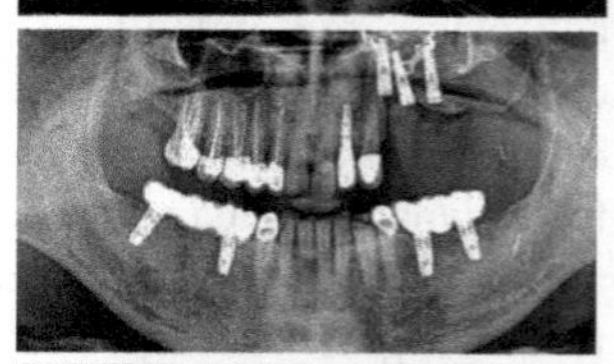
Left mandibular body epidermoid carcinoma	Segmental mandibulectomy and Neck dissection	Double-barrel fibula flap + 70 Gy	dCAIS and sCAIS	3 flap 6 mx	Fixed screw retained (Pending)	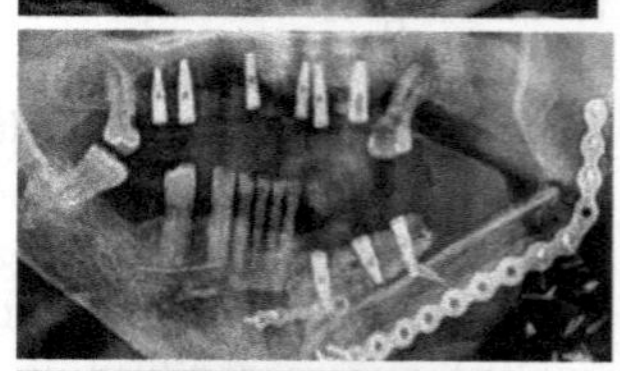
Left mandibular body epidermoide carcinoma	Segmental mandibulectomy and Neck dissection	Fibula flap	dCAIS and sCAIS	3 flap	Fixed screw retained (pending)	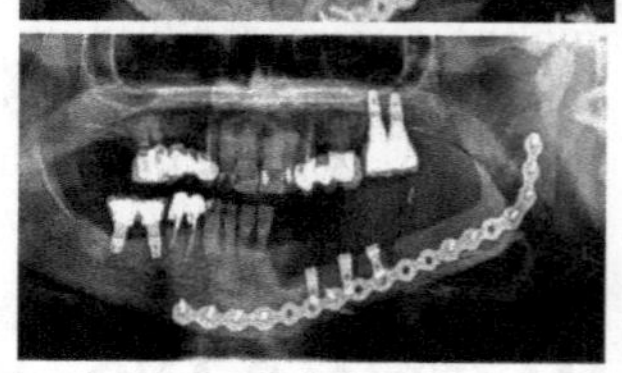

(Continued)

TABLE 1 | Continued

Localization and tumor	Surgery	Reconstruction	Guided method	Implants	Prosthesis	Results
Right hemitongue epidermoid carcinoma	Hemiglosectomy, bilateral neck dissection	Alt+ Vastus Lateralis Flap + 70 Gy	dCAIS	6 mx 6 mdb	Fixed screw retained (pending)	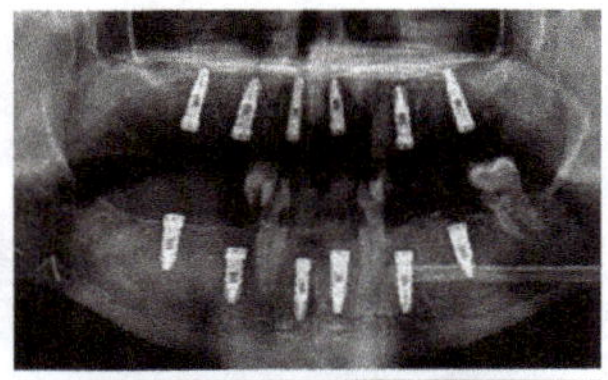
Left hemimandible ameloblastoma	Segmental mandibulectomy	Failed Fibula flap and pectoralis major	sCAIS	5 mx	Fixed screw retained (pending)	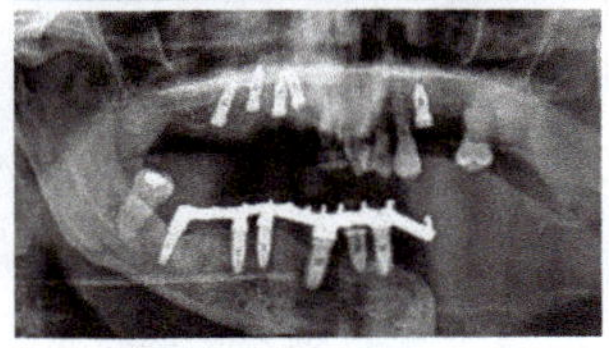

plaster impressions on a semi-adjustable articulator. Registration was based on fiducial markers and in some previous foreign bodies attached to the oncologic patient, including *in-situ* osseointegrated implant heads or fixed osteosynthesis devices, screws, and reconstructive plates.

In the third patient, we encountered a problem with the stability of the silicone tooth-supported jig intraoperatively. This finding forced us to end that procedure in a conventional non-guided freehand way. From this third patient, we decided to stop using the silicone jig as the retention method for the dynamic reference frame.

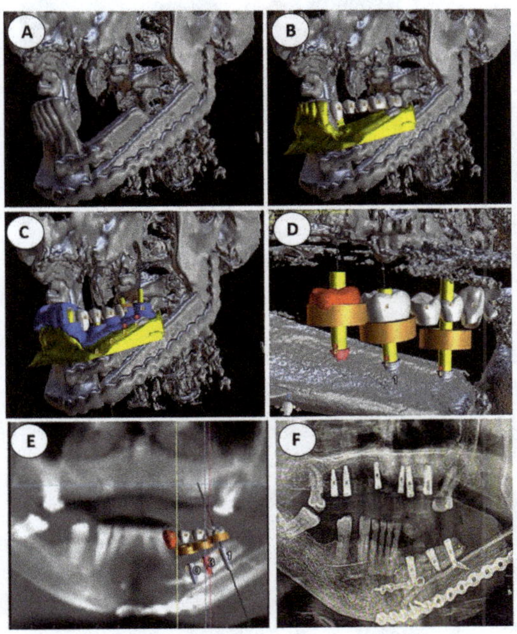

FIGURE 1 | (A) Double barrel fibula flap CBCT 16 months after irradiation with 70 Gy. A basal reconstructive plate and a crestal miniplate. **(B)** Scanned lower jaw plaster model merged with the CBCT and virtual tooth design. **(C)** Prosthetically driven implant planning and in blue the teeth supported rigid splint designed with windows for insertion verification. **(D)** Lingual view seen from the floor of the mouth of the crestal fibula segment and the prosthetically driven implant placement. **(E)** VSP, preoperative implant planned position superimposed in the CBCT **(F)** Postoperative orthopantomogram.

Therefore, for the subsequent seven cases, rigid resin tooth-supported guides were designed with 3D CAD (Blue Sky Bio software) and manufactured by 3D printing technology, seeking intraoperative stability. With this approach, the 3D-printed surgical guide provided excellent stability and was also used for intraoperative registration, avoiding the need for anatomical landmarks. For that purpose, the 3D CAD conventional rigid guide design was imported in Meshmixer software (Autodesk Inc., San Rafael, CA, USA) for design modifications. Several pinholes were added to the surgical guide surface to be used as reference landmarks during patient-to-image registration (**Figure 3A**). A specifically designed socket was also included to attach the dynamic reference frame during navigation or a 3D-printed marker during AR visualization. This socket was positioned on the same jaw as the planned implant but on the opposite side of the arch to avoid interference with the surgical instruments (**Figure 3B**). In general, our rigid guides were designed with a 9- to 12-mm offset between implant head and surgical guide for a 23- or 28-mm drill length. In addition, guiding tubes with a 5.2-mm diameter without metallic sleeves were included to mark the trajectories of the defined implants. Surgical guides were manufactured by the stereolithographic technique with a Formlab Form 2 3D printer and using BioMed Clear V1 biocompatible resin (Formlabs Inc., USA). Finally, surgical guides' stability was evaluated by fitting them on the cast models and on the patient before surgery. With the advantageous rigid guide in place, holding the registration tracers, we could consider dynamic- or static-guided surgery, augmented reality, or a combination of all of them.

Therefore, VSP surgical translation was individualized in each patient. For example in two of them presenting almost an ideal restored anatomy, or when treating a non-reconstructed jaw, we applied a close transmucosal surgical technique with conventional static-guided surgery concept. In one patient, the mandible was treated with dCAIS and the maxilla with sCAIS. In four patients, we mixed both concepts in the same jaw, starting with a half-guided sCAIS, drilling with the static guide and then placing the implant with dynamic navigation.

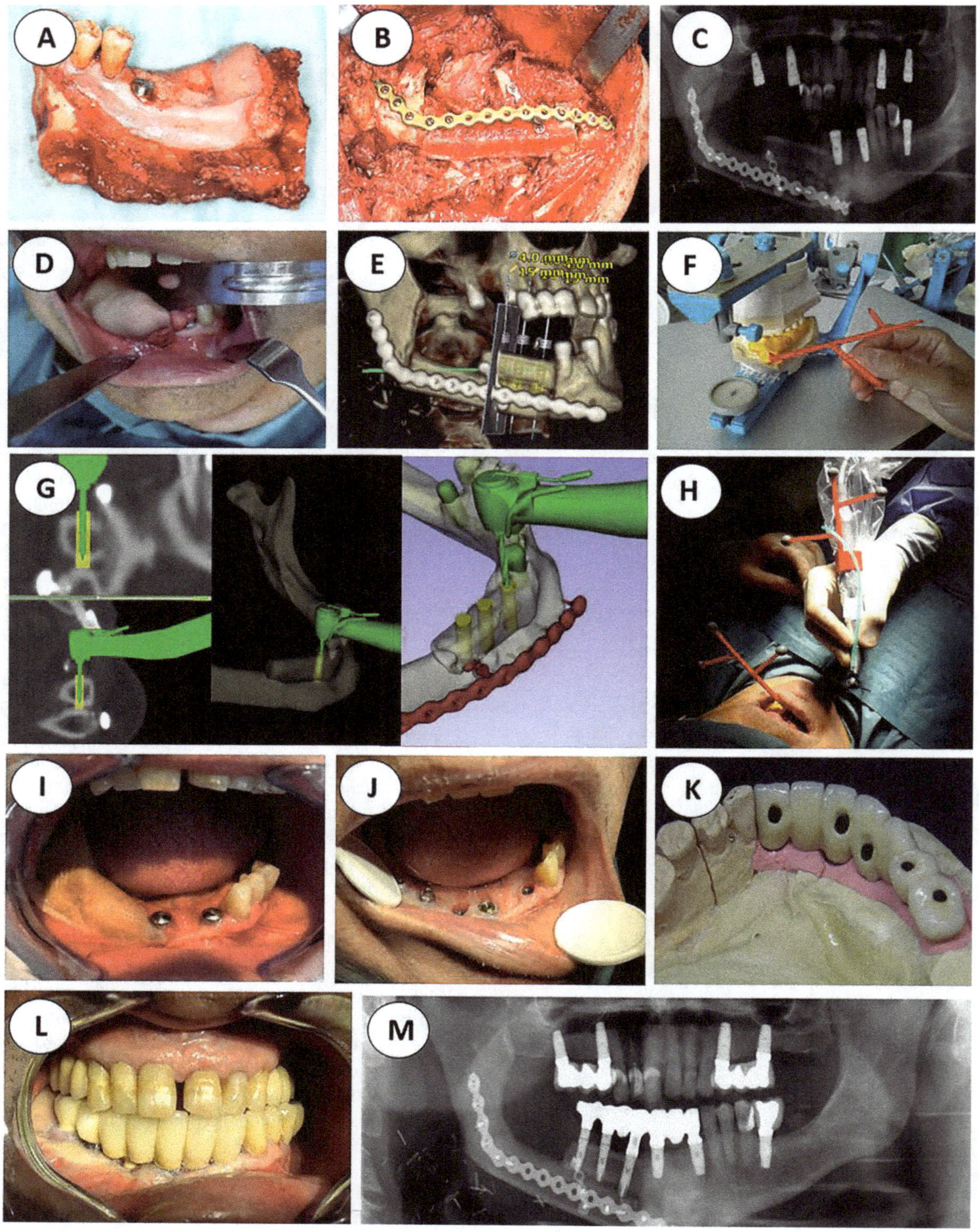

FIGURE 2 | Initial protocol example, from the ablative surgery to the final orthopantomogram **(A)** Right segmental mandibulectomy. **(B)** Double-barrel fibula flap in place. **(C)** Postoperative orthopantomography. **(D)** Redundant fibula skin paddle. **(E)** Implant placement virtual surgical planning with Nobel Clinician-DivX software. **(F)** Teeth supported silicone jig holding the 3D-printed dynamic reference frame. **(G)** Intraoperative screen view of the navigated handpiece and the real-time drilling trajectory. **(H)** Handpiece and patient's optical markers ready for dynamic navigation. **(I)** Still redundant skin paddle after implant surgery. **(J)** Intraoral view after vestibuloplasty and implant second phase. **(K)** Screw retained porcelain fused to metal fixed prosthesis lingual view. **(L)** Final occlusion. **(M)** Final panorex with the prosthesis in place.

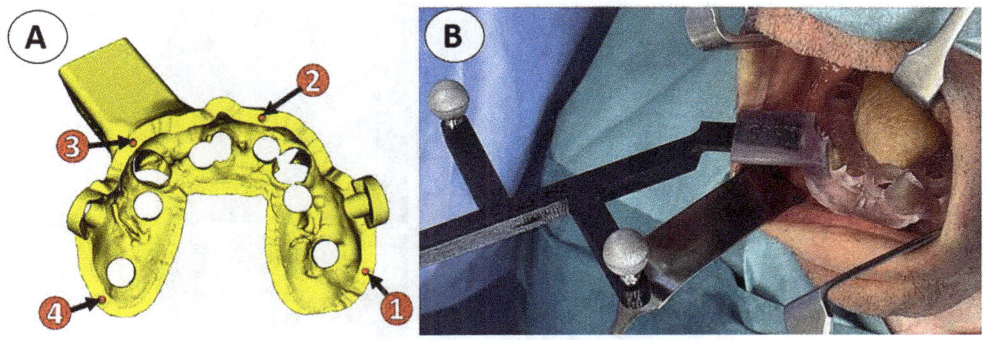

FIGURE 3 | **(A)** Virtual model of the surgical guide with four pinholes (red) for intraoperative registration and a socket for the attachment of the dynamic reference frame. **(B)** 3D-printed biocompatible teeth-supported resin guide holding the dynamic reference frame during computer-assisted surgery in a right hemotingue epidermoid carcinoma reconstructed by means of an ALT with vastus lateralis free flap.

A customized in-house software application was developed in 3D Slicer to assist surgeons during dental implant placement. A Polaris Spectra (Northern Digital Inc., Waterloo, ON, Canada) optical tracking system was used for real-time positioning of the surgical instruments with respect to the patient's anatomy, attaching a dynamic reference frame to the surgical guide. Patient-to-image registration was computed by recording the pinholes included on the surgical guide. This approach ensures an accurate registration when the surgical guide is correctly fixed on the patient. In addition, optical markers were included in the handpiece to track the movements of the tool and guide the drilling trajectory. A calibration step is required to compute the position of the tip of the handpiece with respect to the optical markers. This calibration was performed by fitting the handpiece tool on a specifically designed calibration platform and recording a total of six pinholes located on the platform (**Figure 4**). Head immobilization is no more a requisite for accurate navigation with this workflow due to real-time positioning.

The developed software application displayed the real-time position of the handpiece with respect to the preoperative CT images, anatomical 3D models, and VSP. Optimal drilling trajectory was controlled through constant visual and acoustic feedback to ensure accurate matching with the VSP (**Figure 5A**). The navigation software displayed two target images: one to visualize the linear deviation of the insertion point of the implant (**Figure 5B**), and the other to control the angular deviation of the drilling trajectory (**Figure 5C**, **Video 1**).

AR visualization was also available for the surgical team and applied in five cases as a tool to verify the final position of the implants. A customized AR smartphone application was developed to project the patients' virtual models onto the real-world image. This application uses the smartphone camera to detect and track the position of a 3D-printed cubic reference marker for real-time positioning of the virtual models (**Figure 6**). The tracking marker was designed to contain unique black and white patterns on each face (29). This cubic reference was 3D printed in polylactic acid and sterilized with ethylene oxide at low temperature (37°C) before surgery (25).

The developed application was deployed on an iPhone 6 (Apple Inc., Cupertino, CA, USA) and used after the implants were placed on the patient to verify their final position. Once the reference marker was attached to the surgical guide socket, an automatic registration was performed. Then, the smartphone was introduced in a sterilized case (CleanCase, SteriDev Inc., Lansing, MI, USA) and held by one physician. The surgeon pointed with the smartphone camera to the cubic marker, and once it was detected, the virtual models were projected on the smartphone display (**Figure 6A**). The AR device enabled the surgeons to visualize VSP directly on the patient's anatomy,

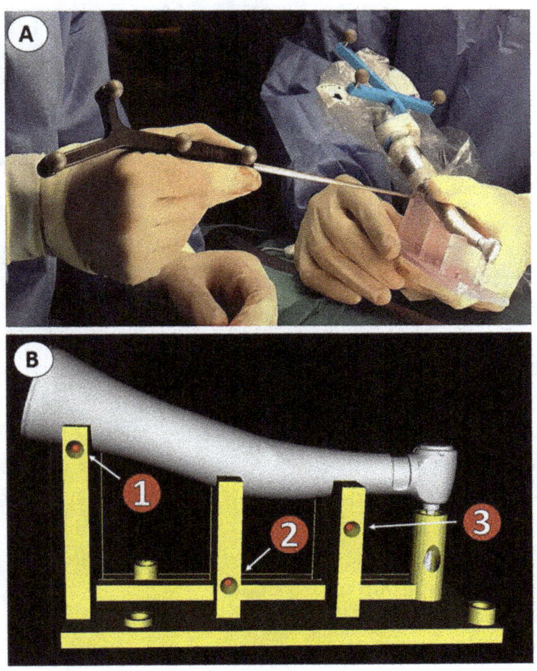

FIGURE 4 | Calibration of handpiece tool prior to dynamic navigation. **(A)** Surgeons recording reference points in the tool calibration platform. **(B)** 3D model of the calibration platform.

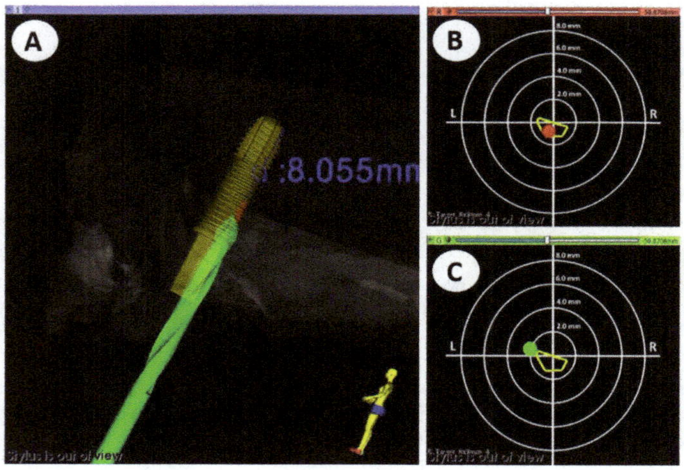

FIGURE 5 | Visualization layout during dynamic navigation. **(A)** 3D view of the handpiece position during drilling with respect to the virtual surgical plan. **(B)** 2D target view to control linear deviation of the handpiece tip at the entry crestal point. **(C)** 2D target view to control angular deviation of the drilling trajectory.

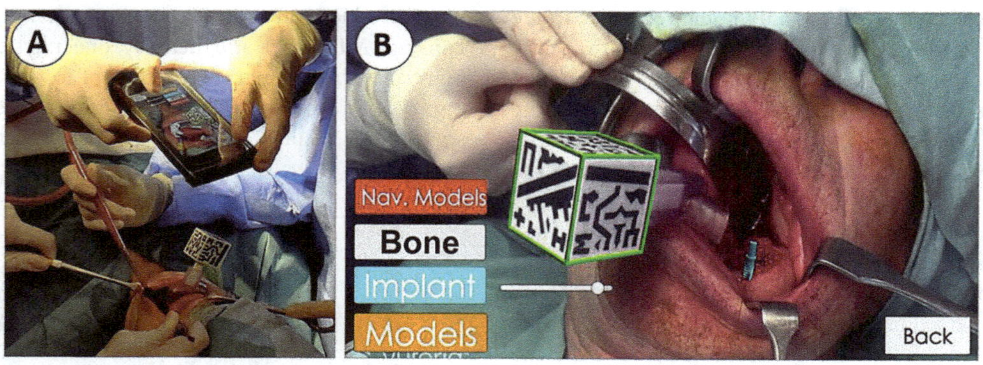

FIGURE 6 | Verification of implant position using augmented reality visualization. **(A)** Surgeon using a smartphone inserted into a sterile cover. **(B)** Augmented reality visualization of the virtual surgical plan overlaid on the patient's anatomy.

showing the bone, target implant location, and the optimal drilling trajectories in their expected position (**Figure 6B**), (**Video 2**).

Postoperative CBCT scans were acquired to evaluate surgical outcomes and navigation accuracy. Implants were segmented from the postoperative CT study, comparing their position with the VSP. Accuracy evaluation metrics included (1) linear deviation of the implant entry point (platform or crestal point of insertion) (2), linear deviation of the implant apex or apical endpoint, and (3) absolute angular deviation (**Figure 7**). We calculated the mean and standard deviation values of these metrics for each group under study.

RESULTS

We placed a total of 56 implants, 25 in the upper jaw, and 31 in the lower jaw. 18 implants were inserted into the fibula bone (conventional or double barrel), 6 into the iliac crest, and 32 in the patient remnant bone; 15 implants were placed in irradiated bone (1 fibula and the ALT with vastus lateralis case).

In those eleven patients, we treated 14 jaws, 3 jaws exclusively with sCAIS (closed transmucosal technique, 13 implants), 4 jaws with dCAIS (13 implants), and the other 7 with a combination of both methods (30 implants). In those 11 navigated jaws, we opened a flap for proper bone visualization and soft tissue remodeling. Adequate bone width control is advisable in extremely narrow alveolar bone cases. Vestibular cortical plate fenestration was noticed in three implants, so we extracted the implants and placed them again in different locations. Those three freehand implants were visually oriented and placed in the best-quality bone that was found available intraoperatively without considering the virtual planning. That is why they were withdrawn from the statistical analysis. We also withdrew our third patient (3 implants) from the analysis, since we did not achieve enough stability of the optical markers. Hence, the

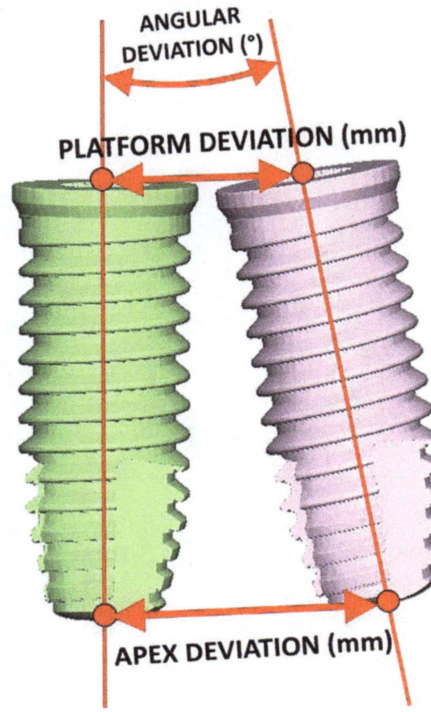

FIGURE 7 | Metrics used to compare the final position of implants with the preoperative virtual surgical plan.

navigation procedure was not accurate enough, ending the surgery in a conventional non-guided freehand method. Consequently, the implants were placed with an eye-oriented insertion axis and without considering the prosthetically driven surgical planning. Despite the intraoperative complication, the osseointegration was uneventful in the fibula and we ended with the planned fixed screw-retained prosthesis (**Table 1**, patient 5, orthopantomogram with the prosthesis in place). Therefore, we withdrew a total of 6 freehand placed implants from our data analysis

All implants except one achieved a successful osseointegration measured during follow-up by ISQ stability (frequency of resonance), resulting in a 98% osseointegration success rate. This follow-up is, however, too short to extract conclusions.

Figure 8 shows an example of the comparison between the virtual surgical planning and the final intraoperative position. Complete data are provided as supplementary material, including patient information, angular deviation, crestal point of insertion, and apical deviation.

The average crestal point insertion error (**Table 2**) was 1.96 mm, with values between 0.35 and 4 mm (standard deviation 0.95 mm). The combination of static and dynamic navigation offers the best accuracy with an average error of 1.52 mm. Static alone has a 1.56-mm average error, and only-dynamic procedures raise the error to 2.7 mm.

The endpoint or apical deviation error (**Table 3**) was 2.66 mm, with a range from 0.62 to 7.5 mm (standard deviation 1.33 mm). Considering different guiding techniques, static shows the best accuracy (1.27 mm), followed by the combination with a 2.94-mm error and dynamic alone (3.94 mm).

The angular deviation (**Table 4**) average error was 8.98°, ranging from 1.4° to 30° (standard deviation 5.38°). The combination of static and dynamic and the static alone shows a similar accuracy (8.07 and 8.1 degrees, respectively). Only-dynamic navigation has a 10.5° average error.

Table 5 summarizes the results for angular deviation and crestal and apical deviation. Each variable is subdivided into three groups for descriptive data analysis: static-guided surgery or dynamic navigation alone, and the combination of both.

A fixed screw-retained prosthesis has already been placed in five patients as planned, while the last six patients are waiting to complete the osseointegration period. We duplicate the period of osseointegration in irradiated bone.

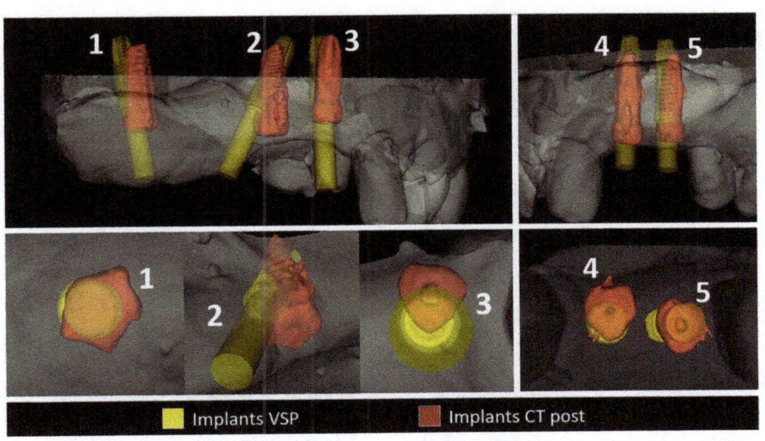

FIGURE 8 | Virtual surgical planning in yellow comparison with final intraoperative position. Excellent accuracy in implants 1,2,4,5, mismatch error in implant 2. Implant 2 while inserting into an extremely narrow alveolar bone developed a vestibular complete fenestration. We intraoperatively corrected the position freehand seeking adequate bone volume. Since this implant is not guided, we withdrew the final result from our study.

TABLE 2 | Results of the insertion point deviation in mm.

PATIENT ID	SUP/INF	IMPLANT ID						AVERAGE	TECHNIQUE
		1	2	3	4	5	6		
ION0001	INFERIOR	3.50	2.47	1.26				2.41	DYNAMIC
ION0002	INFERIOR	2.23	1.99	1.67				1.96	DYNAMIC
ION0003	INFERIOR	*6,42*OUT*	*5,23*OUT*	*1,89* OUT*				OUT	DYNAMIC
ION0004	INFERIOR	3.70	3.11	2.89	4.14			3.46	DYNAMIC
ION005	INFERIOR	2.17	4.37					3.27	STATIC
ION0006	INFERIOR	0.37	0.75	0.35	0.67			0.54	STATIC + DYNAMIC
ION0006	SUPERIOR	0.71	*3,11*OUT*	1.61	1.04	0.37		0.93	STATIC + DYNAMIC
ION0007	SUPERIOR	3.50	1.78	2.52				2.60	STATIC + DYNAMIC
ION0008	INFERIOR	2.11	3.31	*3,99* OUT*				2.71	STATIC + DYNAMIC
ION0009	INFERIOR	1.12	3.47	2.93				2.51	STATIC + DYNAMIC
ION0009	SUPERIOR	0.96	0.54	1.28	1.08	2.02	0.80	1.11	STATIC
ION0010	INFERIOR	0.66	1.59	1.76	1.34	0.50	1.10	1.16	STATIC + DYNAMIC
ION0010	SUPERIOR	1.88	1.88	0.81	2.80	0.44	1.20	1.50	STATIC + DYNAMIC
ION0011	SUPERIOR	1.59	1.58	1.89	*2,51*OUT*	0.43		1.37	STATIC
								1.96	

OUT. Freehand implant placement, data excluded from analysis*

GUIDED TECHNIQUE	STATIC	DYNAMIC	STATIC+DYNAMIC	TOTAL
AVG	**1.56**	**2.70**	**1.52**	**1.96**
STD	**1.01**	**0.88**	**0.97**	**0.95**
MAX	**4.37**	**4.14**	**3.50**	**4.00**
MIN	**0.43**	**1.26**	**0.35**	**0.68**

TABLE 3 | Results of the end point deviation in mm.

PATIENT ID	SUP/INF	IMPLANT ID						AVERAGE
		1	2	3	4	5	6	
ION0001	INFERIOR	5.14	3.74	1.73				3.54
ION0002	INFERIOR	3.22	2.13	3.18				2.84
ION0003	INFERIOR	*3,6*OUT*	*7,45*OUT*	*4,11*OUT*				OUT
ION0004	INFERIOR	3.16	5.67	3.97	7.50			5.08
ION005	INFERIOR	1.35	1.01					1.18
ION0006	INFERIOR	1.30	0.75	0.66	3.03			1.44
ION0006	SUPERIOR	2.41	*1,97*OUT*	2.41	0.85	1.05		1.68
ION0007	SUPERIOR	7.11	6.75	4.82				6.23
ION0008	INFERIOR	2.75	2.97	*2,3*OUT*				2.86
ION0009	INFERIOR	2.05	4.54	4.47				3.69
ION0009	SUPERIOR	1.19	0.70	0.90	1.80	2.46	2.30	1.56
ION0010	INFERIOR	0.90	1.95	0.77	1.00	1.07	1.40	1.18
ION0010	SUPERIOR	4.39	3.41	1.86	0.87	2.82	1.44	2.47
ION0011	SUPERIOR	0.62	0.97	1.19	*7,91*OUT*	0.71		0.87
								2.66

OUT. Freehand implant placement, data excluded from analysis*

GUIDED TECHNIQUE	STATIC	DYNAMIC	STATIC+DYNAMIC	TOTAL
AVG	**1.27**	**3.94**	**2.49**	**2.66**
STD	**0.59**	**1.64**	**1.76**	1.33
MAX	**2.46**	**7.50**	**7.11**	
MIN	**0.62**	**1.73**	**0.66**	

At the end of the surgical procedure, we were able to display planned implant placement intraoperatively with the AR app on our mobile phone in five patients. The final platform and the insertion point deviation were visually verified in 30 implants. The match between virtual planning and final surgical results was observed and recorded.

DISCUSSION

Virtual computerized implant surgery has opened a new horizon in the management of complex cases when the anatomy of the jaw bones has been altered due to trauma or pathology (30). In free flap oncologic reconstructed patients, there are several

TABLE 4 | Results of the angular deviation in degrees.

PATIENT ID	SUP/INF	IMPLANT ID						AVERAGE
		1	2	3	4	5	6	
ION0001	INFERIOR	13.60	11.37	5.75				10.24
ION0002	INFERIOR	9.78	4.19	10.58				8.18
ION0003	INFERIOR	*8,18*OUT*	*10,18*OUT*	*14,51*OUT*				OUT
ION0004	INFERIOR	3.90	9.54	5.76	30.70			12.48
ION005	INFERIOR	16.01	14.21					15.11
ION0006	INFERIOR	5.57	5.57	1.42	13.28			6.46
ION0006	SUPERIOR	10.13	*23*OUT*	5.14	1.74	3.57		5.15
ION0007	SUPERIOR	15.91	20.90	9.72				15.51
ION0008	INFERIOR	4.79	6.77	*15,74*OUT*				5.78
ION0009	INFERIOR	7.90	11.95	7.26				9.04
ION0009	SUPERIOR	6.41	2.27	6.12	11.86	6.29	11.77	7.45
ION0010	INFERIOR	7.86	6.25	4.66	1.58	6.08	2.71	4.86
ION0010	SUPERIOR	12.59	13.11	4.72	12.44	12.01	10.44	10.89
ION0011	SUPERIOR	6.55	6.07	5.50	*33,07*OUT*	4.11		5.56
								8.98

OUT. Freehand implant placement, data excluded from analysis*

GUIDED TECHNIQUE	STATIC	DYNAMIC	STATIC+DYNAMIC	TOTAL
AVG	**8.10**	**10.52**	**8.07**	**8.90**
STD	**4.09**	**7.40**	**4.63**	5.38
MAX	**16.01**	**30.70**	**20.90**	
MIN	**2.27**	**3.90**	**1.42**	

TABLE 5 | Average, standard deviation and maximum and minimum values of the results for angular deviation, insertion point deviation, and end point deviation.

		AVG	STD	MAX	MIN
ANGULAR DEVIATION (degrees) 8.98°	**STATIC**	8.10	4.09	16.01	2.27
	DYNAMIC	10.52	7.40	30.70	3.90
	STATIC+DYNAMIC	8.07	4.63	20.90	1.42
INSERTION POINT (mm) 1.96	**STATIC**	1.56	1.01	4.37	0.43
	DYNAMIC	2.70	0.88	4.14	1.26
	STATIC+DYNAMIC	1.52	0.97	3.50	0.35
END POINT DEVIATION (mm) 2.66	**STATIC**	1.27	0.59	2.46	0.62
	DYNAMIC	3.94	1.64	7.50	1.73
	STATIC+DYNAMIC	2.49	1.76	7.11	0.66

reports regarding guided static surgery-based implant placement (8, 16, 17) but only a few about dynamic navigation and none reporting a combination of both or augmented reality guidance.

There is a gap between surgical planning and interventional procedures in oral and maxillofacial surgery. Medical CAD/CAM technologies ensure a precise virtual plan. However, their translation to the operating room cannot be guaranteed due to the lack of accurate surgical guidance and anatomical visualization during the procedure (31).

The deviation range of an ideal surgical navigation system to meet the clinical requirements should be between 0.5 and 1.5 mm. The more complicated the surgical procedure is, the greater the error should be expected (32–34). The literature seems to indicate that one has to accept a dynamic unavoidable inaccuracy of 2.0 mm in any guided surgery procedure (35). The accuracy of the registration process between the virtual image and the surgical site has the most significant impact on the precision of the navigation system since subsequent tasks depend on that step. Several registration methods have been proposed in craniofacial surgery: bone implants (plates and screws), occlusal splint fitted to the teeth, anatomical landmarks, and laser surface scanning. Occlusal splints provide a non-invasive, highly accurate registration method that is steadily fitted to stable bony landmark-dental cusps (33).

The position of the dynamic reference frame in relation to the surgical site requires consideration. The aim is to position the reference frame as close as possible to the surgical field to maximize navigation accuracy, but considering that it should not limit the surgeon's maneuvers during the intervention. Jiang et al. (33) found that the closer (further) the distance from the reference frame, the smaller (larger) the positional deviation, showing a similar trend for the angular error. They concluded that an occlusal splint might be sufficient for the navigation of maxillary and mandible surgery.

Nevertheless, our first four cases were splintless dynamic-guided surgeries (one iliac crest, one fibula double barrel, and two conventional fibula flaps). We applied the tooth-supported silicone jig dCAIS concept for patient registration, which was the most inaccurate method (linear crestal insertion error 2.7 mm, apical deviation 3.94 mm, and 10° of angular mismatch). These values are similar to those reported in the literature for conventional freehand non-guided placement in simple non-oncological cases. Vercruyssen et al. (35) revealed a crestal error of 2.7 mm, an apical error of 2.9 mm, and an angular deviation of 9.9°. For the same features, Block et al. (36) reported 1.67 mm, 2.51 mm, and 7.69°, respectively. In our study, the tooth-supported silicone jig provided an adequate registration. However, it resulted unstable during surgery. Consequently, the cases with large anatomical distortion (fibula cases patients 3 and 4 with a basal fibula bone placement and a thick skin paddle) showed the lowest accuracy. Moreover, we had to stop the navigation procedure in the third patient and continue with a conventional freehand method. Despite the mismatch, osseointegration was uneventful and the initial group of four patients ended with adequate screw-retained implant-supported prosthesis.

To overcome this stability problem, we introduced the sCAIS in our study, based on a 3D-printed teeth-supported surgical guide that not only stabilized the fiducial markers for accurate registration and navigation but also demonstrated to be a good alternative for implant placement if needed.

Static CAIS systems are limited due to undesirable cooling methods, restricted direct visual contact with the working surgical site (blind technique), and the impossibility of modifying the planned position intraoperatively. Placement and stability of the guide during the surgical procedure are critical to achieving precision. Some sources of error, in oncological reconstructed patients, could be the following: limited mouth opening in patients, nature of the guide support, tooth availability, tooth position or mobility, template fabrication process or flap approach, in particular concerning posterior surgical sites, and the need of long drills in restricted mouth opening patients (37). Previous studies have shown that tooth-supported guides provide better results than mucosa or bone-supported guides. Implants in distal extension gaps resulted in more significant deviation when compared to implants placed in posterior areas with adjacent bilateral teeth support due to possible intraoperative guide movement, tilting, and bending, particularly in long cantilever lengths. Although the mismatch between the planned and final achieved positions can be measured, no information on the source of inaccuracy can be assessed (38). Most of our patients belonged to the group of long posterior extension gaps prone to bending and tilting of the static guide. Therefore, we expected difficulties with static guide accuracy in most of our cases. In addition, sCAIS needs specific surgical drills and instruments.

We restricted the use of static surgery to three patients, 13 implants, carefully choosing the jaws with minimal anatomical distortion, ideal tooth support for splint stabilization, non-restricted mouth opening, and almost average mucosal or soft tissue flap thickness.

sCAIS accuracy results in a healthy population (partially edentulous non-oncological cases) were analyzed by two systematic reviews, Tahmaseb et al. (39) and Jung et al. (40). They reported an entry point error ranging from 1.04 to 1.45 mm, apex mean error between 1.38 and 2.99 mm, and angular error around 4°. Therefore, it is considered a highly accurate method, but many studies are biased reporting single-unit cases with ideal tooth support on both sides of the edentolous space. Our results after a careful selection of patients are respectively 1.56 mm, 1.27 mm, and 8°, similar to non-oncological series. sCAIS usefulness is limited in oncologic patients due to the aforementioned restrictions. It should be considered in irradiated patients when feasible because it allows a close surgical approach. Flapless surgery is a less invasive and traumatic procedure, avoiding raising a flap and detaching undamaged soft and hard tissue from its vascularization, which could be crucial in irradiated patients (8).

On the other hand, open dynamic image-guided navigation techniques enable real-time surgical tool tracking and visualization with respect to surrounding anatomical structures, allowing the surgeon to accurately place the implant on the position defined during preoperative virtual planning. The surgeon's perception of the drilling sequence and implant placement is not affected by a splint. There is no need for a specific set of drills or instruments and can be used in almost all patients, even in cases with limited mouth opening. Kalaivani et al. (13) stated that the major value of the dynamic design is the ability to adjust the planned implant positioning intraoperatively.

dCAIS tracking depends on the registration procedure. Errors in that step could be detected and corrected with continuous recalibration paying attention to reference fixation and position stability. Nevertheless, there are some limitations to evaluate since the registration process is technically sensitive and requires time. In addition, the surgeons need a steep learning curve and the cost of the equipment is high (41). Sun et al. (42) reported that the learning curve plateau is not reached until the surgeon has placed at least 15 dental implants with these systems. Our group created a workflow based on open software, avoiding extra costs, and included laboratory practice with biomodels to reduce the learning curve.

dCAIS in healthy non-oncological case results are excellent, and similar to the sCAIS, Yimarj et al. (19) reported a 1.24-mm crestal insertion error, 1.58-mm apical mismatch, and 3.78° angular deviation. In another systematic review and meta-analysis, Wei et al. (17) reported that the average global platform deviation, global apical deviation, and angular deviation were 1.02 mm, 1.33 mm, and 3.59°, respectively. Our subgroup of five patients, 30 implants, placed by means of a splint-based registration dynamic navigation technique yielded values of 1.52 mm, 2.49 mm, and 8°, respectively, slightly higher than in non-oncological patients.

When comparing sCAIS with dCAIS, Kaewsiri et al. (21), Mischkowski et al. (22), and Block et al. (36) concluded that dynamic navigation provided higher accuracy than any static guide system but without statistical significance. On the other hand, Jorba-García et al. (43) considered that not all commercial dynamic systems are suitable for treating difficult fully edentulous cases, suggesting the use of static systems as the first-line option in guided implant surgery.

Our workflow shares the best capabilities from both methods. Assuming that the surgical template is difficult to use alone in anatomically altered reconstructed oncologic patients and that dynamic navigation information allows intraoperative real-time modifications, we combine both techniques. The rigid tooth-supported acrylic 3D-printed splint provides a stable platform for patient registration and optical marker display. It also holds all the information for guided surgery and the cylinders for static drilling. In our last five patients, we placed the tip of the drill inside the cylinder using dynamic navigation to find the virtually planned crestal insertion point and the best handpiece axis orientation before starting to drill. The main difference with a conventional static drilling technique is that we have a certain degree of freedom within the guiding 5.2-mm-diameter tube, to slightly change the drill insertion point and axis as suggested by the intraoperative dynamic navigation display in order to match the virtual surgical plan. With this combined approach, our results in the last three oncologic patients resemble those achieved in healthy non-oncological patients.

In many implants, we noticed an intraoperative mismatch in the crestal insertion point between the static surgical guide and the dynamic navigation. We give more credit to the position provided by the navigation technique, and the postoperative implant position analysis reveals that dynamic navigation based on a stable splint offers superior accuracy to translate the virtual surgical planning into the operating room (**Figure 9**).

Considering the image-guided surgery learning curve, it is difficult to draw conclusions because all our oncologic patients are different and each case should be individualized while planning (**Table 6**). Our series showed a progressive increase in accuracy and indeed a learning curve despite preclinical laboratory training. The combination of a modified navigation static 3D-printed splint and infrared optical navigation yielded the best results in all the measured variables.

Clinical studies about augmented reality in maxillofacial implantology are scarce with very few publications investigating this technology. Pellegrino et al. (24) presented two cases where they evaluated the feasibility of adopting Hololens glasses-guided AR as a means of facilitating the use of dynamic navigation. Pellegrino placed just one implant on each patient and found a 0.5–0.53-mm deviation at the entry point, a 0.46–0.48-mm deviation at the apical portion, and an angular deviation between 2.19° and 3.05°. They concluded that AR overcomes one of the disadvantages of the dynamic guided system: the need to simultaneously pay attention to the patient and the output from the navigation system display. However, when a 3D virtual layer is displayed and laid over the real environment, there is often a discrepancy between the real and virtual images due to an overlay or positional error. In their opinion, the main limits of AR are the inconvenient virtual window positioning and orientation together with the working distance of the glasses, which could force the surgeon to operate in an uncomfortable position, and the lack of depth perception. In addition, when comparing visual perception of depth on a 3D image with a 2D screen projection, stereo and motion parallax are two missing essential cues (34). These reasons explain why AR is still a field of *in vitro* investigation in maxillofacial surgery with few clinical reports.

We developed a smartphone-based AR navigation system combining an AR application with a 3D-printed reference marker. One of the main advantages of our approach is that there is no need to wear special heavy and bulky head-mounted displays or divert surgeons' eyes from the surgical site, since the smartphone display could overlap the operating area. Another advantage is the automatic patient-to-image registration method, thanks to the reference marker placed into the surgical guide socket. Wang et al. (31) presented an interesting alternative with a stereo camera marker-less image registration method where the only requirement to generate correct AR scenes is to expose the patient's teeth to the camera.

The smartphone was easy to use in the surgical field thanks to the sterilized case. The proposed smartphone app could display the bone, virtual implant planning, and plaster model holding the fixed screw-retained planned prosthesis in the real position on top of the patient. Regarding the implants, it was easy to superimpose, with different degrees of translucency, the planned virtual implant over the final intraoperative position. We applied this in five patients as a final validation method of the guided surgery with favorable results. However, depth perception is still a limitation in AR. Therefore, we believe that using AR technology for surgical guidance is still challenging, and further research and laboratory practice are needed to overcome barriers.

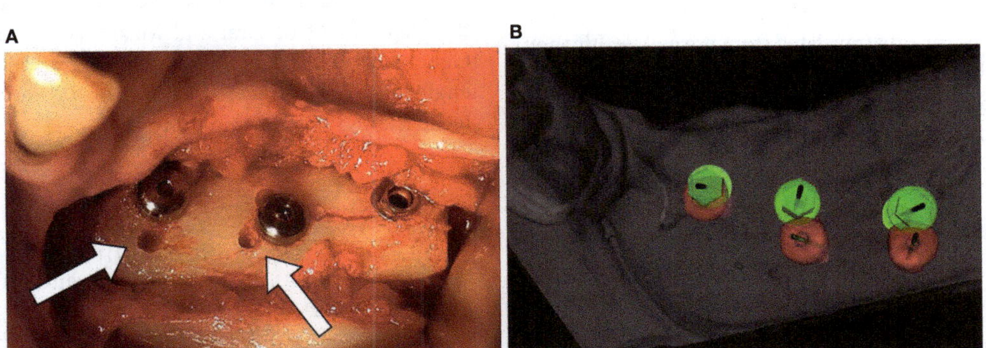

FIGURE 9 | **(A)** Mismatch between the initial 2-mm drilled holes suggested by the static splint (see white arrows) and the final intraoperative implant position achieved with dynamic navigation guidance. **(B)** Static splint-based dynamic navigation accuracy is higher than static navigation alone in this double-barrel fibula case. Postoperative implant position analysis, the achieved position in red, the virtual surgical planned position in green.

TABLE 6 | Learning curve, from the initial jig dynamic navigation to combined, static-dynamic-AR, guided surgery.

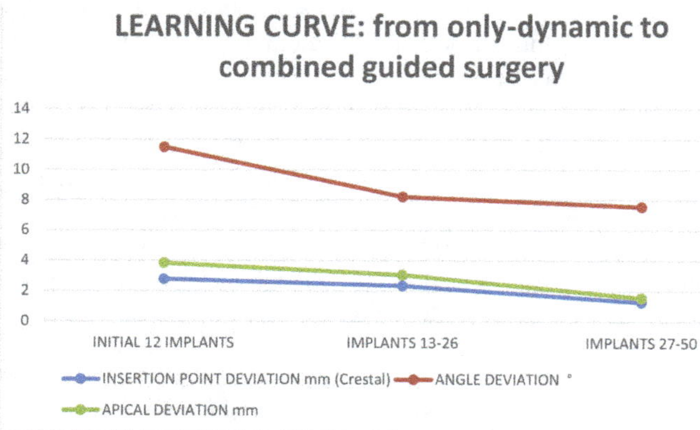

Increasing economic costs and operating time should be mentioned as potential limitations. There are no extra costs in our proposal since planning and splint design is based on free software. We establish a negligible 20 Euros cost for splint exportation and printing. The software allows subsequent splint modifications and impression for a bimaxillary splint without new extra fees for each patient. Regarding surgical time, we calculate that 15 min of extra time are needed for subsequent iterative registration procedures during a three-implant-guided placement.

Despite that, non-oncological implant placement is gradually becoming a navigated surgery. Dental implantologists are increasingly applying this method due to the undoubted advantages. As stated by Michael S. Block in 2017: "Clinicians placing implants should consider routinely using dynamic navigation on daily basis to improve their accuracy and not just for special cases" (41). In our experience, any guided method, even the most inaccurate, yielded at least similar results when compared to the freehand technique.

CONCLUSION

Oncologic patients reconstructed with free flaps represent a challenge for implant treatment. Image-guided implant surgery should be used with caution, since previous results from these techniques cannot be directly translated from normal healthy non-oncologic cases. The static surgery concept could be easily used in non-reconstructed jaws or when the anatomical distortion is minimal and good tooth support ensures surgical guide stability.

Combining a modified static-guided surgery tooth-supported 3D-printed resin guide with dynamic navigation (modified for accurate registration and optical markers display) in oncologic patients could achieve equivalent results to those obtained with guided methods in healthy non-reconstructed patients.

Furthermore, intraoperative flexibility allowing alignment and orientation modifications during implant placement is a significant advantage of VSP and dynamic guided surgery. Augmented reality is a valuable tool for intraoperative verification but needs further research to be considered an alternative guided method for implant surgery.

Computer-aided implant surgery based on dynamic navigation and 3D-printed surgical modified guides is an accurate and valuable technique for prosthetically driven implant placement in free flap oncologic reconstructed patients.

AUTHOR CONTRIBUTIONS

SO, DG-M, and JP conceived and designed the study. SO, DG-M, JP, and AG wrote the main manuscript. SO defined the virtual surgical plan and designed the surgical guides and dental rehabilitations for all patients. DG-M developed the navigation software, performed the data analysis, and edited the supplementary videos, DG-M and AG manufactured the surgical guides and navigation tools. DG-M and AG prepared the figures and tables. SO, MT, CN-C, IN-C, and JS were the surgeons at the ablative, reconstructive free flap procedures and at implant placement. They also made the implant supported fixed dental rehabilitation at the outpatient clinic. RM-M designed the workflow for augmented reality visualization, designed the APP for the mobile phone, and intraoperatively collected the data and images. All authors reviewed the manuscript. All authors contributed to the article and approved the submitted version.

ACKNOWLEDGMENTS

The authors would like to thank Miss Bettina Cortés, from Cortes-Bergmann dental prosthesis laboratory, for her dedication, support, and hard work in building our oncologic patients' dental restorations. We also thank all the surgeons of the Department of Oral and Maxillofacial Surgery at Hospital General Universitario Gregorio Marañón and biomedical engineers from Universidad Carlos III de Madrid for their feedback and help in this study.

REFERENCES

1. Urken ML. Composite Free Flaps in Oromandibular Reconstruction: Review of the Literature. *Arch Otolaryngol Neck Surg* (1991) 117(7):724–32. doi: 10.1001/archotol.1991.01870190036009
2. Riediger D. Restoration of Masticatory Function by Microsurgically Revascularized Iliac Crest Bone Grafts Using Enosseous Implants. *Plast Reconstr Surg* (1988) 81(6):861–77. doi: 10.1097/00006534-198806000-00007
3. Urken ML, Buchbinder D, Weinberg H, Vickery C, Sheiner A, Biller HF. Primary Placement of Osseointegrated Implants in Microvascular Mandibular Reconstruction. *Otolaryngol Neck Surg Off J Am Acad Otolaryngol Neck Surg* (1989) 101(1):56–73. doi: 10.1177/019459988910100111
4. Schoen PJ, Raghoebar GM, Bouma J, Reintsema H, Burlage FR, Roodenburg JLN, et al. Prosthodontic Rehabilitation of Oral Function in Head-Neck Cancer Patients With Dental Implants Placed Simultaneously During Ablative Tumour Surgery: An Assessment of Treatment Outcomes and Quality of Life. *Int J Oral Maxillofac Surg* (2008) 37(1):8–16. doi: 10.1016/j.ijom.2007.07.015

5. Roumanas ED, Garrett N, Blackwell KE, Freymiller E, Abemayor E, Wong WK, et al. Masticatory and Swallowing Threshold Performances With Conventional and Implant-Supported Prostheses After Mandibular Fibula Free-Flap Reconstruction. *J Prosthet Dent* (2006) 96(4):289–97. doi: 10.1016/j.prosdent.2006.08.015
6. Sato N, Koyama S, Mito T, Izumita K, Ishiko R, Yamauchi K, et al. Changes in Oral Health-Related Quality of Life After Oral Rehabilitation With Dental Implants in Patients Following Mandibular Tumor Resection. *J Oral Sci* (2019) 61(3):406–11. doi: 10.2334/josnusd.18-0234
7. Wijbenga JG, Schepers RH, Werker PMN, Witjes MJH, Dijkstra PU. A Systematic Review of Functional Outcome and Quality of Life Following Reconstruction of Maxillofacial Defects Using Vascularized Free Fibula Flaps and Dental Rehabilitation Reveals Poor Data Quality. *J Plast Reconstr Aesthet Surg* (2016) 69(8):1024–36. doi: 10.1016/j.bjps.2016.05.003
8. Meloni SM, Tallarico M, De Riu G, Pisano M, Deledda A, Lolli FM, et al. Guided Implant Surgery After Free-Flap Reconstruction: Four-Year Results From a Prospective Clinical Trial. *J Craniomaxillofac Surg* (2015) 43 (8):1348–55. doi: 10.1016/j.jcms.2015.06.046
9. Smolka K, Kraehenbuehl M, Eggensperger N, Hallermann W, Thoren H, Iizuka T, et al. Fibula Free Flap Reconstruction of the Mandible in Cancer Patients: Evaluation of a Combined Surgical and Prosthodontic Treatment Concept. *Oral Oncol* (2008) 44(6):571–81. doi: 10.1016/j.oraloncology.2007.07.005
10. Cuesta-Gil M, Ochandiano Caicoya S, Riba-García F, Duarte Ruiz B, Navarro Cuéllar C, Navarro Vila C. Oral Rehabilitation With Osseointegrated Implants in Oncologic Patients. *J Oral Maxillofac Surg* (2009) 67(11):2485–96. doi: 10.1016/j.joms.2008.03.001
11. Ochandiano SJ, Navarro Cuellar C, Acero Sanz J, Navarro Vila C. Functional Implant-Supported Dental Rehabilitation in Oncologic Patients. In: Navarro Vila C, editor. *Reconstructive Oral and Maxillofacial Surgery*. Cham: Springer International Publishing (2015). p. 163–202. doi: 10.1007/978-3-319-20487-1_6
12. Clark D, Barbu H, Lorean A, Mijiritsky E, Levin L. Incidental Findings of Implant Complications on Postimplantation CBCTs: A Cross-Sectional Study. *Clin Implant Dent Relat Res* (2017) 19(5):776–82. doi: 10.1111/cid.12511
13. Kalaivani G, Balaji VR, Manikandan D, Rohini G. Expectation and Reality of Guided Implant Surgery Protocol Using Computer-Assisted Static and Dynamic Navigation System at Present Scenario: Evidence-Based Literature Review. *J Indian Soc Periodontol* (2020) 24(5):398–408. doi: 10.4103/jisp.jisp_92_20
14. Kraeima J, Glas HH, Merema BBJ, Vissink A, Spijkervet FKL, Witjes MJH. Three-Dimensional Virtual Surgical Planning in the Oncologic Treatment of the Mandible. *Oral Dis* (2021) 27(1):14–20. doi: 10.1111/odi.13631
15. Fortin T, Loup Coudert J, Champleboux G, Sautot P, Lavallée S. Computer-Assisted Dental Implant Surgery Using Computed Tomography. *J Image Guid Surg* (1995) 1(1):53–8. doi: 10.1002/(SICI)1522-712X(1995)1:1<53::AID-IGS8>3.0.CO;2-L
16. Cebrian-Carretero J-L, Guiñales-Díaz de Cevallos J, Sobrino J-A, Yu T, Burgueño-García M. Predictable Dental Rehabilitation in Maxillomandibular Reconstruction With Free Flaps. The Role of Implant Guided Surgery. *Med Oral Patol Oral Cir Bucal* (2014) 19(6):e605–11. doi: 10.4317/medoral.19116
17. Wei S-M, Zhu Y, Wei J-X, Zhang C-N, Shi J-Y, Lai H-C. Accuracy of Dynamic Navigation in Implant Surgery: A Systematic Review and Meta-Analysis. *Clin Oral Implants Res* (2021) 32(4):383–93. doi: 10.1111/clr.13719
18. Gargallo-Albiol J, Barootchi S, Salomó-Coll O, Wang H-L. Advantages and Disadvantages of Implant Navigation Surgery. A Systematic Review. *Ann Anat = Anat Anzeiger Off Organ Anat Gesellschaft* (2019) 225:1–10. doi: 10.1016/j.aanat.2019.04.005
19. Yimarj P, Subbalekha K, Dhanesuan K, Siriwatana K, Mattheos N, Pimkhaokham A. Comparison of the Accuracy of Implant Position for Two-Implants Supported Fixed Dental Prosthesis Using Static and Dynamic Computer-Assisted Implant Surgery: A Randomized Controlled Clinical Trial. *Clin Implant Dent Relat Res* (2020) 22(6):672–8. doi: 10.1111/cid.12949
20. Smitkarn P, Subbalekha K, Mattheos N, Pimkhaokham A. The Accuracy of Single-Tooth Implants Placed Using Fully Digital-Guided Surgery and Freehand Implant Surgery. *J Clin Periodontol* (2019) 46(9):949–57. doi: 10.1111/jcpe.13160
21. Kaewsiri D, Panmekiate S, Subbalekha K, Mattheos N, Pimkhaokham A. The Accuracy of Static vs. Dynamic Computer-Assisted Implant Surgery in Single Tooth Space: A Randomized Controlled Trial. *Clin Oral Implants Res* (2019) 30(6):505–14. doi: 10.1111/clr.13435
22. Mischkowski RA, Zinser MJ, Neugebauer J, Kübler AC, Zöller JE. Comparison of Static and Dynamic Computer-Assisted Guidance Methods in Implantology. *Int J Comput Dent* (2006) 9(1):23–35.
23. Berryman DR. Augmented Reality: A Review. *Med Ref Serv Q* (2012) 31 (2):212–8. doi: 10.1080/02763869.2012.670604
24. Pellegrino G, Mangano C, Mangano R, Ferri A, Taraschi V, Marchetti C. Augmented Reality for Dental Implantology: A Pilot Clinical Report of Two Cases. *BMC Oral Health* (2019) 19(1):158. doi: 10.1186/s12903-019-0853-y
25. García-Mato D, Moreta-Martínez R, García-Sevilla M, Ochandiano S, García-Leal R, Pérez-Mañanes R, et al. Augmented Reality Visualization for Craniosynostosis Surgery. *Comput Methods Biomech BioMed Eng Imaging \& Vis* (2020) 0(0):1–8. doi: 10.1080/21681163.2020.1834876
26. García-Mato D, Ochandiano S, García-Sevilla M, Navarro-Cuéllar C, Darriba-Allés JV, García-Leal R, et al. Craniosynostosis Surgery: Workflow Based on Virtual Surgical Planning, Intraoperative Navigation and 3D Printed Patient-Specific Guides and Templates. *Sci Rep* (2019) 9(1):17691. doi: 10.1038/s41598-019-54148-4
27. Moreta-Martinez R, García Mato D, García-Sevilla M, García-Leal R, Perez-Mañanes R, Calvo-Haro J, et al. CARS 2020 — *Computer Assisted Radiology and Surgery International Congress and Exhibition*. (2020) 15(1). doi: 10.1007/s11548-020-02171-6
28. García-Mato D, Pascau J, Ochandiano S. *New Technologies to Improve Surgical Outcome During Open-Cranial Vault Remodeling*. Madrid, Spain: Spina Bifida - New Perspectives and Clinical Applications (2020).
29. Moreta-Martinez R, García-Mato D, García-Sevilla M, Pérez-Mañanes R, Calvo-Haro JA, Pascau J. Combining Augmented Reality and 3D Printing to Display Patient Models on a Smartphone. *JoVE* (2020) 155):e60618. doi: 10.3791/60618
30. Ayoub A, Pulijala Y. The Application of Virtual Reality and Augmented Reality in Oral & Maxillofacial Surgery. *BMC Oral Health* (2019) 19(1):238. doi: 10.1186/s12903-019-0937-8
31. Wang J, Shen Y, Yang S. A Practical Marker-Less Image Registration Method for Augmented Reality Oral and Maxillofacial Surgery. *Int J Comput Assist Radiol Surg* (2019) 14(5):763–73. doi: 10.1007/s11548-019-01921-5
32. Meyer U, Wiesmann HP, Runte C, Fillies T, Meier N, Lueth T, et al. Evaluation of Accuracy of Insertion of Dental Implants and Prosthetic Treatment by Computer-Aided Navigation in Minipigs. *Br J Oral Maxillofac Surg* (2003) 41(2):102–8. doi: 10.1016/S0266-4356(02)00297-8
33. Jiang T, Zhu M, Chai G, Li Q. Precision of a Novel Craniofacial Surgical Navigation System Based on Augmented Reality Using an Occlusal Splint as a Registration Strategy. *Sci Rep* (2019) 9(1):501. doi: 10.1038/s41598-018-36457-2
34. Jiang W, Ma L, Zhang B, Fan Y, Qu X, Zhang X, et al. Evaluation of the 3D Augmented Reality-Guided Intraoperative Positioning of Dental Implants in Edentulous Mandibular Models. *Int J Oral Maxillofac Implants* (2018) 33 (6):1219–28. doi: 10.11607/jomi.6638
35. Vercruyssen M, Cox C, Coucke W, Naert I, Jacobs R, Quirynen M. A Randomized Clinical Trial Comparing Guided Implant Surgery (Bone- or Mucosa-Supported) With Mental Navigation or the Use of a Pilot-Drill Template. *J Clin Periodontol* (2014) 41 7:717–23. doi: 10.1111/jcpe.12231
36. Block MS, Emery RW, Cullum DR, Sheikh A. Implant Placement Is More Accurate Using Dynamic Navigation. *J Oral Maxillofac Surg* (2017) 75 (7):1377–86. doi: 10.1016/j.joms.2017.02.026
37. Brief J, Edinger D, Hassfeld S, Eggers G. Accuracy of Image-Guided Implantology. *Clin Oral Implants Res* (2005) 16(4):495–501. doi: 10.1111/j.1600-0501.2005.01133.x
38. Pessoa R, Siqueira R, Li J, Saleh I, Meneghetti P, Bezerra F, et al. The Impact of

Surgical Guide Fixation and Implant Location on Accuracy of Static Computer-Assisted Implant Surgery. *J Prosthodont Off J Am Coll Prosthodont* (2021) 1–10. doi: 10.1111/jopr.13371

39. Tahmaseb A, Wismeijer D, Coucke W, Derksen W. Computer Technology Applications in Surgical Implant Dentistry: A Systematic Review. *Int J Oral \& Maxillofac Implant* (2014) 29 Suppl:25–42. doi: 10.11607/jomi.2014suppl.g1.2
40. Jung R, Schneider D, Ganeles J, Wismeijer D, Zwahlen M, Hammerle C, et al. Computer Technology Applications in Surgical Implant Dentistry: A Systematic Review. *Int J Oral Maxillofac Implants* (2009) 24 Suppl:92–109.
41. Block MS, Emery RW, Lank K, Ryan J. Implant Placement Accuracy Using Dynamic Navigation. *Int J Oral Maxillofac Implants* (2017) 32(1):92–9. doi: 10.11607/jomi.5004
42. Sun T-M, Lan T-H, Pan C-Y, Lee H-E. Dental Implant Navigation System Guide the Surgery Future. *Kaohsiung J Med Sci* (2018) 34(1):56–64. doi: 10.1016/j.kjms.2017.08.011
43. Jorba-García A, González-Barnadas A, Camps-Font O, Figueiredo R, Valmaseda-Castellón E. Accuracy Assessment of Dynamic Computer-Aided Implant Placement: A Systematic Review and Meta-Analysis. *Clin Oral Investig* (2021) 25(5):2479–94. doi: 10.1007/s00784-021-03833-8

5

Adherence to Computer-Assisted Surgical Planning in 136 Maxillofacial Reconstructions

Hongyang Ma[1,2], *Sohaib Shujaat*[1,2], *Jeroen Van Dessel*[1,2], *Yi Sun*[1,2], *Michel Bila*[1,2], *Jan Vranckx*[3], *Constantinus Politis*[1,2] *and Reinhilde Jacobs*[1,2,4*]

[1] OMFS IMPATH Research Group, Department of Imaging & Pathology, Faculty of Medicine, KU Leuven, Leuven, Belgium, [2] Department of Oral and Maxillofacial Surgery, University Hospitals Leuven, Leuven, Belgium, [3] Department of Plastic, Reconstructive, and Aesthetic Surgery, University Hospitals Leuven, Leuven, Belgium, [4] Department of Dental Medicine, Karolinska Institutet, Stockholm, Sweden

***Correspondence:**
Reinhilde Jacobs
reinhilde.jacobs@kuleuven.be

Objective: To investigate the adherence to initially planned maxillofacial reconstructions using computer-assisted surgery (CAS) and to identify the influential factors affecting its compliance for maxillofacial reconstruction.

Patients and Methods: A retrospective analysis of 136 computer-assisted maxillofacial reconstructive surgeries was conducted from January 2014 to June 2020. The categorical parameters involved age, gender, disease etiology, disease site, defect size, bone flap segments, and flap type. Apart from descriptive data reporting, categorical data were related by applying the Fisher-exact test, and a p-value below 5% was considered statistically significant ($P < 0.05$).

Results: The main reasons for partial or non-adherence included unfitness, patient health condition, and other subjective reasons. Out of the total patient population, 118 patients who underwent mandibular reconstruction showed higher CAS compliance (83.9%) compared to the 18 midface reconstruction (72.2%) without any statistically significant difference ($p = 0.361$). Based on the size of the defect, a significantly higher CAS compliance ($p = 0.031$) was observed with a minor defect (80.6%) compared to the large-sized ones (74.1%). The bone flaps with two or more segments were significantly ($p = 0.003$) prone to observe a partial (15.4%) or complete (12.8%) discard of the planned CAS compared to the bone flaps with less than two segments. The malignant tumors showed the lowest CAS compliance when compared to other disorders without any significant difference ($p = 0.1$).

Conclusion: The maxillofacial reconstructive surgical procedures offered optimal compliance to the initially planned CAS. However, large-sized defects and multiple bone flap segments demonstrated a higher risk of partial or complete abandonment of the CAS.

Keywords: computer-assisted surgery (CAS), treatment adherence and compliance, patient-specific model, virtual surgical planning (VSP), 3D printing, oral and maxillofacial reconstruction, head and neck

INTRODUCTION

Reconstructive maxillofacial surgery following tumor resection, trauma, osteonecrosis, and other infectious diseases is vital for restoring facial aesthetics, function, oral rehabilitation and improving the patient's quality of life (QOL) (1). Depending on the complexity of the defect, the reconstruction might range from a local flap with secondary bone grafting to microvascular free flap surgery. The maxillofacial region mandates special care from a surgeon as it occupies a central position concerning the aesthetics and functionality, as an inadequate reconstruction might negatively influence the final outcome (2).

Previously, maxillofacial reconstruction with the traditional freehand technique offered a challenge for optimally repositioning the grafted segments and maintaining facial symmetry. However, with the advent of computer-assisted surgery (CAS) and three-dimensional (3D) printing, the reconstructive surgical accuracy and patient- and surgery-related outcomes have significantly improved (3, 4). Additionally, CAS has also played a vital role in improving the oral rehabilitation by increasing the predictability of replacing missing teeth with both first- and second-stage dental implant placement in the grafted region (5). Thereby, making CAS an indispensable tool for reconstructive surgery.

Over the past few years, the significant technological advancements and availability of surgeon-friendly software programs have led to the domination of CAS for maxillofacial reconstruction compared to its conventional counterpart by offering multiple advantages, which commonly include, improved resection accuracy, reduction in the operation, ischemia and hospitalization time, improved functional and aesthetic outcomes and minimization of the intersegmental gap size (6–8). At the same instance, the disadvantages such as preparation and planning time, and cost aspects cannot be ignored (9–11). Although, multiple centers now offer in-house CAS services for decreasing the time to therapy initiation (TTI) (12). However, an issue still exists where certain centers with low-volume of reconstruction cases rely on out-of-house services, which might cause a delay in the delivery and treatment time, in turn leading to further growth of the tumor (13). All these limiting CAS factors should be taken into consideration, as TTI has been known to be an influential factor for pathologic tumor upstaging, where an untimely intervention might lead to further tumor progression and increased mortality (14, 15).

Various studies have focussed on the accuracy and reproducibility of the CAS for maxillofacial reconstruction. However, a lack of evidence exists pertaining to the CAS compliance during the reconstructive procedures. It is questionable whether a surgeon completely adheres to the planned CAS (16). Previous studies reporting on the CAS compliance have only briefly reported whether the planning was executed entirely, partially, or abandoned and also failed to assess the factors which might influence its adherence.

Therefore, the present study was conducted to investigate the CAS compliance for initially planned maxillofacial reconstruction and to identify potential influential factors that might affect its adherence to the initially planned CAS.

MATERIAL AND METHODS

The Local Ethics Committee approved the study (reference no.: S63615) and was conducted in compliance with the World Medical Association Declaration of Helsinki on medical research (clinicaltrials.gov, NCT04895319). A total of 210 patients who underwent CAS-based maxillofacial reconstruction were screened from January 2014 to June 2020. The inclusion criteria involved patients undergoing maxillofacial reconstruction with CAS, which included virtual surgical planning, CAD-CAM surgical guides/templates, and pre-bent plates on 3D printed models. The workflow in our single-center was illustrated in **Figure 1**.

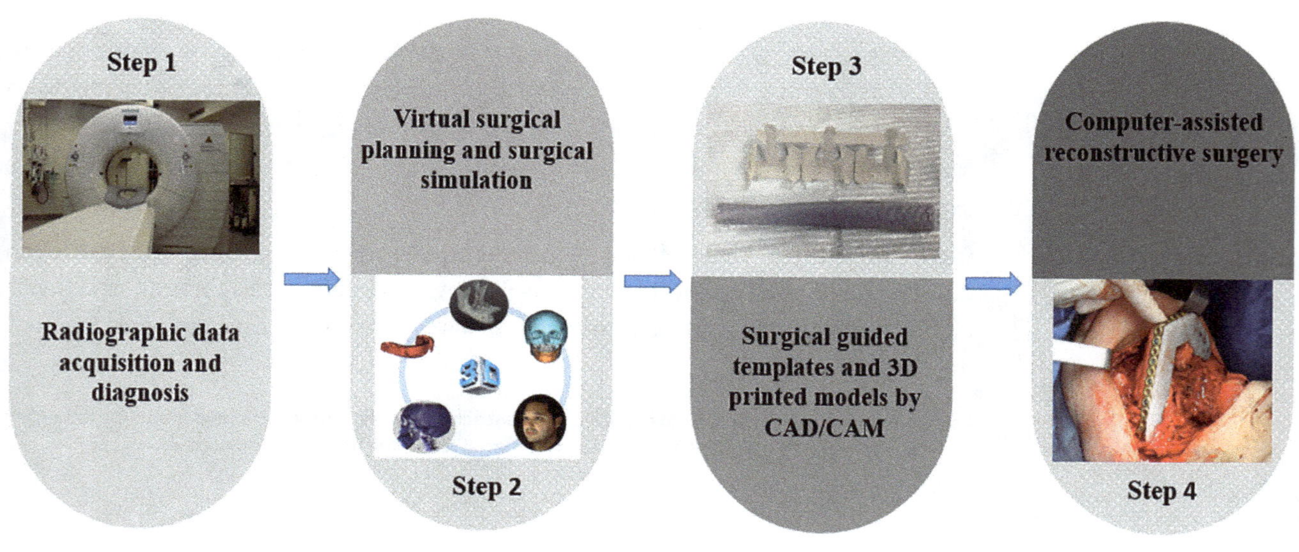

FIGURE 1 | Workflow of Computer-assisted surgery in our single center.

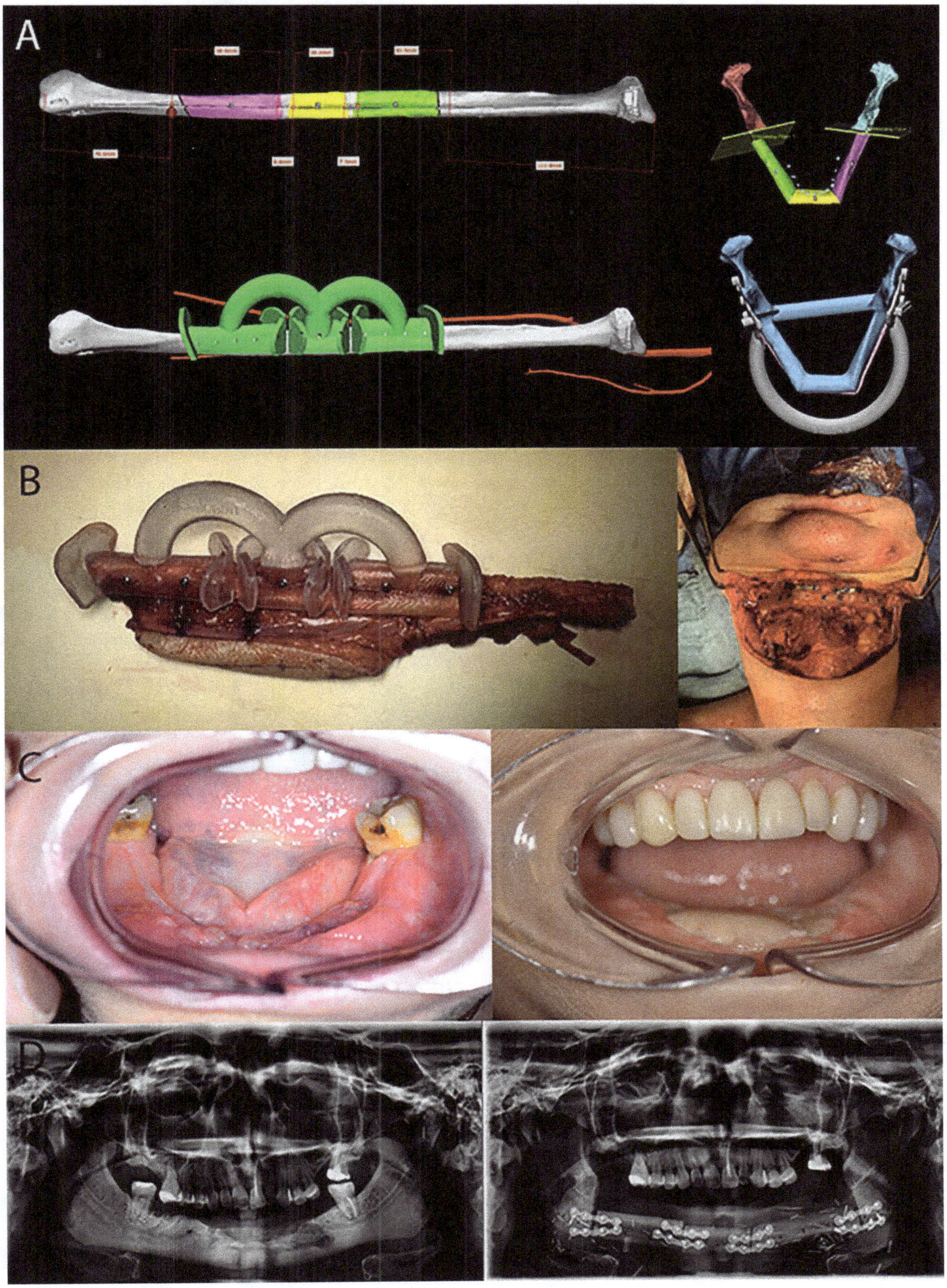

FIGURE 2 | Computer-assisted surgical planning and execution for a squamous cell carcinoma reconstruction. **(A)** Preoperative virtual analysis and planning. **(B)** Fibular graft fabrication assisted by guided templates. **(C)** Preoperative and postoperative intraoral photos of squamous cell carcinoma resection with mandibular reconstruction. **(D)** Preoperative and postoperative panoramic radiographs.

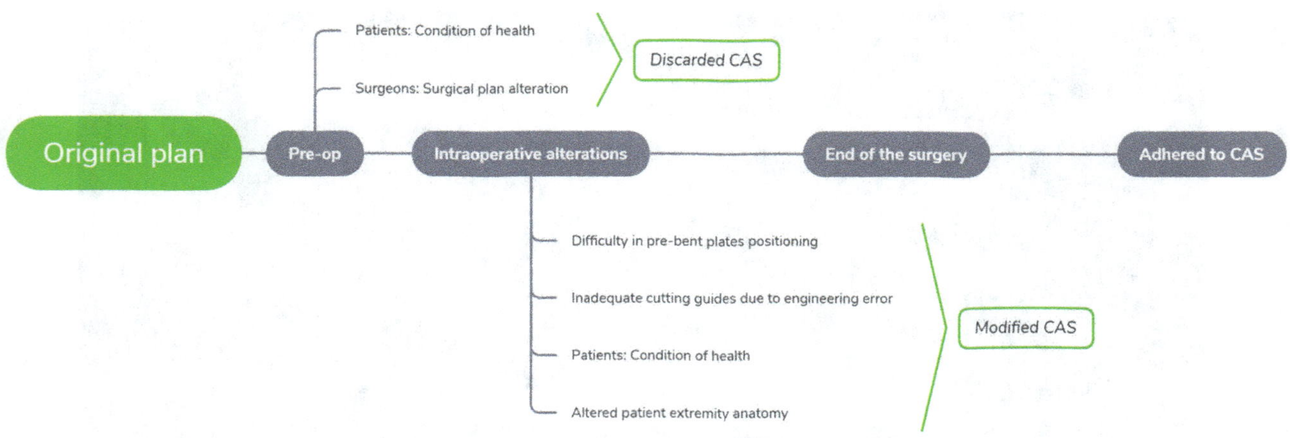

FIGURE 3 | Flowchart of surgical adherence to computer-assisted surgery.

Reasons for reconstruction were oncologic, osteoradionecrosis, trauma, and osteoporosis. Patients undergoing computer-assisted implant surgery and orthognathic surgery were excluded.

All computer-assisted surgeries were planned by an experienced clinical engineer in discussion with the oral and maxillofacial surgical team. The virtual planning was performed to determine the resection, cut margins, and localize the optimal angles for performing osteotomies. After that, surgical cutting guides were designed utilizing a 3D designing software (3-Matic, Version 9.0-13.0, Materialise, Leuven, Belgium). The generated virtual templates and the planned 3D skeletal model were exported in a Standard Tessellation Language (STL) format and printed with a professional 3D printer (Connex 350 3D printer, Stratasys, Eden Prairie, MN, USA). The reconstructive plates were pre-bent on the 3D-printed model. A fixation tray was applied for the guided placement of the reconstructive plates. The screw holes' locations were drilled and marked onto the surgical template by the surgeon (**Figure 2**).

The patients were divided into three groups depending on the CAS compliance either during the pre-operative or intra-operatively, which included; complete adherence, partial adherence, and no adherence (**Figure 3**). The recorded categorical parameters involved disease etiology classified by either malignant or non-malignant tumor, disease site (mandible or midface), bone flap segments (< 2 or ≥ 2 segments), and flap type (bone flap or others). (The defects were classified based on Brown classification, where class I, II of mandibular defect and class I, II, V, VI of maxillary and midface defect were defined as a small defect; Class III, IV of the mandibular defect and class III, IV of maxillary and midface defect were defined as a large defect (17, 18).

Statistical Analysis

Data were analyzed using IBM SPSS Statistics version 25.0 (IBM Corp., Armonk, NY: IBM Corp, USA). Mean values and standard deviation were recorded for all parameters. The categorical data were compared by applying the Fisher-exact test. A p-value below 5% was considered statistically significant ($p < 0.05$).

RESULTS

Following inclusion and exclusion criteria, clinical and image data of 136 consecutive patients (58 females, 78 males, mean age: 55.8 ± 18 years) undergoing CAS-based maxillofacial reconstruction were served further analysis. **Table 1** describes

TABLE 1 | Patients characteristics.

Parameters	Classification	Numbers (N)	Percentage (%)
Gender (M/F)		78/58	57.4/42.6
Age (mean, SD)		55.8 ± 18	/
Adherence of CAS	Complete	112	82.4
	Partial	14	10.3
	Discarded	10	7.4
Etiology	Malignant tumor	72	52.9
	Benign tumor/cyst of jaw	13	9.6
	Trauma	16	11.8
	ORN	25	18.4
	Others	10	7.4
Disease site	Mandible	118	86.8
	Midface	18	13.2
Defect size	Small	72	52.9
	Large	64	47.1
Bone graft segments	0	20	14.7
	1	38	27.9
	2	39	28.7
	>2	39	28.7
Flap type	Fibula	88	64.7
	Iliac	22	16.2
	Scapula	6	4.4
	Plates or prosthesis only	20	14.7

CAS, Computer-assisted surgery; ORN, Osteoradionecrosis.

the patient- and surgery-related characteristics, where the majority of the patients were diagnosed with malignant tumor (n = 72) followed by maxillofacial trauma (n=16), benign tumor or odontogenic keratocyst (n=13), osteoradionecrosis (n=25) and temporomandibular joint ankyloses/congenital maxillofacial defect (n=10). The main reasons for partial abandonment of the planned CAS included unfitness of the cutting guide (n = 4) and pre-bent plates (n = 2), patients health condition (n=7). **Figure 4** illustrates an example of a case showing partial CAS compliance. In contrast, the complete discard of CAS was mainly attributed to subjective reasoning (**Table 2**).

Table 3 describes the factors influencing the compliance to the planned CAS. When evaluating the CAS compliance based on the defect site, patients who underwent mandibular reconstruction showed higher complete adherence (83.9%) compared to the midface reconstruction (72.2%) without any statistically significant difference (p = 0.361). Based on the size of the defect, a significantly higher conformity to the CAS (p = 0.031) was observed for patients with a minor defect (80.6%) compared to the large-sized ones (74.1%). The bone flaps with more than two segments were significantly (p=0.003) prone to observe partial (15.4%) or complete discard of the CAS (12.8%). The malignant tumors showed the lowest conformity to the CAS when compared to other disorders without any significant difference (p=0.1). As for the patients treated with a bone flap, complete adherence was significantly higher (85.3%, p=0.016) when compared with the non-bony flap group (65.0%).

DISCUSSION

The present study explored the conformity to CAS for maxillofacial reconstructive procedures and investigated the influence of the parameters to identify the reasons it was partially executed or wholly discarded.

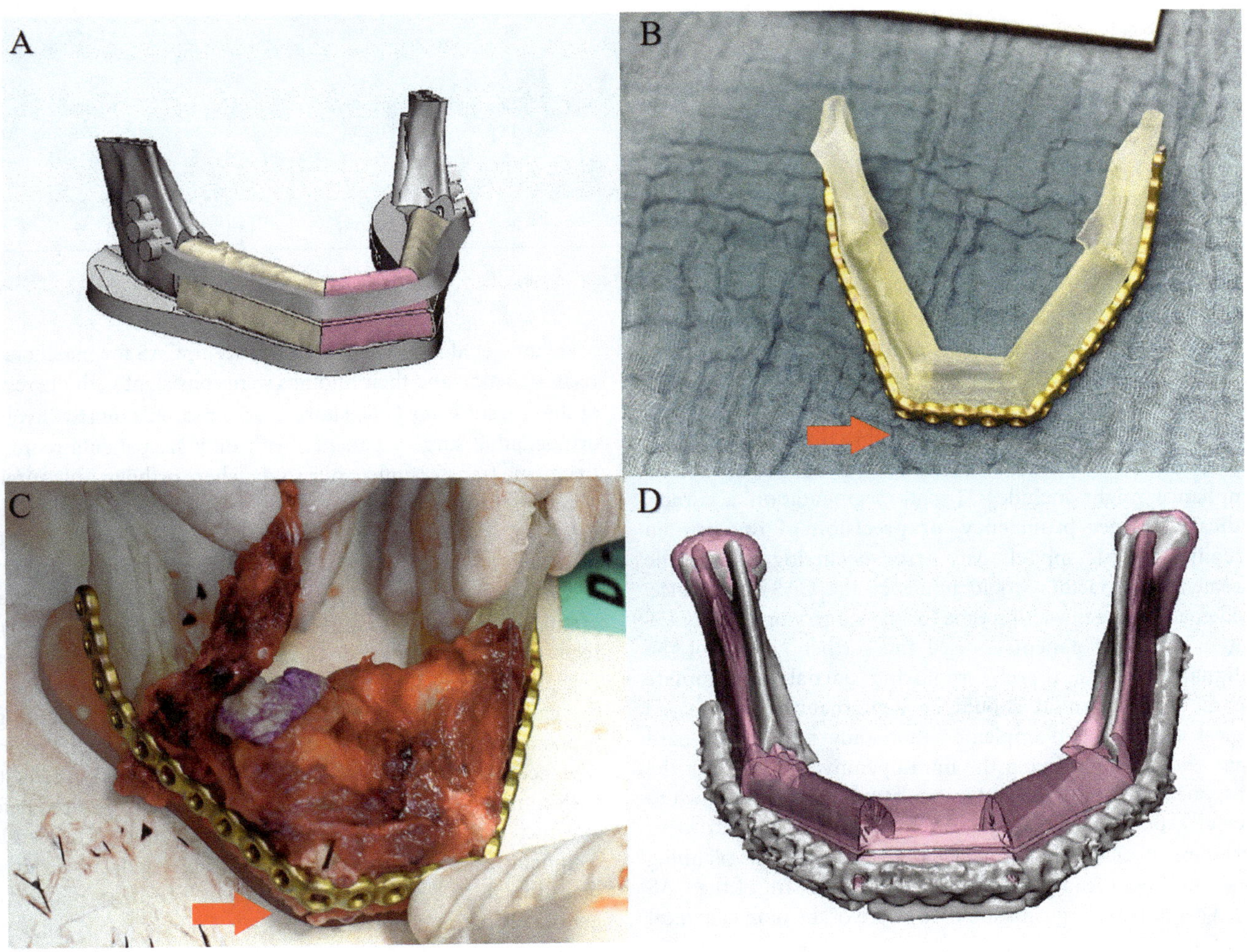

FIGURE 4 | A 56-year-old patient with mandibular squamous cell carcinoma showing partial computer-assisted surgical compliance. **(A)** Virtual surgical planning for mandibular reconstruction. **(B)** Plate prebending on the 3D printed model. **(C)** Intra-operative plate bending modified due to unfitness. **(D)** Postoperative superimposition verifying the 3-D deviation of the reconstructed region compared with the original virtual surgical plan.

TABLE 2 | Partially executed or discarded plan with reasons.

Influential factors	Reason	Numbers	Outcome
Unfitness	Guided templates	4	Partially executed plan
	Pre-bent plates	2	Partially executed plan
Patients' health conditions	Tumor growth	2	Partially executed plan
	Tumor growth	1	Discarded plan
	Bone displacement	1	Partially executed plan
	Altered extremity	2	Partially executed plan
	Complex maxillary defect	1	Partially executed plan
	Death	1	Discarded plan
Subjective reasons	Surgical protocol changes	2	Partially executed plan
	Treatment plan alteration	3	Discarded plan
	Unaffordable cost	2	Discarded plan
	Patients' non-compliance	3	Discarded plan

TABLE 3 | Influential parameters on the adherence of CAS.

Parameters	Classification	Total (n)	Complete adherence (n)	Percentage	Partial adherence (n)	Percentage	Not adherence (n)	Percentage	P-value
Site	Mandible	118	99	83.9%	11	9.3%	8	6.8%	0.361
	Midface	18	13	72.2%	3	16.7%	2	11.1%	
Defect size	Small	72	58	80.6%	6	8.3%	8	11.1%	0.031
	Large	64	99	74.1%	8	9.3%	2	6.8%	
Segments	<2	58	56	96.6%	2	3.4%	0	0.0%	0.003
	≥2	78	56	71.8%	12	15.4%	10	12.8%	
Aetiology	Malignant tumor	72	55	76.4%	11	15.3%	6	8.3%	0.1
	Non-malignant tumor	64	57	89.1%	3	4.7%	4	6.3%	
Flap type	Bone flap	116	99	85.3%	8	6.9%	9	7.8%	0.016
	Others	20	13	65.0%	6	30.0%	1	5.0%	

The present study's findings suggested that the unfitness of the guided templates and patients' health condition were most commonly observed in the partially abandoned CAS, whereas complete CAS discard was based on subjective reasoning. The factors which could have attributed to the reduced CAS compliance might include CT data segmentation accuracy, medical engineer proficiency, or precision of the printed stereolithographic model. Any error occurring due to the aforementioned factors would influence the CAS compliance. Besides, a prolonged waiting time for the surgery or an early CT scan in oncology patients caused the further growth of the malignant tumors, thereby requiring partial or complete discard of the plan. It should be kept that the CAS-based surgical planning and implementation only rely on the hard tissue, without considering the intra-operative influence of the soft tissue. The soft tissue and musculature have been known to forcefully position the bone flap in complex reconstructive procedures, which is not considered at the treatment planning phase and might lead to partial or complete discard of the CAS (19). Therefore, a surgeon should be aware of the biomechanical deformation of the soft tissue during CAS, and a patient-specific soft tissue predictive model should be generated based on the CT data, and finite element analysis at the planning phase improved planning (20).

Efanov et al. assessed the adherence to CAS for maxillofacial reconstruction and their findings were consistent with the results of the current study (21). However, their sample mostly involved orthognathic surgery patients, with only six patients requiring free tissue transfer, unlike our study where orthognathic surgical procedures were excluded to reduce the risk of bias. Hanken et al. reported a relationship between surgical accuracy and the number of bone flap segments for the maxillofacial reconstruction, where higher deviations occurred between virtual and real segment position in patients requiring reconstruction with two or three fibular or iliac crest segments compared to a single segment (22). The accuracy of CAS decreases with the increased number of segments, which might explain the partial adherence or complete discard. Previous evidence failed to report whether the defect size decreases the CAS compliance. Our findings suggested that a large-sized defect and increased bone segments were more prone to lower CAS compliance, especially in cases involving condylar region or mandibular angle where unfitness of pre-bent plates was mainly observed.

A variety of approaches can establish the improvement in CAS. Effective and constant communication between the surgeon and medical engineer might significantly improve the planned CAS. As the incomplete adherence not only leads to an increased risk of intra-operative complications but is also associated with higher financial costs if the plan is changed at the pre-operative stage (23). For improving the virtual planning and CAS, it is recommended to utilize a CT image with a slice thickness of less than 1mm and to advocate a professional 3D printing for printing the skull model to improve the contouring of the pre-bent plates (6). Another option could be the 3D printing of the patient-specific titanium plates which offers improved accuracy compared to the traditional pre-bent plates (24). Regarding the cutting guides, patient-specific titanium alloy cutting guides could be an alternative to improve fitness. These guides are thinner than the polyamide guides, allowing easier intraoral placement and decrease the amount of periosteal stripping and cutaneous resection (25).

The study had certain limitations. Firstly, the quantitative accuracy of the CAS was not assessed. Secondly, the retrospective nature of the study could have acted as a medium of bias. Thirdly, sample distribution was heterogeneous, mainly involving reconstruction following resection of the malignant tumors. Future studies should investigate the amount of error induced at each step of the planning to understand better and improve complex reconstructive procedures.

CONCLUSION

CAS-based maxillofacial reconstructive surgery offered optimal conformity to the initially executed plan. However, large-sized defects and an increased number of bone flap segments led to a higher rate of partial or complete abandonment of CAS. Thereby, a surgeon should be aware of the possibility of non-adherence to the planned CAS for complex reconstructive procedures.

AUTHOR CONTRIBUTIONS

HM and SS: study design, manuscript preparation, statistical analysis, data analysis, and interpretation. RJ and CP: study supervision. JD and YS: data collection. MB, JD, SS, JV, RJ, and CP: contributed to the manuscript review, critical revision for important intellectual content. All authors contributed to the article and approved the submitted version.

ACKNOWLEDGMENTS

The authors thank the statistician Mr. Wim Coucke for his assistance regarding the statistics applied in this research.

REFERENCES

1. Yu P, Chang DW, Miller MJ, Reece G, Robb GL. Analysis of 49 Cases of Flap Compromise in 1310 Free Flaps for Head and Neck Reconstruction. *Head Neck* (2009) 31(1):45–51. doi: 10.1002/hed.20927
2. Wijbenga JG, Schepers RH, Werker PM, Witjes MJ, Dijkstra PU. A Systematic Review of Functional Outcome and Quality of Life Following Reconstruction of Maxillofacial Defects Using Vascularized Free Fibula Flaps and Dental Rehabilitation Reveals Poor Data Quality. *J Plast Reconstr Aesthet Surg* (2016) 69(8):1024–36. doi: 10.1016/j.bjps.2016.05.003
3. Largo RD, Garvey PB. Updates in Head and Neck Reconstruction. *Plast Reconstr Surg* (2018) 141(2):271e–85e. doi: 10.1097/PRS.0000000000004070
4. Harrison P, Patel A, Cheng A, Bell RB. Three-Dimensional Computer-Assisted Surgical Planning, Manufacturing, and Intraoperative Navigation in Oncologic Surgery. *Atlas Oral Maxillofac Surg Clin North Am* (2020) 28 (2):129–44. doi: 10.1016/j.cxom.2020.06.001
5. Ma H, Shujaat S, Bila M, Sun Y, Vranckx J, Politis C, et al. Computer-Assisted Versus Traditional Freehand Technique for Mandibular Reconstruction With Free Vascularized Fibular Flap: A Matched-Pair Study. *J Plast Reconstr Aesthet Surg* (2021). doi: 10.1016/j.bjps.2021.03.121. in press.
6. van Baar GJC, Forouzanfar T, Liberton N, Winters HAH, Leusink FKJ. Accuracy of Computer-Assisted Surgery in Mandibular Reconstruction: A Systematic Review. *Oral Oncol* (2018) 84:52–60. doi: 10.1016/j.oraloncology.2018.07.004
7. van Baar GJC, Schipper K, Forouzanfar T, Leeuwrik L, Winters HAH, Ridwan-Pramana A, et al. Accuracy of Computer-Assisted Surgery in Maxillary Reconstruction: A Systematic Review. *J Clin Med* (2021) 10 (6):1226. doi: 10.3390/jcm10061226
8. D'Haese J, Ackhurst J, Wismeijer D, De Bruyn H, Tahmaseb A. Current State of the Art of Computer-Guided Implant Surgery. *Periodontol 2000* (2017) 73 (1):121–33. doi: 10.1111/prd.12175
9. Mazzola F, Smithers F, Cheng K, Mukherjee P, Hubert Low TH, Ch'ng S, et al. Time and Cost-Analysis of Virtual Surgical Planning for Head and Neck Reconstruction: A Matched Pair Analysis. *Oral Oncol* (2020) 100:104491. doi: 10.1016/j.oraloncology.2019.104491
10. Rommel N, Kesting MR, Rohleder NH, Bauer FMJ, Wolff KD, Weitz J. Mandible Reconstruction With Free Fibula Flaps: Outcome of a Cost-Effective Individual Planning Concept Compared With Virtual Surgical Planning. *J Craniomaxillofac Surg* (2017) 45(8):1246–50. doi: 10.1016/j.jcms.2017.04.010
11. Fatima A, Hackman TG, Wood JS. Cost-Effectiveness Analysis of Virtual Surgical Planning in Mandibular Reconstruction. *Plast Reconstr Surg* (2019) 143(4):1185–94. doi: 10.1097/PRS.0000000000005418
12. Bosc R, Hersant B, Carloni R, Niddam J, Bouhassira J, De Kermadec H, et al. Mandibular Reconstruction After Cancer: An in-House Approach to Manufacturing Cutting Guides. *Int J Oral Maxillofac Surg* (2017) 46(1):24–31. doi: 10.1016/j.ijom.2016.10.004
13. Mottini M, Jafari SMS, Shafighi M, Schaller B. New Approach for Virtual Surgical Planning and Mandibular Reconstruction Using a Fibula Free Flap. *Oral Oncol* (2016) 59:E6–9. doi: 10.1016/j.oraloncology.2016.06.001
14. Graboyes EM, Garrett-Mayer E, Sharma AK, Lentsch EJ, Day TA. Adherence to National Comprehensive Cancer Network Guidelines for Time to Initiation of Postoperative Radiation Therapy for Patients With Head and Neck Cancer. *Cancer* (2017) 123(14):2651–60. doi: 10.1002/cncr.30651
15. Knitschke M, Bäcker C, Schmermund D, Böttger S, Streckbein P, Howaldt H-P, et al. Impact of Planning Method (Conventional Versus Virtual) on Time to Therapy Initiation and Resection Margins: A Retrospective Analysis of 104 Immediate Jaw Reconstructions. *Cancers* (2021) 13(12):3013. doi: 10.3390/cancers13123013
16. Tarsitano A, Battaglia S, Ricotta F, Bortolani B, Cercenelli L, Marcelli E, et al. Accuracy of CAD/CAM Mandibular Reconstruction: A Three-Dimensional, Fully Virtual Outcome Evaluation Method. *J Craniomaxillofac Surg* (2018) 46 (7):1121–5. doi: 10.1016/j.jcms.2018.05.010
17. Brown JS, Barry C, Ho M, Shaw R. A New Classification for Mandibular Defects After Oncological Resection. *Lancet Oncol* (2016) 17(1):e23–30. doi: 10.1016/S1470-2045(15)00310-1
18. Brown JS, Shaw RJ. Reconstruction of the Maxilla and Midface: Introducing a New Classification. *Lancet Oncol* (2010) 11(10):1001–8. doi: 10.1016/S1470-2045(10)70113-3
19. Kim RY, Bae SS, Feinberg SE. Soft Tissue Engineering. *Oral Maxillofac Surg Clin North Am* (2017) 29(1):89–104. doi: 10.1016/j.coms.2016.08.007

20. Mollemans W, Schutyser F, Nadjmi N, Maes F, Suetens P. Predicting Soft Tissue Deformations for a Maxillofacial Surgery Planning System: From Computational Strategies to a Complete Clinical Validation. *Med Image Anal* (2007) 11(3):282–301. doi: 10.1016/j.media.2007.02.003
21. Efanov JI, Roy AA, Huang KN, Borsuk DE. Virtual Surgical Planning: The Pearls and Pitfalls. *Plast Reconstr Surg Glob Open* (2018) 6(1):e1443. doi: 10.1097/GOX.0000000000001443
22. Hanken H, Schablowsky C, Smeets R, Heiland M, Sehner S, Riecke B, et al. Virtual Planning of Complex Head and Neck Reconstruction Results in Satisfactory Match Between Real Outcomes and Virtual Models. *Clin Oral Invest* (2015) 19(3):647–56. doi: 10.1007/s00784-014-1291-5
23. Lou Y, Cai L, Wang C, Tang Q, Pan T, Guo X, et al. Comparison of Traditional Surgery and Surgery Assisted by Three Dimensional Printing Technology in the Treatment of Tibial Plateau Fractures. *Int Orthop* (2017) 41(9):1875–80. doi: 10.1007/s00264-017-3445-y
24. Yang WF, Choi WS, Wong MC, Powcharoen W, Zhu WY, Tsoi JK, et al. Three-Dimensionally Printed Patient-Specific Surgical Plates Increase Accuracy of Oncologic Head and Neck Reconstruction Versus Conventional Surgical Plates: A Comparative Study. *Ann Surg Oncol* (2021) 28(1):363–75. doi: 10.1245/s10434-020-08732-y
25. Gigliotti J, Ying Y, Morlandt AB. Titanium Alloy Cutting Guides in Craniomaxillofacial Surgery-A Minimally Invasive Alternative to Synthetic Polymer Guides. *J Oral Maxillofac Surg* (2020) 78(11):2080–9. doi: 10.1016/j.joms.2020.06.010

6

Frozen Section Analysis and Real-Time Magnetic Resonance Imaging of Surgical Specimen Oriented on 3D Printed Tongue Model to Assess Surgical Margins in Oral Tongue Carcinoma: Preliminary Results

Caterina Giannitto[1†], Giuseppe Mercante[2,3†], Luca Disconzi[1,3], Riccardo Boroni[4], Elena Casiraghi[5], Federica Canzano[2], Michele Cerasuolo[2], Francesca Gaino[2], Armando De Virgilio[2,3], Barbara Fiamengo[6], Fabio Ferreli[2,3], Andrea Alessandro Esposito[7], Paolo Oliva[4], Flavio Ronzoni[3], Luigi Terracciano[3,6], Giuseppe Spriano[2,3‡] and Luca Balzarini[1‡]*

[1] Department of Diagnostic Radiology, Humanitas Clinical and Research Center Istituti di Ricovero e Cura a Carattere Scientifico (IRCCS), Milan, Italy, [2] Otorhinolaryngology Unit, Humanitas Clinical and Research Centre Istituti di Ricovero e Cura a Carattere Scientifico (IRCCS), Milan, Italy, [3] Department of Biomedical Sciences, Humanitas University, Milan, Italy, [4] Department of Supply Chain, Humanitas Clinical and Research Center Istituti di Ricovero e Cura a Carattere Scientifico (IRCCS), Rozzano, Milan, Italy, [5] Department of Computer Science (DI), Università degli Studi di Milano, Milan, Italy, [6] Department of Pathology, Humanitas Clinical and Research Center Istituti di Ricovero e Cura a Carattere Scientifico (IRCCS), Milan, Italy, [7] Department of Radiology, Azienda Socio Sanitaria Territoriale di Bergamo Ovest, Treviglio, Italy

***Correspondence:**
Caterina Giannitto
caterina.giannitto@humanitas.it*

[†]These authors share first authorship

[‡]These authors share senior authorship

Background: A surgical margin is the apparently healthy tissue around a tumor which has been removed. In oral cavity carcinoma, a negative margin is considered ≥ 5 mm, a close margin between 1 and 5 mm, and a positive margin ≤ 1 mm. Currently, the intraoperative surgical margin status is based on the visual inspection and tissue palpation by the surgeon and intraoperative histopathological assessment of the resection margins by frozen section analysis (FSA). FSA technique is limited and susceptible to sampling errors. Definitive information on the deep resection margins requires postoperative histopathological analysis.

Methods: We described a novel approach for the assessment of intraoperative surgical margins by examining a surgical specimen oriented through a 3D-printed specific patient tongue with real-time Magnetic Resonance Imaging (MRI). We reported the preliminary results of a case series of 10 patients, prospectively enrolled, with oral tongue carcinoma who underwent surgery between February 2020 and April 2021. Two radiologists with 5 and 10 years of experience, respectively, in Head and Neck radiology in consensus evaluated specimen MRI and measured the distance between the tumor and the specimen surface. We performed intraoperative bedside FSA. To compare the performance of bedside FSA and MRI in predicting definitive margin status we computed the weighted sensitivity (SE), specificity (SP), accuracy (ACC), area under the ROC curve (AUC), F1-score, Positive Predictive Value (PPV), and Negative Predictive Value (NPV). To express the concordance between FSA and *ex-vivo* MRI we reported the jaccard index.

Results: Intraoperative bedside FSA showed SE of 90%, SP of 100%, F1 of 95%, ACC of 0.9%, PPV of 100%, NPV (not a number), and jaccard of 90%, and *ex-vivo* MRI showed SE of 100%, SP of 100%, F1 of 100%, ACC of 100%, PPV of 100%, NPV of 100%, and jaccard of 100%. These results needed to be validated in a larger sample size of 21- 44 patients.

Conclusion: The presented method allows a more accurate evaluation of surgical margin status, and the first clinical experiences underline the high potential of integrating FSA with *ex-vivo* MRI of the fresh surgical specimen.

Keywords: head and neck, virtual surgical planning, 3D printing, tumor, resection, surgical margins, *ex-vivo*

INTRODUCTION

A surgical margin is the apparently healthy tissue around a tumor that has been surgically removed. Most commonly, in oral cavity carcinoma, a margin larger than or equal to 5 mm is considered as "negative", a margin between 1 and 5 mm as "close", and a margin less than 1 mm as "positive" (1, 2). Radicality and negative margin status represent the most successful outcome in oral cancer surgery. Close or positive margins require re-resection or adjuvant (chemo)radiotherapy contributing to costs, morbidity, and reduced quality of life of the patients who have to undergo these treatments. Mitchell et al. (3) showed that in oral carcinoma five-year survival was 81%, 75%, and 54% for clear, close, and involved margins, respectively, which highlights the importance of clear margins.

Currently, the intraoperative surgical margin status is based on the visual inspection and tissue palpation by the surgeon during surgery and intraoperative histopathological assessment of the resection margins by frozen section analysis (FSA). FSA technique is limited and susceptible to sampling errors (4, 5). Definitive information on the deep resection margins requires postoperative histopathological analysis.

The margin revision of initially positive margins to "clear" based on FSA guidance does not equate to an initially negative margin and does not significantly improve local control. Prospective studies should determine what system of resected specimen analysis best predicts completeness of resection (6).

Real-time Magnetic Resonance Imaging (MRI) on surgical specimen has been used in a few previous studies (7, 8). In particular, Heidkamp et al. (8) showed a positive predictive value (PPV) and negative predictive value (NPV) for Oral Squamous Cell Carcinoma (OSCC) localization of 87-96% and 75-79%, respectively, and a PPV and NPV for identification of margins <5 mm of 5-38% and 87-91%.

When studying correlations between imaging and histological data, the different spatial resolution of the two methods can increase bias, and the evaluation of the piece of the organ as opposed to the whole organ without orientation references could be challenging for the pathologist. The introduction of a 3D-printed anatomic model of the tongue of the patient, obtained from staging MRI for surgical specimen orientation, reproducing the anatomic context from which the specimen has been excised could improve surgeon, pathologist, and radiologist communication in the assessment of margins.

The employment of MRI to examine the surgical specimen oriented through the 3D model could allow for a better macroscopic radial margin evaluation and measurement of the distance to all margins, avoiding sampling errors of FSA.

The purpose of this paper was to report the preliminary results of the diagnostic accuracy of FSA and MRI in evaluating intraoperative surgical margins in oral tongue carcinoma, by examining the surgical specimen oriented through the 3D-printed specific patient tongue model.

MATERIALS AND EQUIPMENT

We described the steps of the process in a sequential workflow, diagrammed in a flow chart (**Figure 1**), to clarify how these steps have been executed.

Pre-Operative Workflow: Design and Implementation of 3D Printed-Tongue Model

We obtained a 3D-printed model of the patient's tongue on which the area which should have been resected has been reproduced. We implemented the model by the 3D post-contrast fat suppressed gradient-echo T1weighted sequence (VIBE) of staging MRI

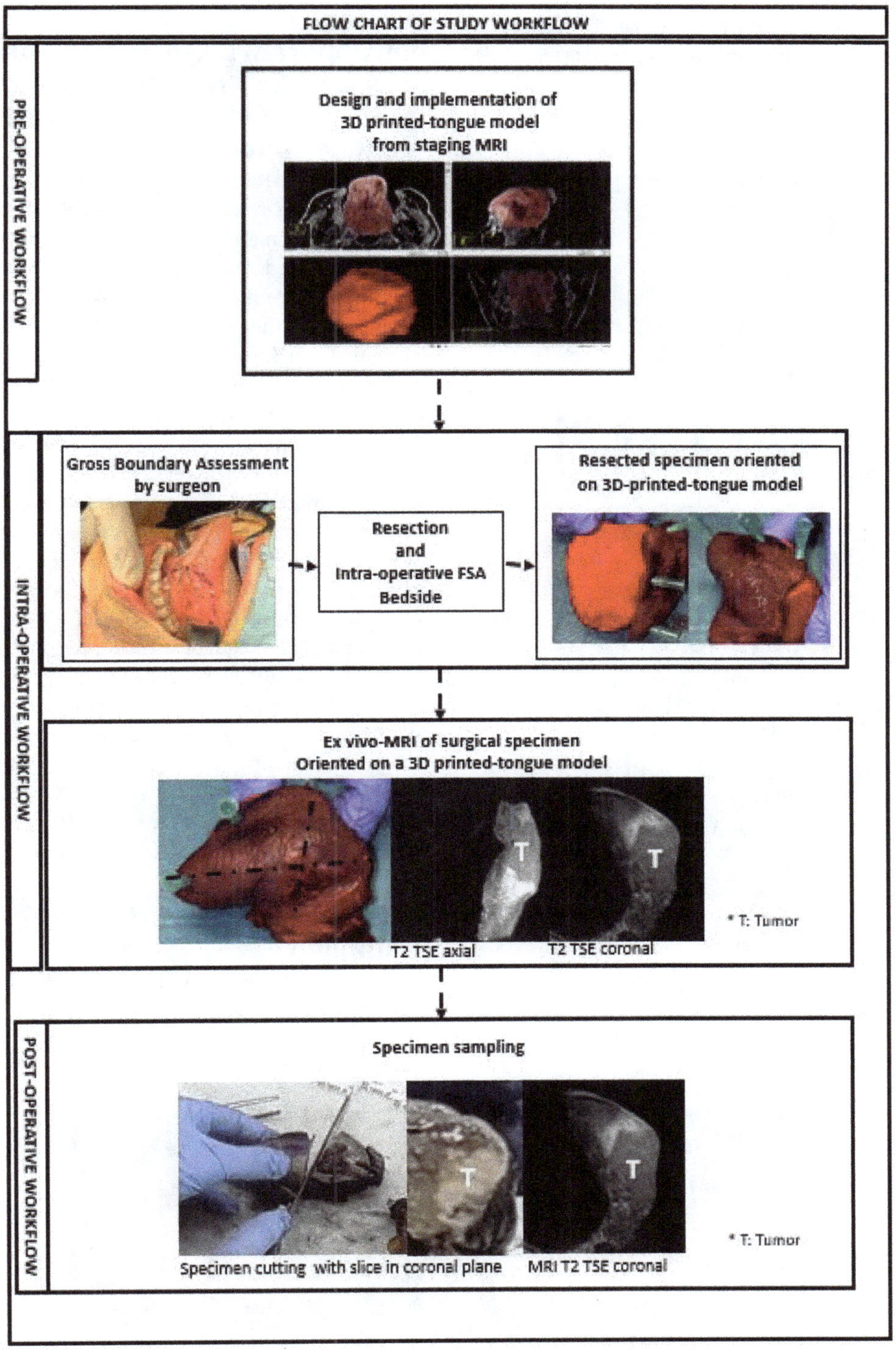

FIGURE 1 | This figure shows pre-operative, intra-operative and post-operative steps of the study workflow.

examinations on a 1.5T MRI System (Magnetom Aera, Siemens Healthineers, Erlangen, Germany) using a phased array surface coil. 3D post-contrast anonymized images demonstrating a good contrast between the tumor and the tongue parenchyma were selected and transferred into ITK-SNAP, a software application used to segment structures in 3D medical images (http://www.itksnap.org/pmwiki/pmwiki.php). The tongue tumor and tongue parenchyma were segmented as separate anatomical regions of interest (ROIs). For all ROIs, both threshold and manual editing were performed to ensure that only the anatomy of interest would be selected. Each ROI was converted to a separate 3D object and combined into a 3D virtual model. The segmentation data, in DICOM format, were converted to STL format so that the 3D printer could recognize them. Surgeons and radiologists segmented tongue tumor, and a 3D virtual model (**Figure 2**) of the tongue with the pathological area was printed by a 3D printer (VERVE, Kentstrapper, Florence Italy).

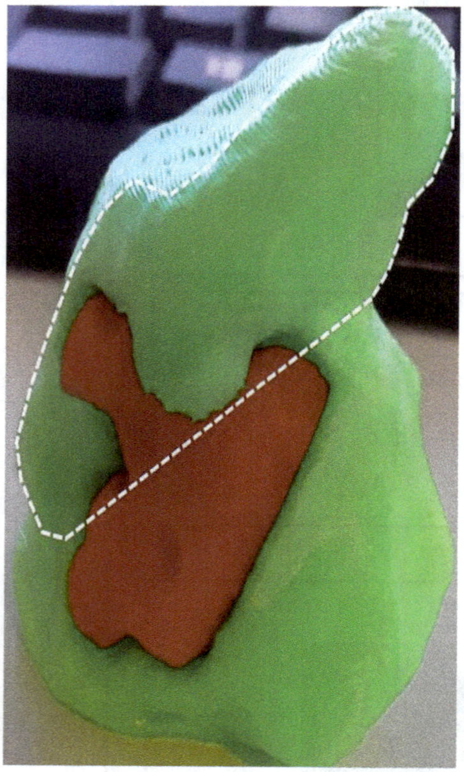

FIGURE 2 | Lateral view of the 3D-printed model shows the protuted tongue (inside the dotted line), the floor of the mouth (outside the dotted line), and the tumor in red.

Intraoperative Workflow: Intraoperative FSA and *Ex Vivo*-MRI of Surgical Specimen Oriented on a 3D Printed-Tongue Model

The surgeon determined the intended boundaries of resection and, following resection, sampled the tumor bed to establish intraoperative margin status. The positive margins at FSA have been radicalized. While maintained at the operating room, fresh specimens were fixed on the 3D-printed model for the correct orientation of the resected surgical specimen (**Figures 3, 4**). The specimen was immersed in perfluoropolyether (Galden, Solvay Solexis, Thorofare, New Jersey) to eliminate magnetic susceptibility artifacts arising from the air tissue transition (7).The specimen oriented on the 3D model was placed on an MRI phantom with a reference placed on the tumor. A four channel phased array surface carotid coil (Magnetom Aera, Siemens, Erlangen, Germany) was mounted underneath and on top of the 3D model which was positioned in a 1.5 T clinical MRI system (Magnetom Aera, Siemens, Erlangen, Germany). Axial, Coronal, Sagittal T2-weighted (T2W) turbo spin echo (TSE) sequences (using Field of View (FoV) read 130 mm, FoV phase 100.0%, slice thickness 3.0 mm, TR 3430.0 ms, TE 92.0 ms, Averages 3) and Diffusion weighted spin-echo echo planar images (using FoV read 140 mm, FoV phase 100.0%, slice thickness 3.0 mm, TR 3500 ms,TE 55.0 ms) were acquired. Apparent diffusion coefficient (ADC) maps were calculated based on acquired b values of 50, 500, and1000 s/mm2 using the standard post processing available on the MRI system.

Post-Operative Workflow: Specimen Sampling

Following MRI acquisition, surgical specimen oriented on the 3D-printed tongue model was transported to the pathology

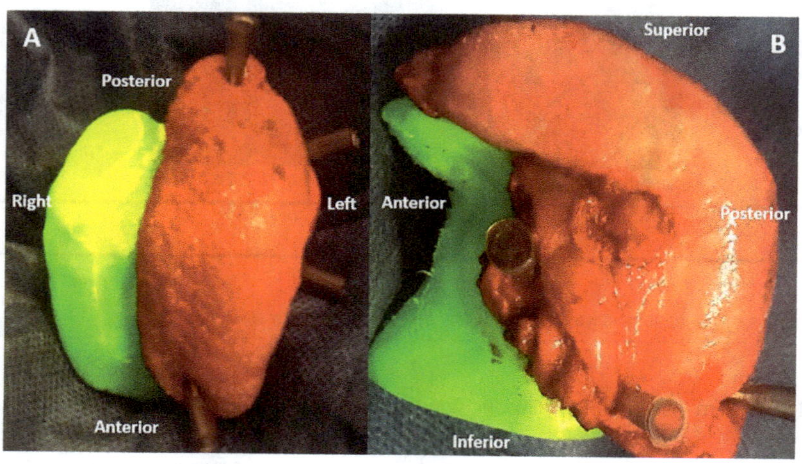

FIGURE 3 | Superior **(A)** and Lateral **(B)** views of surgical specimen of a left hemiglossectomy oriented on a 3D-printed model of the protuted tongue and the floor of the mouth obtained from the staging MRI of the patient.

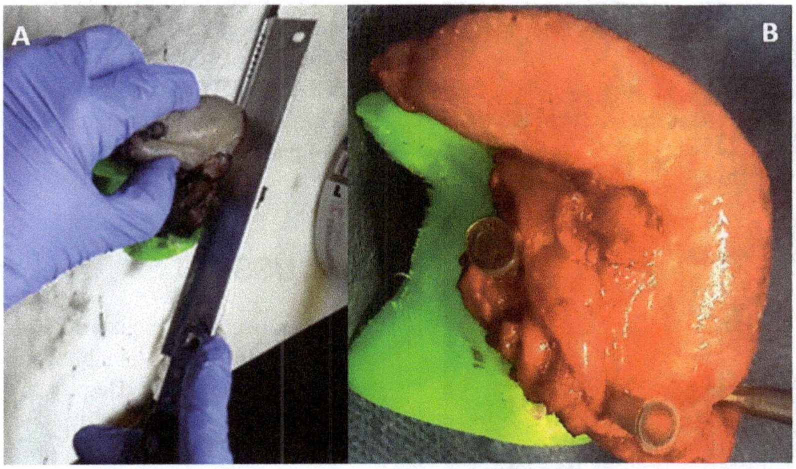

FIGURE 4 | Dissection of the specimen into 3–5 mm slices **(A, B)** parallel to MRI planes to evaluate the distance from the tumour to the surface of the specimen.

laboratory for formalin fixation. Next, the specimen oriented on the 3D model was completely cut up into 4 mm thick slices parallel to the coronal plane of MRI evaluation (**Figure 4**) and whole-mount paraffin was embedded to evaluate the macroscopic depth of invasion of the tumor and the radial distance of the tumor to all of the margins. In addition to this, the radial margin at the periphery has been submitted. The serial slices of the specimen were sequentially laid out, numbered, and photographed.

METHODS

Study Design and Patients

This was a pilot observational prospective mono-institutional cohort study including all consecutive adult patients with a histological diagnosis of OSCC who underwent a primary surgical treatment of lingual resection (hemiglossectomy or partial glossectomy) between February 2020 and April 2021. We prospectively included all the cases with an intraoperative margin status evaluation by FSA and *ex-vivo* MRI. Institutional review board approval and informed consent for all the patients enrolled were obtained.

Qualitative and Quantitative Analysis of *Ex-Vivo* MRI

The mean time duration of *Ex-vivo* MRI examination was 22.7 minutes (range 16-40 minutes).

For the qualitative analysis, two radiologists (CG and LB, dedicated head and neck radiologists with respectively 5 and more than 20 years experience), in consensus, evaluated the image quality of the acquired MRI series, enabling visualization of even small structures.

They, blinded to histological results, radially measured the distance (in millimeters) from all the margins to the tumor (**Figure 5**).

To differentiate tumor from edema they calculated ADC values within ROI drawn on the tumor and surrounding tissue.

They considered a margin clear if > 5mm, close if =1-5 mm, and involved if <1 mm.

The patients were stratified into three groups depending on the analysis of their margins. The three groups were negative, close, and involved.

Reference Standard: Radio-Pathological Correlation

A dedicated head and neck pathologist with more than of ten years of experience (BF) without knowledge of the MRI results annotated tumor location and measured the distance from the tumor to the margins, which was considered the gold standard.

The serial coronal slices were correlated with the T2 coronal sequences of *ex-vivo* MRI of specimen oriented on the 3D-printed tongue model (**Figures 1, 4**).

The patients were stratified into three groups depending on the final analysis of their margins on the specimen. The three groups were negative, close, and involved.

Statistical Analysis

Diagnostic Accuracy

To compare the performance of the initial bedside FSA and *ex-vivo* MRI in predicting definitive negative, close, and involved margins we computed the weighted sensitivity(SE), specificity(SP), accuracy (ACC), area under the ROC curve (AUC), F1-score, Positive Predictive Value (PPV), and Negative Predictive Value (NPV), where the weights are proportional to the cardinality of each class.

In addition to this, to express the concordance between FSA and *ex-vivo* MRI, we reported the jaccard index, computed as the number of equal classifications, divided by the number of total samples. Final pathological diagnosis was the gold standard.

Intended Sample Size for Conclusive Results

In a study published in the literature (6), 640 consecutive patients over an 11-year period with at least five years' follow up were

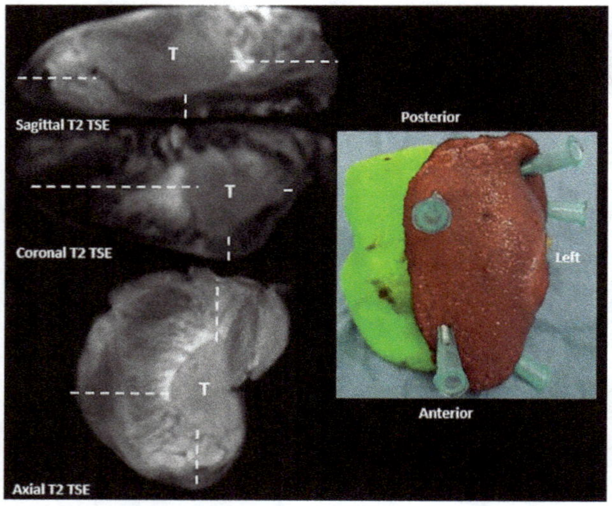

FIGURE 5 | Coronal, sagittal, and axial T2 TSE MRI sequences of the surgical specimen oriented on a 3D-printed model. Multiplanar MRI sequences show the tumor (T) and its macroscopic radial distance (dotted line) from the surface of the specimen in all the planes.

studied. A total of 213 patients (33%) had resection margins that were clear (5 mm or more), 314 (49%) were close (1 - 4.9 mm), and 113 (18%) were involved (0 - 0.9 mm). The required sample size was determined in order to detect a significant difference with an accuracy 0.2-0.3 times greater than 0.50 (which practically corresponds to a random classifier) with a power of 0.90. Assuming equal variance, a total of 21-44 patients should be enrolled to report conclusive results.

RESULTS

Participants

We enrolled 10 patients (6 females and 4 males with a median age 53.1 years, range 30-89) with a histological diagnosis of squamous cell carcinoma of the oral cavity (OSCC) who underwent surgery (5 hemiglossectomies and 5 partial glossectomies) for oral tongue squamous carcinoma between February and April 2021. The definitive margin status was negative in nine cases and positive in one case. In *ex-vivo* MRI, margin status was negative in nine cases and positive in one case (revision was not performed in this case because FSA was negative). The final pathological T status was T1 in one case, T2 in seven cases, and T3 in two cases. In the 10 cases, the mean maximum diameter of the tumor at the final histological diagnosis was 22.3 (range 10-37 mm). The average time taken for each MRI examination was 24.7 minutes (range 16-38 minutes). The T2 series of MRI was therefore the series that was matched to histology and was subsequently annotated.

Preliminary Results

MRI succeeded in margin prediction in all the cases, and FSA failed in one case.

In this group of patients initial bedside FSA showed SE of 90%, SP of 100%, F1 of 95%, ACC of 90%, PPV of 100%, NPV (not a number), and jaccard of 90%, and *ex-vivo* MRI showed SE of 100%, SP of 100%, F1 of 100%, ACC of 100%, PPV of 100%, NPV of 100%, and jaccard of 100%.

These results needed to be validated in a larger sample size of 21- 44 patients.

DISCUSSION

Intraoperative assessment of the resection margins can provide valuable information, enabling additive resection to obtain negative margin status. Despite this, the clinical value and the method of assessing the intraoperative margin are not well defined (5, 9, 10). Many factors influence the evaluation of surgical margins, making it more or less adequate; these include the sampling of the margins (from the block sample compared to the surgical defect alone), the ability and methods used to determine the distance to margins, the communication between the surgeon and the pathologist involving the specimen, orientation and areas of concern, and the subsite in the head and neck (11).

Several techniques aiming for intraoperative assessment of surgical margins in oral cavity/tongue squamous cell carcinoma have been investigated. These include elastic scattering spectroscopy (12) fluorescence (13–15), hyperspectral imaging (16), optical coherence tomography (17), spectroscopy (18), ultrasound (19, 20) and intraoperative slicing of the whole specimen by the pathologist (21). Only MRI, ultrasound, and intraoperative slicing of the whole specimen by the pathologist can allow sampling of the entire specimen and/or probing depth of the lesion.

With our study, we have found it helpful to report and demonstrate to our surgical team the gross distance to all margins by using the intraoperative *ex- vivo* MRI, and to improve surgeon and pathologist communication by introducing a 3D-printed tongue model to allow pathologists to understand specimen orientation and to learn what margins will be revised based on gross impression.

To our knowledge this is the first study in which a surgeon provided orientation of the specimen on the 3D-printed model of the tongue with the reproduced bed of resection. Generally, the surgeon provides orientation by designating one or two points on the specimen.

The specimen orientation on the 3D-printed model from patient MRI facilitates review and correlation.

By maintaining the orientation of the specimen, the pathologist is facilitated in noting the distance of the tumor from each margin and in communicating the site of positive and close margins to the submitting surgeon.

While most surgeons sample margins only from the surgical bed without margin assessment from the resection specimen, as demonstrated by a survey of American Head and Neck Society members (22), we introduced *ex-vivo* MRI to outcome the limit of the lack of a true measurement of the distance of the invasive tumor from the resection margin. According to FSA, a margin can only be determined as positive or negative and the margin presented separately can be thin <5 mm in thickness. Additionally, without a defined margin orientation it is not clear how the separately submitted margins reflect the true areas of the en block specimen that are noted to be close or positive. In our preliminary experience, *ex vivo* MRI was more accurate than intraoperative FSA in predicting margin status.

The results of a previous study (7) showed high specificity and low sensitivity of MRI in identifying margins less than 5 mm. According to these results, *ex-vivo* MRI assessment of the pathologic en bloc specimen could direct intra-operative defect-derived FSA margin assessment and margin revision, determining the closest margins on gross assessment and requiring separately submitted tissues of correct size to have negative margins. The orientation of the specimen on the 3D model could allow a better match between the separately submitted margins and the true areas of the en bloc specimen that are noted to be close or positive. This could be because the revised margin is not taken from the correct location (23).

Some limitations of our study should be discussed. First, the sample size was small and heterogeneous. Our cohort contained a broad range of cases with various T classifications. Furthermore, a relatively small proportion of the margins were less than 5 mm. As established in our statistical analysis on intended sample size, our preliminary results should be validated in a larger cohort of patients.

The limitation of *ex- vivo* MRI could be the lack of identification of microscopic tissue changes. Conventional MRI could not eneable thin differentiations between tumor and surrounding tissue in the presence of edema. Diffusion weighted imaging (DWI) can be used to evaluate the rate of microscopic water diffusion within tissues. DWI may be measured by means of apparent diffusion coefficient (ADC). Areas of decreased ADC values within tumors could be used as a powerful imaging biomarker of cancer (24, 25).

Tumor shrinkage after formalin fixation could lead to an underestimation of tumor margins (26). This could be demonstrated by performing *ex-vivo* MRI of the specimen after formalin fixation. We performed MRI after formalin fixation in one case but the changes of the signal intensity of the specimen did not allow us to evaluate the effect of shrinkage.

Other limitations were the inexperience of the MRI readers, who had experience with *in vivo* applications of MRI but not in *ex-vivo* MRI of tongue resection specimens, and the fact that only one pathologist evaluated histopathology.

Ex-vivo MRI is a costly and time consuming process. It requires the use of MRI equipment, subtracting time for performing diagnostic tests. It also requires excellent communication and coordination between surgeons, operating room staff, pathologists, and radiologists to avoid additional operating time. Considering that the operating times for these types of complex resections and reconstructions, with the maximum operating time of 160 minutes in which flap reconstruction was not required and 700 minutes of microvascular reconstruction, MRI does not unreasonably lengthen the time in the operating room (21). This intervention has the potential to both reduce rates of close pathological margins and the need for postoperative radiotherapy, as shown in our preliminary experience with the detection of positive margins not detected by intraoperative FSA.

In conclusion, considering the staffing and expensive nature of integrating FSA with *ex-vivo* MRI of the fresh specimen for evaluation on macroscopic proximity of the tumor to the margins of resection, this intervention can be performed with some planning and coordination between the radiologists, pathologists, and surgeons in a selected subset of patients most likely to benefit by avoiding adjuvant radiotherapy. Finally, we would recommend consideration of intraoperative MRI tumor margin assessment for selected cases potentially be cured with surgery alone, i.e. T1/T2N0 tumor.

AUTHOR CONTRIBUTIONS

CG, LB, GS, and GM conceived of the presented idea. CG developed the theory and performed the computations. CG, GM, LB, and FF verified the analytical methods. GS encouraged CG to investigate margin status and supervised the findings of this work. All authors discussed the results and contributed to the final manuscript. CG, GM, LD, FC, MC, FG, RB, and BF carried out the experiment. CG wrote the manuscript with support from GM. RB and PO fabricated the 3D model sample. AD, FR, AE, FF, and LT helped supervise the project. CG and EC developed the theoretical formalism, performed the analytic calculations and performed the numerical simulations and contributed to the interpretation of the results. All authors contributed to the article and approved the submitted version.

ACKNOWLEDGMENTS

We would like to acknowledge our radiology technicians for the acquisition of MRI examinations (Giuseppe Morrone, Pasquala Ragucci, Giacomo Marconi, Riccardo Ramberti, Giulio Belice, Riccardo Fabbri) coordinated by Simona Superbi and Antonio Spinillo; all the ENT surgeons of Humanitas Clinical and Research Center IRCCS; Clarissa Nigro of the nursing staff for the coordination of the workflow between the operating room and the MRI room; and Giovanna Giannitto for English language editing and Massimiliano Battaglia and Federica Fici for editing.

REFERENCES

1. Helliwell T, Woolgar J. Standards and Datasets for Reporting Cancers [Internet]. In: *Dataset for Histopathology Reportingofmucosal Malignancies of the Oral Cavity*. Carlton House Terrace, London: The Royal College of Pathologists 2. (2013). Available at: https://www.rcpath.org/uploads/assets/c4a9faf7-393a-4ba8-9532f719d8cdff3b/Dataset-for-histopathology-reporting-of-mucosal-malignancies-of-the-oral-cavity.pdf.
2. Hinni ML, Ferlito A, Brandwein-Gensler MS, Takes RP, Silver CE, Westra WH, et al. Surgical Margins in Head and Neck Cancer: A Contemporary Review. *Head Neck* (2013) 35(9):1362–70. doi: 10.1002/hed.23110
3. Mitchell DA, Kanatas A, Murphy C, Chengot P, Smith AB, Ong TK. Margins and Survival in Oral Cancer. *Br J Oral Maxillofac Surg* (2018) 56(9):820–9. doi: 10.1016/j.bjoms.2018.06.021
4. DiNardo LJ, Lin J, Karageorge LS, Powers CN. Accuracy, Utility,and Cost of Frozen Section Margins in Head and Neck Cancersurgery. *Laryngoscope* (2000) 110(10):1773–6. doi: 10.1097/00005537-200010000-00039
5. Gerber S, Gengler C, Grätz KW, Kruse AL. The Impact of Frozensections on Final Surgical Margins in Squamous Cell Carcinoma of the Oral Cavity and Lips: A Retrospective Analysis Over an 11 Years Period. *Head Neck Oncol* (2011) 3(1):56. doi: 10.1186/1758-3284-3-56
6. Azzopardi S, Lowe D, Rogers S. Audit of the Rates of Re-Excision for Close or Involved Margins in the Management of Oral Cancer. *Br J Oral Maxillofacial Surg* (2019) 57(7):678–81. doi: 10.1016/j.bjoms.2019.05.006
7. Steens SCA, Bekers EM, Weijs WLJ, Litjens GJS, Veltien A, Maat A, et al. Evaluation of Tongue Squamous Cell Carcinoma Resection Margins Using *Ex-Vivo* MR. *Int J Comput Assist Radiol Surg* (2017) 12(5):821–8. doi: 10.1007/s11548-017-1524-6
8. Heidkamp J, Weijs WLJ, van Engen-van Grunsven ACH, de Laak-de Vries I, Maas MC, Rovers MM, et al. Assessment of Surgical Tumor-Free Resection Margins in Fresh Squamous-Cell Carcinoma Resection Specimens of the Tongue Using a Clinical MRI System. *Head Neck* (2020) 42(8):2039–49. doi: 10.1002/hed.26125
9. Gokavarapu S, Chandrasekhara Rao LM, Patnaik SC, Parvataneni N, Raju KVVN, Chander R. Prognostic Value of Frozen Section in T1, T2 Carcinoma of Oral Cavity. *Indian J Otolaryngol Head Neck Surg* (2015) 67(Suppl 1):86–90. doi: 10.1007/s12070-014-0783-6
10. Chaturvedi P, Datta S, Nair S, Nair D, Pawar P, Vaishampayan S, et al. Gross Examination by the Surgeon as an Alternative to Frozen Section for Assessment of Adequacy of Surgical Margin in Head and Neck Squamous Cell Carcinoma: Gross Examination Versus Frozen Section for Assessing Surgical Margin of HNSCC. *Head Neck* (2014) 36(4):557–63. doi: 10.1002/hed.23313
11. MD. Determining Adequate Margins in Head and Neck Cancers: Practice and Continued Challenges. *Curr Oncol Rep* (2016) 18(9):54. doi: 10.1007/s11912-016-0540-y
12. Grillone GA, Wang Z, Krisciunas GP. The Color of Cancer: Margin Guidance for Oral Cancer Resection Using Elastic Scatteringspectroscopy. *Laryngoscope* (2017) 127(suppl 4):S1–9. doi: 10.1002/lary.26763
13. JM, de Boer E, van Dam GM, Moore LS, Bevans SL, Walsh EM, et al. Fluorescence Imaging to Localize Head and Neck Squamous Cell Carcinoma for Enhanced Pathological Assessment: Fluorescence-Guided Pathology. *J Pathol Clin Res* (2016) 2(2):104–12. doi: 10.1002/cjp2.40
14. van Keulen S, Nishio N, Birkeland A, Fakurnejad S, Martin B, Forouzanfar T, et al. The Sentinel Margin: Intraoperative *Ex Vivo* Specimen Mapping Using Relative Fluorescence Intensity. *Clin Cancer Res* (2019) 25(15):4656–62. doi: 10.1158/1078-0432.CCR-19-0319
15. RW, Teraphongphom NT, Berg NS. Determinationof Tumor Margins With Surgical Specimen Mapping Using Near-Infrared Fluorescence. *Cancer Res* (2018) 78(17):5154. doi: 10.1158/0008-5472.CAN-18-0878
16. Fei B, Lu G, Wang X, Zhang H, Little JV, Patel MR, et al. Label-Free Reflectance Hyperspectral Imaging for Tumor Margin Assessment: A Pilot Study on Surgical Specimens of Cancer Patients. *J BioMed Opt* (2017) 22(8):1–7. doi: 10.1117/1.JBO.22.8.086009
17. Hamdoon Z, Jerjes W, McKenzie G, Jay A, Hopper C. Opticalcoherence Tomography in the Assessment of Oral Squamous Cell Carcinoma Resection Margins. *Photodiagnosis Photodyn Ther* (2016) 13:211–7. doi: 10.1016/j.pdpdt.2015.07.170
18. Barroso EM, Smits RWH, van Lanschot CGF, Caspers PJ, Ten Hove I, Mast H, et al. Water Concentration Analysis by Raman Spectroscopy to Determine the Location of the Tumor Border in Oral Cancer Surgery. *Cancer Res* (2016) 76 (20):5945–53. doi: 10.1158/0008-5472.CAN-16-1227
19. O, Kanumuri V, Juliano AF, Faquin WC, Cunnane ME, Varvares MA. Intraoperative Ultrasound in Oral Tongue Cancer Resection: Feasibility Study and Early Outcomes. *Otolaryngol Head Neck Surg* (2018) 158(4):645–8. doi: 10.1177/0194599817742856
20. de Koning KJ, Koppes SA, de Bree R, Dankbaar JW, Willems SM, van Es RJJ, et al. Feasibility Study of Ultrasound-Guided Resection of Tongue Cancer With Immediate Specimen Examination to Improve Margin Control - Comparison With Conventional Treatment. *Oral Oncol* (2021) 116 (105249):105249. doi: 10.1016/j.oraloncology.2021.105249
21. Smithers FAE, Haymerle G, Palme CE, Low T-HH, Froggatt C, Gupta R, et al. A Prospective Study of Intraoperative Assessment of Mucosal Squamous Cell Carcinoma Margins in the Head and Neck. *Head Neck* (2021) 43(2):590–600. doi: 10.1002/hed.26517
22. Meier JD, Oliver DA, Varvares MA. Surgical Margin Determination in Head and Neck Oncology: Current Clinical Practice. The Results of an International American Head and Neck Society Member Survey. *Head Neck* (2005) 27 (11):952–8. doi: 10.1002/hed.20269
23. Scholl P, Byers RM, Batsakis JG. Microscopic Cut-Through of Cancer in the Surgical Treatment of Squamous Carcinoma of Thetongue. *Prognostic Ther Implications Am J Surg* (1986) 152(4):354–60. doi: 10.1016/0002-9610(86) 90304-1
24. Hermans R, de keyzer F, Vandecaveye V, Carp L. Imaging Techniques. In: *Head and Neck Cancer Imaging*. Berlin/Heidelberg, Germany: Springer (2012). p. 33–54.
25. Bonello L, Preda L, Conte G, et al. Squamous Cell Carcinoma of the Oral Cavity and Oropharynx: What Does the Apparent Diffusion Coefficient Tell Us About Its Histology? *Acta Radiol* (2016) 57(11):1344–51. doi: 10.1177/0284185115587734
26. Chen C-H, Hsu M-Y, Jiang R-S, Wu S-H, Chen F-J, Liu S-A. Shrinkage of Head and Neck Cancer Specimens After Formalin Fixation. *J Chin Med Assoc* (2012) 75(3):109–13. doi: 10.1016/j.jcma.2012.02.006

7

Simultaneous Resection of Bone Tumor and CAD/CAM Titanium Cranioplasty in Fronto-Orbital Region

Konstantin S. Yashin[1*], Anton Yu. Ermolaev[1], Mikhail V. Ostapyuk[1], Marina A. Kutlaeva[2], Marina V. Rasteryaeva[2], Sergey G. Mlyavykh[3] and Igor A. Medyanik[1]

[1] Department of Oncology and Neurosurgery, Institute of Traumatology and Orthopedics, Privolzhsky Research Medical University, Nizhny Novgorod, Russia, [2] Department of Radiation Diagnostics, Institute of Traumatology and Orthopedics, Privolzhsky Research Medical University, Nizhny Novgorod, Russia, [3] Institute of Traumatology and Orthopedics, Privolzhsky Research Medical University, Nizhny Novgorod, Russia

***Correspondence:**
Konstantin S. Yashin
jashinmed@gmail.com

Background: Simultaneous resection of bone tumors in the fronto-naso-orbital region is a great challenge due to the need for adequate reconstruction of the facial skeleton. Pre-operative virtual planning of resection margins and the simultaneous fabrication of the cranioplasty using computer-aided design/computer-aided manufacturing (CAD/CAM) technology could allow combining the tumor resection and cosmetic restoration steps into a single procedure.

Methods: We present five consecutive cases of patients with bone tumors of the fronto-naso-orbital region. The indications for surgery included: (1) the presence of a major cosmetic defect; (2) progressive tumor growth. The histological examination revealed vascular malformation, hemangioma, and fibrous dysplasia in two cases. Tumor resection was performed with the help of a drilling template in form of a tumor. The computer-designed cranioplasty formed based on the non-involved side of the skull of the patient was manufactured. In one patient, the reconstruction was performed using two separate implants.

Results: The position of the implant fits in with pre-operative planning in two cases; in those cases, the additional trimming of the implant or bone defect was required. Good cosmetic outcomes were noted in all patients, and no complications occurred. No repeat surgery was necessary. The template has proved to have high application potential.

Conclusion: Simultaneous resection and CAD/CAM cranioplasty in the case of bone tumors in the fronto-orbital region is a promising technique with the aim of minimizing operation time and achieving a good esthetic outcome.

Keywords: CAD/CAM, cosmetic outcome, drilling template, single-step resection and reconstruction, skull bone tumors, titanium cranioplasty, custom-made implants, skull reconstruction

INTRODUCTION

In patients with skull bone tumors, it was demonstrated that not only the oncological but also the cosmetic result has a significant influence on the long-term outcome (1, 2). It becomes more significant in the case of lesions in the fronto-orbital area, having an important functional and aesthetic role.

The adequate reconstruction of facial contours after craniofacial traumas is a great challenge due to the unique sophisticated spatial complexity of this region (3). A more challenging task is a restoration of facial symmetry during a one-step resection of lesions in the craniofacial region, following a skull reconstruction, where contour and shape may be difficult to achieve with intraoperative modeling of autogenous bone grafts, titanium, or another synthetic material (4). Thus, the two-step procedure has been proposed: a pre-operative-performed patient specific implant (PSI) is inserted in a second surgery. However, two-step-technology determinates to weigh the pros and cons, with calculation, the risk of surgery-associated complications in relation to the profit for the patient, which, most of all, is a cosmetic improvement.

To improve the precision of surgical resection and reconstruction procedures, computer pre-operative planning and intraoperative navigation can be used (4–6). The next step is performing a one-step template-assisted resection of bone tumor following a cranioplasty with the PSI based on the virtual planning of the resection margins, which has already been reported in the cases of fibrous dysplasia and intraosseous skull base meningiomas (7, 8).

In this article, we present the results of simultaneous resection and computer-aided design/computer-aided manufacturing (CAD/CAM) titanium cranioplasty in four consecutive treating patients with bone tumors in the fronto-orbital region. This technology looks most promising in this group of patients, with the aim of minimizing operation time and achieving a good esthetic outcome.

METHODS

Patients

Four surgical cases with a pathology involving the fronto-orbital region were included in the study. The general characteristics of patients are summarized in **Table 1**. The indications for surgery were: (1) the presence of a major cosmetic defect; (2) progressive tumor growth. The histological examination revealed vascular malformation, hemangioma, and fibrous dysplasia in two cases. The details of the surgical procedure were discussed before hospitalization, and informed consent was obtained from the patients. Written informed consent was obtained from the individuals for the publication of any potentially identifiable images or data included in this article. This study was carried out in accordance with the recommendations of the World Medical Association's Declaration of Helsinki. The protocol was approved by the Ethical Committee of the Privolzhsky Research Medical University of the Ministry of Health of the Russian Federation. The post-operative follow-up was up to 5 years.

Pre-operative Planning and Manufacturing of the Cranioplasty

Resection planning and manufacturing of the cranioplasty in one session were planned in several steps in collaboration with the specialists of two manufacturing companies: Endoprint Innovation and Technology Company (Endoprint ITK LLC, Moscow, Russian Federation) and LOGEEKS DM (Logix LLC, Novosibirsk, Russian Federation). Using 0.5-mm computer tomography (CT) scan slices, the surgeon drew a digital resection line (**Figures 1a1–a3**). Based on this resection line, the reconstruction of future defect margins was performed using CAD software (**Figures 1b1–b3**). The skull surface in the resection area is generated as a CAD surface by mirroring the opposite side of the skull.

Corresponding to this CAD surface, the computer modeling of the implant was performed, and screw holes over the non-affected bone are integrated (**Figures 1c1–c3**). In three cases, a resection template was constructed for the defect using the identical geometric data of the resected bone with tumor. When both the implant and the template are constructed completely, the design has to be released by the neurosurgeons.

Based on the results of virtual surgical planning of the proposed skull defect after lesion resection, the implants were growing by the 3D metal printing method—direct metal laser sintering (DMLS). After that, during manufacturing, the implants go through stages such as sandblasting, ultrasonic washing, and disinfection.

Surgical Procedure

The procedures were performed under general anesthesia according to the pre-operative virtual plan (**Figure 2**). The part of the cranium that matched the interior surface of the template was identified, and the osteotomy line was drawn along the edge of the template. An osteotomy was performed along the line,

TABLE 1 | Patient profiles, surgery, and results.

Patient no.	Age/gender	Diagnosis	Indication for surgery	Using template	Number of implants
1	36, F	Fibrous dysplasia	Growth	No	Two
2	35, F	Vascular malformation	Cosmetic	Yes	One
3	44, F	Fibrous dysplasia	Cosmetic	Yes	One
4	40, F	Hemangioma	Cosmetic/growth	Yes	One

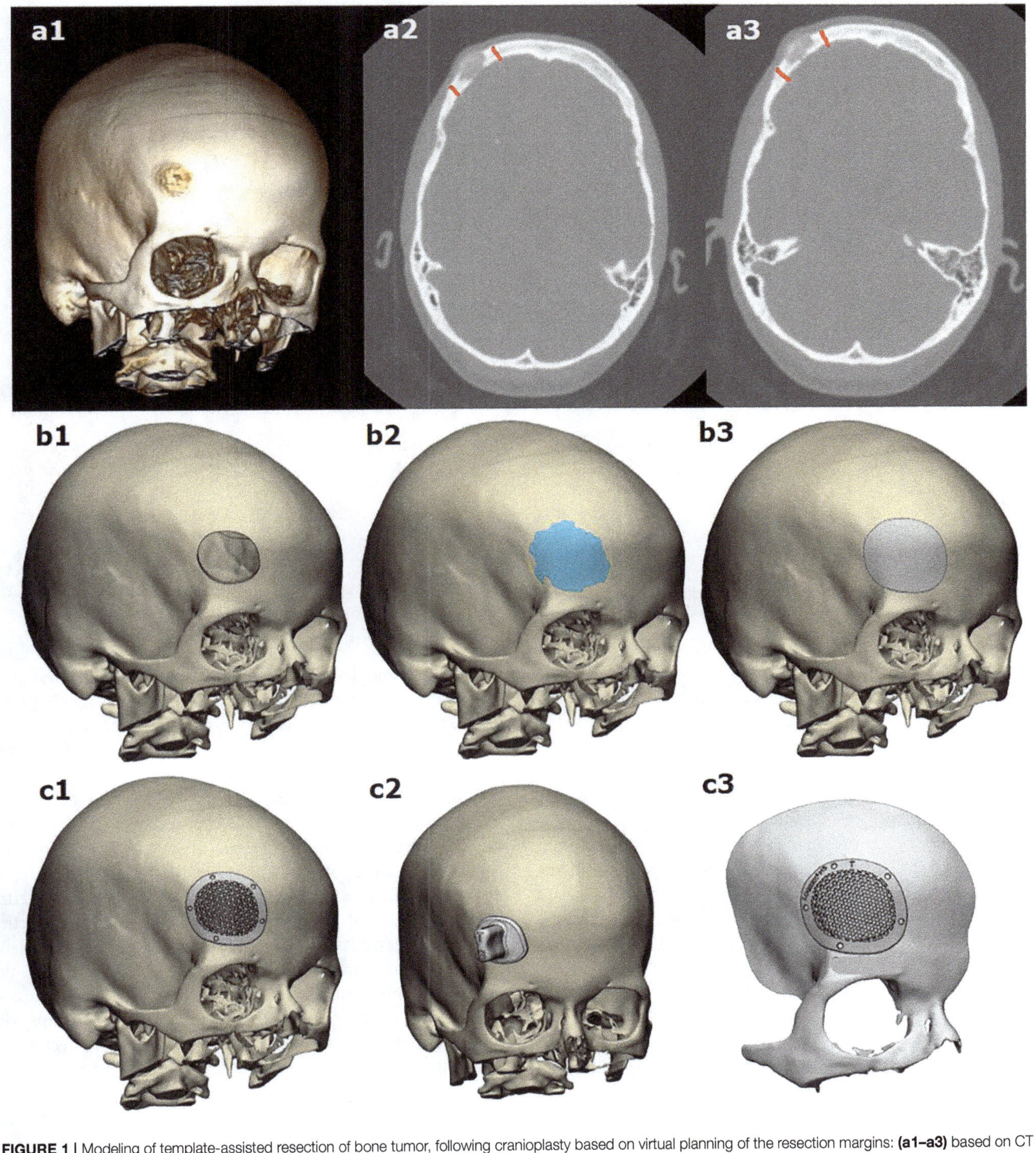

FIGURE 1 | Modeling of template-assisted resection of bone tumor, following cranioplasty based on virtual planning of the resection margins: **(a1–a3)** based on CT scans, planning of resection margins made by the surgeon; **(b1–b3)** 3D modeling of tumor resection and the anatomical shape of the resected part of the bone; **(c1, c2)** 3D modeling of the implant and resection template; **(c3)** a pre-operative planning template.

resulting in the removal of the tumor with the bone. In no one case, the reconstruction of the dura was necessary to perform. The implant was then placed in the skull defect and fixed with screws. In one patient, the reconstruction was performed using two separate implants.

RESULTS

The position of the implant fits in with pre-operative planning. In three cases, the complete resection confirmed on post-operative CT scans of the lesion was achieved. In one case of

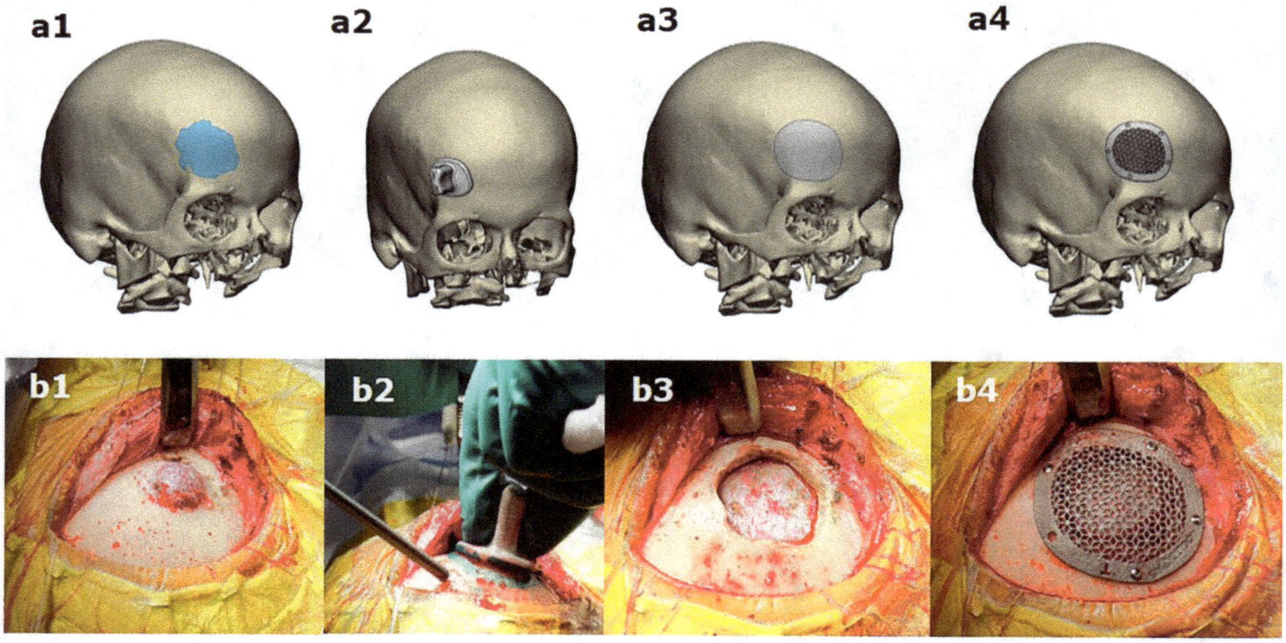

FIGURE 2 | Simultaneous resection of bone tumor and titanium cranioplasty in patients with a lesion in the fronto-orbital region **(b1–b4)** according to pre-operative virtual planning of resection margins **(a1)**, using a drilling template **(a2)** and the simultaneous fabrication of the cranioplasty **(a3,a4)**.

fibrous dysplasia, the subtotal resection was performed. On post-operative CT scans, no continued growth was detected at up to 5-year follow-up. Good cosmetic outcomes were noted in all patients, and no complications occurred (**Figures 3a1–c4**). No repeat surgery was necessary. The usage of the template was highly practicable. Perioperative trimming of the implant or bone defect was not required in two patients. In one patient, the implant was additionally modeling during the procedure, preserving the branches of nervus supraorbitalis (**Figures 3b1–b4**). The template used was not possible in the case of severe fibrous dysplasia due to the shape and the size of resection (**Figures 3a1–a4**). Therefore, additional bone drilling was required for adequate implant positioning.

DISCUSSION

Individual CAD/CAM cranioplasty for the reconstruction of extensive and complex skull defects has been a recently actively developing field of neurosurgery and craniomaxillofacial surgery (9, 10). The patient-specific reconstruction of a bone flap becomes a preferred method in clinical practice due to a favorable functional and cosmetic outcome compared with the other methods. Pre-operative computer modeling and using CAD/CAM technologies have expanded the possibilities of surgery for achieving good cosmetic and functional results in the treatment of bone tumors. It allows abandoning the conventional techniques of reconstruction or two-step procedures that are particularly important in the case of tumor resection in the fronto-orbital region.

The one-step template-assisted resection of bone tumor following cranioplasty has been already reported in the cases of including fibrous dysplasia and intraosseous meningiomas (7, 8, 11). This method looks promising for intraosseous tumors compared with other modalities, such as intraoperatively modeling an artificial bone flap without a template (1, 12) or manufacturing the custom-made implant based on the stereolithographic model (13). It has several advantages over other reported methods: (1) pre-operative time and costs benefits, all steps of modeling are performed virtually, so no additional production steps are needed; (2) operation time, the using of the template allows to perform resection and cranioplasty fast and precisely; (3) the best available cosmetic and functional result for resection of fronto-orbital region tumors. This corresponds to the results of the application of CAD/CAM custom implants in patients with skull defects with satisfactory aesthetic results, technically simplicity, reducing surgery times, and surgical blood loss (14).

In most cases of bone tumor location, the skull reconstruction would have not required a patient specific implant since a standard titanium cranioplasty could have been easily adapted. However, we believe that in the case of the location of the tumor in the bones forming the facial region of the skull, using PSI will be the method of choice, achieving the best congruence and cosmetic results. Moreover, using the customized template can help with the resection and reduce the time of the procedure even when the reconstruction does not require a PSI. Using a template as an alternative to navigation systems, especially in the case of the poorly visible extracranial component, is

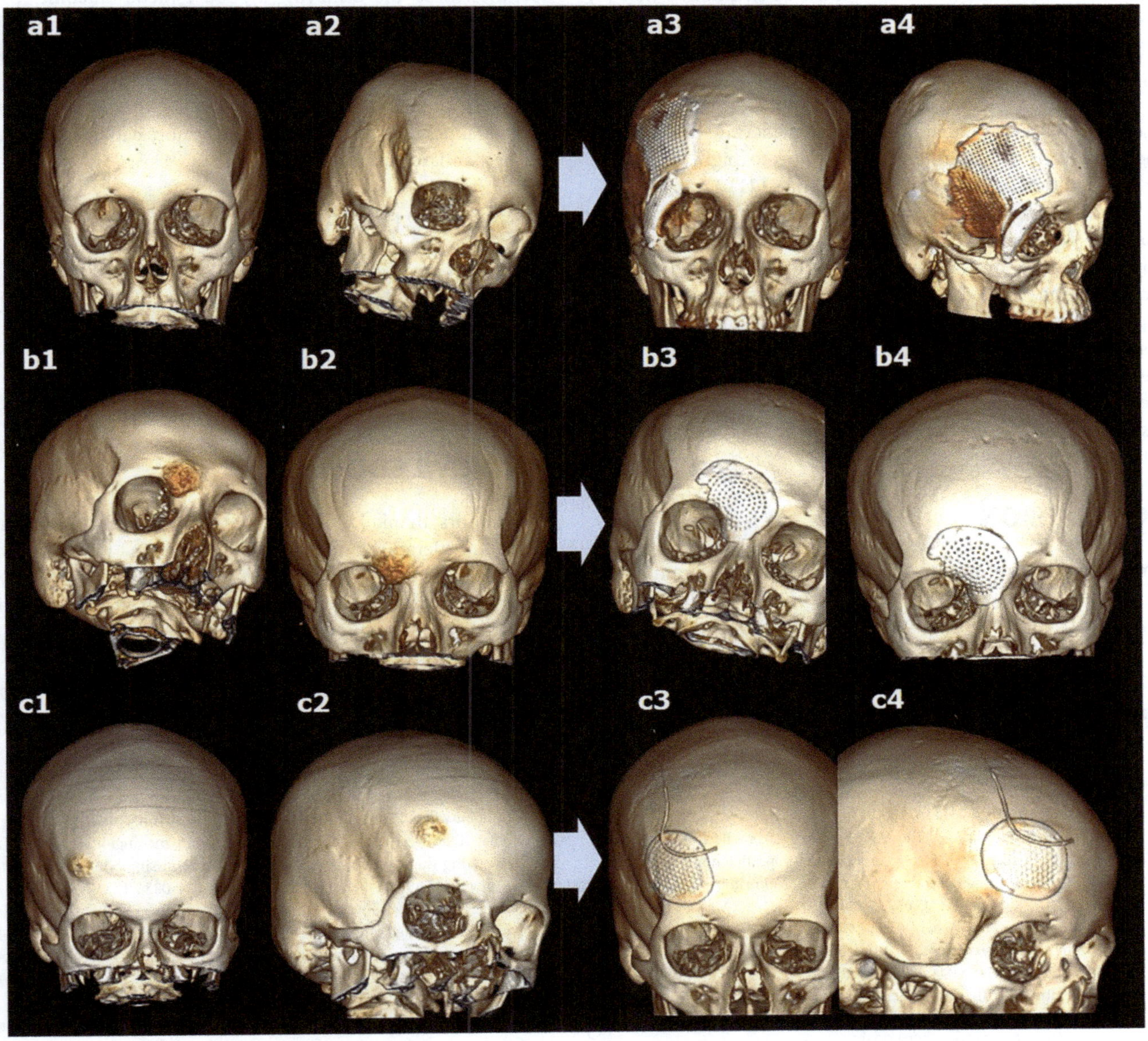

FIGURE 3 | The 3D reconstructions of CT scans before **(a1–c1,a2–c2)** and after **(a3–c3,a4–c4)** simultaneous resection of bone tumor and titanium cranioplasty in different cases of lesions in the fronto-orbital region, using two **(a1–a4)** or one **(b1–b4,c1–c4)** implants.

controversial. It is obvious that navigation can be very useful for contouring tumors (6, 15). Also, the specific approach combining "mirroring" virtual computational planning with intraoperative-guided surgical navigation was suggested (5). We believe that the combination of navigation and a drilled template provides the best results since navigation can be used for the planning of the site and the size of skin resection and clarification of the resection margins.

For cranioplasty, a variety of alloplastic biomaterials can be used, including standard hydroxyapatite (HA), polymethylmethacrylate (PMMA), polyetheretherketone (PEEK), titanium, and actively developing new substances (16–18). Each has its own advantages and disadvantages; most of them are suitable for CAD/CAM pre-fabrication, and all of them are potentially biologically toxic, with the likely exception of hydroxyapatite (14). For simultaneous tumor resection and cranioplasty, titanium seemed to be the most suitable, overcovering the area of resection and allowing correction of the resection area. In the case of other biomaterials, the exact match of the resection area and the implant is more challenging. However, several studies have shown good results after one-step bone lesions resection and cranioplasty (8, 19).

Another important issue is the tumor nature. As we mentioned above, single-stage cranioplasty with a template is usually performed for benign tumors since the surgical resection is potentially curative. However, this method can be used for malignant tumors (20). In this, it must be mentioned that (1) the time between CT scanning, cranioplasty manufacturing, and performing surgery should be minimized due to interim growth of the tumor; (2) presence of malignant tumors may require further radiation therapy; therefore, the implants material should be chosen to prevent radiation ulcers. Considering this, titanium does not seem to be the best choice due to high backscatter radiation to the scalp among other materials (21).

The limitation of our study is the small number of patients. However, skull lesions are not frequent, and reconstruction in the fronto-orbital region is not a surgery performed often. Including for this reason, up to date, there is no consensus on the optimal approach for simultaneous tumor resection and cranioplasty based on virtual surgical planning. The approaches differ by the modeling and manufacturing technologies and materials used. The general problem is difficulties in the evaluation of the cosmetic result. In our study, we based on the feelings of the patients themselves.

CONCLUSION

Simultaneous resection and CAD/CAM titanium cranioplasty in the case of benign bone tumors in the fronto-orbital region is also a promising technique, with the aim of minimizing operation time and achieving a good esthetic outcome. Using a resection template allows to perform a practicable and precise craniotomy; however, in the case of large tumors with compound contours, it can be difficult. Unfortunately, there are a limited number of studies reproducing this approach with individualities. Future studies including more patients are needed for the standardization of this technique.

AUTHOR CONTRIBUTIONS

KY, IM, and SM: study concept and design. KY, AE, MO, MK, and MR: data acquisition and quality control of data. KY and IM: data analysis and interpretation. KY and AE: manuscript preparation. IM and SM: manuscript review. All authors contributed to the article and approved the submitted version.

ACKNOWLEDGMENTS

The authors thank LOGEEKS DM (Logix LLC, Novosibirsk, Russian Federation) for the assistance in preparing this manuscript and Dr. Nikolay N. Karyakin (rector of PRMU, Nizhny Novgorod, Russia) for active support in the translation of additive technologies into clinical usage.

REFERENCES

1. Bloch O, McDermott MW. *In situ* cranioplasty for hyperostosing meningiomas of the cranial vault. *Can J Neurol Sci.* (2011) 38:59–64. doi: 10.1017/S0317167100011082
2. Marbacher S, Coluccia D, Fathi AR, Andereggen L, Beck J, Fandino J. Intraoperative patient-specific reconstruction of partial bone flap defects after convexity meningioma resection. *World Neurosurg.* (2013) 79:124–30. doi: 10.1016/j.wneu.2011.05.057
3. Chen SH, Ko AT, Chen HC, Roan TL, Tang YB. Fronto-naso-orbital reconstructions. *Ann Plast Surg.* (2018) 81(Suppl. 1):S10–4. doi: 10.1097/SAP.0000000000001606
4. Ricalde P, Horswell BB. Craniofacial fibrous dysplasia of the fronto-orbital region: a case series and literature review. *J Oral Maxillofac Surg.* (2001) 59:157–68. doi: 10.1053/joms.2001.20487
5. Guatta R, Scolozzi P. Bone Recontouring by guided surgical navigation integrating "mirroring" computational planning in the management of severe fronto-orbital asymmetry in fibrous dysplasia. *J Neurol Surg A Cent Eur Neurosurg.* (2018) 79:181–5. doi: 10.1055/s-0037-1615286
6. Gui H, Zhang S, Shen SG, Wang X, Bautista JS, Voss PJ. Real-time image-guided recontouring in the management of craniofacial fibrous dysplasia. *Oral Surg Oral Med Oral Pathol Oral Radiol.* (2013) 116:680–5. doi: 10.1016/j.oooo.2013.07.012
7. Broeckx CE, Maal TJJ, Vreeken RD, Bos RRM, Ter Laan M. Single-step resection of an intraosseous meningioma and cranial reconstruction: technical note. *World Neurosurg.* (2017) 108:225–9. doi: 10.1016/j.wneu.2017.08.177
8. Carolus A, Weihe S, Schmieder K, Brenke C. One-step CAD/CAM titanium cranioplasty after drilling template-assisted resection of intraosseous skull base meningioma: technical note. *Acta Neurochir (Wien).* (2017) 159:447–52. doi: 10.1007/s00701-016-3053-4
9. Ghai S, Sharma Y, Jain N, Satpathy M, Pillai AK. Use of 3-D printing technologies in craniomaxillofacial surgery: a review. *Oral Maxillofac Surg.* (2018) 22:249–59. doi: 10.1007/s10006-018-0704-z
10. Chobulov SA, Kravchuk AD, Potapov AA, Likhterman LB, Maryakhin AD, Sinbukhova EV. Sovremennye aspekty rekonstruktivnoi khirurgii defektov cherepa [Modern aspects of reconstructive surgery of skull defects]. *Zh Vopr Neirokhir Im N N Burdenko.* (2019) 83:115–24. doi: 10.17116/neiro201983021115
11. Schebesch KM, Höhne J, Gassner HG, Brawanski A. Preformed titanium cranioplasty after resection of skull base meningiomas - a technical note. *J Craniomaxillofac Surg.* (2013) 41:803–7. doi: 10.1016/j.jcms.2013.01.030
12. Velnar T, Pregelj R, Limbaeck-Stokin C. Brain meningioma invading and destructing the skull bone: replacement of the missing bone *in vivo*. *Radiol Oncol.* (2011) 45:304–9. doi: 10.2478/v10019-011-0036-1
13. Saringer W, Nöbauer-Huhmann I, Knosp E. Cranioplasty with individual carbon fibre reinforced polymere (CFRP) medical grade implants based on CAD/CAM technique. *Acta Neurochir (Wien).* (2002) 144:1193–203. doi: 10.1007/s00701-002-0995-5
14. Zanotti B, Zingaretti N, Verlicchi A, Robiony M, Alfieri A, Parodi PC. Cranioplasty: review of materials. *J Craniofac Surg.* (2016) 27:2061–72. doi: 10.1097/SCS.0000000000003025
15. Ahmed M, Soliman S, Noman SA, Ali S. Computer-guided contouring of craniofacial fibrous dysplasia involving the zygoma using a patient-specific surgical depth guide. *Int J Oral Maxillofac Surg.* (2020) 49:1605–10. doi: 10.1016/j.ijom.2020.04.009
16. Cavalu S, Antoniac IV, Mohan A, Bodog F, Doicin C, Mates I, et al. Nanoparticles and nanostructured surface fabrication for innovative cranial and maxillofacial surgery. *Materials (Basel).* (2020) 13:5391. doi: 10.3390/ma13235391
17. Kolmogorov YN, Uspensky IV, Maslov AN, Novikov AE, Tarasov DA, Myachin NL, et al. Rekost-M bone replacement implants based on 3D modeling for closing post-craniotomy skull defects: pre-clinical and clinical studies. *Sovrem Tehnol v Med.* (2018) 10:95–101. doi: 10.17691/stm2018.10.3.11
18. Korytkin AA, Orlinskaya NY, Novikova YS, Gerasimov SA, Davydenko DV, Kulakova KV, et al. Biocompatibility and osseointegration of calcium phosphate-coated and non-coated titanium implants with various porosities. *Sovrem Tehnol Med.* (2021) 13:52–8. doi: 10.17691/stm2021.13.2.06
19. Wu CT, Lu TC, Chan CS, Lin TC. Patient-specific three-dimensional printing guide for single-stage skull bone tumor surgery: novel software workflow with manufacturing of prefabricated jigs for bone resection and reconstruction.

World Neurosurg. (2021) 147:e416–27. doi: 10.1016/j.wneu.2020.12.072

20. Berli JU, Thomaier L, Zhong S, Huang J, Quinones A, Lim M, et al. Immediate single-stage cranioplasty following calvarial resection for benign and malignant skull neoplasms using customized craniofacial implants. *J Craniofac Surg.* (2015) 26:1456–62. doi: 10.1097/SCS.0000000000001816
21. Sakamoto Y, Koike N, Takei H, Ohno M, Miwa T, Yoshida K et al. Influence of backscatter radiation on cranial reconstruction implants. *Br J Radiol.* (2017) 90:20150537. doi: 10.1259/bjr.20150537

8

Development and Application of Digital Maxillofacial Surgery System Based on Mixed Reality Technology

Rong Yang[1†], Chenyao Li[1†], Puxun Tu[2], Abdelrehem Ahmed[3], Tong Ji[1*] and Xiaojun Chen[2*]

[1] Shanghai Key Laboratory of Stomatology/Shanghai Institute of Stomatology, Department of Oral and Maxillofacial Head and Neck Oncology, National Clinical Research Center for Oral Diseases, School of Medicine, The Ninth People's Hospital, Shanghai Jiao Tong University, Shanghai, China, [2] School of Mechanical and Engineering, Shanghai Jiaotong University, Shanghai, China, [3] Department of Craniomaxillofacial and Plastic Surgery, Faculty of Dentistry, Alexandria University, Alexandria, Egypt

***Correspondence:**
Tong Ji
jitong70@hotmail.com
Xiaojun Chen
xiaojunchen@sjtu.edu.cn

† These authors share first authorship

Objective: To realize the three-dimensional visual output of surgical navigation information by studying the cross-linking of mixed reality display devices and high-precision optical navigators.

Methods: Applying quaternion-based point alignment algorithms to realize the positioning configuration of mixed reality display devices, high-precision optical navigators, real-time patient tracking and calibration technology; based on open source SDK and development tools, developing mixed reality surgery based on visual positioning and tracking system. In this study, four patients were selected for mixed reality-assisted tumor resection and reconstruction and re-examined 1 month after the operation. We reconstructed postoperative CT and use 3DMeshMetric to form the error distribution map, and completed the error analysis and quality control.

Results: Realized the cross-linking of mixed reality display equipment and high-precision optical navigator, developed a digital maxillofacial surgery system based on mixed reality technology and successfully implemented mixed reality-assisted tumor resection and reconstruction in 4 cases.

Conclusions: The maxillofacial digital surgery system based on mixed reality technology can superimpose and display three-dimensional navigation information in the surgeon's field of vision. Moreover, it solves the problem of visual conversion and space conversion of the existing navigation system. It improves the work efficiency of digitally assisted surgery, effectively reduces the surgeon's dependence on spatial experience and imagination, and protects important anatomical structures during surgery. It is a significant clinical application value and potential.

Keywords: maxillofacial surgery, digital surgery, surgical navigation, mixed reality, three-dimensional visual output

BACKGROUND

The combination of surgery and digital navigation technology is the international mainstream and frontier development trend in this field. In the oral and maxillofacial regions, the rigidity characteristics of the skull base and maxillofacial bones provide an anatomical basis for the clinical application of digital navigation technology (1). Existing digital technologies such as surgical planning, intraoperative real-time navigation, and others have significantly improved oral and maxillofacial surgery accuracy. They can avoid secondary injuries to the greatest extent on the premise of completing the established resection goals of the operation (2). The advantages of current digital navigation technology are summarized as follows: (1) Precisely locate the anatomical structures and pathological tissues of the operation area; (2) Perfect surgical planning and approach before surgery; (3) Precisely control the resection range to protect important anatomical structures; (4) Accurate Repair the morphology of maxillofacial defect (3).

Although the existing digital navigation system-assisted surgical system has matured day by day, there are still some problems. (1) There is no direct spatial relationship between the patient and the surgical planning and the output image of the navigation system. The surgeon needs to watch the tomographic image output by the surgical planning and the navigation system through the display screen. When using images to locate anatomical structures, the surgeon needs to imagine the actual relationship between the image and the patient's anatomy, which requires a solid anatomical foundation and robust spatial imagination ability, which raises the technical threshold (4). (2) The existing navigation system is single-point navigation. It means that it can see only a particular point of navigation information during the operation but not a full grasp of the surgical area (5). (3) The existing navigation system is a display screen output. During use, the surgeon needs to repeatedly switch the field of vision between the display screen and the operation area. In addition to affecting the operation process and reducing the operation efficiency, it also quickly causes the doctor's visual fatigue and affects the operation effect (6). The above problems limit the further promotion and development of the existing navigation system in oral and maxillofacial surgery.

With improved computing capabilities and image processing technology, it has become possible to introduce augmented reality and mixed reality technologies into the medical field. Mixed reality technology integrates the technical advantages of augmented reality and virtual reality, can present virtual model information in natural scenes, integrate virtual models and real locations, and create a better realistic experience through stage superimposition (7). Intraoperative navigation is one of the best application scenarios of mixed reality technology in the medical field. Mixed reality equipment can assist the navigation system in integrating the surgical planning three-dimensional model with the actual patient's anatomy during the operation and complete the continuous spatiotemporal registration of the patient's surgical area anatomy and the planned three-dimensional model. Mixed reality technology can extend the surgeon's field of vision, enhance the visual system, and obtain the internal structure of organs invisible to the naked eye. The accurate spatial information of the surgical site and surrounding critical anatomical structures are further obtained (8).

Therefore, the introduction of mixed reality technology into the navigation system of oral and maxillofacial surgery can realize three-dimensional visual navigation and better solve spatial imagination and graphic conversion of existing navigation systems. The following introduces the project team's cross-linking of mixed reality display equipment with high-precision optical navigators, developing a digital maxillofacial surgery system based on mixed reality technology, and successfully implemented mixed reality-assisted tumor resection and reconstruction in 4 cases.

METHODS

MR Display Equipment and Patient Tracking Calibration Technology

The dynamic tracking of the optical positioner mainly realizes the change from real space to MR space. The process has two steps: the change from the real space to the space of the optical positioner and the change from the distance of the optical positioner to the MR display device. The reference frame fixed on the patient's head and the reflective ball on the MR display device's positioning frame can define the real space and the MR space. Using the optical positioner to track the reflective balls on the two positioning frames can directly obtain the change from the positioner to the MR space. Sum these two changes can get the transformation relationship from the real space to the MR space. Moreover, the MR equipment can scan the operating room environment through the depth camera for auxiliary calibration, further improving the accuracy of the tracking calibration.

Development of Maxillofacial Digital Surgery System Based on Mixed Reality Technology

The hardware used in this system includes HoloLens, a commercial head-mounted mixed reality display device from Microsoft Corporation in the United States, Passive Polaris Spectra, an infrared positioning tracking device from NDI Corporation in Canada, and infrared-reflective balls and reference frames.The software architecture used in this system includes HoloLens application development kit Mixed Reality Toolkit, Unity3D game engine for middleware development, open-source toolkit IGSTK developed by the National Institute of Biomedical Imaging and Bioengineering, National Institutes of Health, cross-platform QT, and communication-based on TCP protocol. The software used in this system is a commercial development kit or an open-source kit.

Preliminary Clinical Application of Maxillofacial Digital Surgery System Based on Mixed Reality Technology

A total of four patients who were treated at the Ninth People's Hospital of Shanghai Jiaotong University were selected. All patients had mandibular tumors that needed resection and reconstruction. We collected the patient's original CT data, completed the patient's preoperative three-dimensional reconstruction and surgical planning, and used the mixed reality technology of the maxillofacial digital surgery system to assist the surgery (**Table 1**).

The patients were re-examined 1 month after the operation, the postoperative CT data of the patient were collected, and the data were processed through the 3DMeshMetric to form the

TABLE 1 | Information of the 4 patients and surgical results.

Case	Gander	Age/years	Number of fibula bone segments	Maximum error/mm	Type of defect	Cause of defect	Benign or Malignant
A	Female	37	2	5.46	Metal and body	Mandible tumor	Benign
B	Male	46	1	5.80	Metal and body	Mandible tumor	Benign
C	Male	45	2	6.08	Metal and body	Mandible tumor	Benign
D	Female	54	3	4.79	Bilateral	Mandible tumor	Malignant

error distribution map, and completed the error analysis and quality control.

RESULTS

MR Display Equipment and Patient Tracking Calibration Technology

The preoperative CT or MRI inspection data can be transformed into a virtual visual model through three-dimensional modeling. Select the anatomical landmarks accurately identified in the surgical site as the marker points. Calculate the coordinates of the marked points on the virtual model in the original coordinate system of the virtual model, denoted as {Mi}, which is the coordinates of the patient's accurate anatomical marked points in the actual model coordinate system. During the operation, the navigation system tracks the surgical probe. The anatomical landmarks preset as the marker points on the actual model are sequentially selected to obtain the position of the marker point in the coordinate system of the navigation device. Click the anatomical landmarks preset as marker points on the actual model in turn to obtain the position of the marker point in the coordinate system of the navigation device, and further calculate the coordinates of the marker point in the reference frame coordinate system of the actual model, denoted as {Ni}.

Use the least-square method to find the optimal transformation matrix NTM to make the transformed coordinates NTM (Mi) to (Ni) closer to complete the tracking calibration of the MR display device and the patient. When performing point registration, as the number of marker points increases, the registration error will decrease. However, too many marker points in the actual operation will prolong the registration time and affect the efficiency of the process (9). Based on the research data, we set the number of marking points to six and control the point registration error within 1 mm, which achieves a balance of accuracy and efficiency (**Figure 1**).

Development of Maxillofacial Digital Surgery System Based on Mixed Reality Technology

The surgical system software system includes MR image processing and selection module, registration module, control module, target area depth calculation module. The design interface of the software system is simple and straightforward. It can display the MR virtual three-dimensional model and CT/MRI cross-section conditions simultaneously, switch arbitrarily, and realize the distance measurement and real-time display of the target area and the position of the surgical instrument.

MR image processing and selection module: including 3D model rendering optimization algorithm, image segmentation selection algorithm and display, mainly used for MR image processing optimization and separate production; registration module: assists the virtual and actual matching of the MR 3D model and the patient's factual anatomical structure Accuracy, including the extraction and matching of virtual and real landmarks, and the identification of landmarks and positioning frames by the navigator; control module: the surgeon mainly operates and sets the entire navigation system through this module, including the hardware interface program of the navigator and MR display equipment; Target area depth calculation module: Calculate the depth of the surgical instrument and the target area, and optimize the navigation accuracy of the target area. The hardware system required for the prototype includes MR image display equipment, navigator, reference system (probe, positioning frame, reflector...). The MR image display device completes the real-time communication with the navigator through the data transmission interface based on the TCP/UDP transmission protocol.

The MR image display device is the key to the navigation system. This article uses the finished head-mounted wireless MR display device-HoloLens as the display device. The image rendering optimization, intraoperative registration, tracking calibration algorithm, and hardware real-time communication protocol involved are all designed and developed by this project team (**Figure 2**).

Preliminary Clinical Application of Maxillofacial Digital Surgery System Based on Mixed Reality Technology

The operation of the four patients went smoothly. During the operation, the surgeon could observe the operation plan and virtual three-dimensional model in the operation field in real time, and adjust it through voice and gesture operations. In all cases, the mandible and other anatomical structures were well displayed, and the information response of the reconstructed fibula was accurate.By comparing the CT and surgical planning models before and after the operation, and through the error analysis chart, the maximum error of all patients is not more than 6.08 mm, and the error in most areas is $<$4.79 mm. Besides, The errors in all cases are mainly concentrated in the chin, which may be caused by the difference between the surface of the chin and the shape of the fibula. The error of the selected case in this article meets the requirements, and the patient's surgical wound were

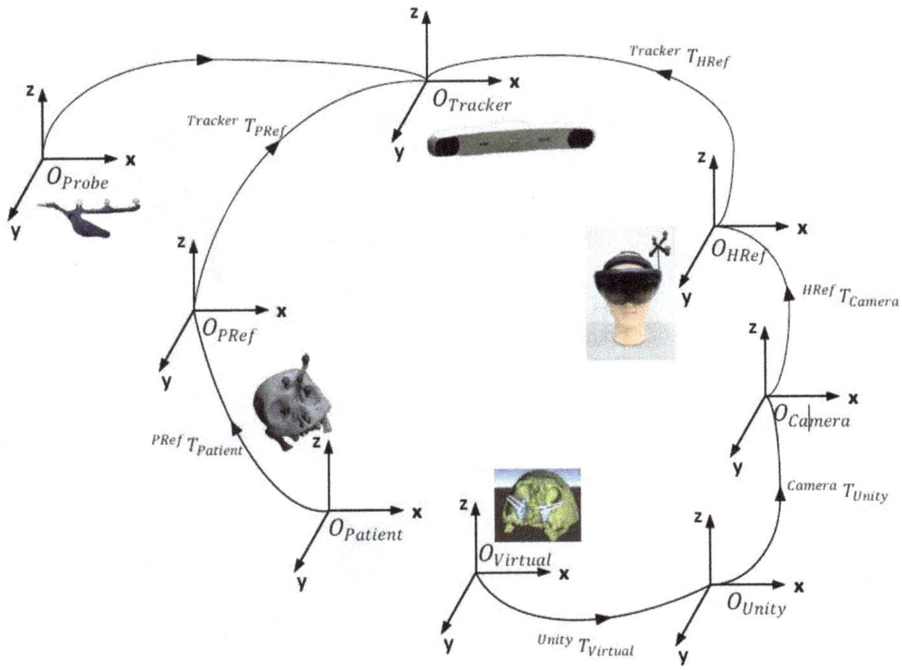

FIGURE 1 | Tracking calibration of MR display equipment, navigation system, and actual patients.

normal healing according to the Southampton scoring system without related complications (**Figure 3**).

DISCUSSION

The existing navigation system is a single-point display screen output mode, which cannot establish an effective spatial connection between the surgical planning image and the patient's actual anatomical structure. The surgeon needs to view the output of the tomographic image by the surgical planning and navigation system through the display screen and then imagine the actual relationship between the image x'and the patient's anatomical structure. There is a problem with the spatial conversion. The doctor's repeated switching of the field of view between the operation area and the display screen will reduce the operating efficiency and affect the operation effect (6).

This paper introduces mixed reality technology into the existing navigation system, so the navigation system can output three-dimensional images and display them together with the patient's actual anatomy in real-time. Mixed reality equipment can assist the navigation system in integrating the surgical planning three-dimensional model with the actual patient's anatomy during the operation and complete the continuous spatiotemporal registration of the patient's surgical area anatomy and the planned three-dimensional model (8). The whole process includes importing the preoperative planning 3D model, the fusion registration of the 3D projection of the intraoperative planning model, and the patient's actual anatomical structure. And surgeon can see the patient's anatomical structure and the 3D model simultaneously in the operation field. Therefore, the introduction of mixed reality technology into the navigation system of oral and maxillofacial surgery can realize three-dimensional visual navigation, better solve spatial imagination and graphic conversion of existing navigation systems (10) (**Figure 4**).

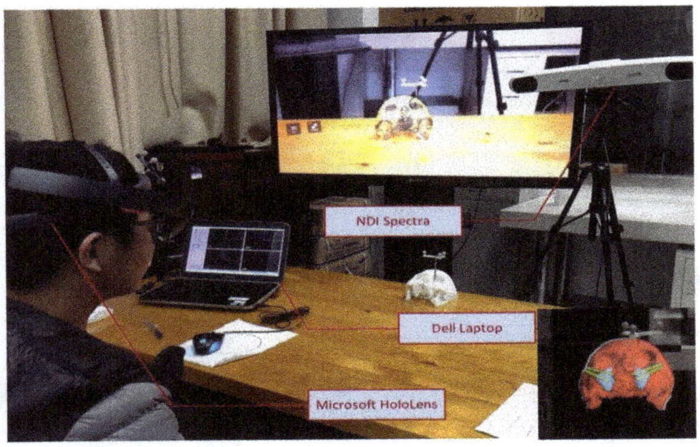

FIGURE 2 | Construction of a prototype of a digital maxillofacial surgery system based on mixed reality technology.

The mixed reality display device used in this study is a commercial wireless headset (Hololens) developed by Microsoft Corporation in the United States. As the most advanced mixed reality display device, its display technology is optical transmission (near-eye 3D diffraction) display. Unlike the more researched video-based display technology, the visual

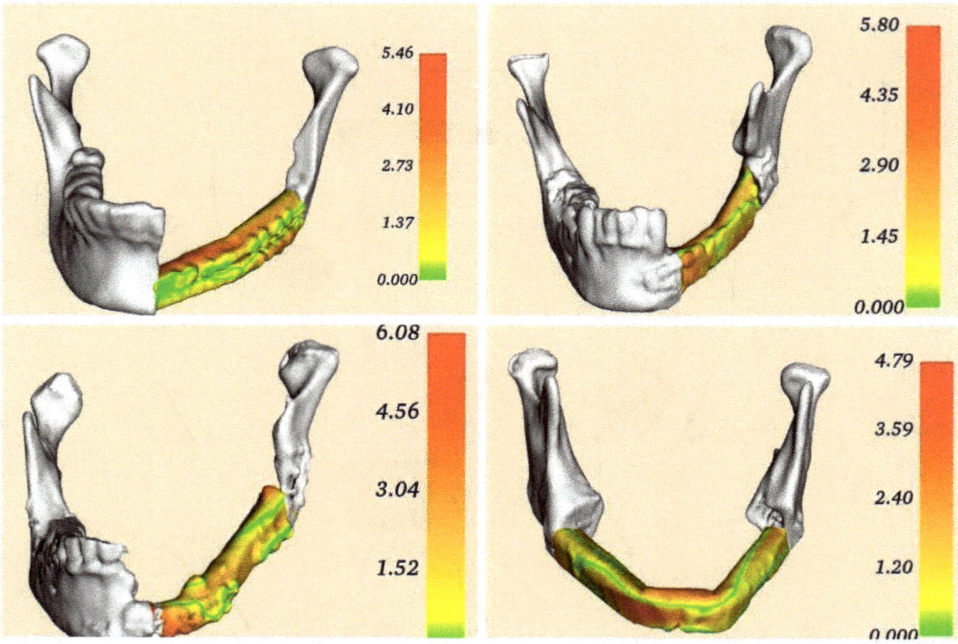

FIGURE 3 | Error distribution diagram formed by point-to-point comparison between preoperative planning and model postoperative CT reconstruction model. The bar graph on the right represents the value of the error (unit: mm). The color in the figure corresponds to the point error.

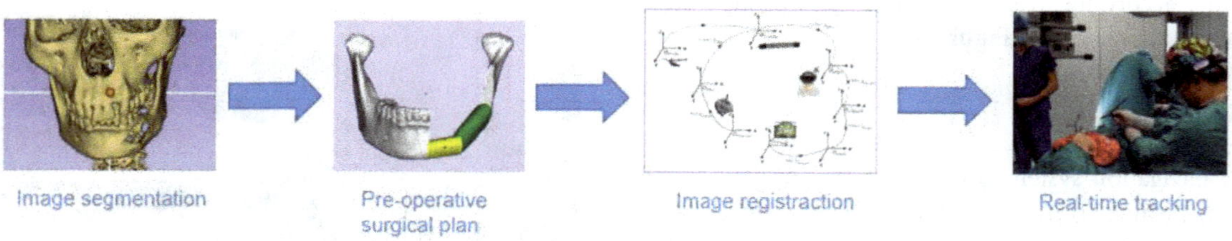

FIGURE 4 | The main procedures of MR-based surgical navigation.

transmissive display can integrate the three-dimensional model image and the natural ambient light in the translucent lens, thereby completely restoring the three-dimensional human vision (11). The three-dimensional model is directly superimposed on the patient's actual surgical area and maintains consistency with the patient's corresponding anatomical structure through continuous Spatio-temporal registration. Therefore, the surgeon can visually observe the patient's internal anatomy in the surgical field of view, accurately determine the resection range, and avoid secondary injuries. In addition, the device is operated through gesture recognition and voice control, avoiding physical contact during use, providing conditions for its application in surgery. The US Microsoft Corporation launched a commercial head-mounted mixed reality display device (Hololens) in 2015 and used it in mechanical processing and manufacturing. Due to its excellent three-dimensional display performance quickly gained clinical applications in the medical, especially the surgical field. Scholars such as Sun et al. (12) first reported using mixed reality technology to assist accurate breast tumor resection in a domestic journal in 2017; Tepper et al. (13) also said using mixed reality technology to help jaw reconstruction surgery in the same year. Based on the excellent optical performance of HoloLens and the open software development environment, more and more scholars have begun to use this device for mixed reality technology-assisted surgery-related research in the past 2 years (**Figure 5**).

In the research of Chinese scholars, mixed reality technology has been reported in neurosurgery, orthopedics, thoracic surgery and other fields for preoperative planning and doctor-patient communication. Scholar Yang Dezhen used mixed reality technology to holographically display individualized 3D virtual models of tumors, blood vessels, brain tissues, and others. They were used for preoperative planning, intraoperative guidance, preoperative talks, and teaching rounds. Research shows that mixed reality technology can display individualized holographic images of patients in a three-dimensional and intuitive manner

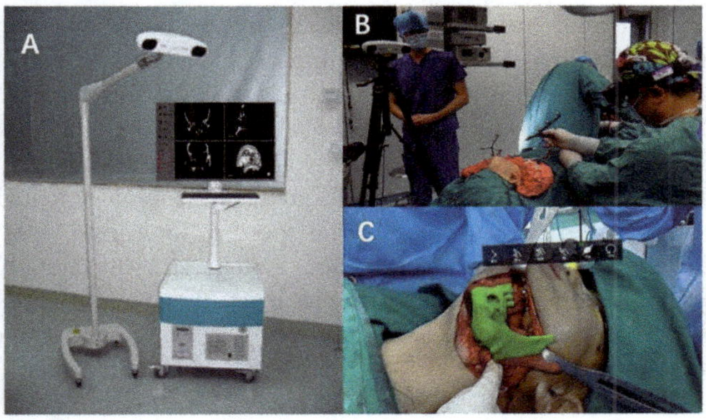

FIGURE 5 | (A) The existing navigation system is a single-point display screen navigation. According to the tomographic image on the display screen, the surgeon needs to imagine the space independently and cannot observe the surgical field and the display screen simultaneously. **(B)** The working model of the mixed reality navigation system, which can directly display the surgical planning plan and three-dimensional virtual model in the surgical field, and the surgeon can adjust it through voice and gesture operations. **(C)** The head-mounted device uses the navigator to perform continuous intraoperative temporal and spatial configuration, directly realizing the superimposed display of the patient's anatomical structure and the virtual model in the surgical field.

in any scene. So that surgeons, patients and family members can have a comprehensive understanding of the lesion and surrounding anatomical structures, which improves surgeons' understanding of the anatomy of the operation area and the efficiency of doctor-patient communication. Huang et al. (14) Scholars use mixed reality technology to assist surgical treatment of osteoporotic femoral neck fractures. This technology can shorten the operation time while optimizing the femoral neck nail passage, increasing the femoral neck cortical support, and improving the efficacy; Ma et al. (15) Scholars have introduced mixed reality technology in the percutaneous kyphoplasty of the spine, which accurately displays the compression fracture site and surrounding anatomical structures in three dimensions during the operation. The operation path is clear, and the compression fracture forming site can be accurately located; Tang et al. (16) and Ma et al. (17) tried to introduce mixed reality technology in the field of thoracic surgery and achieved good results in the precise resection and reconstruction of chest wall tumors and the precise positioning and resection of small pulmonary nodules. Tang et al. (18) has completed preoperative three-dimensional reconstruction, intraoperative three-dimensional display and postoperative evaluation for eight patients with head and neck tumors. Although they successfully completed the operations with a control error of 5 mm, their system is mainly used for intraoperative display and lacks an effective positioning tracking system.

Mixed reality technology-assisted surgical navigation is also a hot topic in this field by international scholars in the past 2 years. In 2018, García-Vázquez and other scholars from the University of Lübeck in Germany (19) discussed the possibility of using mixed reality technology to assist endovascular aortic repair (EVAR) in the field of vascular surgery, and found that three-dimensional visual display can be a better alternative Intraoperative angiography reduces radiation exposure and the use of contrast agents, but its calculation speed and intraoperative registration accuracy cannot meet clinical needs; in 2019, Checcucci and other scholars from the University of Turin, Italy (20) performed nephron-preserving surgery in the urology department (NSS) tried to use mixed reality display equipment for three-dimensional visual surgery planning. Research shows that using mixed reality display equipment to assist surgery planning has better performance in plan display and anatomical accuracy, which helps surgeons better understand surgery Complexity, but the research is limited to preoperative planning and presentation and does not involve intraoperative navigation; in the field of Otorhinolaryngology-Head and Neck Surgery, American Rose and other scholars (21) affirmed the superiority of mixed reality display technology in a three-dimensional display. And its potential value in improving surgical efficiency and patient safety also pointed out the need to further enhance the computing speed and registration accuracy of head-mounted devices to meet clinical needs.

Worldwide scholars agree that mixed reality technology-assisted surgery has broad application prospects, and it is becoming a hot research topic in digital surgery. However, although the current mixed reality display device (Hololens) can scan the surrounding environment in real-time through a depth camera for positioning, it is limited by hardware conditions. Its positioning accuracy and speed cannot meet the needs of surgical operations. Pepe et al. (22) tried to improve the system's accuracy by improving the registration algorithm. The average error in the three-dimensional direction was reduced to 3–5 mm, but it still could not meet the needs of oral and maxillofacial surgery. Therefore, it is necessary to improve further the response speed of mixed reality equipment and the accuracy of intraoperative registration in the following research.

At this stage, the related research involving improving the registration accuracy of mixed reality devices is trying to improve the system response speed and intraoperative registration accuracy through the software development and algorithm optimization of the mixed reality display device (Microsoft's HoloLens) (22, 23). Scholars such as Faith (24) tried to use manual registration methods to improve the registration accuracy of mixed reality display devices. Studies have shown that the deviation from standard neurosurgical navigation systems reaches 4 mm, which still cannot meet clinical needs. At present, it is generally believed that the mixed reality display device (HoloLens) is an essential factor that limits its registration accuracy. Because the volume and weight of the head-mounted device are strictly limited, the accuracy of the depth camera and the computing power of the processor used is far inferior to that of the desktop Class equipment (25). The limitation of hardware restricts the improvement of the mixed reality system's overall registration accuracy and operation speed by this research idea. This paper innovatively proposes and realizes the research idea of combining mixed reality display devices with high-precision optical navigation systems.

By leveraging the advantages of the existing optical navigation system's computing power and positioning accuracy, the overall registration accuracy of the mixed reality navigation system is improved. And computing speed (10). Moreover, the maxillofacial surgery planning software and navigation system involved in this article are all independently developed by the project team, with critical technologies and systems with independent intellectual property rights, which have broad clinical transformation and application prospects (26–28). However, the system still needs some preliminary data preparation work. The overall registration speed and overall accuracy cannot fully meet the clinical needs, that is, the target average error for bone tissue is controlled at 1 mm. There is still room for improvement in real-time registration and tracking and the surgeon has certain equipment learning requirements.

CONCLUSIONS

The maxillofacial digital surgery system based on mixed reality technology can superimpose and display three-dimensional navigation information in the doctor's surgical field of vision, which solves the problem of visual conversion and space conversion of the existing navigation system work efficiency of digitally assisted surgery. It improves the work efficiency of digitally assisted surgery, effectively reduces the surgeon's dependence on spatial experience and imagination, and protects important anatomical structures during surgery. It is a significant clinical application value and potential. However, the current cross-linking speed of the mixed reality display device and the navigation system and the system's overall accuracy still cannot fully meet the clinical needs. Further research is needed to improve the system accuracy and response speed.

AUTHOR CONTRIBUTIONS

TJ and XC designed the experiments. RY and CL collected the data. PT and AA did the calculation. RY wrote the main manuscript text and all authors approved the manuscript.

REFERENCES

1. Juergens P, Beinemann J, Zandbergen M, Raith S, Kunz C, Zeilhofer HF, et al. computer-assisted diagnostic and treatment concept to increase accuracy and safety in the extracranial correction of cranial vault asymmetries. *J Oral Maxillofac Surg.* (2012) 70:677–84. doi: 10.1016/j.joms.2011.02.046
2. Yu H, Wang X, Zhang S, Zhang L, Xin P, Shen SG. Navigation-guided en bloc resection and defect reconstruction of craniomaxillary bony tumours. *Int J Oral Maxillofac Surg.* (2013) 42:1409–13. doi: 10.1016/j.ijom.2013.05.011
3. Rudman K, Hoekzema C, Rhee J. Computer-assisted innovations in craniofacial surgery. *Facial Plast Surg.* (2011) 27:358–65. doi: 10.1055/s-0031-1283054
4. Blackwell M, Morgan F, DiGioia AM 3rd. Augmented reality and its future in orthopaedics. *Clin Orthop Relat Res.* (1998) 354:111–22. doi: 10.1097/00003086-199809000-00014
5. Chytas D, Malahias MA, Nikolaou VS. Augmented reality in orthopedics: current state and future directions. *Front Surg.* (2019) 6:38. doi: 10.3389/fsurg.2019.00038
6. Ma LF, Zhao Z, Chen F, Zhang B, Fu L, Liao H. Augmented reality surgical navigation with ultrasound-assisted registration for pedicle screw placement: a pilot study. *Int J Comput Assist Radiol Surg.* (2017) 12:2205–15. doi: 10.1007/s11548-017-1652-z
7. Chen B, Qin X. Composition of virtual-real worlds and intelligence integration of human-computer in mixed reality. *Scientia Sinica (Informationis).* (2016) 46:1737–47. doi: 10.1360/N112016-00249
8. Chen G. Application and Prospect of Augmented/Mixed Reality in Head and Neck Surgery. *J Tissue Eng Reconstruct Surg.* (2018) 1:21–3. doi: 10.3969/j.issn.1673-0364.2018.01.006
9. Bai J, Ding H, Wang G, Xu D, Zhao L. A study on the registration method and precision in image guided surgery. *J Biomed Eng.* (2008) 25:1242–8.
10. Sun PJ, Chen XJ, Yang R, Ji T. A pilot study of mandibular reconstruction surgery based on augmented reality using Microsoft HoloLens. *Int J CARS.* (2018) 13:S270–2.
11. Langlotz T, Cook M, Regenbrecht H. Real-Time radiometric compensation for optical see-through head-mounted displays. *IEEE Trans Vis Comput Graph.* (2016) 22:2385–94. doi: 10.1109/TVCG.2016.2593781
12. Sun T, Deng F, Li J, Tang J. Application of mixed reality technology in precise surgery of breast neoplasms. *Chin J Surg Oncol.* (2017) 03:145–8. doi: 10.3969/j.issn.1674-4136.2019.03.003
13. Tepper OM, Rudy HL, Lefkowitz A, Weimer KA, Marks SM, Stern CS, et al. Mixed reality with HoloLens: where virtual reality meets augmented reality in the operating room. *Plast Reconstr Surg.* (2017) 140:1066–70. doi: 10.1097/PRS.0000000000003802
14. Huang X, Wan L, Liang D. Study on optimization of femoral neck nail channel assisted by CAD based on osteoporosis MR model. *J Pract Med.* (2019) 35:2090–3. doi: 10.3969/j.issn.1006-5725.2019.13.013
15. Ma X, Lin Y, Huang Y, Sun W, Shen J, Sun M, et al. Application and exploration of mixed reality technology in accurate operation of percutaneous vertebroplasty of spine. *J Shanghai Jiaotong Univ (Medical Science).* (2019) 39:637–41+36. doi: 10.3969/j.issn.1674-8115.2019.06.012
16. TangY, Xiao G, Chen Y. Application of virtual reality, augmented reality and mixed reality technology in chest wall tumor resection and reconstruction of precise surgical treatment. *Chin J Thorac Surg.* (2018) 5:129–133. doi: 10.3877/cma.j.issn.2095-8773.2018.02.12
17. Ma Y, Li Y, Zhang T, Feng C, Pan J, Liu Y. Accurate localization and resection of small pulmonary nodules assisted by mixed reality technique. *Chin J Laparosc Surg.* (2019) 12:179–181. doi: 10.3877/cma.j.issn.1674-6899.2019.03.012
18. Tang ZN, Hui Y, Hu LH Yu Y, Zhang WB, Peng X. Application of mixed reality technique for the surgery of oral and maxillofacial tumors. *Beijing Da Xue Xue Bao Yi Xue Ban.* (2020) 52:1124–9. doi: 10.19723/j.issn.1671-167X.2020.06.023
19. García-Vázquez V, von Haxthausen F, Jäckle S, Schumann C, Kuhlemann I, Bouchagiar J, et al. Navigation and visualisation with HoloLens in endovascular aortic repair. *Innov Surg Sci.* (2018) 3:167–77. doi: 10.1515/iss-2018-2001
20. Checcucci E, Amparore D, Pecoraro A, Peretti D, Aimar R, De Cillis S, et al. 3D mixed reality holograms for preoperative surgical planning of nephron-sparing surgery: evaluation of surgeons' perception. *Minerva Urol Nefrol.* (2019). doi: 10.23736/S0393-2249.19.03610-5
21. Rose AS, Kim H, Fuchs H, Frahm JM. Development of augmented-reality applications in otolaryngology-head and neck surgery. *Laryngoscope.* (2019) 129 (Suppl 3):S1–S11. doi: 10.1002/lary.28098
22. Pepe A, Trotta GF, Mohr-Ziak P, Gsaxner C, Wallner J, Bevilacqua V, et al. Marker-less registration approach for mixed reality-aided maxillofacial surgery: a pilot evaluation. *J Digit Imaging.* (2019) 32:1008–18. doi: 10.1007/s10278-019-00272-6
23. Nguyen NQ, Cardinell J, Ramjist JM, Lai P, Dobashi Y, Guha

D, et al. An augmented reality system characterization of placement accuracy in neurosurgery. *J Clin Neurosci.* (2019) 72:392–6. doi: 10.1016/j.jocn.2019.12.014

24. Incekara F, Smits M, Dirven C, Vincent A. Clinical feasibility of a wearable mixed-reality device in neurosurgery. *World Neurosurg.* (2018) 118:e422–7. doi: 10.1016/j.wneu.2018.06.208
25. Mitsuno D, Ueda K, Hirota Y, Ogino M. Effective application of mixed reality device HoloLens: simple manual alignment of surgical field and holograms. *Plast Reconstr Surg.* (2019) 143:647–65. doi: 10.1097/PRS.0000000000005215
26. Chen X, Xu L, Wang H, Wang F, Wang Q, Kikinis R. Development of a surgical navigation system based on 3D Slicer for intraoperative implant placement surgery. *Med Eng Phys.* (2017) 41:81–9. doi: 10.1016/j.medengphy.2017.01.005
27. Chen X, Xu L, Wang Y, Wang H, Wang F, Zeng X, et al. Development of a surgical navigation system based on augmented reality using an optical see-through head-mounted display. *J Biomed Inform.* (2015) 55:124–31. doi: 10.1016/j.jbi.2015.04.003
28. Chen X, Xu L, Yang Y, Egger J. A semi-automatic computer-aided method for surgical template design. *Sci Rep.* (2016) 6:20280. doi: 10.1038/srep20280

9

High Precision Bone Cutting by Er: YAG Lasers Might Minimize the Invasiveness of Navigated Brain Biopsies

Thanh Tu Ha[1], *Florian M. Thieringer*[3,4], *Martin Bammerlin*[2] *and Dominik Cordier*[1*]

[1] Department of Neurosurgery, University Hospital Basel, Basel, Switzerland, [2] Advanced Osteotomy Tools AG, Basel, Switzerland, [3] Department of Oral and Cranio-Maxillofacial Surgery, University Hospital Basel, Basel, Switzerland, [4] Medical Additive Manufacturing Research Group, Department of Biomedical Engineering, University of Basel, Allschwil, Switzerland

***Correspondence:**
Dominik Cordier
dominik.cordier@usb.ch

Biopsies of brain tissue are sampled and examined to establish a diagnosis and to plan further treatment, e.g. for brain tumors. The neurosurgical procedure of sampling brain tissue for histologic examination is still a relatively invasive procedure that carries several disadvantages. The "proof of concept"-objective of this study is to answer the question if laser technology might be a potential tool to make brain biopsies less invasive, faster and safer. Laser technology might carry the opportunity to miniaturize the necessary burr hole and also to angulate the burr hole much more tangential in relation to the bone surface in order to take biopsies from brain regions that are usually only difficult and hazardous to access. We examined if it is possible to miniaturize the hole in the skull bone to such a high extent that potentially the laser-created canal itself may guide the biopsy needle with sufficient accuracy. The 2-dimensional, i.e. radial tolerance of the tip of biopsy needles inserted in these canals was measured under defined lateral loads which mimic mechanical forces applied by a surgeon. The canals through the skull bones were planned in angles of 90° (perpendicular) and 45° relative to the bone surface. We created a total of 33 holes with an Er : YAG laser in human skull bones. We could demonstrate that the achievable radial tolerance concerning the guidance of a biopsy needle by a laser created bone canal is within the range of the actual accuracy of a usual navigated device if the canal is at least 4 mm in length. Lateral mechanical loads applied to the biopsy needle had only minor impact on the measurable radial tolerance. Furthermore, in contrast to mechanical drilling systems, laser technology enables the creation of bone canals in pointed angles to the skull bone surface. The latter opens the perspective to sample biopsies in brain areas that are usually not or only hazardous to access.

Keywords: diagnostic, brain lesion, Er : YAG laser, laser osteotomy, cold ablation, brain biopsies

INTRODUCTION

In case of unclear brain lesions in imaging studies, tissue biopsies are mandatory for a definitive histologic diagnosis and adequate treatment planning, e.g. for brain tumors. In many of these cases, navigated brain biopsies are routinely performed by directing a biopsy needle in the brain's affected area. Depending on the institution and the surgeon's preferences, this kind of biopsy often includes a skin incision of up to more than 4 centimeters and a burr hole of up to 14 millimeters in diameter. Furthermore, an incision of the dura mater and the insertion of the biopsy needle, often through functional brain tissue, are necessary. The guidance of the biopsy needle by a navigation system warrants the necessary accuracy (1–7).

The depicted current method is relatively invasive, often time-consuming and carries several risks and side effects. In general, symptomatic intracerebral hemorrhages are reported in 1 - 10% of cases and are among the main risks because they may be associated with permanent morbidity or mortality (2, 3, 5, 8, 9). The reported rate of asymptomatic hemorrhages ranges from 8 - 54% (4, 8, 10). The accuracy of navigated brain biopsies is dependent on the used methodology and lies between 1 and 3 millimeters but may be impaired by the phenomenon of brain shift after the opening of the dura mater. The size of the bone opening, respectively, the opening of the dura mater and the duration of the procedure may be associated with the observed degree of brain shift (7, 11, 12). A further disadvantage of the current method is cosmetic impairment by a relatively large scar (13, 14).

The "proof of concept"-objective of this study is to answer the question if laser technology might be a suitable tool to make brain biopsies less invasive, perhaps also faster and safer. Laser technology might potentially enable us to miniaturize the necessary burr hole and also to angulate the burr hole much more tangential in relation to the bone surface in order to take biopsies from brain regions that are usually only difficult and hazardous to access.

We examined if it is possible to miniaturize the hole in the skull bone to such a high extent that potentially the laser-created canal itself may guide the biopsy needle with sufficient tolerance. The 2-dimensional, radial tolerance of the tip of the biopsy needles inserted in these canals was measured under defined lateral loads which mimic the mechanical forces applied by a surgeon during the procedure.

The use of pulsated Er : YAG lasers in bone ablation has been shown to produce precise hole geometries and chemical surface characteristics comparable to conventional drilling (15).

Due to the pulsation and the ER : YAG laser parameters in the "cold ablation" range (16), melting or carbonization typically associated with CO_2-laser ablation can be avoided. Moreover, bone healing, under certain conditions, was found to be similar for osteotomies performed with Er : YAG lasers and piezoelectric osteotomes (17, 18). Bone healing might be improved in comparison to mechanical trepanation (10–21).

Furthermore, in contrast to conventional rotating drilling systems, lasers offer the possibility to create holes in pointed angles relative to the bone surface. The latter offers the opportunity to position the entry point of the biopsy needle in, e.g., hair-covered regions that are virtually invisible after the biopsy or to obtain biopsies from areas of the brain that are otherwise inaccessible or at least difficult and hazardous to reach.

Taken together, laser technology could have the potential to improve several aspects of the current practice of brain biopsies.

This proof of concept study examines if an Er : YAG laser can cut holes in different angles to the surface in native human skull bones with such a high level of precision that the created canal in the bone itself might act as a useable guide for the biopsy needle along the predefined trajectory. The radial tolerance of guidance of the tip of the inserted needle was measured under different predefined lateral loads applied to the "outside part" of the needle (i.e. at the outer surface of the skull bone) which mimic mechanical forces applied by a surgeon.

MATERIAL AND METHODS

Skull Bone

Vital human skull bone was immediately cryoconserved at -80° C after explantation. Frontal, temporal and parietal parts of human skull bones have been used to experiment with a realistic reconstruction of a usual brain biopsy setup. The thickness of the skull bone samples ranged from 1.5 - 11.2 millimeters. For the experiments, the skull bone samples were thawed to room temperature.

According to the responsible ethics committee, formal ethical approval was not required due to anonymized bone material from deceased donors.

Laser Osteotome

To create the holes in the bone samples for the biopsy needle along predefined trajectories, the CARLO®-system (Cold Ablation Robot-guided Laser Osteotome; AOT, Basel, Switzerland) was used. CARLO® consists of an Er : YAG laser which is mounted on a navigated multiaxial robotic arm. The used Er : YAG laser is designed to perform "cold ablation" with a pulse energy of 650 mJ and a pulse duration of 200 µs as described in (16, 22).

The Er : YAG laser-emitted light has a wavelength of 2943 nanometers with a pulse repetition frequency of 10 Hertz. The achievable bone ablation of the used laser osteotome is around 1 millimeter in depth and 0.8 millimeters in width per pulse.

Experimental Setup

The skull bone samples were securely fastened on a workbench. The canals through the skull bones were planned in angles of 90° (perpendicular) and 45° relative to the bone surface. After referencing the navigation system, the robotic arm with the attached Er : YAG laser was programmed concerning the planned trajectories and the 1.8-millimeter diameter of the hole, i.e. the diameter of the biopsy needle (BrainPro, PAJUNK®, Germany), and activated (**Figures 1A–C**)

Following the creation of the hole, the biopsy needle was inserted up to a predefined depth (5.0 cm), and the axis of the

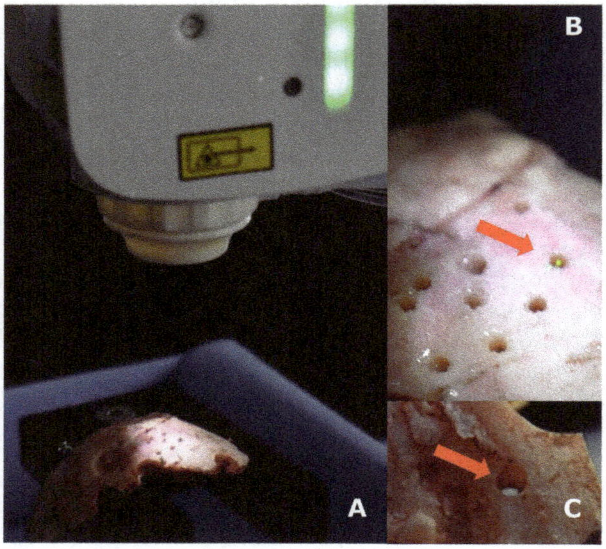

FIGURE 1 | Experimental setup with navigated Er : YAG laser and skull bone **(A)**, detailed photos of the laser in action **(B)**, and a laser-created hole in skull bone **(C)**.

biopsy needle was oriented perpendicularly to a scale paper with millimeter-division. By using a tension spring balance, lateral forces of 0.05 N, 0.1 N, 0.2 N, 0.5 N, and 1 N were applied to the proximal part (i.e. at the outer surface of the skull bone, 10.0 cm distance from the bone surface) of the biopsy needle and the correlating radial tolerance, as reflected by the measured deflection, of the tip of the biopsy needle was measured (**Figure 2**).

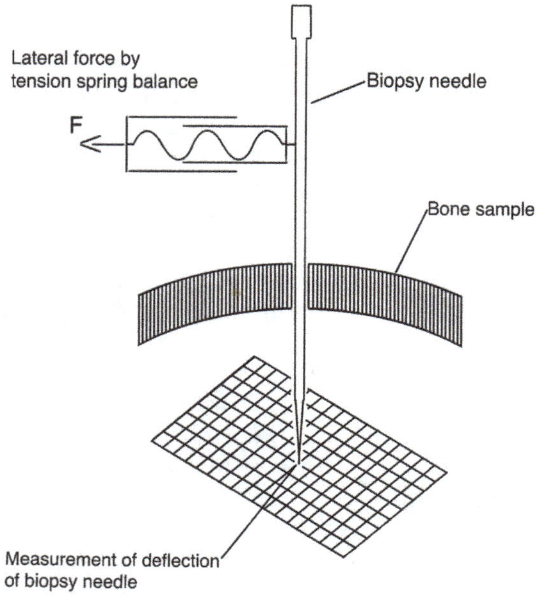

FIGURE 2 | Schematic drawing of the experimental setup to measure the deflection of the tip of the biopsy needle under different lateral loads.

These applied lateral forces represent different forces during the handling of the biopsy needle by the neurosurgeon. The radial tolerance of the distal tip of the biopsy needle, i.e. at the inside of the skull bone at the different applied forces was then recorded by using the underlying scale paper with an accuracy of 0.5 millimeters.

RESULTS

In three skull bone samples, 33 holes were created by the Er : YAG laser. The planned diameter of the bone canals was 1.8 millimeters which equals the outer diameter of the biopsy needle. 13 holes had been created at an angle of 45°, 20 holes at an angle of 90° to the outer bone surface.

The first eight holes were utilized to identify the appropriate laser parameters to cut skull bone. These eight holes have not been used for the further examinations.

In all of the the next 25 holes, the biopsy needles could be introduced with low resistance with a perceptible defined guidance along the trajectory due to the holes' exact fit. These 25 holes have been used for further examinations.

In the following, measurement of the radial tolerance of the tip of the biopsy needle after lateral load application as described above, has been performed. An increase of the applied lateral force was generally associated with a slightly increased deflection of the tip of the biopsy needle. **Figure 3** displays the deflection of the tip of the biopsy needle at 5.0 cm distance from the skull bone sample's inner surface. The colored dots represent the deflection at different defined lateral forces (0.05 N, 0.1 N, 0.2 N, 0.5 N, 1.0 N). Correlated to the applied loads, no differences in the deflection values were found for the holes in 45°- and 90°-orientation to the surface. A longer canal through the bone was associated with less deflection, i.e. a more accurate guidance of the needle along the trajectory. The bone canal's length is influenced by the thickness of the bone and the angle of the hole in relation to the bone surface. It is notable that forces of more than 0.2 N cause a visible bending of the biopsy needle on the outside part of the needle, where the load was applied.

DISCUSSION

Brain biopsies are a routinely used diagnostic tool, but the usual current brain biopsy procedure is still a relatively invasive intervention that carries several disadvantages and risks.

The ongoing evolution of laser technology might carry the opportunity to improve the procedure of brain biopsies regarding aspects of invasiveness, safety and surgery time. Lasers have been shown to cut biologic tissue such as bone, fascia, or soft tissue with high precision and less thermal strain to adjacent tissue than mechanical bone drilling techniques and good or even superior postoperative wound healing (20, 21, 23, 24). Concerning Er : YAG lasers, the absorption of the transmitted energy is nearly exclusively by the water molecules in the tissue, resulting in only minimal thermal stress of

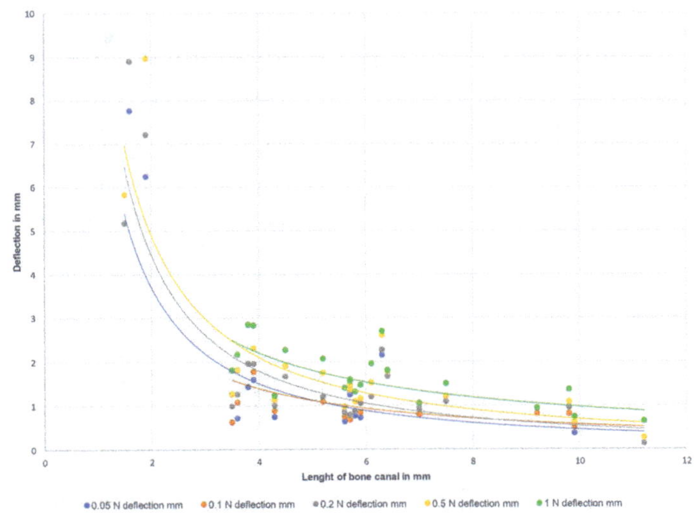

FIGURE 3 | Deflection of the tip of the biopsy needle in 5.0 cm distance from the inner bone surface to the bone canal's length. Different colors represent the applied lateral loads at the outer part of the biopsy needle (10.0 cm distance from outer bone surface): blue – 0.05 N; orange – 0.1 N; grey – 0.2 N; yellow – 0.5 N; green - 1.0 N.

surrounding tissue (21, 25, 26). In contrast to conventional drills, lasers do not leave metal debris at their site of action, which might produce artifacts in subsequent MR-imaging studies (22, 27).

Finally aiming at the further development of less invasive brain biopsy techniques, the presented study aims to evaluate as a first "proof of principle"-step if it is possible to miniaturize the hole in the skull bone to such a high extent that potentially the laser-created canal itself may guide the biopsy needle with acceptable tolerance.

A potential future scenario could be the use of high-precision holes in the skull bone as a guidance for the biopsy needle without the need for an additional and error prone mechanical navigated guiding system.

In our examinations, we at first established knowledge about high-precision cutting of the skull bone with an Er : YAG laser. Subsequently, with the adequate laser parameters, we found that the laser provided reproducible and exact fitting apertures in the skull bone to insert the biopsy needle. The needle was inserted to a depth of 5.0 cm distance to the inner surface of the skull bone. By applying defined lateral forces to the part of the biopsy needle at the skull's outer surface, we simulated the manipulation of the needle by the neurosurgeon during a biopsy. A trained neurosurgeon will not exceed forces of 0.2 N during insertion resp. manipulation of the needle. However, we also examined excessive forces up to 1.0 N of lateral load. In 87 of 93 measurements, the deflection, i.e. the radial tolerance, of the tip of the biopsy needle was less than 3 millimeters.

Assuming a usual scenario with bone canal lengths of more than 4 millimeters and the expectable lateral loads during the procedure, the deflection of the tip of the biopsy needle was less than 2.5 millimeters. In clinical application, the accuracy of a mechanical navigated guiding system would be the equivalent to the observed radial tolerance.

Notably, the observed primary determinant for the biopsy needle's deflection was the bone canal's length and not the lateral force applied to the biopsy needle (see **Figure 3**). However, bone canal lengths of less than 3 millimeters did not provide sufficient guidance if one presumes that a maximum deviation of 3 millimeters in 5 centimeters distance from the inner skull surface is sufficient for the planned biopsy. This tolerance is within the range of reported accuracy-values of different conventional navigation systems (28).

The depicted results demonstrate the potential that lies in this technology. Regarding the whole procedure of brain biopsies, these results can be regarded as a first and groundbreaking step in the further development of brain biopsies that use laser technology. There are several other steps of the whole biopsy procedure that need to be re-thought. The necessary short skin incision itself could potentially also be created by a laser or, if using a conventional scalpel, at least substantially be shortened to introduce a small speculum-like device to keep the incision open. In practical use, when creating the canal through the skull bone by laser technology, the laser energy transmission needs to be terminated when the thickness of the skull bone is traversed, and the dura mater is the only remaining firm mechanical barrier to the brain. The technique of optical coherence tomography can terminate the transmission of laser energy at precisely this point and is part of current research (29, 30). A laser could also perform the puncture and hemostasis of the dura mater with adapted parameters. The corticotomy at the entry site of the biopsy needle in the brain could be done by laser or by electrocautery. After obtaining the biopsy, an appropriate laser could be employed to improve the subcutaneous wound closure.

Regarding this wide range of potential applications, laser technology could be a tool to make the procedure of brain biopsies much faster because the usual multiple change of instruments becomes unnecessary. A shorter surgical procedure time and the smaller operative situs might lower the perioperative risk profile. Furthermore, the much smaller incision and smaller hole in the bone would improve patient satisfaction due to better cosmetic results.

CONCLUSION

Laser technology might be a valuable tool to improve the procedure of brain biopsies regarding invasiveness, procedure time and finally risk profile. In this "proof of principle"-study with an Er : YAG laser we could show, as a prerequisite for further research, that this technology can create canals in skull bone with such a high degree of precision that these canals alone could act as a sufficient guide for the biopsy needles.

AUTHOR CONTRIBUTIONS

DC, initiation and realization of project, overall responsibility for project, literature work, planning of experimental setup, evaluation of results, manuscript compilation, and ethical issues. TH, planning of experimental setup, execution of experiments, evaluation of results, and literature work. MB, planning of experimental setup and execution of experiments. FT, project expertise, literature work, and revision of manuscript. All authors contributed to the article and approved the submitted version.

ACKNOWLEDGMENTS

This work was made possible with the friendly support of Advanced Osteotomy Tools AG (Basel, Switzerland), who provided the Cold Ablation Robot-guided Laser Osteotome (CARLO®) for the experiments. No financial support was received.

REFERENCES

1. Grossman R, Sadetzki S, Spiegelmann R, Ram Z. Haemorrhagic Complications and the Incidence of Asymptomatic Bleeding Associated With Stereotactic Brain Biopsies. *Acta Neurochir (Wien)* (2005) 147 (6):627–31; discussion 31. doi: 10.1007/s00701-005-0495-5
2. Georgiopoulos M, Ellul J, Chroni E, Constantoyannis C. Efficacy, Safety, and Duration of a Frameless Fiducial-Less Brain Biopsy Versus Frame-Based Stereotactic Biopsy: A Prospective Randomized Study. *J Neurol Surg A Cent Eur Neurosurg* (2018) 79(1):31–8. doi: 10.1055/s-0037-1602697
3. Minchev G, Kronreif G, Ptacek W, Dorfer C, Micko A, Maschke S, et al. A Novel Robot-Guided Minimally Invasive Technique for Brain Tumor Biopsies. *J Neurosurg* (2019) 132:1–9. doi: 10.3171/2018.8.JNS182096
4. Chen CC, Hsu PW, Erich Wu TW, Lee ST, Chang CN, Wei KC, et al. Stereotactic Brain Biopsy: Single Center Retrospective Analysis of Complications. *Clin Neurol Neurosurg* (2009) 111(10):835–9. doi: 10.1016/j.clineuro.2009.08.013
5. Malone H, Yang J, Hershman DL, Wright JD, Bruce JN, Neugut AI. Complications Following Stereotactic Needle Biopsy of Intracranial Tumors. *World Neurosurg* (2015) 84(4):1084–9. doi: 10.1016/j.wneu.2015.05.025
6. Gralla J, Nimsky C, Buchfelder M, Fahlbusch R, Ganslandt O. Frameless Stereotactic Brain Biopsy Procedures Using the Stealth Station: Indications, Accuracy and Results. *Zentralbl Neurochir* (2003) 64(4):166–70. doi: 10.1055/s-2003-44620
7. Ivan ME, Yarlagadda J, Saxena AP, Martin AJ, Starr PA, Sootsman WK, et al. Brain Shift During Bur Hole-Based Procedures Using Interventional MRI. *J Neurosurg* (2014) 121(1):149–60. doi: 10.3171/2014.3.JNS121312
8. Mizobuchi Y, Nakajima K, Fujihara T, Matsuzaki K, Mure H, Nagahiro S, et al. The Risk of Hemorrhage in Stereotactic Biopsy for Brain Tumors. *J Med Invest* (2019) 66(3.4):314–8. doi: 10.2152/jmi.66.314
9. Purzner T, Purzner J, Bernstein M. Outpatient Brain Biopsy and Craniotomy for Supratentorial Tumor. In: *Tumors of the Central Nervous System.* Hayat MA. editor. Dordrecht: Springer (2012) 9:85–9. doi: 10.1007/978-94-007-5488-1_11
10. Marcus HJ, Vakharia VN, Ourselin S, Duncan J, Tisdall M, Aquilina K. Robot-Assisted Stereotactic Brain Biopsy: Systematic Review and Bibliometric Analysis. *Childs Nerv Syst* (2018) 34(7):1299–309. doi: 10.1007/s00381-018-3821-y
11. Giamouriadis A, Perera D, Safdar A, Vergani F, Bhangoo R, Gullan R, et al. Safety and Accuracy of Frameless Electromagnetic-Navigated (AXIEM. *Acta Neurochir (Wien)* (2019) 161(12):2587–93. doi: 10.1007/s00701-019-04093-y
12. Nimsky C, Ganslandt O, Cerny S, Hastreiter P, Greiner G, Fahlbusch R. Quantification of, Visualization of, and Compensation for Brain Shift Using Intraoperative Magnetic Resonance Imaging. *Neurosurgery* (2000) 47 (5):1070–9; discussion 9-80. doi: 10.1097/00006123-200011000-00008
13. Im TS, Lee YS, Suh SJ, Lee JH, Ryu KY, Kang DG. The Efficacy of Titanium Burr Hole Cover for Reconstruction of Skull Defect After Burr Hole Trephination of Chronic Subdural Hematoma. *Korean J Neurotrauma* (2014) 10(2):76–81. doi: 10.13004/kjnt.2014.10.2.76
14. Dujovny M, Aviles A, Cuevas P. Bone-Like Polyethelyne Burr-Hole Cover. *Neurol Res* (2005) 27(3):333–4. doi: 10.1179/016164105X22138
15. Sasaki KM, Aoki A, Ichinose S, Yoshino T, Yamada S, Ishikawa I. Scanning Electron Microscopy and Fourier Transformed Infrared Spectroscopy Analysis of Bone Removal Using Er:YAG and CO2 Lasers. *J Periodontol* (2002) 73(6):643–52. doi: 10.1902/jop.2002.73.6.643
16. Lukac M, Marincek M, Grad L. Dental Laser Drilling: State of the Art With the Latest Generation of Variable Square Pulse Erbium Dental Laser Systems. *J Laser Health Acad* (2007) 2007(7/2):1–5.
17. Stübinger S, Nuss K, Pongratz M, Price J, Sader R, Zeilhofer HF, et al. Comparison of Er:YAG Laser and Piezoelectric Osteotomy: An Animal Study in Sheep. *Lasers Surg Med* (2010) 42(8):743–51. doi: 10.1002/lsm.20946
18. Stübinger S, Biermeier K, Bächi B, Ferguson SJ, Sader R, von Rechenberg B. Comparison of Er:YAG Laser, Piezoelectric, and Drill Osteotomy for Dental Implant Site Preparation: A Biomechanical and Histological Analysis in Sheep. *Lasers Surg Med* (2010) 42(7):652–61. doi: 10.1002/lsm.20944
19. Baek KW, Deibel W, Marinov D, Griessen M, Dard M, Bruno A, et al. A Comparative Investigation of Bone Surface After Cutting With Mechanical Tools and Er:YAG Laser. *Lasers Surg Med* (2015) 47(5):426–32. doi: 10.1002/lsm.22352
20. Baek KW, Dard M, Zeilhofer HF, Cattin PC, Juergens P. Comparing the Bone Healing After Cold Ablation Robot-Guided Er:YAG Laser Osteotomy and Piezoelectric Osteotomy-A Pilot Study in a Minipig Mandible. *Lasers Surg Med* (2020) 53(3):291–9. doi: 10.1002/lsm.23281
21. Ohsugi Y, Aoki A, Mizutani K, Katagiri S, Komaki M, Noda M, et al. Evaluation of Bone Healing Following Er:YAG Laser Ablation in Rat Calvaria Compared With Bur Drilling. *J Biophotonics* (2019) 12(3): e201800245. doi: 10.1002/jbio.201800245
22. Burgner J, Müller M, Raczkowsky J, Wörn H. Ex Vivo Accuracy Evaluation for Robot Assisted Laser Bone Ablation. *Int J Med Robot* (2010) 6(4):489–500. doi: 10.1002/rcs.366
23. Nguendon Kenhagho H, Shevchik S, Saeidi F, Faivre N, Meylan B, Rauter G, et al. Characterization of Ablated Bone and Muscle for Long-Pulsed Laser Ablation in Dry

and Wet Conditions. *Mater (Basel)* (2019) 12(8):1338. doi: 10.3390/ma12081338

24. Onisor I, Pecie R, Chaskelis I, Krejci I. Cutting and Coagulation During Intraoral Soft Tissue Surgery Using Er: YAG Laser. *Eur J Paediatr Dent* (2013) 14(2):140–5. doi: 10.1016/j.ijom.2019.05.012
25. Suter VGA, Altermatt HJ, Bornstein MM. A Randomized Controlled Trial Comparing Surgical Excisional Biopsies Using CO. *Int J Oral Maxillofac Surg* (2020) 49(1):99–106. doi: 10.1016/j.ijom.2019.05.012
26. Augello M, Baetscher C, Segesser M, Zeilhofer HF, Cattin P, Juergens P. Performing Partial Mandibular Resection, Fibula Free Flap Reconstruction and Midfacial Osteotomies With a Cold Ablation and Robot-Guided Er:YAG Laser Osteotome (CARLO. *J Craniomaxillofac Surg* (2018) 46(10):1850–5. doi: 10.1016/j.jcms.2018.08.001
27. Romeo U, Del Vecchio A, Palaia G, Tenore G, Visca P, Maggiore C. Bone Damage Induced by Different Cutting Instruments–An *In Vitro* Study. *Braz Dent J* (2009) 20(2):162–8. doi: 10.1590/S0103-64402009000200013
28. Stieglitz LH, Fichtner J, Andres R, Schucht P, Krähenbühl AK, Raabe A, et al. The Silent Loss of Neuronavigation Accuracy: A Systematic Retrospective Analysis of Factors Influencing the Mismatch of Frameless Stereotactic Systems in Cranial Neurosurgery. *Neurosurgery* (2013) 72(5):796–807. doi: 10.1227/NEU.0b013e318287072d
29. Yashin KS, Kravets LY, Gladkova ND, Gelikonov GV, Medyanik IA, Karabut MM, et al. [Optical Coherence Tomography in Neurosurgery]. *Zh Vopr Neirokhir Im N N Burdenko* (2017) 81(3):107–15. doi: 10.17116/neiro2017813107-115
30. Katkar RA, Tadinada SA, Amaechi BT, Fried D. Optical Coherence Tomography. *Dent Clin North Am* (2018) 62(3):421–34. doi: 10.1016/j.cden.2018.03.004

10

Comparison of the Accuracy and Clinical Parameters of Patient-Specific and Conventionally Bended Plates for Mandibular Reconstruction

Henriette L. Möllmann, Laura Apeltrath, Nadia Karnatz, Max Wilkat, Erik Riedel, Daman Deep Singh and Majeed Rana*

Department of Oral and Maxillofacial Surgery, University Hospital Duesseldorf, Duesseldorf, Germany

***Correspondence:** Henriette L. Möllmann, henriettelouise.moellmann@med.uni-duesseldorf.de*

Objectives: This retrospective study compared two mandibular reconstruction procedures—conventional reconstruction plates (CR) and patient-specific implants (PSI)—and evaluated their accuracy of reconstruction and clinical outcome.

Methods: Overall, 94 patients had undergone mandibular reconstruction with CR (n = 48) and PSI (n = 46). Six detectable and replicable anatomical reference points, identified *via* computer tomography, were used for defining the mandibular dimensions. The accuracy of reconstruction was assessed using pre- and postoperative differences.

Results: In the CR group, the largest difference was at the lateral point of the condyle mandibulae (D2) -1.56 mm (SD = 3.8). In the PSI group, the largest difference between preoperative and postoperative measurement was shown at the processus coronoid (D5) with +1.86 mm (SD = 6.0). Significant differences within the groups in pre- and postoperative measurements were identified at the gonion (D6) [$t(56) = -2.217$; $p = .031 < .05$]. In the CR group, the difference was 1.5 (SD = 3.9) and in the PSI group -1.04 (SD = 4.9). CR did not demonstrate a higher risk of plate fractures and post-operative complications compared to PSI.

Conclusion: For reconstructing mandibular defects, CR and PSI are eligible. In each case, the advantages and disadvantages of these approaches must be assessed. The functional and esthetic outcome of mandibular reconstruction significantly improves with the experience of the surgeon in conducting microvascular grafts and familiarity with computer-assisted surgery. Interoperator variability can be reduced, and training of younger surgeons involved in planning can be reaching better outcomes in the future.

Keywords: mandibular reconstruction, CAS, PSI, reconstruction plate, virtual planning

INTRODUCTION

After continuity resections of the lower jaw in case of carcinoma, osteonecrosis, osteomyelitis, or trauma, a mandibular reconstruction is essential to restore function and esthetics (1, 2). The size of the defect is determined by the preoperative extent, the entity of the pathology, and the resulting radicality of the resection.

Defects of the mandible are reconstructable using either a reconstruction plate without bony reconstruction or immediately with a combination of reconstruction plate and primary bone flap. For reconstructing with a fibula flap, hand-bended (conventional reconstruction) plates (CR) or patient-specific implants (PSI) can be used. Despite the considerable progress in microvascular surgery, complications, such as tissue necrosis, failure of the graft, infections (donor site or recipient), prolonged hospital stay, and a long recovery process, occur (3, 4).

Advancements in computer-assisted surgery (CAS), particularly with regard to computer-aided design/computer-aided manufacturing (CAD/CAM) technology, are beneficial compared to the traditional method of mandibular reconstruction with hand-bent plates (5–15). The accuracy of CAD/CAM or selective laser melting plates is superior to the manually bent reconstruction plates. These plates provide greater results in terms of strength and intraoperative positioning (16). The decisive factors for this procedure are anatomical and symmetrical bone shaping, restoration of a stable dental occlusion, and condylar repositioning into a centric relation (5, 17–19).

In the conventional technique, in contrast to CAS, the plates are bent intraoperatively or preoperatively manually before their adaptation. Depending on the complexity of the case and the skills as well as experience of the surgeon, this procedure might be very time-consuming. The standard plates offered by manufacturers do not always possess the required size and number of holes for the intraoperative situation. An advantage is offered by the PSI, which are more resistant to fracture while normally being thinner than CR. PSI do not need to be bent to fit the mandible of the patient and do not require predefined bending points such as with CR (20, 21). With the advancement of CAD/CAM technology, it is possible to accurately plan the reconstruction of craniofacial defects preoperatively, manufacture precise patient-specific implants, and place them in shorter operating times. The implant can be designed and shaped by the surgeon according to the defect size, shape, and morphology (22, 23). By selecting the appropriate design method, manufacturing process, and implant material, it is possible to perform a precise surgical procedure and reduce complications (24–31). The integration of this technology in the pre- and intraoperative workflow has simplified the production of cutting guides and has been shown to shorten the operation time and the length of stay and to improve osseus consolidation, symmetry, and morphology (10, 29, 32). Recent research demonstrated additional advantages, for instance, minimized interoperator variability caused by the experience of the surgeon and improved teaching possibilities for younger colleagues involved in the planning procedures/sessions with a senior consultant and/or biomedical engineer (33).

The preoperative planning of the exact position of dental implants is enabled for an early satisfying functional outcome (22). In contrast to the reported advantages, the time-consuming preoperative planning and associated costs need to be considered. With precise preoperative planning, it is challenging to react to unexpected intraoperative changes. Implementing changes in virtual planning is complicated (33, 34) and might increase the risk of R1 resections in tumor surgery in cases of primary reconstruction. An R1 resection is the macroscopic removal of the tumor. In histopathology, however, smaller portions of the tumor can be detected in the resection margin. The aim of this study was, on the one hand, to compare the results of patients regarding surgical technique and, on the other hand, to evaluate the accuracy and reproducibility of virtual surgical planning.

The use of modern technologies offers novel possibilities in the treatment of complex defect situations. With the development of preoperative virtual planning as well as PSI, another possibility emerged for achieving a true-to-the-original contour of the resected bone. Surgeons and users can use IPS Gate® to request, plan, and complete patient-specific products. The PSI, planning guidance, and anatomical models are manufactured using various materials with the help of the latest construction technologies. Through computer-based planning and functionalized PSI, preoperative planning can be transferred to higher precision of surgeries. For case creation, patient data and case-related information are uploaded to the web-based IPS Gate® platform. Based on the information and requirements of the users, the IPS® developer prepares the case planning in close collaboration with the surgeon. Once the resection margins have been defined, the donor region is virtually projected onto the recipient region, and the graft is designed for the best possible esthetic and functional restoration. Drilling and marking templates as well as a case-specific optimized implant are created. The type, diameter, and length of the osteosynthesis screws are defined. Finally, the surgeon approves the design for production.

In the study at hand, we analyze the restoration of the mandible with a PSI or with the conventional technique regarding their accuracy of reconstruction, the associated complication rate, and the outcome. To evaluate the reconstruction, six clinically relevant distances of the preoperative and postoperative conditions were evaluated. This is a less-followed approach but highly suitable for determining pre- and post-operative dimensions. With our research, clinicians comprehend the extent to which a PSI or conventional reconstruction is advisable for recovery with low complication rates and improved outcomes.

MATERIALS AND METHODS

This study was approved by the local ethics committee at the University of Düsseldorf, Germany (approval number 2018-250). In this retrospective study, the results of mandibular reconstructions of osseous defects treated with patient-specific or conventional implants in 2014–2019 in the Department of

Oral and Maxillofacial Plastic Surgery at the University Hospital Düsseldorf were evaluated.

Inclusion Criteria

All patients who underwent mandibular reconstruction at the Center for Operative Medicine II Clinic for Oral and Maxillofacial Plastic Surgery at the University Hospital Düsseldorf between 2014 and 2019 were included. Both alloplastic reconstructions and free microvascular grafts were included in this study. All cases operated on using the standard method with CR (hand-bended reconstruction plates) and those who received a PSI were included, as well as cases from secondary reconstruction.

Acquisition of Patient Data

Based on patient data, the course, the healing process, and the postoperative quality of life are compared. A group of 46 patients (PSI) were compared to 48 patients who were treated with a conventional procedure (CR). The following patient- and implant-related data were collected from clinical documentation, surgical reports, and findings:

- patient data (name, age, date of birth, and gender)
- preoperative findings (previous operations, concomitant diseases/pretreatments with possible effect on wound healing, etiology of the defect, histology of the defect, preoperative radiological findings, localization of the defect, and size of the defect)
- surgery (date, type of graft resection limits, ischemia time, duration of surgery, surgical technique, implant material, intraoperative fitting accuracy, complications during insertion and fixation of the implant, and necessary adjustment of the bony graft bed or the implant)
- inpatient stay (wound healing process, postoperative imaging, position of the implant, symmetry of the reconstruction, signs of loosening, complications, and length of stay)
- postoperative course (sensitivity disorders, pain, pressure sensitivity, skin conditions, scar conditions, and complications)
- preoperative and postoperative intercondylar distance

Selection of CT Data Sets

The preoperative CT image should accurately depict the current condition before partial mandibular resection and allow the measurement of the defined measurement distances. The postoperative dataset was the first postoperative image to show all relevant anatomical structures. For evaluation, the distances of the corresponding points were measured pre- and postoperatively and tabulated. In addition, the differences of the distances were determined by subtracting the postoperative value from the value determined preoperatively.

Determination of the Defect Extent and Size

To localize the osseous defect or lesion, the bony and soft tissue portions of the mandible were divided into sections. In the bony portion, four areas were defined according to the anatomy: the alveolar process (pars alveolaris mandibulae), the ascending branch (ramus mandibulae), the mandibular angle (angulus mandibulae), and the mandibular body (corpus mandibulae). If partial resection of the mandible is indicated, the sections can be resected individually or in combination, as well as unilaterally or bilaterally. The soft tissue portion of the mandible was divided into the tongue, floor of the mouth, cheek, and lip for localization in the presence of a lesion. With the aid of histopathology, radiology, or surgical reports, the defect size and localization were documented.

Measuring Points and Distances

To evaluate the reconstruction, six clinically relevant distances of the preoperative and postoperative situation were compared. The dataset was oriented according to the Frankfurt horizontal plane and mid-sagittal plane. Measurements were conducted from the capitulum (most lateral and most medial points), incisura (most caudal points), mandibular foramina, to the coronoid process (most cranial points), dorsal tip of the mandible closest to the gonion point) using preoperative and postoperative CT or CBCT. They run between the following bilateral anatomical structures: D1, capitulum mandibulae lateralmost point; D2, capitulum mandibulae medialmost point; D3, incisura mandibulae; D4, foramen mandibulae; D5, processus coronoideus; and D6, gonion dorsalmost tip of the mandible (cf. **Figure 1**). The measurements were captured using dicomPACS®.

To evaluate the accuracy of the reconstruction, the distances measured pre- and postoperatively were compared. This enables verifying whether the original position of the condyles and the symmetry of the mandible have been restored for ensuring functionality and esthetics. The restoration of the individual dimensions is a key quality factor after resection and the reconstruction of the mandible. Whether a narrowing or widening of the respective measured distance between the corresponding anatomical points has occurred postoperatively is reflected in the sign of the calculated difference. A deviation into the negative range means a narrowing of the section in question, while a deviation into the positive range is to be interpreted as a widening in this area. If the differences calculated for a patient have positive and negative signs, this means that opposing movements have taken place during the reconstruction, *i.e.*, the mandibular segments have rotated.

Statistical Analysis

The determined values of the measurements as well as the clinical data were statistically analyzed using jamovi (version 1.6.9). The Shapiro–Wilk test was conducted to check the data for normal distribution, and the Mann–Whitney *U*-test and Student's *t*-test were used to compare the means of the two groups. The Mann–Whitney *U*-test is a parameter-free statistical test that compares two independent samples that are not normally distributed. Thus, it is used to test the significance of the consistency between two distributions. A *p*-value of <.05 was defined as significant, a value of <.01 as very significant, and a value of <.001 as highly significant. A significance level of $p > .05$ is set for hypothesis testing. For associations between two variables, like A and B, Pearson's product–moment correlation

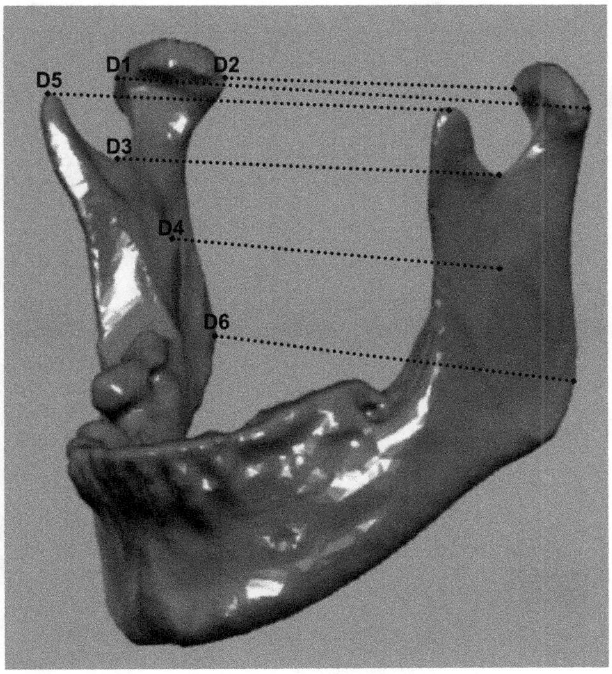

FIGURE 1 | Representation of the measurement distances. D1, lateralmost point of condyle mandibulae right to the lateralmost point of condyle mandibulae left; D2, medialmost point of condyle mandibulae right to the medialmost point of condyle mandibulae left; D3, most caudal point of the incisura mandibulae on the right to the most caudal point of the incisura mandibulae on the left; D4, foramen mandibulae on the right to the foramen mandibulae on the left, D5, processus coronoideus on the right to processus coronoideus on the left; D6, gonion on the right to gonion on the left.

(r) is calculated if the assumptions of linear relationship and exclusion of outliers tested by visual inspection of scatterplots and normal distribution of data, assessed with Shapiro-wilk test, were met. For non-normal data, Spearman's rank-order correlation (ρ) is calculated. Mean differences are tested with independent t-test when significant outliers, identified with boxplots, were excluded and normal distribution of the dependent variable, tested with Shapiro–Wilk test, and homoscedasticity, tested with Levene's test, were met. Mean differences of non-normal dependent variable data were analyzed with Mann–Whitney U-test.

RESULTS

Descriptive Statistics

The patient collective was distributed in two groups and analyzed according to age at the time of surgery, gender, clinical picture, and resection size. The collective consists of 94 patients. Forty-six patients received a PSI, and forty-eight patients were treated with a CR. (cf. **Table 1**).

The age of the patients was between 37 and 90 years (MD = 66.3; SD = 12.5) and distributed as normal. In the PSI group, the age ranged between 42 and 82 years (MD = 66.2; SD = 11.3), with 28 (60.9%) being male. Within the group of patients receiving the CR, the patients were between 37 and 90 years old (MD = 66.5; SD = 13.6), of which 54 (57.4%) were male. The mean age of groups PSI and CR did not differ significantly.

All patients were divided according to medical conditions that led to the indications of partial mandibular resection and subsequent reconstruction. Forty-five subjects were diagnosed with squamous cell carcinoma (SCC) (47.8%), and 20 received reconstruction with a PSI (44.4%). In each case, eight of 18 patients (44.4%) followed a diagnosis of maxillary necrosis with reconstruction using a PSI. A pathologic fracture was present in 17.0% (n = 16) of cases. Fracture was diagnosed in 2.0%, (n = 2), secondary reconstruction in 9.0% (n = 9), and osteomyelitis in 3.1% (n = 3) of patients. One patient developed basal cell carcinoma. In the patient population treated with PSI, four diagnoses occurred: SCC, osteomyelitis, secondary reconstruction, and pathological fracture.

Of the total of 46 patients who received a PSI, 20 (43.5%) had a resection indication based on the diagnosis of squamous cell carcinoma. In contrast, 25 patients with the same diagnosis were treated conventionally. Of the total of 18 patients diagnosed with mandibular necrosis, eight (44.4%) were treated with PSI, and 10 (55.6%) patients received a conventional reconstruction plate.

To investigate associations between a previous disease and a specific diagnosis, a differentiation was made between seven relevant previous diseases. These included cardiovascular, pulmonary, and metabolic diseases, nicotine and alcohol abuse, mental and neurological diseases, and the occurrence of another carcinoma. Considering the presence of previous diseases in each diagnostic group, it was found that 41 of 45 (91.1%) patients who developed squamous cell carcinoma had one or more previous diseases. All patients diagnosed with osteonecrosis of the jaw (n = 18) had a preexisting disease prior to this diagnosis. Patients with osteomyelitis (n = 3) or basal cell carcinoma (n = 1) had one or more prior diseases. In 33.3% (n = 3) of the cases, no previous disease was present in the secondary reconstructions. Using χ^2 test, no stochastic dependence between the general presence of a previous disease and a specific diagnosis was demonstrated [$\chi^2(1{,}94) = 10.9$; $p = .09$].

Fourteen of 18 patients diagnosed with osteonecrosis of the jaw, another carcinoma, were already present in terms of medical history, and a stochastic dependency between a prior disease and diagnosis was found [$\chi^2(1;94) = 11.3$; $p = .002$]. There was a stochastic dependence likewise between the diagnosis of pathologic fracture and the prior disease of nicotine abuse [$\chi^2(1;94) = 6.2$; $p = .013$]. In the sample, an average of M = 1.78 complications occurred (SD = 1.8).

On average, patients who received a PSI had two complications in the postoperative course (SD = 1.9). Patients who received a CR developed an average of 1.5 complications (SD = 1.7). The maximum number of complications was six in the PSI patient group and five in the CR patient group. No significant mean difference was tested with an achieved power of 15.8%.

The documented and possible complications that may occur after reconstruction include dehiscence, the development of

TABLE 1 | Descriptive statistics [conventional reconstruction plates (CR) *vs.* patient-specific implants (PSI)].

	CR	PSI	Total
Patients			
N	48	46	94
Age			
Years (mean ± SD)	66.5 ± 13.6	66.2 ± 11.3	66.3 ± 12.5
>60 years	64.6%	67.7%	65.9%
<60 years	35.4%	32.3%	34.1%
Gender			
Male	26 (54.2%)	28 (60.8%)	54 (57.4%)
Female	22 (45.8%)	18 (39.1%)	40 (42.6%)
Diagnosis			
SCC	25	20	45 (47.8%)
Maxillary necrosis	10	8	18 (16.1%)
Pathological fracture	10	6	16 (17.0%)
Fracture	0	2	2 (2.0%)
Osteomyelitis	0	3	3 (3.1%)
Basal cell carcinoma	0	1	1 (1.06%)
Secondary reconstruction	2	6	8 (8.0%)
Complications			
Mean ± SD	1.5 ± 1.7	2 ± 1.9	1.78 ± 1.8
N with complications	31 (48.0%)	33 (51.0%)	64 (68.1%)
Defect size (mm)			
Mean ± SD	58.8 ± 28.1	64.7 ± 29.2	61.7 ± 28.7
Maximum	120	120	120
Minimum	8	12	8
Operative time (min)			
Mean ± SD	397 ± 229	467 ± 240	431 ± 236
Maximum	1000	878	1000
Minimum	143	73	73
Hospital stay (days)			
Mean ± SD	26.4 ± 22.4	34.6 ± 32.4	
Maximum	97	125	
Minimum	4	6	
No reconstruction			
Mean ± SD	10.7 ± 8.4	27.1 ± 43.4	16.4 ± 26.5
Local reconstruction			
Mean ± SD	16.3 ± 8.8	27.1	15 ± 8.8
Microvascular reconstruction			
Mean ± SD	35.4 ± 24	36.7 ± 30.6	36.1 ± 27.8
Reconstruction group			
No reconstruction			20 (21.3%)
N complications (mean ± SD)			0.9 ± 1.39
Local reconstruction			7 (7.4%)
N complications (mean ± SD)			1.29 ± 1.8
Microvascular reconstruction			67 (71.3%)
N complications (mean ± SD)			2.07 ± 1.81
Tumor patients			
N (% of total)	25 (26.3%)	18 (19.1%)	43 (45.7%)
N complications (mean ± SD)	2.2 ± 1.8	2.56 ± 2.04	Tumor: 2.35 ± 1.9 No tumor: 1.3 ± 1.5

hematoma, exposed reconstruction plate, dysphagia, necrosis, infection, flap congestion, chyle fistula, restricted mouth opening, recurrence, revision, patient death, dislocation of the reconstruction plate, fistulation, and wound healing problems at the graft harvest site. The mean number of complications in the PSI and CR groups was not significantly different ($U = .57$; $p > .05$).

Overall, postoperative complications occurred in 64 of 94 patients (68.1%), and no complications occurred during follow-up in 30 patients (31.0%) after the use of PSI or CR. Of the patients with documented complications during the postoperative course, 48.4% ($n = 31$) had received a CR and 51.6% ($n = 33$) a PSI. No stochastic dependence could be determined between the occurrence of complications and the use of a PSI or CR. The probability of revision is not statistically dependent on diagnosis in the sample.

Mortality

Of the 45 patients diagnosed with SCC, 22.2% ($n = 10$) died. A stochastic dependence between the diagnosis of squamous cell carcinoma and the complication death could not be demonstrated using the chi-square test [$\chi^2(1;94) = 3.7$; $p = .056$]. The complication death was also not dependent on any of the diagnoses. Statistically, in patients in whom the complication of revision was documented, reconstruction ended lethally in the further course [$\chi^2(1;94) = 5.6$; $p = .018$].

Defect Size

The defect size of the collective varies from the minimum extension of 8 mm to a maximum of 120 mm (M = 61.7; SD = 28.7). In the patient-specific implant group, the size varies from the minimum extension of 12 mm to a maximum size of 120 mm (M = 64.7; SD = 29.2), which was not significantly different to the defect size of the conventional reconstruction plate group that varies from 8 to 120 mm (M = 58.8, SD = 28.1) (cf. **Figure 2**).

Operating Time

The mean operating time (OR) time of the sample was 431 min (SD = 236 min), the maximum OR time was 1,000 min, and the shortest OR time was 73 min. The mean OR time of PSI (M = 467 min, SD = 240 min) did not differ significantly to the OR time of CR (M = 397 min, SD = 229 min) [t (89) = -1.42; p = .159) (cf. **Figure 3**).

Length of Stay

The average length of stay of the group with PSI was 34.6 days (SD = 32.4) and was not significantly different to the group with CR which was 26.4 days (SD = 22.4; U = -1.4; p = .154). The shortest length of stay for the group with PSI was 6 days, and the longest length of stay was 125 days. For the patients with CR, the shortest length of stay was 4 days, and the longest was 97 days.

The mean values of the lengths of stay of the groups PSI and CR are not significantly different. Comparing the length of stay, the mean length of stay of patients with a microvascular graft is highest at 36.1 days (SD = 27.8). Patients who did not receive reconstruction stayed on the ward for an average of 16.4 days (SD = 26.5) and those with local reconstruction for 15 days (SD = 8.8).

In the group of PSI patients who received a microvascular graft, the mean inpatient length of stay was 36.7 days (SD = 30.6)

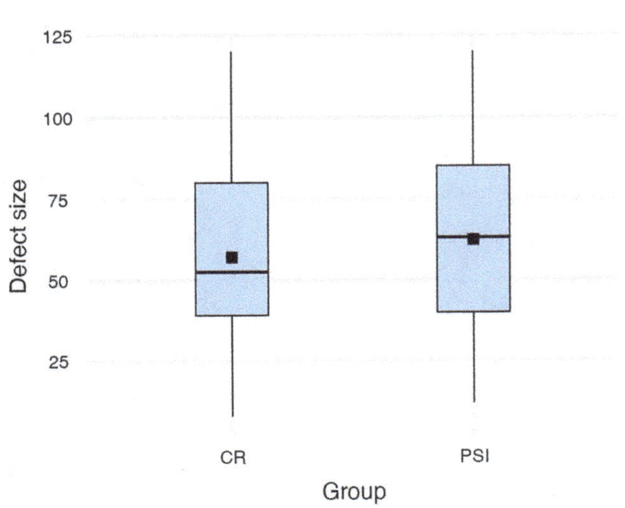

FIGURE 2 | Defect sizes in both groups (conventional reconstruction plates *vs*. patient-specific implants).

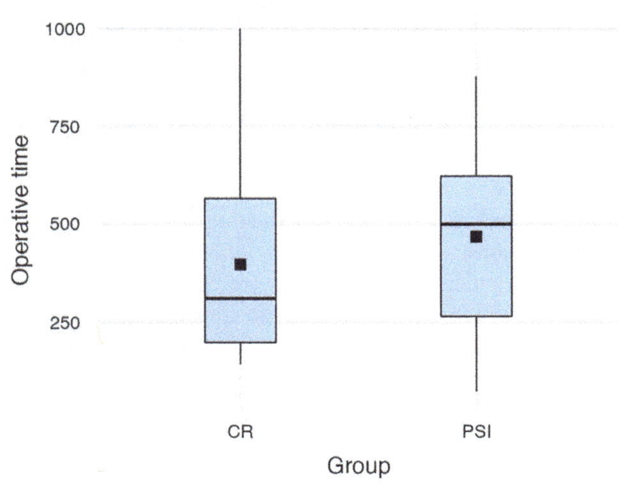

FIGURE 3 | Operation times in both groups (conventional reconstruction plates *vs*. patient-specific implants).

and in CR patients 35.4 days (SD = 24.0). Thus, length of stay for patients in the microvascular reconstruction group did not differ between those who received a patient-specific implant and those who received a conventional reconstruction plate.

Reconstruction Groups

Three reconstruction groups and seven reconstruction types are differentiated. The three groups consist of patients who received no reconstruction, local reconstruction, and microvascular reconstruction. Reconstruction options include grafts in the form of lingual, radial, pectoralis, and latissimus dorsi flaps as well as fibula grafts. In addition, combinations of grafts are possible for more complex defects.

In the sample, 21.3% (n = 20) of patients did not receive any reconstruction, 7.4% (n = 7) took place locally, and most reconstructions were microvascular at 71.3% (n = 67). On average, patients who received a microvascular graft developed the most complications (M = 2.1; SD = 1.8), followed by those who received local reconstruction (M = 1.3; SD = 1.8). Patients who did not receive reconstruction developed the least number of complications on average 0.9 (SD = 1.4).

Of the 45 patients diagnosed with SCC, 88.9% (n = 40) received a microvascular graft, two received no reconstruction, and three received local reconstruction, with a dependence between diagnosis and the use of a microvascular graft. In patients with the diagnosis of osteonecrosis of the jaw (n = 18), in 80% of these cases (n = 8), a microvascular graft was used. When considering complications in the postoperative course, a stochastic dependence was determined between the use of a microvascular graft and the development of dehiscence as a postoperative complication [χ^2 (1;94) = 6.3; p = .012]. Dehiscence was documented in 31 of the 67 patients who received a microvascular graft. Examination of the dependence between preexisting disease and reconstruction type revealed a stochastic dependence between preexisting disease in the form of alcohol abuse and the use of a microvascular graft

[χ^2(1;94) = 4.8; p = .029]. There were 15 patients diagnosed with the preexisting condition of alcohol abuse who received a microvascular graft. In the local reconstruction group, most patients had a prior cardiovascular disease (n = 5), four patients had a history of another CA, and three each were affected by nicotine abuse and metabolic disease. The most common prior disease in patients with microvascular reconstruction was also cardiovascular (n = 33), followed by nicotine abuse (n = 26), another carcinoma (n = 25), mental/neurological disease (n = 18), and alcohol abuse (n = 15).

Of the 94 patients included in the study, 45.7% (n = 43) were patients with a tumor disease. Of these 43 patients, 18 received a PSI, and 25 patients received a conventional reconstruction plate. No stochastic dependence was demonstrated between a tumor disease and the use of a PSI [χ^2(1;94) = 1.6; p = .208].

Squamous Cell Carcinoma

The number of complications between the group of tumor patients (M = 2.2, SD = 1.8) and the group with no tumor diagnosed (M = 1.4, SD = 1.6) does not differ significantly (U = 855, p = .051, r = .255). Thus, on average, significantly more complications develop in patients with a tumor disease. The mean number of complications in group PSI (M = 2.6; SD = 2.0) and in group CR (M = 2.2; SD = 1.8) did not differ significantly.

Differences Between the Measurements for PSI and Conventional Restorations

The defined measurement distances run between the following bilateral anatomical structures: D1, capitulum mandibulae lateralmost point; D2, capitulum mandibulae medialmost point; D3, incisura mandibulae; D4, foramen mandibulae; D5, processus coronoideus; and D6, gonion dorsalmost tip of mandible. Post-operative CT scans were, on average, taken 69.6 days after the surgery. Considering the differences of the measurement distances of the group supplied with PSI, on average, the smallest deviations occurred at the measurement point D4 (M = -.341; SD = 3.2) and the largest differences, on average, occurred at the measurement point D5 (M = 1.9; SD = 6.0). On average, the measurement points at the coronoid process seem to undergo the greatest change in position during repositioning of the resection parts. In group CR, the largest dimensional changes are drawn at D2 (M = -1.6; SD = 3.8) and the smallest postoperative changes at D5 (M = -.217; SD = 4.2). A direct comparison of the differences in the respective measured distances reveals the following: at D1, an average change of -.48 (SD = 4.4) is shown in group CR and -.585 (SD = 4.2) in group PSI. D2 showed an average change of -1.56 (SD = 3.6) for CR and -1.66 (SD = 4.1) for PSI, and D3 showed an average change of.838 (SD = 5.9) for group CR and -1.2 (SD = 3.8) for group PSI. In D5, group PSI experienced a mean postoperative difference of -1.86 (SD = 6.0) and group CR -.22 (SD = 4.2). The mean differences of the differences are significantly different at D6 [t(56) = -2.217; p = .031, d = .0286]. In all other measurement stretches, the mean postoperative differences are not significantly different between groups. Point D6 shows the mean postoperative differences of -1.04 (SD = 4.9) in group PSI and differences of 1.52 (SD = 3.9), on average, in group CR. Thus, there are significantly lower average postoperative differences between the measurement points at the gonion (cf. **Figure 4**).

Localization

For a more precise localization of the defect, nine sections were defined. These sections are divided into the tongue, floor of the mouth, alveolar process, mandibular ramus, mandibular angle, mandibular corpus, cheek, lip, and combinations of these localizations. The most frequent complications occurred in patients whose defect was localized to the mandibular corpus. A dependency between defects in the mandibular angle and the postoperative complication of wound healing disorders at the extraction site was found [χ^2(1;94) = 11.90; p = .049] Another dependency exists between the complication in the form of exposed plates and combined defects [χ^2(1;94) = 4.39; p = .036]. Complications most frequently occur in patients with defects localized to the floor of the mouth.

Defect Size Quartile

To validly compare defect sizes and examine them with respect to complications and dependencies on diagnosis, four quartiles were defined. Quartile 1 includes all patients whose defect is in the range of 0–30 mm, quartile 2 includes defects from 31 to 60 mm, all defects from 61 to 90 mm are in the third quartile, and all defects from 91 to 120 mm are in the fourth quartile. A statistical dependence between defects located in the first quartile and the diagnosis of pathologic fracture was determined [χ^2(1;94) = 8.87;

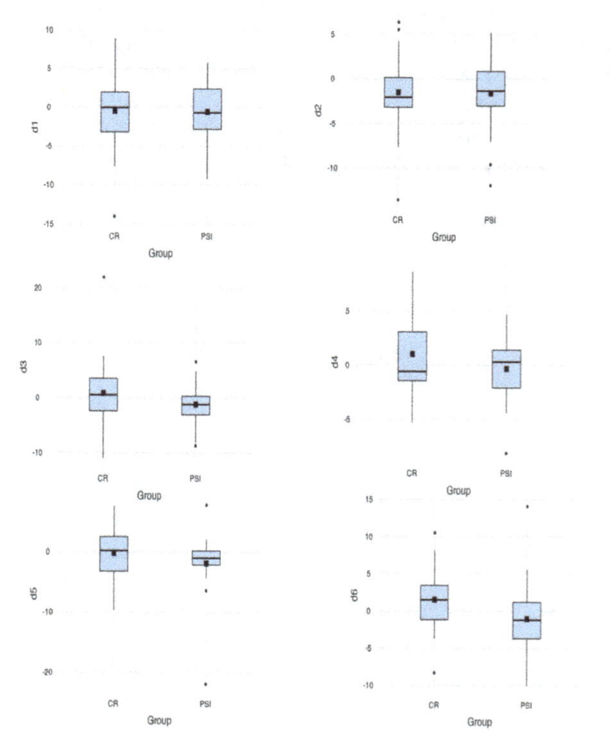

FIGURE 4 | Differences between the measurements (D1–D6) for conventional reconstruction plates and patient-specific implants; D6 [t(56) = -2.217; p = .031 <. 05].

p = .003]. Patients diagnosed with a pathologic fracture statistically had post-resection defects ranging in size from 0 to 30 mm. Similarly, patients had defect sizes in the range of 31-60 mm in 24% of cases because of a diagnosis of squamous cell carcinoma and subsequent resection. A statistical dependence between diagnosis and defect size was demonstrated again [χ^2 (1;94) = 3.77; p = .046]. Regarding the complications occurring post-resection, statistical dependencies between resection size and a complication exist in the first three quartiles. Patients with defect sizes in the range of up to 30 mm developed wound healing disorders at the donor site more frequently in the postoperative course [χ^2(1;94) = 8.57; p = .003].

DISCUSSION

Clinical parameters were retrospectively evaluated for obtaining differences in CR and PSI. The virtual planning is intended to support the surgeon in adhering resection limits. The use of computer-assisted planning and manufacturing of PSI should prevent oversizing the extent of resection while achieving R0 status. We investigated how the success of the operation is influenced by pre-existing diseases, previous operations, the size and etiology of the defect, localization, and occurring complications. The question arises as to whether the extensive preoperative virtual planning of the resection procedure leads to certain benefits: a reduced operation time, an optimal fit of the implants without dimensional changes of the bony mandible, and a reduction of the postoperative complication rates for patients.

The results further identified that there is no preferred approach when the defect exceeds a certain size. In the CR group, the mean defect size was 58.8 mm (SD = 28.1) and in the PSI group 64.7 mm (SD = 29.2). There was no significant difference regarding the mean defect size. The decision for or against a PSI is thus not linked to the size of the defect but rather depends on the discretion of the surgeon and the overall complexity of each case in this study. PSI are used primarily for extensive reconstruction (*i.e.*, multi-fragmentary fibula graft), multi-fragmentary fractures, or pseudarthrosis (35–38). Virtual preoperative planning might simplify the selection of a flap suitable for covering a defect as well as provide the basis for the design, shape, and positioning of the graft based on the previously produced three-dimensional model (39).

In CAD/CAM implants, intraoperative steps can be performed more effectively and efficiently compared to conventional methods in terms of minimizing the burden for patients as well as the risks of postoperative complications (1, 14, 15, 39–41). This approach was also followed by Rustemeyer et al. in their investigation of intraoperative times in osseous reconstructions with free fibular grafts. No significant differences were found between the CAD/CAM group and the conventional implant group (42). This was also shown by Ritschl et al. (43) who also revealed no significant differences between these groups (43). In contrast, other researchers reported shorter operation times in patients with CAD/CAM implants compared to conventionally performed operations (14, 15, 40). The results of this study are consistent with the current literature by Rustemeyer and Ritschl who determined no significant differences in operating times. On average, operations lasted 467 min (SD = 240 min) for patients who received PSI compared to 397 min (SD = 229 min) in the CR group. An exact prefabricated fit for reducing the insertion time of the implant as well as the overall duration of the surgery was not given. However, in case of a more complex operation with a pronounced defect and complex reconstruction, the step of dimensioning the resection margins and the graft can take place preoperatively. Intraoperatively, the prefabricated template makes these steps considerably easier for the surgeon and leads to shorter operation times in the long term (1, 44). In future studies, operations of equivalent complexity should be compared in terms of required time for the individual steps between the two groups—for example, tumor resections in which a radical neck dissection is also performed increase the time required compared to less complex resections. According to a recent study by Vaira et al., unilateral neck dissections require an average operative time of 71.2 min (SD = 27.2 min) (45). Accordingly, the time required doubles for bilateral operations, although variability can be assumed depending on the surgeon. Another component worth to be considered are consolidated workflows through the repeated use of PSI between 2014 and 2020. The growing experience with computer-planned and manufactured implants leads to minimized time for the individual steps. A comparable hypothesis was pursued in a study by Cho et al. who investigated the use of CAD/CAM-assisted surgery for craniosynostosis and concluded that even less experienced surgeons achieved equivalent long-term results with this method (46). Accordingly, gaining knowledge when performing computer-assisted surgery could be proportional to experience.

Comparing the inpatient length of stay of the two groups showed no significant differences. The same conclusion was reached by other researchers who examined the hospital stay between PSI and CR (12, 15, 43). The average length of stay of patients with PSI was approximately 9 days longer compared to patients with CR. Including all patients without differentiation might not yield significant results since, depending on whether reconstruction or resection was performed, the patients require longer recovery under inpatient monitoring. Therefore, a distinction was needed between patients who received a local reconstruction, microvascular reconstruction, and no reconstruction. The group of microvascular grafts showed the longest mean length of stay, followed by the local grafts and the group without reconstruction. Due to the higher complexity of the microvascular reconstructions, this group was divided into PSI and CR patients to compare the healing process and duration based on the inpatient length of stay. However, there were no significant differences between the two groups; this has also been shown by other researchers (13). The healing process might thus be independent of the type of reconstruction used.

The three reconstruction groups were examined regarding dependencies on different diagnoses. A total of 88.9% of patients diagnosed with squamous cell carcinoma received a microvascular reconstruction. An equally high proportion of microvascular grafts (80.0%) is found in patients who underwent resection due to osteonecrosis of the jaw. There is a statistical dependence on the use of a microvascular graft for both the diagnosis of SCC and the diagnosis of osteonecrosis of the jaw (p <.05). During the postoperative course, 46.3% of patients who received a microvascular graft developed dehiscence. Considering whether any of the documented pre-existing conditions predisposed to a particular graft, it was found that patients received a microvascular graft after C2 abuses in most cases (n = 15). Cardiovascular pathologies were recorded as the most frequent previous disease in the microvascular group. However, this association can also be attributed to the increasing morbidity in older age which also results in a higher susceptibility to developing cardiovascular diseases (47–49).

A total of 45.7% of all patients had a tumor disease, and 41.8% of these tumor patients received a PSI. Especially for patients with complex tumors in the jaw region, preoperative virtual planning can be very important for restoring function and contour (40). Thus, with the help of stereolithic models, the resection margins are precisely dimensioned so that these are tumor-free and less bone is resected (40). Oversizing and resection of healthy bone should be avoided by the CAD/CAM method. Moreover, the implant does not have to be bent to the osseous conditions intraoperatively but is already existing for exact insertion (50). In addition, a statistical dependency showed that patients with a tumor disease developed more complications regardless of whether they were treated with a PSI or a CR.

When looking at the measurement distances, significant differences were found in one measurement point. The difference between the gonion (defined as point 6) experienced an average dimensional change of 1.52 mm (SD = 3.9) in the group of CR patients and differed significantly from the group PSI, which only showed average differences of -1.04 mm (SD = 4.9). Recent research identified additional dimensional changes in patients who were restored with CR (31). A changed distance between the mandibular and the intercondylar angle after using intraoperatively bended plates was documented (51). This goes in line with previous research indicating that better three-dimensional precision is achieved when using PSI (1, 16, 31, 44, 51). Dimensional changes due to rotation errors of the resection parts are avoided by prescribing exact positioning in the preoperative planning aiming at restoring the physiological position (51).

The division into four quartiles allowed a more specific examination of the extent to which the size of the defect depends on the diagnosis and predisposes to certain complications. In 24.0% of SCC patients, the resection extent was between 31 and 60 mm, thus in the second size quartile. Tumor size in oral squamous cell carcinoma is a risk factor for the development of systemic inflammation and postoperative complications (52). In size quartile two, where the patients with SCC are located, an increased incidence of dehiscence in the postoperative course was identified. In defect size quartile three, between 61 and 90 mm, most frequent complications were exposed plates in the healing process. The literature indicates that a low number of residual teeth is a significant prognostic factor for reconstruction plate loss (53). The results of this study are consistent with the literature as bone loss in the 61–90-mm range is associated with loss of dentition. The choice of reconstruction has no impact on plate exposure in the healing process (54). Other risk factors are rather intraoperative blood loss and the choice of reconstruction flap (55).

CONCLUSION

For the reconstruction of mandibular defects, regardless of their etiology, the options available to the treating surgeon include CR and reconstruction using PSI. In each case, the advantages and disadvantages of the options must be weighed. Regardless of the method of fixation, the functional and esthetic outcomes of mandibular reconstruction have been significantly improved by the experience of the surgeon with microvascular grafts along with preoperative planning. In line with extant research, we highlighted that three-dimensional precision seems to be superior with a PSI. Interoperator variability can be reduced, and the training of younger surgeons involved in planning can be improved for better outcomes.

In future research, scholars might be interested in not only comparing the two methods used in this study but also validating the individual procedures. Thereby, the comparison of pre- and postoperative CT scans might be validated within the planning software (merging images). In a prospective study design, the required time for the individual virtual planning might be assessed along with relevant economic aspects, such as cost and time spent on patients receiving different surgical procedures.

AUTHOR CONTRIBUTIONS

MR and HM designed and coordinated this study. HM and LA collected data. HM, LA, ER, and MW analyzed the data. HM and LA wrote this paper. MR, DS, and NK general supervised the research group. All authors contributed to the article and approved the submitted version.

ACKNOWLEDGMENTS

The use of **Figure 1** was allowed with kind permission from the KLS Martin Group, Tuttlingen.

REFERENCES

1. Essig H, Rana M, Kokemueller H, von See C, Ruecker M, Tavassol F, et al. Pre-Operative Planning for Mandibular Reconstruction - A Full Digital Planning Workflow Resulting in a Patient Specific Reconstruction. *Head Neck Oncol* (2011) 3(1):45. doi: 10.1186/1758-3284-3-45
2. Zhou L, Shang H, He L, Bo B, Liu G, Liu Y, et al. Accurate Reconstruction of Discontinuous Mandible Using a Reverse Engineering/Computer-Aided Design/Rapid Prototyping Technique: A Preliminary Clinical Study. *J Oral Maxillofac Surg* (2010) 68(9):2115–21. doi: 10.1016/j.joms.2009.09.033
3. U V, Mehrotra D, Howlader D, Singh PK, Gupta S. Patient Specific Three-Dimensional Implant for Reconstruction of Complex Mandibular Defect.

J Craniofac Surg (2019) 30(4):e308–11. doi: 10.1097/SCS.0000000000005228

4. Chaine A, Pitak-Arnnop P, Hivelin M, Dhanuthai K, Bertrand J-C, Bertolus C. Postoperative Complications of Fibular Free Flaps in Mandibular Reconstruction: An Analysis of 25 Consecutive Cases. *Oral Surg Oral Med Oral Pathol Oral Radiol Endod* (2009) 108(4):488–95. doi: 10.1016/j.tripleo.2009.05.043
5. Eckardt A, Swennen GRJ. Virtual Planning of Composite Mandibular Reconstruction With Free Fibula Bone Graft. *J Craniofac Surg* (2005) 16 (6):1137–40. doi: 10.1097/01.scs.0000186306.32042.96
6. Hallermann W, Olsen S, Bardyn T, Taghizadeh F, Banic A, Iizuka T. A New Method for Computer-Aided Operation Planning for Extensive Mandibular Reconstruction. *Plast Reconstr Surg* (2006) 117(7):2431–7. doi: 10.1097/01.prs.0000219076.83890.e8
7. Adolphs N, Haberl E-J, Liu W, Keeve E, Menneking H, Hoffmeister B. Virtual Planning for Craniomaxillofacial Surgery – 7 Years of Experience. *J Craniomaxillofac Surg* (2014) 42(5):e289–95. doi: 10.1016/j.jcms.2013.10.008
8. Wilde F, Cornelius CP, Schramm A. Computer-Assisted Mandibular Reconstruction Using a Patient-Specific Reconstruction Plate Fabricated With Computer-Aided Design and Manufacturing Techniques. *Craniomaxillofac Trauma Reconstr* (2014) 7(2):158–66. doi: 10.1055/s-0034-1371356
9. Rodby KA, Turin S, Jacobs RJ, Cruz JF, Hassid VJ, Kolokythas A, et al. Advances in Oncologic Head and Neck Reconstruction: Systematic Review and Future Considerations of Virtual Surgical Planning and Computer Aided Design/Computer Aided Modeling. *J Plast Reconstr Aesthet Surg* (2014) 67 (9):1171–85. doi: 10.1016/j.bjps.2014.04.038
10. Gil RS, Roig AM, Obispo CA, Morla A, Pagès CM, Perez JL. Surgical Planning and Microvascular Reconstruction of the Mandible With a Fibular Flap Using Computer-Aided Design, Rapid Prototype Modelling, and Precontoured Titanium Reconstruction Plates: A Prospective Study. *Br J Oral Maxillofac Surg* (2015) 53(1):49–53. doi: 10.1016/j.bjoms.2014.09.015
11. Antony AK, Chen WF, Kolokythas A, Weimer KA, Cohen MN. Use of Virtual Surgery and Stereolithography-Guided Osteotomy for Mandibular Reconstruction With the Free Fibula. *Plast Reconstr Surg* (2011) 128 (5):1080–4. doi: 10.1097/PRS.0b013e31822b6723
12. Powcharoen W, Yang W-F, Yan Li K, Zhu W, Su Y-X. Computer-Assisted Versus Conventional Freehand Mandibular Reconstruction With Fibula Free Flap: A Systematic Review and Meta-Analysis. *Plast Reconstr Surg* (2019) 144 (6):1417–28. doi: 10.1097/PRS.0000000000006261
13. Barr ML, Haveles CS, Rezzadeh KS, Nolan IT, Castro R, Lee JC, et al. Virtual Surgical Planning for Mandibular Reconstruction With the Fibula Free Flap: A Systematic Review and Meta-Analysis. *Ann Plast Surg* (2020) 84(1):117–22. doi: 10.1097/SAP.0000000000002006
14. Serrano C, van den Brink H, Pineau J, Prognon P, Martelli N. Benefits of 3D Printing Applications in Jaw Reconstruction: A Systematic Review and Meta-Analysis. *J Craniomaxillofac Surg* (2019) 47(9):1387–97. doi: 10.1016/j.jcms.2019.06.008
15. Nilsson J, Hindocha N, Thor A. Time Matters - Differences Between Computer-Assisted Surgery and Conventional Planning in Cranio-Maxillofacial Surgery: A Systematic Review and Meta-Analysis. *J Craniomaxillofac Surg* (2020) 48(2):132–40. doi: 10.1016/j.jcms.2019.11.024
16. Rana M, Chin S-J, Muecke T, Kesting M, Groebe A, Riecke B, et al. Increasing the Accuracy of Mandibular Reconstruction With Free Fibula Flaps Using Functionalized Selective Laser-Melted Patient-Specific Implants: A Retrospective Multicenter Analysis. *J Craniomaxillofac Surg* (2017) 45 (8):1212–9. doi: 10.1016/j.jcms.2017.04.003
17. Urken ML, Weinberg H, Vickery C, Buchbinder D, Lawson W, Biller HF. Oromandibular Reconstruction Using Microvascular Composite Free Flaps: Report of 71 Cases and a New Classification Scheme for Bony, Soft-Tissue, and Neurologic Defects. *Arch Otolaryngol Head Neck Surg* (1991) 117(7):733–44. doi: 10.1001/archotol.1991.01870190045010
18. Hidalgo DA, Pusic AL. Free-Flap Mandibular Reconstruction: A 10-Year Follow-Up Study. *Plast Reconstr Surg* (2002) 110(2):438–49. doi: 10.1097/00006534-200208000-00010
19. Bak M, Jacobson AS, Buchbinder D, Urken ML. Contemporary Reconstruction of the Mandible. *Oral Oncol* (2010) 46(2):71–6. doi: 10.1016/j.oraloncology.2009.11.006
20. Rendenbach C, Sellenschloh K, Gerbig L, Morlock MM, Beck-Broichsitter B, Smeets R, et al. CAD-CAM Plates Versus Conventional Fixation Plates for Primary Mandibular Reconstruction: A Biomechanical In Vitro Analysis. *J Craniomaxillofac Surg* (2017) 45(11):1878–83. doi: 10.1016/j.jcms.2017.08.024
21. Telschow T, Wilde F, Pietzka S, Schramm A, Mascha F. Unbreakable? – Frakturen Patientenspezifischer Implantate Nach Alloplastischer Unterkieferrekonstruktion. *MKG-Chirurg* (2019) 12(4):263–7. doi: 10.1007/s12285-019-00220-x
22. Wilde F, Hanken H, Probst F, Schramm A, Heiland M, Cornelius C-P. Multicenter Study on the Use of Patient-Specific CAD/CAM Reconstruction Plates for Mandibular Reconstruction. *Int J Comput Assist Radiol Surg* (2015) 10(12):2035–51. doi: 10.1007/s11548-015-1193-2
23. Shan X-F, Chen H-M, Liang J, Huang J-W, Cai Z-G. Surgical Reconstruction of Maxillary and Mandibular Defects Using a Printed Titanium Mesh. *J Oral Maxillofac Surg* (2015) 73(7):1437.e1–9. doi: 10.1016/j.joms.2015.02.025
24. Roser SM, Ramachandra S, Blair H, Grist W, Carlson GW, Christensen AM, et al. The Accuracy of Virtual Surgical Planning in Free Fibula Mandibular Reconstruction: Comparison of Planned and Final Results. *J Oral Maxillofac Surg* (2010) 68(11):2824–32. doi: 10.1016/j.joms.2010.06.177
25. Hanasono MM, Skoracki RJ. Computer-Assisted Design and Rapid Prototype Modeling in Microvascular Mandible Reconstruction. *Laryngoscope* (2013) 123(3):597–604. doi: 10.1002/lary.23717
26. Hsu SS-P, Gateno J, Bell RB, Hirsch DL, Markiewicz MR, Teichgraeber JF, et al. Accuracy of a Computer-Aided Surgical Simulation Protocol for Orthognathic Surgery: A Prospective Multicenter Study. *J Oral Maxillofac Surg* (2013) 71(1):128–42. doi: 10.1016/j.joms.2012.03.027
27. Schendel SA, Jacobson R, Khalessi S. 3-Dimensional Facial Simulation in Orthognathic Surgery: Is it Accurate? *J Oral Maxillofac Surg* (2013) 71 (8):1406–14. doi: 10.1016/j.joms.2013.02.010
28. Stirling Craig E, Yuhasz M, Shah A, Blumberg J, Salomon J, Lowlicht R, et al. Simulated Surgery and Cutting Guides Enhance Spatial Positioning in Free Fibular Mandibular Reconstruction. *Microsurgery* (2015) 35(1):29–33. doi: 10.1002/micr.22229
29. Weitz J, Bauer F, Hapfelmeier A, Rohleder NH, Wolff K-D, Kesting MR. Accuracy of Mandibular Reconstruction by Three-Dimensional Guided Vascularised Fibular Free Flap After Segmental Mandibulectomy. *Br J Oral Maxillofac Surg* (2016) 54(5):506–10. doi: 10.1016/j.bjoms.2016.01.029
30. Farfalli GL, Albergo JI, Ritacco LE, Ayerza MA, Milano FE, Aponte-Tinao LA. What Is the Expected Learning Curve in Computer-Assisted Navigation for Bone Tumor Resection? *Clin Orthop Relat Res* (2017) 475(3):668–75. doi: 10.1007/s11999-016-4761-z
31. Zeller AN, Neuhaus MT, Weissbach LVM, Rana M, Dhawan A, Eckstein FM, et al. Patient-Specific Mandibular Reconstruction Plates Increase Accuracy and Long-Term Stability in Immediate Alloplastic Reconstruction of Segmental Mandibular Defects. *J Maxillofac Oral Surg* (2020) 19(4):609–15. doi: 10.1007/s12663-019-01323-9
32. Tarsitano A, Ciocca L, Scotti R, Marchetti C. Morphological Results of Customized Microvascular Mandibular Reconstruction: A Comparative Study. *J Craniomaxillofac Surg* (2016) 44(6):697–702. doi: 10.1016/j.jcms.2016.03.007
33. Avraham T, Franco P, Brecht LE, Ceradini DJ, Saadeh PB, Hirsch DL, et al. Functional Outcomes of Virtually Planned Free Fibula Flap Reconstruction of the Mandible. *Plast Reconstr Surg* (2014) 134(4):628e–34e. doi: 10.1097/PRS.0000000000000513
34. Moro A, Cannas R, Boniello R, Gasparini G, Pelo S. Techniques on Modeling the Vascularized Free Fibula Flap in Mandibular Reconstruction. *J Craniofac Surg* (2009) 20(5):1571–3. doi: 10.1097/SCS.0b013e3181b0db5c
35. Nocini PF, Saia G, Bettini G, Ragazzo M, Blandamura S, Chiarini L, et al. Vascularized Fibula Flap Reconstruction of the Mandible in Bisphosphonate-Related Osteonecrosis. *Eur J Surg Oncol* (2009) 35(4):373–9. doi: 10.1016/j.ejso.2008.05.002
36. Foster RD, Anthony JP, Sharma A, Pogrel MA. Vascularized Bone Flaps Versus Nonvascularized Bone Grafts for Mandibular Reconstruction: An Outcome Analysis of Primary Bony Union and Endosseous Implant Success. *Head Neck* (1999) 21(1):66–71. doi: 10.1002/(SICI)1097-0347(199901)21:1<66::AID-HED9>3.0.CO;2-Z
37. Pogrel M, Podlesh S, Anthony JP, Alexander J. A Comparison of Vascularized

and Nonvascularized Bone Grafts for Reconstruction of Mandibular Continuity Defects. *J Oral Maxillofac Surg* (1997) 55(11):1200–6. doi: 10.1016/S0278-2391(97)90165-8
38. de Santis G, Pinelli M, Starnoni M. Extended and Unusual Indications in Jaw Reconstruction With the Fibula Flap: An Overview Based on Our 30-Year Experience. *Ann Med Surg* (2021) 62:37–42. doi: 10.1016/j.amsu.2020.12.049
39. Modabber A, Ayoub N, Möhlhenrich SC, Goloborodko E, Sönmez TT, Ghassemi M, et al. The Accuracy of Computer-Assisted Primary Mandibular Reconstruction With Vascularized Bone Flaps: Iliac Crest Bone Flap Versus Osteomyocutaneous Fibula Flap. *Med Devices (Auckl)* (2014) 7:211–7. doi: 10.2147/MDER.S62698
40. Ren W, Gao L, Li S, Chen C, Li F, Wang Q, et al. Virtual Planning and 3D Printing Modeling for Mandibular Reconstruction With Fibula Free Flap. *Med Oral Patol Oral Cir Bucal* (2018) 23(3):e359–66. doi: 10.4317/medoral.22295
41. Tiberio F, Cacciotti I, Frassanito P, Nocca G, Tamburrini G, Arcovito A, et al. Personalized Bone Reconstruction and Regeneration in the Treatment of Craniosynostosis. *Appl Sci* (2021) 11(6):2649. doi: 10.3390/app11062649
42. Rustemeyer J, Sari-Rieger A, Melenberg A, Busch A. Comparison of Intraoperative Time Measurements Between Osseous Reconstructions With Free Fibula Flaps Applying Computer-Aided Designed/Computer-Aided Manufactured and Conventional Techniques. *Oral Maxillofac Surg* (2015) 19(3):293–300. doi: 10.1007/s10006-015-0493-6
43. Ritschl LM, Mücke T, Fichter A, Güll FD, Schmid C, Duc JMP, et al. Functional Outcome of CAD/CAM-Assisted Versus Conventional Microvascular, Fibular Free Flap Reconstruction of the Mandible: A Retrospective Study of 30 Cases. *J Reconstr Microsurg* (2017) 33(4):281–91. doi: 10.1055/s-0036-1597823
44. Modabber A, Legros C, Rana M, Gerressen M, Riediger D, Ghassemi A. Evaluation of Computer-Assisted Jaw Reconstruction With Free Vascularized Fibular Flap Compared to Conventional Surgery: A Clinical Pilot Study. *Int J Med Robot* (2012) 8(2):215–20. doi: 10.1002/rcs.456
45. Vaira LA, de Riu G, Ligas E, Deiana G, Vacca G, Massarelli O, et al. Neck Dissection With Harmonic Instruments and Electrocautery: A Prospective Comparative Study. *Oral Maxillofac Surg* (2021) 25(1):75–9. doi: 10.1007/s10006-020-00897-w
46. Cho RS, Lopez J, Musavi L, Kachniarz B, Macmillan A, Badiei B, et al. Computer-Assisted Design and Manufacturing Assists Less Experienced Surgeons in Achieving Equivalent Outcomes in Cranial Vault Reconstruction. *J Craniofac Surg* (2019) 30(7):2034–8. doi: 10.1097/SCS.0000000000005748
47. Forman DE, Maurer MS, Boyd C, Brindis R, Salive ME, Horne FM, et al. Multimorbidity in Older Adults With Cardiovascular Disease. *J Am Coll Cardiol* (2018) 71(19):2149–61. doi: 10.1016/j.jacc.2018.03.022
48. Barnes PJ. Mechanisms of Development of Multimorbidity in the Elderly. *Eur Respir J* (2015) 45(3):790–806. doi: 10.1183/09031936.00229714
49. Forman DE, Rich MW, Alexander KP, Zieman S, Maurer MS, Najjar SS, et al. Cardiac Care for Older Adults. Time for a New Paradigm. *J Am Coll Cardiol* (2011) 57(18):1801–10. doi: 10.1016/j.jacc.2011.02.014
50. Rana M, Essig H, Eckardt AM, Tavassol F, Ruecker M, Schramm A, et al. Advances and Innovations in Computer-Assisted Head and Neck Oncologic Surgery. *J Craniofac Surg* (2012) 23(1):272–8. doi: 10.1097/SCS.0b013e318241bac7
51. Naros A, Weise H, Tilsen F, Hoefert S, Naros G, Krimmel M, et al. Three-Dimensional Accuracy of Mandibular Reconstruction by Patient-Specific Pre-Bent Reconstruction Plates Using an "in-House" 3D-Printer. *J Craniomaxillofac Surg* (2018) 46(9):1645–51. doi: 10.1016/j.jcms.2018.05.047
52. Kågedal Å, Rydberg Millrud C, Häyry V, Kumlien Georén S, Lidegran M, Munck-Wikland E, et al. Oropharyngeal Squamous Cell Carcinoma Induces an Innate Systemic Inflammation, Affected by the Size of the Tumour and the Lymph Node Spread. *Clin Otolaryngol* (2018) 43(4):1117–21. doi: 10.1111/coa.13122
53. Hirohata H, Yanagawa T, Takaoka S, Yamagata K, Sasaki K, Shibuya Y, et al. A Small Number of Residual Teeth After the Mandibular Resection of Oral Cancer Is Associated With Titanium Reconstruction Plate Exposure. *Clin Exp Dent Res* (2019) 5(5):469–75. doi: 10.1002/cre2.208
54. Nicholson RE, Schuller DE, Forrest LA, Mountain RE, Ali T, Young D. Factors Involved in Long- and Short-Term Mandibular Plate Exposure. *Arch Otolaryngol Head Neck Surg* (1997) 123(2):217–22. doi: 10.1001/archotol.1997.01900020107016
55. Fanzio PM, Chang K-P, Chen H-H, Hsu H-H, Gorantla V, Solari MG, et al. Plate Exposure After Anterolateral Thigh Free-Flap Reconstruction in Head and Neck Cancer Patients With Composite Mandibular Defects. *Ann Surg Oncol* (2015) 22(9):3055–60. doi: 10.1245/s10434-014-4322-1

11

The Learning Curve of Computer-Assisted Free Flap Jaw Reconstruction Surgery using 3D-Printed Patient-Specific Plates: A Cumulative Sum Analysis

*Wang-yong Zhu, Wing Shan Choi, May Chun Mei Wong, Jingya Jane Pu†, Wei-fa Yang and Yu-xiong Su**

Division of Oral and Maxillofacial Surgery, Faculty of Dentistry, The University of Hong Kong, Hong Kong, SAR China

***Correspondence:**
Yu-xiong Su
richsu@hku.hk

†ORCID:
Jingya Jane Pu
orcid.org/0000-0001-8349-4031

Background: Computer-assisted jaw reconstruction (CAJR) has benefits in reducing operation time and improving reconstruction accuracy, compared to conventional freehand jaw reconstruction. However, no information is available regarding learning curves in CAJR with the use of 3D-printed patient-specific surgical plates (PSSP). The purpose of this study was to assess surgical outcomes and learning curve for the first 58 consecutive CAJR using 3D-printed PSSP performed by a single surgical team in a single institution.

Methods: In a prospective study, consecutive patients who underwent free flap CAJR using 3D-printed PSSP were included. The determination of proficiency, based on the cumulative sum of surgical success (no major adjustment of 3D-printed PSSP, flap survival) passing the acceptable boundary line of cumulative sum analysis, was the primary outcome. To find out any potential factors influencing the learning curve, baseline characteristics of patients were compared before and after proficiency achievement. Secondary outcomes included inflexion points of the total operation time, blood loss, length of hospital stay, and bone graft deviation, measured by the cumulative sum analysis.

Results: From December 2016 to November 2020, 58 consecutive cases underwent surgery performed by a single surgical team. The overall surgical success rate was 94.8% (55/58). A three-stage learning curve of primary outcome was observed. The proficiency was achieved after 23 cases. The proportions of advanced tumor staging and concomitant surgery after obtaining proficiency were significantly higher than those before achieving proficiency ($p = 0.046$ and $p < 0.001$, respectively). Mean values of operation time, intraoperative blood loss, length of hospital stay, and bone graft deviation were 532.5 ± 119.2 min, 1,006.8 ± 547.2 ml, 16.1 ± 6.3 days, and 0.9 ± 1.2 mm, respectively. Two trends of learning curve were observed in the CUSUM analyses of total operation time, length of hospital stay, and bone graft deviation, in which the first and second inflexion points occurred between 8 and 17 cases and between 43 and 46 cases, respectively.

Conclusion: Our results revealed a three-stage learning curve of CAJR with the use of PSSP, including initial learning, plateau, and overlearning. Based on CUSUM analysis, the surgical proficiency was achieved after 23 cases, and total operation time, length of hospital stay, and bone graft deviation stabilized after 8–17 cases.

Keywords: computer-assisted jaw reconstruction, virtual surgical planning, patient-specific surgical plate, three-dimensional printing technology, learning curve, cumulative sum analysis

INTRODUCTION

The emerging technique of computer-assisted jaw reconstruction (CAJR), which facilitates preoperative surgery simulation and transfers the virtual plan to a real operation, significantly impacted conventional surgical approaches (1, 2). Studies have reported the benefits of CAJR compared to conventional freehand jaw reconstruction, including reductions of ischemia time, operation time, and related costs, and improvement of reconstruction accuracy (3–10).

With the increasing popularization of CAJR surgery, the needs of standardizing surgical training and optimizing patient outcomes are urgent. The cumulative sum (CUSUM) control chart is a sequential analysis technique in statistical quality control, typically used for monitoring change detection (11). Now, the concept of CUSUM analysis has been used by surgeons to assess the learning curve in complex surgeries, such as robot-assisted surgery and endoscopic surgery (12–14). It allows surgeons to precisely detect potential imperfections and then improve surgical outcomes. However, very sparse data are available on learning curves of free flap jaw reconstruction (15–18). To our best knowledge, there is no study reporting the learning curve in the practice of CAJR.

Our team started performing CAJR using 3D-printed patient-specific surgical plates (PSSP) in December 2016. We reported our first experience in 2018 and indicated that CAJR with PSSP is feasible, safe, and precise (19). This study aimed to analyze the surgical outcomes and learning curve for the first 58 consecutive CAJR cases using 3D-printed PSSP performed by a single surgical team in a single institution.

MATERIALS AND METHODS

This study was approved by the Institutional Review Board of the University of Hong Kong/Hospital Authority Hong Kong West Cluster (No. UW 16-315), registered in ClinicalTrials.gov with a No. of NCT03057223 and in The University of Hong Kong Clinical Trials Centre with a study identifier of HKUCTR-2113 (www.HKUCTR.com).

Surgical Interventions

From December 2016 to November 2020, all consecutive patients who underwent CAJR with 3D-printed PSSP performed by a single surgical team led by the same chief surgeon in the Queen Mary Hospital in Hong Kong were enrolled without dropout. Before December 2016, the surgical team had no previous experience in using PSSP.

The virtual planning, design, and fabrication of 3D-printed PSSP and surgical techniques have been described in our previous publications (19, 20). Patients indicated for jaw surgery were arranged to undertake contrast-enhanced CT scan of head and neck and the donor site. The virtual surgical planning was done using Proplan CMF 3.0 software (Materialise, Leuven, Belgium). To exactly transfer the surgical plan to the operation room, we designed PSSP in line with the planned surgery using the 3-Matic software (Materialise, Leuven, Belgium). The surgical templates were printed using the stereolithography technology from high-strength resin. The plates were printed using Grade 2 pure titanium by selective laser melting technology. All the surgical procedures and perioperative management were conducted in a routine manner, except that osteotomies, bone movements, and flap inset were guided by the prepared 3D-printed patient-specific surgical templates and fixed by the 3D-printed patient-specific pure titanium plate. Patients were followed up regularly. Plain x-ray image and CT/CBCT scanning were done approximately 1 month after surgery.

Outcomes

The primary outcome was the achievement of proficiency. All CAJR cases were recorded chronologically by operation date. Proficiency was based on the cumulative sum of surgical success reaching the acceptable boundary line of the CUSUM analysis. Surgical success was defined as no change of 3D-printed PSSP (major adjustment of plates, including the need for bending plate and conversion to conventional commercialized titanium plates) and flap survival. Cases were divided into two groups according to the achievement of proficiency, and the baseline characteristics were compared to analyze the potential factors influencing the learning curves.

The secondary outcomes were the stabilization of total operation time, intraoperative blood loss, length of hospital stay, and reconstruction accuracy to a steady state. The determination of stabilization was based on the inflection point of the cumulative graph. The accuracy of jaw reconstruction 1 month postoperatively was measured by calculating the deviation distance between preoperative planned and postoperative achieved bone graft positions using the same method described previously (4).

CUSUM Analysis

CUSUM analysis was performed to detect subtle deviations of the surgeon's performance in primary and secondary outcomes (21).

The overall fibula flap failure rate was revealed as 7.0% (n = 161/2,305) by the latest systematic review and meta-analysis (22). Since fibula flaps were used in most of our cases, we utilized 7.0% as the current failure rate of free flap. We reviewed the available studies using PSSP in maxillofacial reconstruction (**Table 1**) and pooled the current failure rate of PSSP as 4.4% (n = 6/136) (19, 23–27). Therefore, the overall success rate of implementing free flap and PSSP was 88.9%, and the acceptable level of surgical failure (p0) was set at 11.1% [100% – (100% – 7.0%) × (100% – 4.4%)] in the CUSUM analysis. A chosen level of surgical failure rate (p1) reflecting a change in surgical performance was set as two times the acceptable level of surgical failure (28). All calculation procedures and intermediate values are shown in **Appendix**. Briefly, with each surgical success obtained, the line would rise by 0.162; with each failure, the line would fall by 0.838. Type 1 and type 2 errors, the probabilities of wrongly accusing the surgeon of unacceptable performance and acceptable performance, were set as 0.10, which were considered rational (28). Boundary lines were calculated to determine whether the surgical performance was acceptable (H_1) or unacceptable (H_0). Once the line reached H_1 or H_0, proficiency was obtained or lost, respectively.

The sequential differences of total operation time, intraoperative blood loss, length of hospital stay, and bone graft deviation between each case and the mean value were also detected by CUSUM (29). The mean values of each variable were calculated and used as the reference. Briefly, with each variable more or less than the mean value, the line would rise or fall by the absolute difference, respectively. The best-fit curve and its corresponding equation were determined with the cftool command in Excel (version 2019; Microsoft Corporation, USA).

Statistical Analysis

All statistics were calculated using SPSS Statistics (version 26.0; IBM Corporation, Chicago, IL, USA). Data were presented as number (percentage) for categorical data and mean ± standard deviation for continuous data. Independent samples t test was used to detect differences in the means in the patients' age and donor bone length. Chi-square test was used to detect differences in the proportions of gender, diagnosis, TNM classification, surgical site, bone segments, and concomitant surgery. $p < 0.05$ was considered statistically significant.

TABLE 1 | Literature review on studies using PSSP in maxillofacial reconstruction.

Author	Total No. of Cases Using PSSP	Failed No. of Cases Using PSSP
Frank Wilde, 2015 (23)	32	6
Majeed Rana, 2017 (24)	22	0
Yang, 2018 (19)	10	0
David Öhman, 2019 (25)	5	0
Philipp Jehn, 2020 (26)	20	0
Zavattero, 2021 (27)	47	0

RESULTS

A total of 58 consecutive patients who underwent CAJR using PSSP were included. Baseline characteristics of total cases are shown in **Table 2**.

Primary Outcome

Altogether, surgical failure occurred in 5.2% of patients (3/58). One was intraoperative flap failure due to sclerotic vessels and recurrent arterial thrombosis. The other two cases were postoperative flap failures caused by venous compromise of flap at postoperative day 4 and late-stage artery thrombosis at postoperative day 10. 3D-printed PSSP were successfully used in all the patients. **Figure 1** shows the CUSUM analysis of the surgical success for the surgeon. After a surgical failure occurred in the 11th case, a steadily climbing line was seen and proficiency was first obtained after 23 cases. A new concomitant surgery of simultaneous dental implant placement with or without immediate loading was added to selective cases from the 23rd case. Two surgical failures occurred in the 26th and 33rd cases

TABLE 2 | Baseline characteristics and surgical details.

Characteristics	Total cases (n = 58)
Gender (n, %)	
Male	26 (44.8%)
Female	32 (55.2%)
Age (years)	59.3 ± 16.0
Diagnosis (n, %)	
Malignant tumor	40 (69.0%)
Benign tumor	13 (22.4%)
Others[a]	5 (8.6%)
TNM classification[b] (40 cases) (n, %)	
Stage I and II	15 (37.5%)
Stage III and IV	25 (62.5%)
Surgical site (n, %)	
Mandible	44 (75.9%)
Maxilla	14 (24.1%)
Donor bone graft (n, %)	
Fibula	54 (93.1%)
Iliac crest	4 (6.9%)
Donor bone length (mm)	89.7 ± 31.0
Bone segments (n, %)	
One	12 (20.7%)
Two	31 (53.4%)
Three and more	15 (25.9%)
Concomitant surgery (n, %)	
None	36 (62.1%)
Simultaneous dental implant	21 (36.2%)
Radial forearm flap	1 (1.7%)

[a]*Others: osteoradionecrosis of the jaw (n = 4) and mandibular defect secondary to malignancy resection (n = 1).*
[b]*According to the AJCC (American Joint Committee on Cancer) Cancer Staging Manual (8th Edition).*

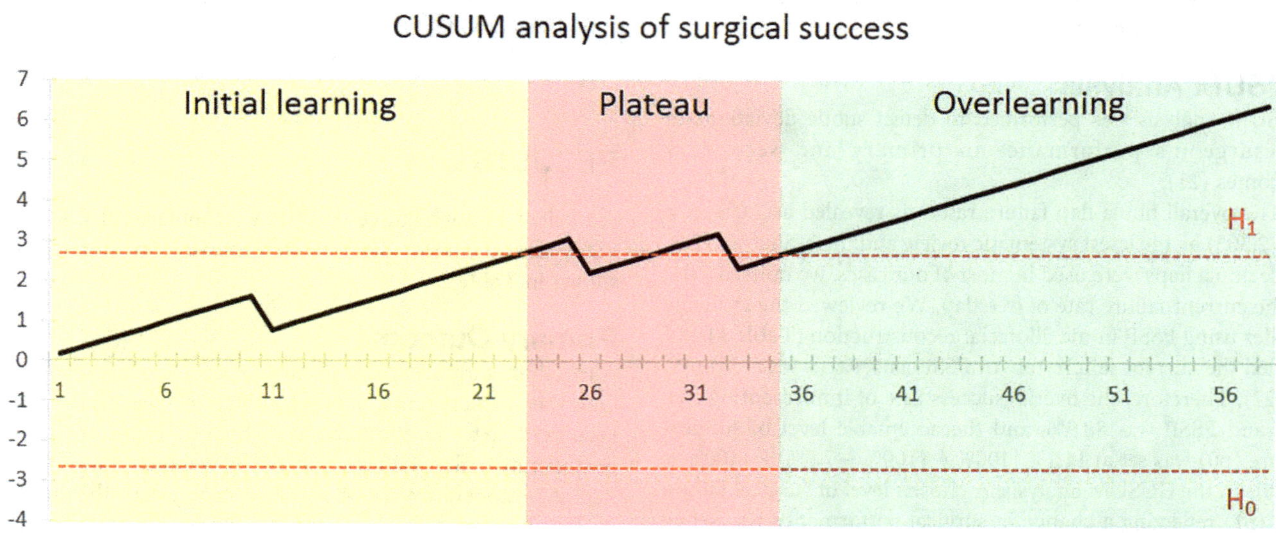

FIGURE 1 | CUSUM analysis of surgical success for the CAJR with PSSP performed by the surgical team. The *x*-axis shows the chronological sequence of cases. The black line indicates the cumulative sum of surgical success. The horizontal red dotted lines represent the acceptable boundary line H_1 and unacceptable boundary line H_0. Proficiency was first achieved after 35 cases.

and the surgical performance line dropped below the acceptable boundary line. After that, proficiency was completely regained after 35 cases.

According to the achievement of proficiency, we divided the patients into two groups. From the baseline characteristics of the two groups in **Table 3**, there was no significant difference in the patient's baseline features, except TNM stage ($p = 0.046$) and concomitant surgery ($p < 0.001$). From the 24th to 58th cases, the proportions of stage III & IV malignancy and concomitant surgery were significantly higher than the first 23 cases, indicating an increased proportion of cases with advanced stage malignancy and more complex surgery after first achieving the proficiency.

Secondary Outcomes

The mean operation time was 532.5 ± 119.2 min. The inflexion point is the 8th case, from which the operation time started to diminish, although there was a slight trend of increasing operation time from the 28th case to the 46th case. The linear and CUSUM analysis graphs of total operation time are shown in **Figure 2**.

Mean intraoperative blood loss was 1,006.8 ± 547.2 ml. There was a trend of decreasing blood loss in the first 22 cases. After that, the intraoperative blood loss was increasing. The linear and CUSUM analysis graphs of intraoperative blood loss are shown in **Figure 3**.

Mean length of hospital stay was 16.1 ± 6.3 days. Four inflexion points were presented at the 5th, 17th, 28th, and 45th cases, respectively. The linear and CUSUM analysis graphs of hospital stay length are shown in **Figure 4**.

Mean bone graft deviation was 0.9 ± 1.2 mm. After 15 cases, the bone graft deviation started to diminish as a general trend. However, from the 31st to 43rd cases, a slightly increasing trend of bone graft deviation was observed. The linear and CUSUM analysis graphs of bone grafts deviation are shown in **Figure 5**.

TABLE 3 | Comparison of baseline characteristics among chronological 2 groups.

Characteristics	Group 1 (Case No.1-23)	Group 2 (Case No.24-58)	P value
Gender (n; %)			
Male	8 (34.8%)	18 (51.4%)	0.212
Female	15 (65.2%)	17 (48.6%)	
Age (years)	58.7±15.0	59.6±16.9	0.831
Diagnosis (n; %)			
Malignant tumor	16 (69.6%)	24 (68.6%)	0.523
Benign tumor	4 (17.4%)	9 (25.7%)	
Others	3 (13.0%)	2 (5.7%)	
TNM classification (40 cases) (n; %)			
Stage I & II	9 (56.3%)	6 (25.0%)	0.046
Stage III & IV	7 (43.8%)	18 (75.0%)	
Surgical site (n; %)			
Mandible	17 (73.9%)	27 (77.1%)	0.779
Maxilla	6 (26.1%)	8 (22.9%)	
Donor bone graft (n; %)			
Fibula	21 (91.3%)	33 (94.3%)	0.522
Iliac crest	2 (8.7%)	2 (5.7%)	
Donor bone length (mm)	89.6±36.5	89.7±27.4	0.982
Bone segments (n; %)			
One	4 (17.4%)	8 (22.9%)	0.771
Two	12 (52.2%)	19 (54.3%)	
Three and more	7 (30.4%)	8 (22.9%)	
Concomitant surgery (n; %)			
No	22 (95.7%)	14 (40.0%)	<0.001
Yes	1 (4.3%)	21 (60.0%)	

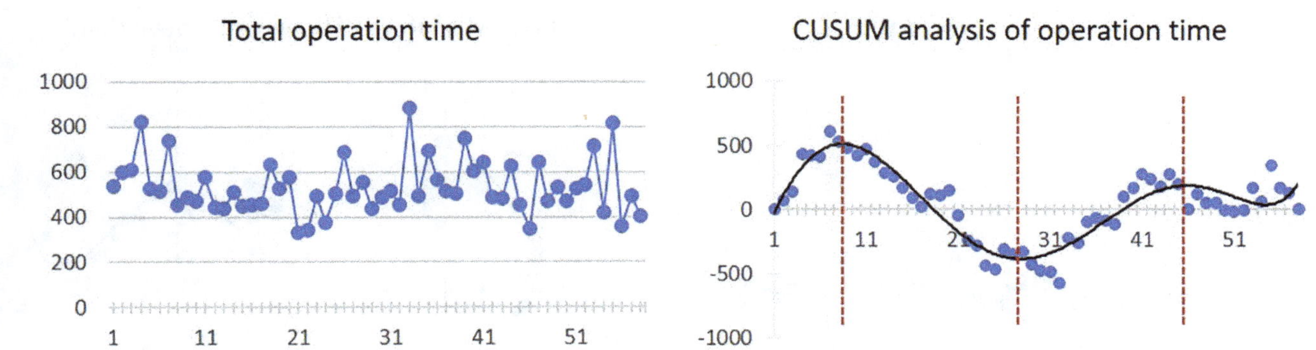

FIGURE 2 | Linear graph and CUSUM analysis of total operation time in CAJR applying patient-specific surgical plates. The black line represents the curve of best fit in a general model with equation, $y = 4E{-}06x^6 - 0.0006x^5 + 0.0299x^4 - 0.3358x^3 - 9.1732x^2 + 168.85x - 187.47$, $R^2 = 0.8506$.

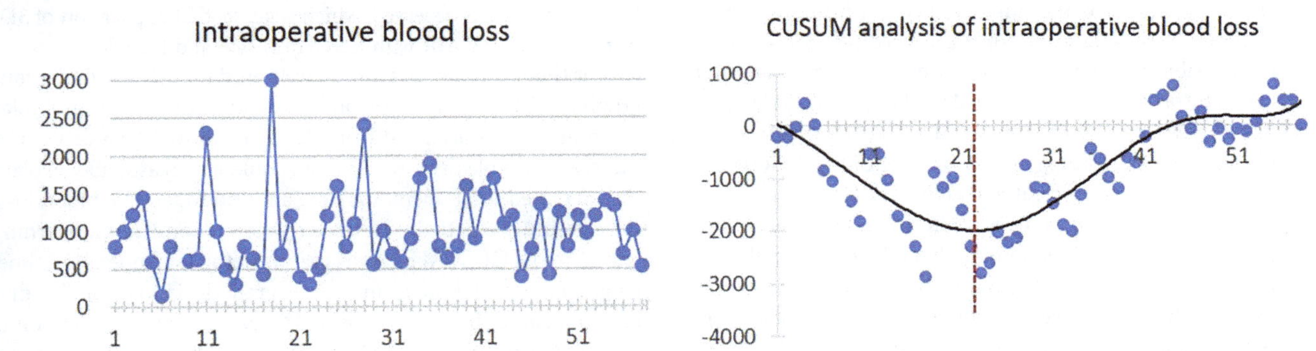

FIGURE 3 | Linear graph and CUSUM analysis of intraoperative blood loss in CAJR applying patient-specific surgical plates. The black line represents the curve of best fit in a general model with equation, $y = 4E{-}06x^6 - 0.0006x^5 + 0.0274x^4 - 0.2982x^3 - 1.1805x^2 - 94.942x + 133.67$, $R^2 = 0.7233$.

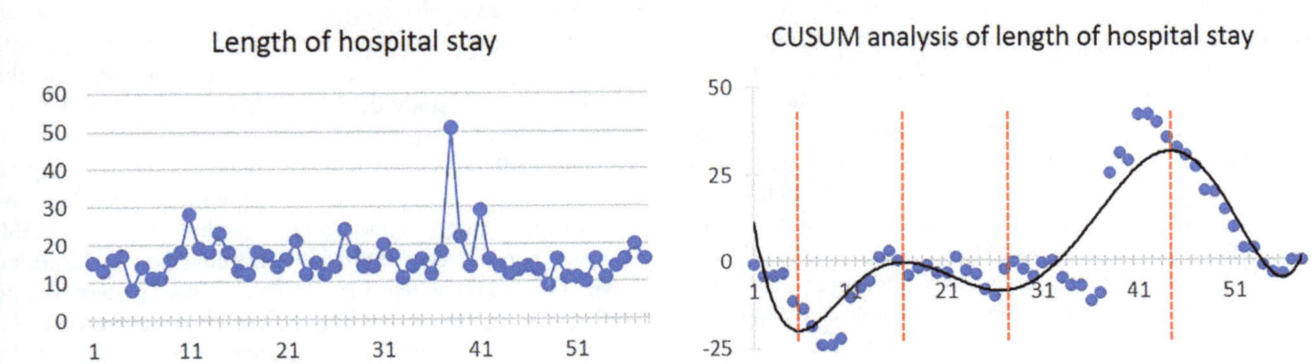

FIGURE 4 | Linear graph and CUSUM analysis of hospital stay length in CAJR applying patient-specific surgical plates. The black line represents the curve of best fit in a general model with equation, $y = 6E{-}07x^6 - 0.0001x^5 + 0.0077x^4 - 0.2461x^3 + 3.7349x^2 - 23.636x + 31.376$, $R^2 = 0.7912$.

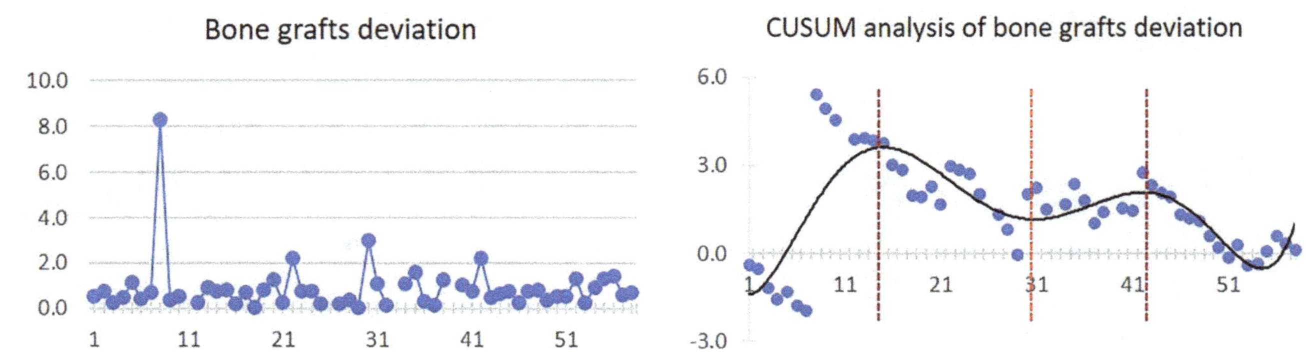

FIGURE 5 | Linear graph and CUSUM analysis of bone grafts deviation in CAJR applying patient-specific surgical plates. The black line represents the curve of best fit in a general model with equation, $y = 5E{-}08x^6 - 8E{-}06x^5 + 0.0005x^4 - 0.0148x^3 + 0.1689x^2 - 0.2517x - 1.307$, $R^2 = 0.5936$.

DISCUSSION

The concept of learning curve in medicine was commonly defined as the time taken and/or the number of procedures an average surgeon needs to be able to perform a procedure independently with a reasonable outcome (30). As modern surgical training is always beset by problems like increased working hours, inadequate training facilities, lack of resources, and medicolegal issues (31), the understanding of learning curves on surgical procedures can make the training more efficient and standard. However, a study reviewed assessments of learning curve in health technologies and indicated that learning curves were rarely evaluated formally with a proper study design and statistical method (32). As a new tool, the CUSUM technique for learning curve has been introduced and proposed as a useful instrument in the field of surgical training, which allows quantitative monitoring of individual performance during the learning process (28, 33).

Nowadays, computer-assisted surgery is increasingly utilized in reconstructive surgery, while no literature has reported the learning curve for this surgical procedure. In the present study, we performed CUSUM analysis on the learning curve of CAJR using 3D-printed PSSP by a single surgical team. Although operation time is the most common determinant for the learning curve on surgery, the assessment on the basis of a single parameter might be simplistic (12, 34). We tried to analyze trends in multidimensional variables in the present study.

For the primary outcome, our study revealed a three-stage learning pattern of CAJR with the use of PSSP, including initial learning, plateau, and overlearning. The first stage is initial learning. The learning curve regarding surgical success stabilized after 11 cases, and first achieved proficiency after 23 cases. The second stage is plateau. When surgeons felt competent in this surgical procedure, the significantly increased proportions of tumor staging and concomitant surgery suggested that the complexity of surgery after 23 cases was higher than the earlier cases. The concomitant surgery, simultaneous dental implant placement with the aid of a "three-in-one" patient-specific surgical guide (35), was also a technically challenging procedure. Accordingly, a fluctuation of proficiency was observed at this stage. The final stage is overlearning. A steady proficiency was completely achieved after 35 cases. Overall, the surgical failures in our cohort were infrequent (5.2%), and no performance of the surgeon below the unacceptable boundary line was observed, which suggests that application of 3D-printed PSSP in CAJR with free flap is safe and feasible.

For the secondary outcomes, we found that although the four graphs of CUSUM analysis had different curve shapes, a similar ascending trend occurred from 23–31 cases to 43–46 cases. The increased complexity after 23 cases could also reasonably explain the increased total operation time and intraoperative blood loss. As a result, we actually observed two phenomena of "learning curve" in the CUSUM analysis graphs of the total operation time, length of hospital stay, and bone graft deviation. In the first learning curve (from 1st to 28th–31st cases), the inflexion points occurred between 8 and 17 cases, from which operation time, length of hospital stay, and bone graft deviation started to diminish. In the second learning curve (from 28th–31st to 58th cases), stabilizations of the operation time, length of hospital stay, and bone graft deviation occurred between 43 and 46 cases.

The main novelty of this study was using the CUSUM technique to analyze the learning curve of CAJR with PSSP. We utilized a chosen level of surgical failure rate as strict as two times the currently acceptable level (11.1%) to determine proficiency, which was one strength of our study (28). The cohort of patients from a prospective clinical trial without dropout was also the strength. Since no study described the learning curve of CAJR surgery, our work can provide the first quantitative assessment on this topic to the literature. It should be noted that our surgical team had previous experience in conventional free flap jaw reconstruction surgery and also CAJR without the use of PSSP (36), which could help shorten the learning process. Learning curve varies from different surgeons, but its stage pattern may be similar. Among three stages, the occurrence and persistence of a plateau depend on many reasons, such as the interference by previous experience, the nature of the task, and the motivation (37). Finding out the correct cause and getting over this period will be an important portion in surgical training.

There are certain limitations of the present study that need to be addressed. First, the CUSUM analysis included different diseases (malignant and benign tumors), surgeries (maxillary and mandibular reconstructions), and free flaps (fibular and iliac flaps), which influenced the homogeneity of enrolled cases. A multi-center clinical trial, with a big enough sample size of the same disease and surgery, might be needed to overcome this limitation. However, it will lead to other limitations of different expertise of multiple surgical teams and hospital setting. Second, post-operative oral function and quality of life are important outcomes for jaw reconstruction. However, there are a lot of confounding factors influencing these outcomes, which will need a well-designed prospective randomized control trial for further investigation. Thus, we did not include them in the present analysis. Last, the learning curve of time spent on preoperative preparation, such as virtual surgical planning and PSSP design, was not reported in this study. Previously, we reported that the time spent on virtual surgery and plate design was 18.8 ± 13.2 h, and the time taken for 3D printing, post-processing, and product delivery was 162.9 ± 55.2 h (38). The consecutive data of the time spent on preoperative preparation with a large sample size would provide a better understanding of the whole learning process of CAJR using PSSP.

CONCLUSION

A three-stage learning pattern of CAJR with the use of PSSP was revealed, including initial learning, plateau, and overlearning, which may guide the clinical teaching and training of CAJR using PSSP. Based on CUSUM analysis, surgical proficiency was obtained after 23 cases. Stabilization of total operation time, length of hospital stay, and bone graft deviation occurred after 8–17 cases. Our study provided evidence to guide the training of this new surgical procedure to ensure patient safety and clinical outcomes.

AUTHOR CONTRIBUTIONS

W-yZ and Y-xS: study design. Y-xS: study supervision. W-yZ, WC, JP and W-fY: data collection. W-yZ and MW: manuscript preparation, statistical analysis, and data interpretation. All authors contributed to the article and approved the submitted version.

REFERENCES

1. Okay D, Al Shetawi AH, Moubayed SP, Mourad M, Buchbinder D, Urken ML. Worldwide 10-Year Systematic Review of Treatment Trends in Fibula Free Flap for Mandibular Reconstruction. *J Oral Maxillofac Surg* (2016) 74 (12):2526–31. doi: 10.1016/j.joms.2016.06.170
2. Kakarala K, Shnayder Y, Tsue TT, Girod DA. Mandibular Reconstruction. *Oral Oncol* (2018) 77:111–7. doi: 10.1016/j.oraloncology.2017.12.020
3. Powcharoen W, Yang WF, Yan Li K, Zhu W, Su YX. Computer-Assisted Versus Conventional Freehand Mandibular Reconstruction With Fibula Free Flap: A Systematic Review and Meta-Analysis. *Plast Reconstr Surg* (2019) 144 (6):1417–28. doi: 10.1097/prs.0000000000006261
4. Yang WF, Choi WS, Wong MC, Powcharoen W, Zhu WY, Tsoi JK, et al. Three-Dimensionally Printed Patient-Specific Surgical Plates Increase Accuracy of Oncologic Head and Neck Reconstruction Versus Conventional Surgical Plates: A Comparative Study. *Ann Surg Oncol* (2021) 28(1):363–75. doi: 10.1245/s10434-020-08732-y
5. Pucci R, Weyh A, Smotherman C, Valentini V, Bunnell A, Fernandes R. Accuracy of Virtual Planned Surgery Versus Conventional Free-Hand Surgery for Reconstruction of the Mandible With Osteocutaneous Free Flaps. *Int J Oral Maxillofac Surg* (2020) 49(9):1153–61. doi: 10.1016/j.ijom.2020.02.018
6. Weitz J, Bauer FJM, Hapfelmeier A, Rohleder NH, Wolff KD, Kesting MR. Accuracy of Mandibular Reconstruction by Three-Dimensional Guided Vascularised Fibular Free Flap After Segmental Mandibulectomy. *Br J Oral Maxillofac Surg* (2016) 54(5):506–10. doi: 10.1016/j.bjoms.2016.01.029
7. Bao T, He J, Yu C, Zhao W, Lin Y, Wang H, et al. Utilization of a Pre-Bent Plate-Positioning Surgical Guide System in Precise Mandibular Reconstruction With a Free Fibula Flap. *Oral Oncol* (2017) 75:133–9. doi: 10.1016/j.oraloncology.2017.11.011
8. De Maesschalck T, Courvoisier DS, Scolozzi P. Computer-Assisted Versus Traditional Freehand Technique in Fibular Free Flap Mandibular Reconstruction: A Morphological Comparative Study. *Eur Arch Otorhinol* (2017) 274(1):517–26. doi: 10.1007/s00405-016-4246-4
9. Ciocca L, Marchetti C, Mazzoni S, Baldissara P, Gatto MRA, Cipriani R, et al. Accuracy of Fibular Sectioning and Insertion Into a Rapid-Prototyped Bone Plate, for Mandibular Reconstruction Using CAD-CAM Technology. *J Cranio-Maxillo-Facial Surg* (2015) 43(1):28–33. doi: 10.1016/j.jcms.2014.10.005
10. Zhang L, Liu Z, Li B, Yu H, Shen SG, Wang X. Evaluation of Computer-Assisted Mandibular Reconstruction With Vascularized Fibular Flap Compared to Conventional Surgery. *Oral Surg Oral Med Oral Pathol Oral Radiol* (2016) 121(2):139–48. doi: 10.1016/j.oooo.2015.10.005
11. Grigg OA, Farewell VT, Spiegelhalter DJ. Use of Risk-Adjusted CUSUM and RSPRT Charts for Monitoring in Medical Contexts. *Stat Methods Med Res* (2003) 12(2):147–70. doi: 10.1177/096228020301200205
12. Barrie J, Jayne DG, Wright J, Murray CJC, Collinson FJ, Pavitt SH. Attaining Surgical Competency and Its Implications in Surgical Clinical Trial Design: A Systematic Review of the Learning Curve in Laparoscopic and Robot-Assisted Laparoscopic Colorectal Cancer Surgery. *Ann Surg Oncol* (2014) 21(3):829–40. doi: 10.1245/s10434-013-3348-0
13. Song X, Wang D, Sun X, Wang J, Liu Z, Liu Q, et al. Cumulative Sum Analysis of the Learning Curve for Endoscopic Resection of Juvenile Nasopharyngeal Angiofibroma. *Surg Endosc* (2018) 32(7):3181–91. doi: 10.1007/s00464-018-6035-1
14. Antoun A, Chau J, Alsharqawi N, Kaneva P, Feldman LS, Mueller CL, et al. P338: Summarizing Measures of Proficiency in Transanal Total Mesorectal Excision-A Systematic Review. *Surg Endosc* (2021) 35(8):4817–24. doi: 10.1007/s00464-020-07935-4
15. Kim H, Jeong WJ, Ahn SH. Results of Free Flap Reconstruction After Ablative Surgery in the Head and Neck. *Clin Exp Otorhinolaryngol* (2015) 8(2):167–73. doi: 10.3342/ceo.2015.8.2.167
16. Ratnagiri R, Jena S, Parvathi P, Srikanth R, Raju GSN. Reconstruction in Head-and-Neck Cancers - Analysis of the Learning Curve. *Natl J Maxillofac Surg* (2018) 9(2):191–5. doi: 10.4103/njms.NJMS_66_17
17. Cariati P, Cabello Serrano A, Monsalve Iglesias F, Roman Ramos M, Fernandez Solis J, Martinez Lara I. Unfavorable Outcomes in Microsurgery: Possibilities for Improvement. *J Plast Surg Handb Surg* (2019) 53(5):279–87. doi: 10.1080/2000656X.2019.1606005
18. Fliss E, Yanko R, Bracha G, Teman R, Amir A, Horowitz G, et al. The Evolution of the Free Fibula Flap for Head and Neck Reconstruction: 21 Years of Experience With 128 Flaps. *J Reconstr Microsurg* (2021) 37(4):372–9. doi: 10.1055/s-0040-1717101
19. Yang WF, Choi WS, Leung YY, Curtin JP, Du R, Zhang CY, et al. Three-Dimensional Printing of Patient-Specific Surgical Plates in Head and Neck Reconstruction: A Prospective Pilot Study. *Oral Oncol* (2018) 78:31–6. doi: 10.1016/j.oraloncology.2018.01.005
20. Pu JJ, Choi WS, Yu P, Wong MCM, Lo AWI, Su YX. Do Predetermined Surgical Margins Compromise Oncological Safety in Computer-Assisted Head and Neck Reconstruction? *Oral Oncol* (2020) 111:104914. doi: 10.1016/j.oraloncology.2020.104914
21. Steiner SH, Cook RJ, Farewell VT, Treasure T. Monitoring Surgical Performance Using Risk-Adjusted Cumulative Sum Charts. *Biostatistics*

(2000) 1(4):441–52. doi: 10.1093/biostatistics/1.4.441
22. Awad ME, Altman A, Elrefai R, Shipman P, Looney S, Elsalanty M. The Use of Vascularized Fibula Flap in Mandibular Reconstruction; A Comprehensive Systematic Review and Meta-Analysis of the Observational Studies. *J Cranio-Maxillo-Facial Surg* (2019) 47(4):629–41. doi: 10.1016/j.jcms.2019.01.037
23. Wilde F, Hanken H, Probst F, Schramm A, Heiland M, Cornelius C-P. Multicenter Study on the Use of Patient-Specific CAD/CAM Reconstruction Plates for Mandibular Reconstruction. *Int J Comput Assist Radiol Surg* (2015) 10(12):2035–51. doi: 10.1007/s11548-015-1193-2
24. Rana M, Chin S-J, Muecke T, Kesting M, Groebe A, Riecke B, et al. Increasing the Accuracy of Mandibular Reconstruction With Free Fibula Flaps Using Functionalized Selective Laser-Melted Patient-Specific Implants: A Retrospective Multicenter Analysis. *J Cranio-Maxillofac Surg* (2017) 45 (8):1212–9. doi: 10.1016/j.jcms.2017.04.003
25. Öhman D, Schaefer C, Nannmark U, Kjeller G, Malmström J. Mandible Reconstruction With Patient-Specific Implants: Case Report of Five Consecutive Patients. *Int J Oral Maxillofac Implants* (2019) 34(1):e7–e11. doi: 10.11607/jomi.6913
26. Jehn P, Spalthoff S, Korn P, Zeller A-N, Dittmann J, Zimmerer R, et al. Patient-Specific Implant Modification for Alloplastic Bridging of Mandibular Segmental Defects in Head and Neck Surgery. *J Cranio-Maxillofac Surg* (2020) 48(3):315–22. doi: 10.1016/j.jcms.2020.01.018
27. Zavattero E, Bolzoni A, Dell'Aversana G, Santagata M, Massarelli O, Ferri A, et al. Accuracy of Fibula Reconstruction Using Patient-Specific Cad/Cam Plates: A Multicenter Study on 47 Patients. *Laryngoscope* (2021) 131(7): E2169–75. doi: 10.1002/lary.29379
28. Bolsin S, Colson M. The Use of the Cusum Technique in the Assessment of Trainee Competence in New Procedures. *Int J Qual Health Care* (2000) 12 (5):433–8. doi: 10.1093/intqhc/12.5.433
29. Kim CW, Kim WR, Kim HY, Kang J, Hur H, Min BS, et al. Learning Curve for Single-Incision Laparoscopic Anterior Resection for Sigmoid Colon Cancer. *J Am Coll Surg* (2015) 221(2):397–403. doi: 10.1016/j.jamcollsurg.2015.02.016
30. Subramonian K, Muir G. The 'Learning Curve' in Surgery: What Is it, How do We Measure It and Can We Influence It? *BJU Int* (2004) 93(9):1173–4. doi: 10.1111/j.1464-410X.2004.04891.x
31. Chikwe J, de Souza AC, Pepper JR. No Time to Train the Surgeons. *BMJ (Clinical Res ed)* (2004) 328(7437):418–9. doi: 10.1136/bmj.328.7437.418
32. Ramsay CR, Grant AM, Wallace SA, Garthwaite PH, Monk AF, Russell IT. Statistical Assessment of the Learning Curves of Health Technologies. *Health Technol Assess* (2001) 5(12):1–79. doi: 10.3310/hta5120
33. Biau DJ, Williams SM, Schlup MM, Nizard RS, Porcher R. Quantitative and Individualized Assessment of the Learning Curve Using LC-CUSUM. *Br J Surg* (2008) 95(7):925–9. doi: 10.1002/bjs.6056
34. Pernar LIM, Robertson FC, Tavakkoli A, Sheu EG, Brooks DC, Smink DS. An Appraisal of the Learning Curve in Robotic General Surgery. *Surg Endosc* (2017) 31(11):4583–96. doi: 10.1007/s00464-017-5520-2
35. Zhu WY, Su YX, Pow EHN, Yang WF, Qin L, Choi WS. "Three-In-One" Patient-Specific Surgical Guides for Simultaneous Dental Implants in Fibula Flap Jaw Reconstruction: A Prospective Case Series. *Clin Implant Dent Relat Res* (2021) 23(1):43–53. doi: 10.1111/cid.12954
36. Zheng G-S, Su Y-X, Liao G-Q, Liu H-C, Zhang S-E, Liang L-Z. Mandibular Reconstruction Assisted by Preoperative Simulation and Accurate Transferring Templates: Preliminary Report of Clinical Application. *J Oral Maxillofac Surg* (2013) 71(9):1613–8. doi: 10.1016/j.joms.2013.02.018
37. N, Pam MS. *LEARNING PLATEAU*. PsychologyDictionary.org (2018). Available at: https://psychologydictionary.org/learning-plateau/ (Accessed September 9, 2021).
38. Yang WF, Zhang CY, Choi WS, Zhu WY, Li DTS, Chen XS, et al. A Novel 'Surgeon-Dominated' Approach to the Design of 3D-Printed Patient-Specific Surgical Plates in Mandibular Reconstruction: A Proof-of-Concept Study. *Int J Oral Maxillofac Surg* (2020) 49(1):13–21. doi: 10.1016/j.ijom.2019.05.005

APPENDIX

Current acceptable failure rate (p0)=0.111

Chosen level of failure rate (p1)=0.222

Type 1 error (α)=0.1

Type 2 error (β)=0.1

P=ln(p1/p0)=ln(0.222/0.111)=ln2 = 0.690

Q=ln[(1-p0)/(1-p1)]=ln[0.889/0.778]=ln1.143 = 0.133

a=In[(1-β)/α]=In(0.9/0.1)=2.197

b=In[(1-α)/β]=In(0.9/0.1)=2.197

s=Q/(P+Q)=0.133/(0.690 + 0.133)=0.162 (With success, graph goes 0.162 upwards, and with failure, graph goes 0.838 [1-s] downwards.)

Unacceptable boundary line: H_0=-b/(P+Q)=-2.197/(0.690 + 0.133)=-2.670

Acceptable boundary line: H_1=a/(P+Q)=2.197/(0.690 + 0.133)=2.670

12

Unexpected Change of Surgical Plans and Contingency Strategies in Computer-Assisted Free Flap Jaw Reconstruction: Lessons Learned from 98 Consecutive Cases

*Jane J. Pu, Wing Shan Choi, Wei-fa Yang, Wang-yong Zhu and Yu-xiong Su**

Division of Oral and Maxillofacial Surgery, Faculty of Dentistry, The University of Hong Kong, Hong Kong, Hong Kong SAR, China

Correspondence:
Yu-xiong Su
richsu@hku.hk

Background: Computer-assisted surgeries (CAS) are increasingly being adopted as the treatment of choice for jaw reconstructions with osseous free flaps. Although unexpected change of surgical plans remains a major concern of CAS, there are few studies focusing on this unfavorable clinical scenario. The aim of the present study was to investigate the rate of unexpected change of surgical plans and potential influential parameters, and to discuss the contingency strategies.

Methods: A retrospective study was performed to evaluate all the patients who underwent computer-assisted jaw resections and osseous free flap reconstructions. The postoperative radiographs were reviewed and compared with the preoperative surgical plans. Operating records were examined to analyze the reasons for unexpected change of surgical plans and the management. The potential influential parameters for the change of surgical plans were analyzed using Fisher-exact test. The difference was regarded as statistically significant for a p-value less than 5%.

Results: From Nov 2014 to Oct 2021, a total of 98 consecutive computer-assisted free flap jaw reconstruction cases with osseous free flaps were included in this study. Our experience showed that 5.1% of the patients (five cases) needed intra-operative change of the surgical plans. We summarized the unexpected change of surgical plans and the contingency strategies as four clinical scenarios, including extended resection and reconstruction, shortened resection and reconstruction, modified resection without changing reconstruction, and modified reconstruction without changed resection. None of the potential influential parameters was identified as significant in relation to unexpected change of surgical plans intraoperatively.

Conclusion: Our experience shows that with the comprehensive methodology for computer-assisted free flap jaw reconstruction surgery planning, we can minimize the possibility of unexpected change of surgical plans during surgery. The lessons learned from our 98 consecutive cases can help beginners prevent unexpected change of surgical plans and rationalize contingency strategies in computer-assisted free flap jaw reconstruction.

Keywords: head & neck, computer-assisted surgery (CAS), reconstruction, fibula free flap, fibula free flap donor site head and neck cancer, unexpected changes

INTRODUCTION

Computer-assisted surgeries (CAS) are increasingly being adopted as the treatment of choice for jaw reconstructions (1, 2). Although unexpected change of surgical plans remains a major concern of CAS, there are few studies focusing on this unfavorable clinical scenario.

Our previous systematic review showed that CAS increased the efficiency of surgery in terms of ischemic time, total operative time, reconstruction time and length of post-operative hospital stay (3). Increased accuracy and reduced interfibular gaps with the use of virtual surgical planning were reported by Pucci et al. and Stirling Craig et al. respectively (4, 5). However, there are also criticisms about CAS in head and neck reconstruction. Although our previous report on oncological safety of CAS proved that with careful clinical examination and proper utilization of imaging modalities, there was no significant difference in margin status and patient survival outcome between CAS and non-CAS groups of patients (6), some authors were still concerned as they found it difficult to accurately determine the resection margins before the real surgeries (7). In CAS, all resection guides and plates are determined pre-operatively. In cases with rapid tumor growth over a short period of time before the operation or uncertain bone margins for osteonecrosis, CAS leaves little room to accommodate the unexpected changes in surgical plans during the operation if the pre-surgical planning was not applicable or needed to be changed (8).

Compared to 'trial and error' in free hand surgery, CAS offers high predictability and repeatability that most surgeons desire. However, when unexpected situations arise intraoperatively, surgeons may have to abandon the virtual surgical planning and convert to free hand surgery. Not only does this waste the effort engaged in the pre-operative planning, but also lengthens the operating time and increases the psychological burden of the surgical team. Several studies briefly mentioned whether changes in surgical plans were needed in CAS (9, 10), but no detailed analysis was provided. Efanov et al. reported the reasons for abandoning the CAS plans (11). However, the paper was mostly focused on orthognathic surgery. The sample size for craniomaxillofacial reconstruction (8 patients) was too small for a more reproducible conclusion. Recent publication by Ma et al. investigated the adherence to CAS in maxillofacial reconstructions (12). However, nonvascular grafts, bridging plates and obturator prosthesis were also included in the study. While surgeons always need to prepare for troubleshooting when things go wrong during surgery, so far, no study comprehensively discussed the detailed contingency strategies for these unfavorable clinical scenarios.

The aim of the current study is to review the CAS free flap reconstruction cases in a single center, investigate the rate of unexpected change of surgical plans and potential influential parameters, and discuss the contingency strategies.

METHODS

Study Design

This study was approved by the institutional review board of the University of Hong Kong Hospital Authority Hong Kong West Cluster (UW 15-315). We conducted a retrospective study on all the CAS head and neck free flap reconstruction cases in our center performed by the same chief surgeon.

The patients' demographic data and operating theater records were obtained from chart review. Pre-operative computer assisted surgical planning files were retrieved from the department database. Post-operative CT scans of the patients were reviewed to verify the execution of the pre-surgical plans.

Inclusion Criteria

Patients with the age of 18 years old or above at the time of diagnosis; Underwent jaw resections and reconstructions by bony free flaps; Computer assisted surgery technique was adopted with predetermined resection margins and reconstruction plans; Treated by the same surgical team in The Division of Oral and Maxillofacial Surgery, The University of Hong Kong.

Exclusion Criteria

Patients below 18 years old at the time of diagnosis; Patients who did not undergo jawbone reconstruction or underwent jaw resection and reconstruction by freehand techniques.

Workflow of CAS

Preoperative Imaging and Building of Models

As described in our previous publications, preoperative CT scan of head & neck and lower extremities was performed for the patients. MRI and PETCT were acquired for the selected cases (6, 13). Digital intraoral scanning was performed when simultaneous dental implants were planned. The patient's CT scan and intraoral scan data were imported to ProPlan CMF 2.0 software (Materialize, Leuven, Belgium) and segmentation was performed to build the 3D virtual models of the lesion in the jaw and the donor site of fibula or iliac crest (**Figure 1**).

A Comprehensive Methodology for Computer-Assisted Free Flap Jaw Reconstruction Surgery Planning

Virtual surgical planning was performed in house by a "surgeon-dominated" approach with pre-determined osteotomies and desired reconstructions with fibula or iliac crest (9). Firstly, the extent of resection and reconstruction depended on the extension of the pathology. When determining resection margins for malignancy cases, the histopathology of the tumor, clinical signs and symptoms and imaging results were taken into consideration and safe distances of 15mm and 10mm were adopted for bone and soft tissue margins respectively. We used three methods to decide the surgical margins. Combining CT scan with careful clinical examination for soft tissue involvement was the most commonly used and straightforward approach. In addition, image fusion of CT, MRI and/or PETCT was performed with the use of iPlan Cranial 2.0 (BrainLAB, Feldkirchen, Germany) in selected cases to further assess the soft tissue and bone invasion of the lesions. Fusion of CT scan with intraoral digital scan in ProPlan software, in particular for superficial mucosa tumors, was a fast, simple, and low-cost technique, which could also provide high resolution images for dentition especially when simultaneous dental implants were planned (**Figure 1**). After the 3D composite model was built, the model was imported back to the CT scan to double check the accuracy of the model. Secondly, the recipient site was carefully assessed. This included the estimated location and size of the soft tissue defect which would determine the inset of the free flap skin paddle. The recipient vessels for anastomosis were planned based on the pedicle length and vessel diameter of the flap. Previous surgeries and radiation therapy to the head and neck were also taken into consideration. Thirdly, CT angiogram was performed for the donor sites. Donor vessel conditions were carefully assessed. Length of the pedicle was traced and matched with the recipient site. Large skin perforators were identified, which would be taken into account when designing the osteotomies.

Designing and Fabrication of Surgical Guides and/or Plates

When designing bony flap reconstruction, considerations were given to the size and shape of the defect, need for dental rehabilitation, location of the recipient vessels, length, and position of the free flap pedicles, and inset of the skin paddle. After the virtual surgical plan was confirmed, the surgical guides and/or plates were designed using 3-matic 13.0 software (Materialise). The guides were printed with biocompatible and autoclavable resin, either MED610 (Stratasys Ltd, Eden Prairie, MN, USA) or NextDent SG (Vertex Dental, The Netherlands). The patient-specific titanium plates were printed using selective laser melting technology. When patient-specific titanium plates were not used, either multiple mini-plates were bent intraoperatively or reconstruction plates pre-bent according to 3D-printed models were fixed intraoperatively.

Confirmation of the Surgical Plan Before the Surgery

When the surgical guides and plate were ready, patients were reviewed and examined right before their scheduled surgeries. The surgical plans were double confirmed by the chief surgeon and the team.

Execution of Surgery

Intraoperatively, osteotomies of jaws were performed with prefabricated osteotomy guides or surgical navigation (Kolibri Navigation Station 2.0, BrainLAB, Feldkirchen, Germany). Donor fibulas and iliac bones were harvested using the prefabricated harvest guides. Donor bones were fixed to the recipient jaw bones with commercially available Titanium plates (DePuy Synthes, United States) or 3D-printed patient-specific Titanium plates. The detailed workflow of the 3D-printed titanium plates of our team was previously described (14). Panoramic radiograph and CT scan of the recipient sites were performed after the surgery to confirm the results of the reconstruction.

Post-Operative Analysis

Operative records were reviewed. Intraoperative photos and post-operative radiographs were retrieved and compared with the preoperative virtual surgical plans. Cases where changes were made intra-operatively were analyzed.

Data analyses were performed using IBM SPSS Statistics version 25.0. Fisher-exact test was adopted to identify the potential risk factors for intraoperative change of surgical plans.

Outcome

The outcome of this study was to evaluate the percentage of unexpected change of plan in computer-assisted free flap jaw reconstruction, and to analyze the potential influential parameters. We also rationalized contingency strategies according to our experience.

RESULTS

Proportion of Unexpected Changes and Potential Influencing Factors

From Nov 2014 to October 2021, there were a total of 98 consecutive computer-assisted bony free flap jaw reconstruction cases in our center. Three free flap failures (3.1%) were recorded due to arterial (2 cases) and venous (1 case) failures. More than three fourths of the patients presented with defects at mandible and the fibula free flap was the workhorse for bony reconstruction (91.8%). Patient-specific plates were used in 73.5% of the patients.

There were five cases where intra-operative adjustments of the surgical plans were recorded. The rate of unexpected change plan in our cohort was only 5.1%. We analyzed the potential influencing factors including patient-specific surgical plates versus conventional plates, gender of the patients, maxilla versus mandible reconstruction, donor site of the osseous free flap, malignancy versus non-malignancy, reasons for reconstruction, number of segments of osseous flaps. The results showed that none of them led to significant difference. The demographic data and statistical analyses are presented in **Table 1**.

TABLE 1 | Demographic data and influencing factor analysis.

	Change plan				Significance
	Yes		No		(p=)
Patient Specific Implant					0.12
No	3	11.5%	23	88.5%	
Yes	2	2.8%	70	97.2%	
Sex					1.00
Female	3	5.5%	52	94.5%	
Male	2	4.7%	41	95.3%	
Site					0.58
Maxilla	0	0.0%	22	100.0%	
Mandible	5	6.6%	71	93.4%	
Donor					1.00
Fibula	5	5.6%	85	94.4%	
DCIA	0	0.0%	7	100.0%	
Medial Femoral Condyle	0	0.0%	1	100.0%	
Malignancy					0.33
Yes	2	3.1%	63	96.9%	
No	3	9.1%	30	90.9%	
Reasons for Reconstruction					0.11
SCC	1	2.0%	50	98.0%	
Other Malignancies	1	7.1%	13	92.9%	
Benign Pathology	2	6.9%	27	93.1%	
Secondary Reconstruction	1	25%	3	75.0%	
Segments					1.00
1	0	0.0%	17	100.0%	
2	4	7.5%	49	92.5%	
3	1	4.8%	20	95.2%	
4	0	0.0%	7	100.0%	

Lessons Learned From the Unexpected Change of Plans

The clinical scenarios of unexpected changes and contingency strategies are summarized as follows.

Clinical Scenario 1: Extended Resection and Reconstruction

In scenario 1, the actual resection margin is extended from the junction between jaw remnant and the flap, leading to a defect that is larger than planned. An extended or an extra segment of bony flap is needed to reconstruct the defect.

Two cases of scenario 1 were recorded, including one adenoid cystic carcinoma and one osteoradionecrosis. **Figure 2** shows a case illustration. The patient was a 65-year-old male presented with osteoradionecrosis of the jaw. The original plan was to resect the affected part of the mandible body with preservation of the angle and reconstruct it with a three-segment fibula free flap. However, after planned resection, the blood supply of the remaining ramus was unsatisfactory, leading to additional resection of the whole ramus. To reconstruct the defect, an additional fibula segment was harvested. 3D-printed patient-specific titanium plates were still able to be used, with the proximal part of the plate fixed to the additional fibula segment instead of ramus. The neo-condylar head was trimmed and reshaped to fit into the condylar fossa.

Clinical Scenario 2: Shortened Resection and Reconstruction

In clinical scenario 2, the planned amount of resection is deemed unnecessary based on the intraoperative findings. The actual resection is shortened compared to the pre-operative planning which requires shorter or less segments of the donor flap.

There was one case of scenario 2 in the series. As shown in **Figure 3**, this was a second-stage mandible reconstruction in a 49-year-old female presented with fracture and displacement of the non-vascular bone graft segments. The original plan was to reconstruct the hemi-mandibulectomy defect with a three-segment fibula free flap. Intraoperatively, the remaining ramus segment was found to be well-vascularized. The decision was made to keep the remaining ramus segment and reconstruct the mandible with two fibula segments.

Clinical Scenario 3: Modified Resection Without Changing Reconstruction

In clinical scenario 3, the resection margin is extended without changing the junction between the remaining jaw and the bone flap. For example, adding a marginal mandibulectomy without involving the lower border of mandible. Reconstruction can still be performed according to the original plan regardless of the extended resection.

One case of scenario 3 was documented (**Figure 4**). A 76-year-old male was diagnosed with squamous cell carcinoma at the right mandibular gingiva. The plan was to perform segmental mandibulectomy and reconstruct the defect with a fibula free flap. However, a very small ulcerative lesion at the left mandibular gingiva was identified during surgery and confirmed malignant with intraoperative frozen section. Accordingly, in addition to originally planned segmental mandibulectomy, an extended marginal mandibulectomy was added. Although the bony defect was extended, the fibula could still be fixed to the remnant of mandible with 3D-printed patient-specific titanium plate without any adjustment.

Clinical Scenario 4: Modified Reconstruction Without Changed Resection

In scenario 4, the planned resection doesn't change. However, the reconstruction may be modified due to different reasons, such as changes in the side of donor bone due to vessel variation, skin paddle inset and the side of recipient vessels in vessel-depleted neck, and compromised vascularity of donor bone segments, etc.

We encountered one case of scenario 4 in our series (**Figure 5**). A 22-year-old girl presented with a benign peripheral nerve sheath tumor at the mandible. The original plan was a three-segment

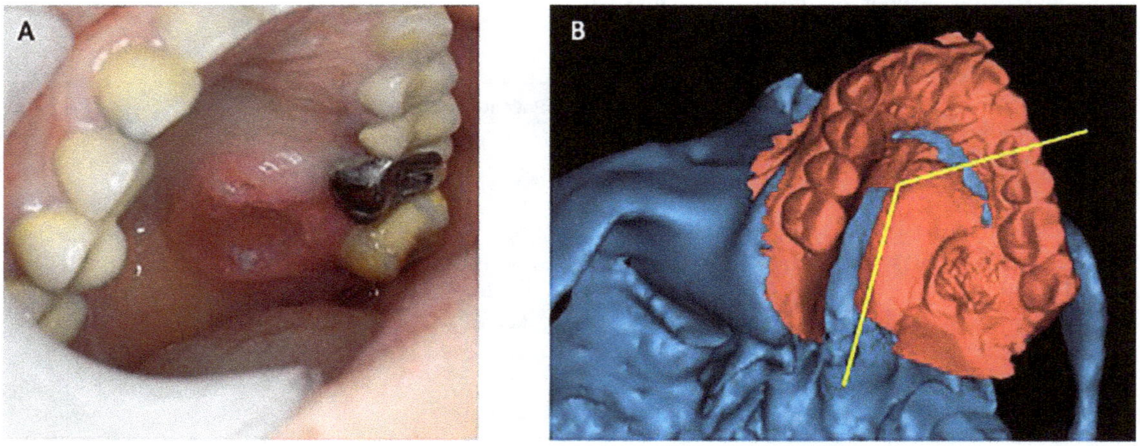

FIGURE 1 | Superimposing intraoral scan to CT data for designing of surgical margin. **(A)** Clinical photo of a patient with squamous cell carcinoma at left palate. **(B)** Intraoral scan superimposed to the digital model built from CT scan. (Yellow line: planned resection margins).

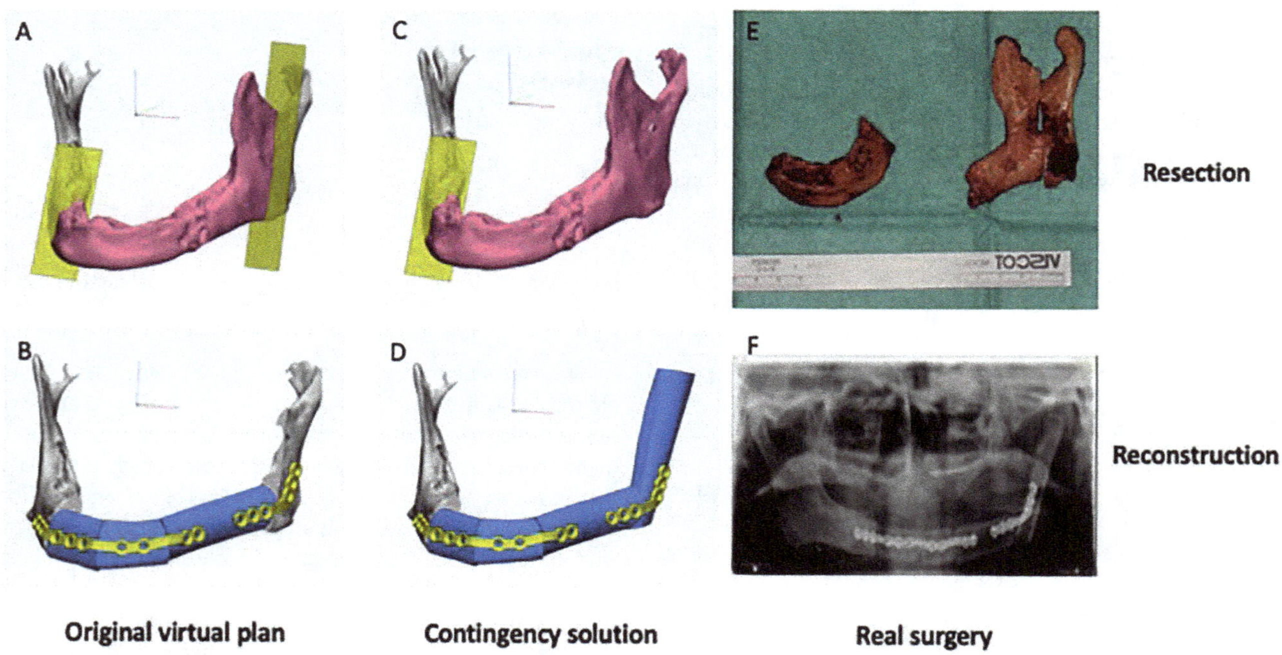

FIGURE 2 | Clinical scenario 1: Extended resection and reconstruction. A case illustration of a 65-year-old male presented with osteoradionecrosis of jaw. **(A)** Original virtual plan of resection. **(B)** Original virtual plan of reconstruction. **(C)** Extended resection. **(D)** Contingency solution for reconstruction. **(E)** Real surgery of resection. **(F)** Real surgery of reconstruction.

fibula reconstruction with a double barrel design for the anterior mandible, followed by a second-stage sagittal split osteotomy at the contralateral side to correct the facial profile. However, arterial spasm was encountered shortly after the vessel anastomosis and the blood supply to the most distal segment was unsatisfactory despite multiple attempts of re-anastomosis. The distal segment which was folded as the upper layer of the double barrel fibula flap was abandoned. The other two segments remained unchanged and fixed at the lower border of mandible according to the original plan.

DISCUSSION

Lack of flexibility during surgery has been considered a main drawback of computer-assisted free flap jaw reconstruction. In

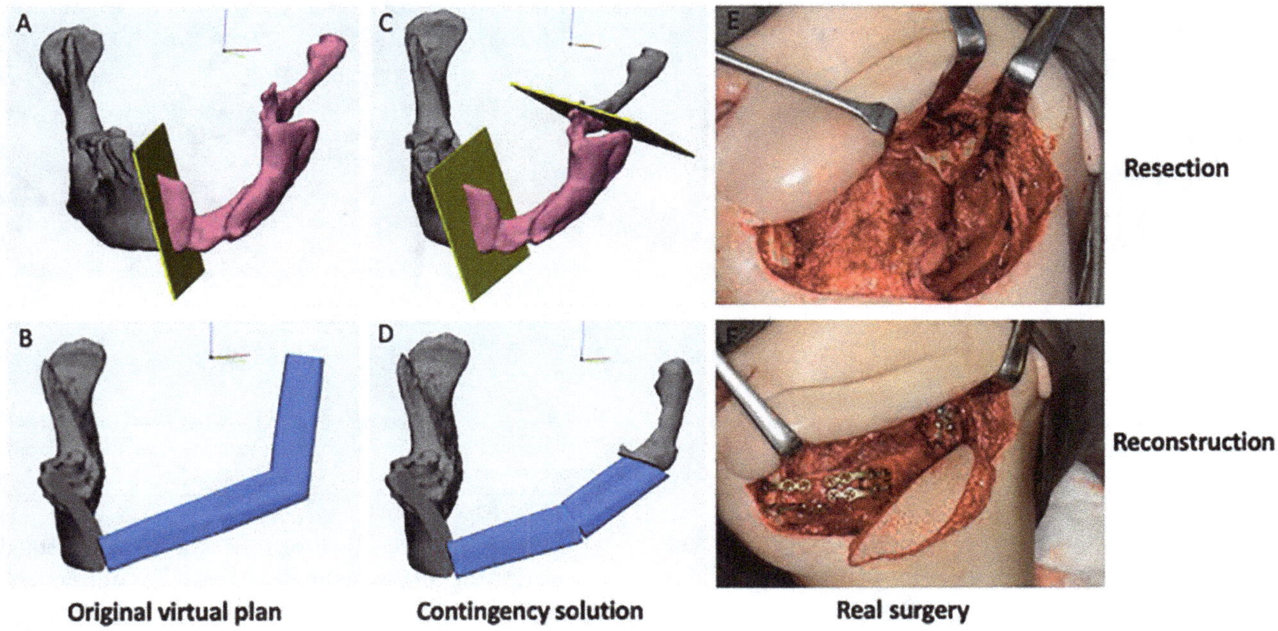

FIGURE 3 | Clinical scenario 2: Shortened resection and reconstruction. A case illustration of a second-stage mandible reconstruction of a 49-year-old female presented with fracture and displacement of the mandible segments. **(A)** Original virtual plan of resection. **(B)** Original virtual plan of reconstruction. **(C)** Shortened resection. **(D)** Contingency solution for reconstruction. **(E)** Real surgery of resection. **(F)** Real surgery of reconstruction.

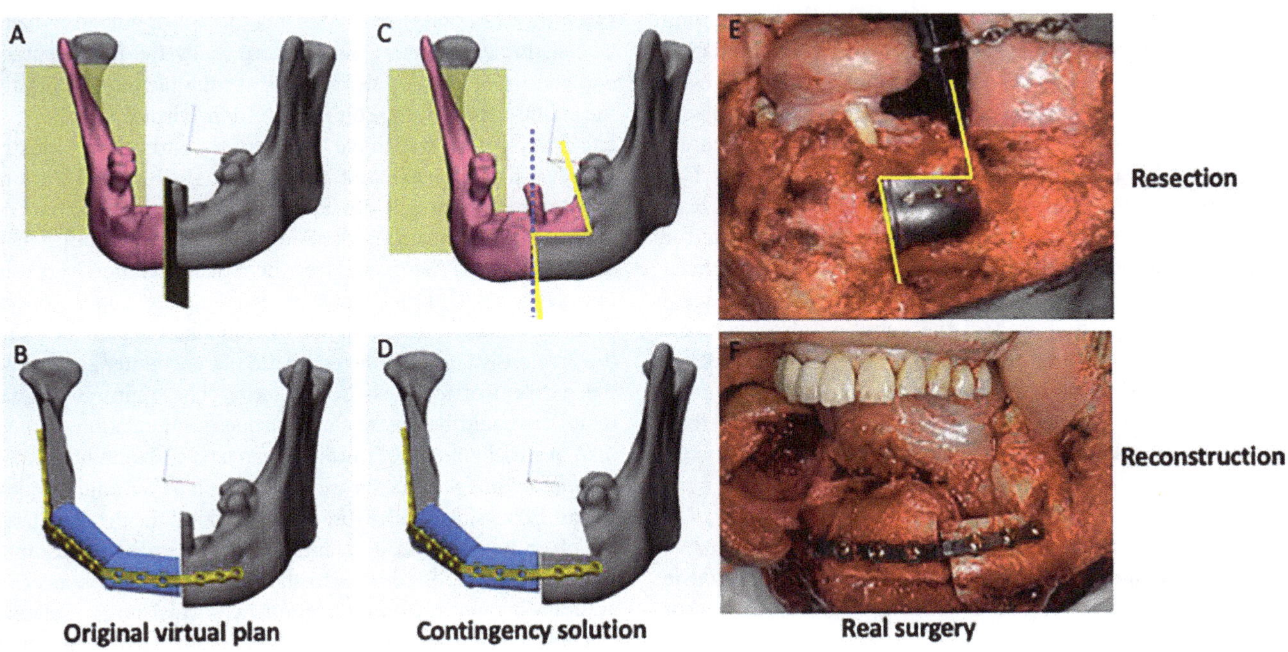

FIGURE 4 | Clinical scenario 3: Modified resection without changing reconstruction. A case illustration of a 76-year-old male presented with lower alveolar squamous cell carcinoma. **(A)** Original virtual plan of resection. **(B)** Original virtual plan of reconstruction. **(C)** Extended resection. (Blue dotted line: planned resection; yellow ling: actual resection.) **(D)** Actual reconstruction. **(E)** Real surgery of resection. **(F)** Real surgery of reconstruction.

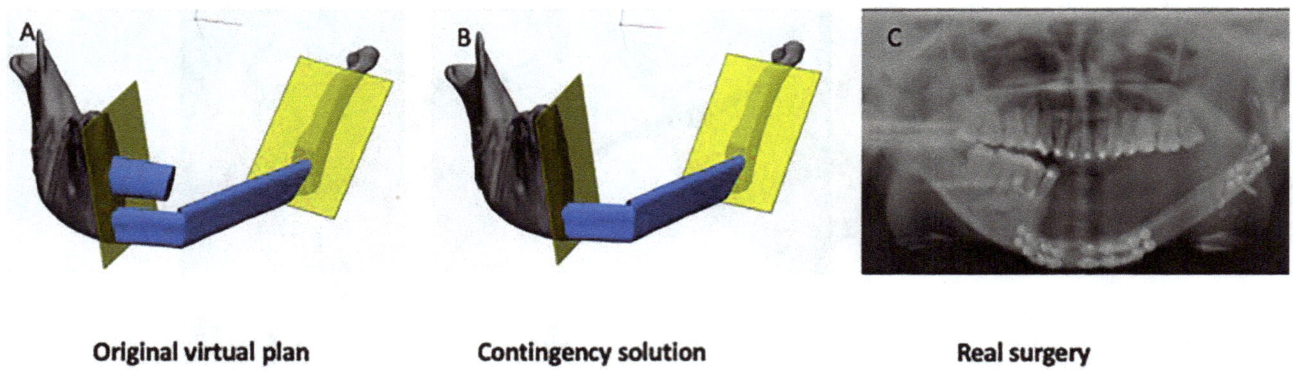

FIGURE 5 | Clinical scenario 4: Modified reconstruction without changed resection. A case illustration of a 22-year-old female presented with benign peripheral nerve sheath tumor. The presentation of open bite was due to the planned sagittal split on the contralateral side to advance the mandible at a later stage to improve facial esthetics. **(A)** Original virtual plan of reconstruction. **(B)** Actual reconstruction. **(C)** Post-operative x-ray.

this study, we analyzed unexpected change of surgical plans and corresponding contingency strategies in computer-assisted free flap jaw reconstruction. In a total of 98 consecutive cases, only 5.1% required intraoperative adjustments of the pre-operative planning, the lowest percentage in the literature so far. With proper contingency management during surgery, no patient-specific plate was abandoned.

Our experiences showed that the three methods for predetermination of surgical margins played an important role in obtaining favorable clinical outcomes. Firstly, a careful history taking and clinical examination helped us assess the clinical behavior of the lesion. For tumors with an aggressive behavior, wider surgical margins are warranted. Multiple imaging techniques might be used together with clinical examination when determining the tumor resection margins. CT scan with contrast was the main imaging modality used, and its fusion with MRI and PETCT was performed in selected cases for accurate assessment of the tumor extension in soft tissue and bone (15, 16). Superimposition of intraoral scan with the skull model built from the patient's CT scan was a useful way to incorporate the clinical presentation of the lesion, especially for superficial mucosa lesion, to the virtual surgical planning process (**Figure 1**). The intraoral scan of the dentition also overcame the limitation of low resolution of teeth in CT model if simultaneous dental implantation was planned. Secondly, careful planning of the vessel condition and soft tissue defects of recipient site was mandatory. This is the difference between free flap reconstruction and other techniques such as non-vascular bone graft and reconstructive plates. Thirdly, CT angiogram of lower extremities was proved to be a valuable tool in predicting the vessel conditions and planning the osteotomies in fibula free flap harvesting (17, 18). In recent years, CT angiogram was performed for all patients when the free fibula or DCIA flap reconstructions were planned in our center. This might have contributed to the fact that in our case series, we never encountered situations where change in the side of donor flaps or recipient vessels were necessary. Our data proved that with careful preoperative planning and proper execution, computer-assisted-surgery is a reliable method in jaw reconstruction with minimal need for intraoperative change of plan.

Wilde 2015 reported 6 cases of change of plan intraoperatively in the series of 32 patients (19%). The reasons for changes included the decision to extend the osseous resection margins, change of side of the donor fibula and the recipient vessels and unknown reasons in two cases. In one case, the upper barrel of the double barrel fibula reconstruction was abandoned with the reason unrevealed (10). The recent publication by Ma et al. also reported the rate of intraoperative change of plans of 17.6% (12). The rate of modification of preoperative surgical plans during real surgery was much lower in our series of patients (5.1%). In our center, all the virtual surgical planning was performed by the junior surgeons and confirmed by the chief surgeon at multiple time points along the planning process. In comparison to the virtual planning by the engineer, this could have avoided the miscommunications between the engineer and the surgeons. This also warranted careful assessment and discussion of the cases among surgeons, accordingly some reasons identified in the previous studies such as surgical protocol change and treatment plan alteration were rare in our case series. Unfitness of the guided templates and the pre-bent plates caused the greatest number of nonadherences to the plans in the previous studies. However, we did not encounter any case with the problem of unfitness in our series. The unfitness of guided templates could be due to the improper segmentation of the CT scan or misalignment of intraoral scan to CT scan to build the 3D composite model. Once the model was built by the engineer, it was almost impossible for the surgeons to pick up the problem later in the planning stages. In our center, for all cases, the 3D composite models were imported back to the CT scan to double check the accuracy before proceeding with further virtual surgical planning. In comparison to the previous studies, in our series of 98 patients, none of them needed extension of bony resections due to tumor growth or positive intraoperative surgical margin from frozen section report. This agrees with the reports by Toto et al. and Azuma et al. of smaller case series of 25 patients and 12 patients respectively (9, 19). Two cases of altered extremities as donor site were reported by Ma et al. This did not happen in our cases. Compared to previous reports (11, 12), our study exclusively included osseous free flap reconstructions which required more considerations of the donor and recipient vessel conditions and skin paddle locations. Our experience shows that most of the unexpected change of surgical plan is preventable by careful and comprehensive presurgical planning.

On the other hand, the clinical scenarios stated in this paper helped us predict those cases at higher risk of changing plan during surgery. For example, for secondary reconstruction and osteoradionecrosis cases, resection margins may be difficult to determine preoperatively without assessing blood supply of the remaining segments. For tumors with perineural invasion tendency such as adenoid cystic carcinoma, wider resection may be encountered intra-operatively depending on the frozen section results of nerve invasion.

When we identify cases with high risk for changing plan, we need to prepare for contingency solutions from the virtual planning stage. With the lesson learned from our 98 consecutive cases, we organized the intraoperative change of plans into four clinical scenarios so as to aid development of proper contingency strategies. The clinical scenarios I-III are related to the change of resection during surgery, while IV is due to the reconstructive reason. In hospitals where head and neck tumor resection and reconstruction are performed by two teams, when intraoperative modification of surgical plans is expected, the communication of the two teams are crucial. Decisions about change in reconstruction plans are better made before segmentation of the donor flaps when any adjustment can be easily incorporated.

For clinical scenario 1, extended resection and reconstruction, either longer or extra bony segments will be needed depending on the extension and location of the extended resection. For mandibular defects, Brown's Classification can be taken for reference when deciding on the contingency strategies (20). Generally speaking, for the extension of defect within one classification, a longer fibula segment will suffice. However, when the modification of resection involves the "corners" of mandible leading to a different Brown's Classification, an extra bony segment shall be needed. For example, the case demonstrated in **Figure 2** changed from Brown's Class III to Class IVc, an extra bony segment was used. To accommodate this in the virtual surgical plan, we should include a longer proximal or distal segment of harvest guide and reserve space for the extra segment that may be needed. At the recipient site, we shall design extra screw fixation holes at the remaining jaw segments and longer patient-specific surgical plate to accommodate the possible need for extended margins. When in doubt, more than one set of computer-assisted surgery plan may be necessary to prepare for different intraoperative scenarios. For cases where pre-determination of margin is extremely difficult, 3D models can be printed and used as guides for bending plates intraoperatively.

For clinical scenario 2, shortened resection and reconstruction, shorter or less segments of the donor flap will be used. For mandibular defects, similar to scenario 1, involving the "corner" of mandible or not will lead to different contingency plans. When a segment is shortened, we may need to avoid compromised vascularity, such as a less than 2cm fibula segment. For major adjustments such as the case shown in **Figure 3**, a fibula segment may need to be abandoned. If patient-specific implants are designed, whether the plate and screw holes originally planned to be fitted onto the fibula segment can still be used onto the remaining jaw depends on the relative position between the two. If there is obvious position discrepancy between the planned fibula segment and the actual remaining jaw, commercial plates may need to be used instead.

For clinical scenario 3, extended resection without changing reconstruction, the patient-specific surgical plates could be designed at the lower border of mandible to allow enough space for the marginal mandibulectomy with no interference to the reconstruction plan (**Figure 4**) although in some cases this might compromise dental rehabilitation.

For clinical scenario 4, modified reconstruction without changed resection, CT angiogram of donor site is helpful to prevent this type of unexpected change in reconstruction. Whenever patient-specific surgical plates are planned, commercial plates shall always be served as an alternative. Three-dimensional model of the jaw can be printed and used as a guide for bending commercial plates.

Computer assisted surgery increases the predictability and repeatability of free flap jaw reconstruction while reducing the uncertainty. With the routine applications of computer assisted surgery, the young generation of surgeons may not have enough chance to get familiar with the traditional techniques. However, even with most thorough preoperative planning, change in surgical plans may still be encountered in certain cases. This requires the young surgeons to get familiarized with the conventional techniques of jaw reconstructions so that they can adapt themselves to unexpected changes.

One limitation was due to the development of techniques with time, more patient-specific implants were used in later stage while commercial plates were used in earlier stage. This could have led to the heterogeneity of data. Another main limitation of the study lies in the limited sample size of the cases with intraoperative changes. With a total number of 98 cases of computer assisted head and neck free-flap reconstructions, only 5 cases of intra-operative changes were encountered, and no case ended up with an abandoned patient-specific surgical plate. The low rate of deviation from planning in our cohort may be viewed as both a strength and a limitation of the current study. On one hand it proves the effectiveness of our comprehensive methodology of surgical planning, on the other hand it makes our conclusion less definitive. A multicenter prospective study with large sample size and a well-controlled study design can better address this important issue in the future, although it will also bring other limitations such as heterogeneity of surgeons' skill and experiences. The stated clinical scenarios and proposed strategies were not meant to be exhaustive. However, the current study made the effort in detailed analysis of the intraoperative changes and contingency strategies, which could be further perfected with more experiences at various centers.

CONCLUSION

With the comprehensive methodology of surgical planning for computer-assisted free flap jaw reconstruction, we can minimize the unexpected change of surgical plans during surgery. The lessons learned from our 98 consecutive cases can help beginners prevent unexpected change of surgical plans and rationalize contingency strategies in computer-assisted free flap jaw reconstruction.

ETHICS STATEMENT

The studies involving human participants were reviewed and approved by the institutional review board of the University of Hong Kong Hospital Authority Hong Kong West Cluster (UW 15-315). The patients/participants provided their written informed consent to participate in this study.

AUTHOR'S NOTE

The results from this article were presented at the Asia Conference of Oral and Maxillofacial Surgery 2021 (Virtual).

AUTHOR CONTRIBUTIONS

JP: Conceptualization, methodology, data curation, formal analysis, writing - original draft, and writing - review and editing. WC, W-fY, and W-yZ: Project administration, supervision, validation and writing - review and editing. Y-xS: Conceptualization, formal analysis, funding acquisition, supervision, validation and writing - review and editing. All authors approved the final manuscript for publication.

REFERENCES

1. Levine JP, Bae JS, Soares M, Brecht LE, Saadeh PB, Ceradini DJ, et al. Jaw in a Day: Total Maxillofacial Reconstruction Using Digital Technology. *Plast Reconstr Surg* (2013) 131(6):1386–1391. doi: 10.1097/PRS.0b013e31828bd8d0
2. Hanasono MM, Matros E, Joseph D. Important Aspects of Head and Neck Reconstruction. *Plast Reconstr Surg* (2014) 134(6):968–80. doi: 10.1097/PRS.0000000000000722
3. Powcharoen W, Yang WF, Li KY, Zhu W, Su YX. Computer-Assisted Versus Conventional Freehand Mandibular Reconstruction With Fibula Free Flap: A Systematic Review and Meta-Analysis. *Plast Reconstr Surg* (2019) 144 (6):1417–28. doi: 10.1097/PRS.0000000000006261
4. Pucci R, Weyh A, Smotherman C, Valentini V, Bunnell A, Fernandes R. Accuracy of Virtual Planned Surgery Versus Conventional Free-Hand Surgery for Reconstruction of the Mandible With Osteocutaneous Free Flaps. *Int J Oral Maxillofac Surg* (2020) 49:1153–61. doi: 10.1016/j.ijom.2020.02.018
5. Stirling Craig E, Yuhasz M, Shah A, Blumberg J, Salomon J, Lowlicht R, et al. Simulated Surgery and Cutting Guides Enhance Spatial Positioning in Free Fibular Mandibular Reconstruction. *Microsurgery* (2015) 35(1):29–33. doi: 10.1002/micr.22229
6. Pu JJ, Choi WS, Yu P, Wong MCM, Lo AWI, Su YX. Do Predetermined Surgical Margins Compromise Oncological Safety in Computer-Assisted Head and Neck Reconstruction? *Oral Oncol* (2020) 111:104914. doi: 10.1016/j.oraloncology.2020.104914
7. Deek NF, Wei FC. Computer-Assisted Surgery for Segmental Mandibular Reconstruction With the Osteoseptocutaneous Fibula Flap: Can We Instigate Ideological and Technological Reforms? *Plast Reconstr Surg* (2016) 137 (3):963–70. doi: 10.1097/01.prs.0000479998.49928.71
8. Mazzoni S, Marchetti C, Sgarzani R, Cipriani R, Scotti R, Ciocca L. Evaluation of the Accuracy of a Surgical Guide and Custom-Made Bone Plate in Oncology Patients After Mandibular Reconstruction. *Plast Reconstr Surg* (2013) 131(6):1376–85. doi: 10.1097/PRS.0b013e31828bd6b0
9. Toto JM, Chang E, Agag R, Devarajan K, Patel SA, Topham NS. Improved Operative Efficiency of Free Fibula Flap Mandible Reconstruction With Patient-Specific, Computer-Guided Preoperative Planning. *Head Neck* (2015) 37(11):1660–4. doi: 10.1002/hed.23815
10. Wilde F, Hanken H, Probst F, Schramm A, Heiland M, Cornelius CP. Multicenter Study on the Use of Patient-Specific CAD/CAM Reconstruction Plates for Mandibular Reconstruction. *Int J Comput Assist Radiol Surg* (2015) 10:2035e2051. doi: 10.1007/s11548-015-1193-2
11. Efanov JI, Roy AA, Huang KN, Borsuk DE. Virtual Surgical Planning: The Pearls and Pitfalls. *Plast Reconstr Surg Glob Open* (2018) 5:e1443. doi: 10.1097/GOX.0000000000001443
12. Ma H, Shujaat S, Van Dessel J, Sun Y, Bila M, Vranckx J, et al. Adherence to Computer-Assisted Surgical Planning in 136 Maxillofacial Reconstructions. *Front Oncol* (2021) 11:713606. doi: 10.3389/fonc.2021.713606
13. Yang WF, Choi WS, Leung YY, Curtin JP, Du R, Zhang CY, et al. Three-Dimensional Printing of Patient-Specific Surgical Plates in Head and Neck Reconstruction: A Prospective Pilot Study. *Oral Oncol* (2018) 78:31–6. doi: 10.1016/j.oraloncology.2018.01.005
14. Yang WF, Zhang CY, Choi WS, Zhu WY, Li DTS, Chen XS, et al. A Novel 'Surgeon-Dominated' Approach to the Design of 3D-Printed Patient-Specific Surgical Plates in Mandibular Reconstruction: A Proof-of-Concept Study. *Int J Oral Maxillofac Surg* (2020) 49:13–21. doi: 10.1016/j.ijom.2019.05.005
15. Grosu AL, Lachner R, Wiedenmann N, Stärk S, Thamm R, Kneschaurek P, et al. Validation of a Method for Automatic Image Fusion (BrainLAB System) of CT Data and 11C-Methionine-PET Data for Stereotactic Radiotherapy Using a LINAC: First Clinical Experience. *Int J Radiat Oncol Biol Phys* (2003) 56:1450–63. doi: 10.1016/S0360-3016(03)00279-7
16. Thani NB, Bala A, Swann GB, Lind CRP. Accuracy of Postoperative Computed Tomography and Magnetic Resonance Image Fusion for Assessing Deep Brain Stimulation Electrodes. *Neurosurgery* (2011) 69, Issue 1:207–14. doi: 10.1227/NEU.0b013e318218c7ae
17. Garvey PB, Chang EI, Selber JC, Skoracki RJ, Madewell JE, Liu J, et al. A Prospective Study of Preoperative Computed Tomographic Angiographic Mapping of Free Fibula Osteocutaneous Flaps for Head and Neck Reconstruction. *Plast Reconstr Surg* (2012) 130(4):541e–9e. doi: 10.1097/PRS.0b013e318262f115
18. Qaisi M, Kolodney H, Swedenburg G, Chandran R, Caloss R. Fibula Jaw in a Day: State of the Art in Maxillofacial Reconstruction. *J Oral Maxillofac Surg* (2016) 74(6):1284. doi: 10.1016/j.joms.2016.01.047
19. Azuma M, Yanagawa T, Ishibashi-Kanno N, Uchida F, Ito T, Yamagata K, et al. Mandibular Reconstruction Using Plates Prebent to Fit Rapid Prototyping 3-Dimensional Printing Models Ameliorates Contour Deformity. *Head Face Med* (2014) 10:45. doi: 10.1186/1746-160X-10-45
20. Brown JS, Barry C, Ho M, Shaw R. A New Classification for Mandibular Defects After Oncological Resection. *Lancet Oncol* (2016) 17(1):e23–30. doi: 10.1016/S1470-2045(15)00310-1

13

A New Strategy for Patient-Specific Implant-Borne Dental Rehabilitation in Patients with Extended Maxillary Defects

*Philippe Korn**†, *Nils-Claudius Gellrich*†, *Philipp Jehn*, *Simon Spalthoff and Björn Rahlf*

Department of Oral and Maxillofacial Surgery, Hannover Medical School, Hannover, Germany

***Correspondence:**
Philippe Korn
korn.philippe@mh-hannover.de

†*These authors have contributed equally to this work and share first authorship*

Purpose of the Study: Patients undergoing ablative tumor surgery of the midface are faced with functional and esthetic issues. Various reconstructive strategies, such as implant-borne obturator prostheses or microvascular tissue transfer, are currently available for dental rehabilitation. The present study shows the first follow-up of patients treated with patient-specific implants (IPS Implants® Preprosthetic) for the rehabilitation of extended maxillary defects following ablative surgery.

Patients and Methods: All patients treated with patient specific implants due to postablative maxillary defects were included. 20 implants were placed in the 19 patients (bilateral implants were placed in one of the cases). In 65.75% of the cases, resection was performed due to squamous cell carcinoma. In addition to the primary stability, the clinical implant stability, soft tissue management, successful prosthodontic restoration, and complications were evaluated at a mean follow-up period of 26 months.

Results: All patient-specific implants showed primary stability and were clinically stable throughout the observation period. Definitive prosthodontic restorations were performed in all patients. No implant loosening was observed. Major complications occurred only in previously irradiated patients with insufficient soft tissue conditions ($p = 0.058$). Minor complications such as exposure of the underlying framework or mucositis were observed, but they never led to failure of restorations or implant loss.

Conclusions: Treatment of postablative maxillary defects with patient-specific implants offers a safe alternative with predictable results for full and rapid dental rehabilitation, avoiding time-consuming augmentation procedures and additional donor-site morbidity.

Keywords: maxillary defect, patient-specific implants, postablative surgery, dental rehabilitation, dental implants

INTRODUCTION

Ablative tumor surgery of the midface often leads to esthetic and functional limitations that burden patients physically as well as psychologically (1). In addition, reconstruction of these defects is challenging, and a wide variety of reconstructive procedures have been described (2–4). Management of extended maxillary defects symbolizes technical achievements in maxillofacial surgery over the last 100 years. It started with obturating intra-oral defects and the use of prosthesis, followed by techniques of pedicled and free tissue transfer (5, 6). However, the overall goal is the full dental rehabilitation of compromised patients with implant-borne prostheses. The technique of subperiosteally placed but not bone-anchored implants was described as early as the 1940s, but was subsequently abandoned due to high complication rates (7, 8). The most technically advanced concept to achieve this goal was introduced by Dennis Rohner and Beat Hammer by combining the idea of immediate dental rehabilitation following a prosthodontic backwards planning protocol with the insertion of conventional dental implants into the fibula; prelaminating the perimplant soft tissues around the fibula with skin grafts and in a second stage, harvesting of the fibula bone flap using patient-specific cutting guides to accomplish the backwards-planned design; and mounting the individual prostheses onto the osseointegrated dental implants with plate fixation of the microvascular bone flap and into the maxillary defect site (9, 10). This technique was first published in 2000 and has only two potential drawbacks: first, microvascular bone transfer is mandatory, and second, to achieve a stable result of the backwards planned dental rehabilitation concept, the patients' biology has to comply without forming pseudarthroses in the area of the fibular "wedge" cuts as well as the contact zones between the bony recipient site and bone flap. However, in cases where the patient is not eligible for harvesting a microvascular bone flap, the whole technique cannot be used. Nevertheless, this concept was unique in times of analogous planning and was benchmarked as the most advanced concept for rehabilitating patients with extended maxillary or mandibular defects. Today, this protocol can be realized using virtual planning and digital 3D printing technology to fabricate patient-specific cutting guides or plates (11–13). In cases where bony reconstruction was either not possible or failed and conventional implants were not an option, the bail-out strategy limited to the lateral maxilla was the insertion of zygomatic implants to enable prosthodontic restoration (14).

Recently, subperiostally placed and multi-vector anchored patient-specific implants with immediate loading for a one-step reconstruction of the maxilla (IPS Implants® Preprosthetic, KLS Martin, Tuttlingen, Germany) have become available (15, 16). The authors present the first follow-up of patients treated with this type of implants following ablative surgery of the maxilla.

PATIENTS AND METHODS

This is a retrospective single-center study, which included patients treated with a patient-specific implant (IPS Implants® Preprosthetic) in course of secondary reconstruction after ablative surgery of the maxilla, at Hannover Medical School (Germany).The exclusion criteria were implant insertion without previous tumor resection, for example due to a failed augmentative procedure or a defect caused by trauma or cleft lip and palate. 20 of these patient-specific implants were included in this study, which were placed in 19 patients (10 males and 9 females) as one bilateral implantation was performed. The mean age of the patients at the time of surgery was 65 years (30–85 years). Most of the defects were due to a malignant tumor; in 65.75% of the cases, resection was performed due to squamous cell carcinoma, but rare tumor entities or benign lesions were also etiological for the defects. Depending on the underlying pathology, five patients received adjuvant radiotherapy prior to implant placement, and in most cases, primary reconstruction included free tissue transfer (**Table 1**). The defects were classified according to Brown's classification, in which the number describes the vertical extent of the defect and the letter indicates the resected part of the alveolar process or palate, as shown in **Figure 1** (17).

The implants used for reconstruction were digitally backwards-planned based on the subsequent prosthodontic restoration as shown in **Figure 2**. The manufacturing process using selective laser melting allows 3D printing of a one-fit-only implant, which is placed subperiostally and anchored multi-vectorially by osteosynthesis screws, especially in the area of the load-bearing paranasal and lateral facial buttresses as well as implementing other features such as functionalization e.g. due to positioning aids in the area of the piriform aperture, tapering implant edges or a protruding pillar alignment to compensate for the maxillary tissue deficit. Depending on the defect or compromise of the load-bearing buttresses, the design of the patient-specific implant has to be adapted. With a higher

TABLE 1 | Synopsis of patients.

Diagnosis	Number of patients	Irradiation	Soft tissuefree flaps	Failed bone reconstruction	Time after primary surgery[1]
Squamous cell carcinoma	11	3	9	2	44.64 (37.10)
Keratocyst	2	–	1	1	20.50 (2.50)
Mucoepidermoid carcinoma	1	–	–	–	150
Adenoid cystic carcinoma	1	1	1	1	47
Adenocarcinoma	1	–	1	–	52
Osteosarcoma	1	–	1	1	91
Malignant Melanoma	1	1	1	–	9
Myxoma	1	–	1	–	39
Total/Mean	19	5	15	5	48.21 (39.72)

[1] *in months; brackets, standard deviation.*

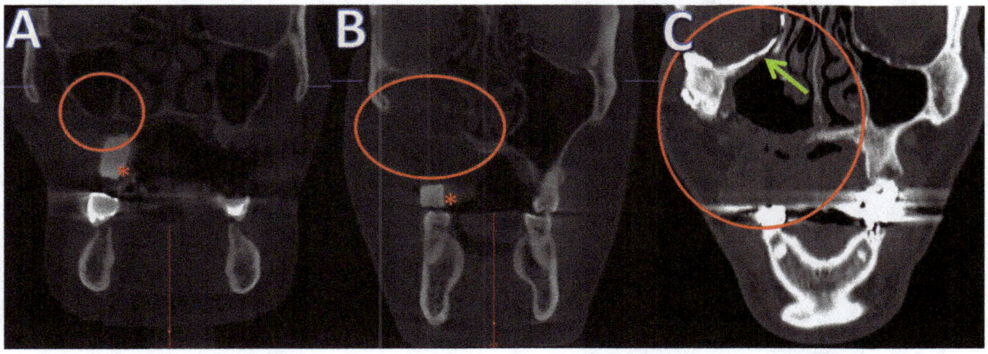

FIGURE 1 | Examples of different Brown's classifications (defect size marked with red circles). **(A)** Class 1 without oroantral fistula. **(B)** Class 2 after resection of parts of the maxillary sinus and covering with microvascular anastomosed soft tissue flaps. **(C)** Class 3 with resection of the orbital floor (arrow: patient-specific orbital implant). *Radiopaque scanning templates for prosthodontic backwards planning of IPS Implants® Preprosthetic.

Brown´s class 1 often a more distant anchorage is required, so that the implant is extended over the zygomatic arch, for example. The implementation of numerous screw holes guarantees multi-vector anchorage even in patients with poor bone quality. The authors prefer not to place under 20 screws, if this is possible.

Using a standardized protocol, the clinical implant stability as well as insertion of the definitive prosthodontic restoration were documented during follow-up as primary outcome variables. The duration of the operation, the number and size of the osteosynthesis screws, and the need for additional soft tissue procedures, such as local flaps, as well and complications were assessed as secondary variables. Descriptive statistical analyses were performed using Microsoft Excel 2010 and SigmaStat 4.0.

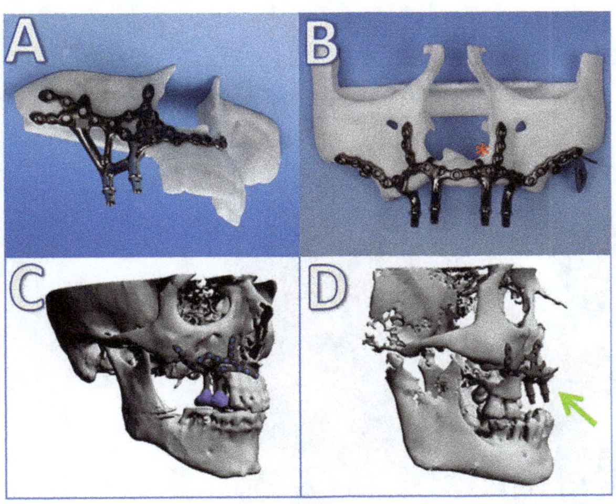

FIGURE 2 | Examples of patient-specific implants from stereolithographic biomodels **(A, B)** as well as digital planning **(C, D)**. *Additional anatomical landmarks are included in the implant design as little flanges on both sides of the piriform aperture. Arrow: protrusion of the antagonizing implant against the massive (pseudo-) class III relationship.

Group comparisons were performed using the Fisher's exact test. Statistical significance was set at $p < 0.05$, based on a 95% confidence interval. Written informed consent from the patients and ethical approval from the institutional ethics committee were obtained (reference number 8552_BO_K_2019).

RESULTS

Most of the patients were assigned to Brown's class 2, suggesting that although the maxillary sinus was affected, the orbital floor remained intact. **Table 2** shows an overview of the extent of defects in the examined patient population.

At the time of surgery, the average age of the patients was 65 years (30–87 years). The observation period was 6–74 months, with an average of 26 months. Adapted to the defect, the implants were designed with 2–4 posts. The average operating time was 127 min (69–205 min). A multivectorial screw-based anchoring of the subperiosteally placed implants was performed using an average of 22 (16–48) partly locking screws sized 1.2–2.0 mm, which always resulted in primary stability. In order to achieve soft tissue coverage of the implants, local flaps (n = 14), such as gingival advancement flaps (n = 11) were used just as regional flaps (n = 8), for example, by mobilization of Bichat's fat pad (n = 6) or by using palatine artery flaps (n = 2) (**Figure 3**).

All implants showed clinical implant stability and were restored prosthetically. There were no clinical signs of implant loosening at any point of time, and no implant was lost. **Figure 4** shows a clinical case, from resection to the final prosthodontic restoration.

TABLE 2 | Defects according to Brown's classification.

		a	b	c
1	3	–	–	–
2	–	6	6	1
3	–	–	3	–
4	–	–	–	–

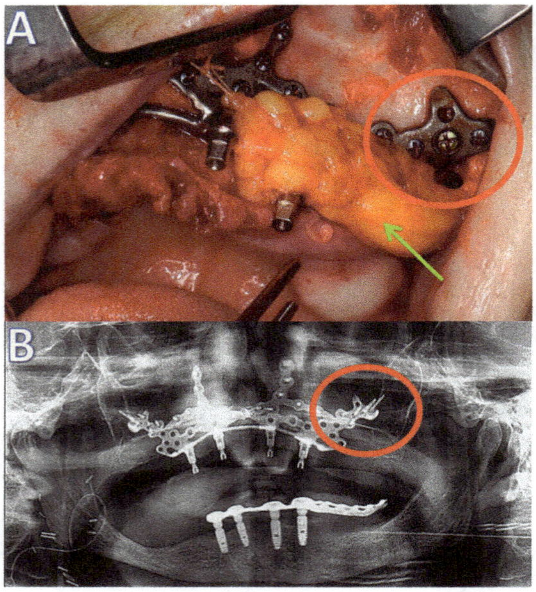

FIGURE 3 | Soft tissue coverage of the left side using the Bichat's fat pad (green arrow) **(A)** and postoperative orthopantomogram of the patient **(B)**. The red circle indicates the same implant area clinically and radiologically.

In two cases, hardware related interventions had to be performed: in one case two exposed screws had to be removed as well as in the second case where in addition to screws a single implant post was reduced without affecting the stability of the implant or the prosthetic restoration per se. The implants are still in place, and patients are free of complaints. Partial exposure of the underlying framework was observed in nine cases (47.36%), without affecting implant stability or compromising a rapid prosthetic restoration (**Figure 5**). An additional soft tissue coverage using a radial free forearm flap was necessary in one case (with a history of radiotherapy in the course of tumor treatment). In the area of the soft tissue surrounding the implant posts that penetrate into the oral cavity, an inflammatory reaction in the form of mucositis was observed in some cases. The denture saddle should shield the soft tissues to prevent movement of the implant posts, especially if separation of the anatomical units is not guaranteed (**Figure 5**). Two postoperative infections in the form of abscesses were observed, both of which occurred in irradiated patients; one of the abscesses progressed to an extraoral fistula. A trend toward a higher rate of major complications in irradiated patients was observed ($p = 0.058$), without any influence on the endpoints, such as implant survival or final prosthetic restoration.

DISCUSSION

Autologous bone grafting and prosthodontic restoration using obturators represent the most commonly used techniques for post-ablative maxillary reconstruction (2). Both treatment options have individual disadvantages: in case of autologous bone grafts, there are issues of donor-site morbidity and risk of graft loss, and in case of obturators, nasal leakage as well discomfort (e.g., instability) may cause problems. Thus, valid recommendations regarding the best therapy, especially those concerning the quality of life, are still missing (18, 19). The use of patient-specific implants (IPS Implants® Preprosthetic) offers a one-step palate-free implant-borne prosthodontic restoration without any donor-site morbidity. In addition, time-consuming and invasive augmentative procedures, which pose a risk of graft loss and are often refused by patients, are avoided. The only prerequisite for this approach to rehabilitate patients with extended maxillary defects is that the compromised anatomical units should be separated by soft tissue reconstruction prior to IPS preprosthetic implant placement. Depending on the individual defect size and extent of tissue damage, including

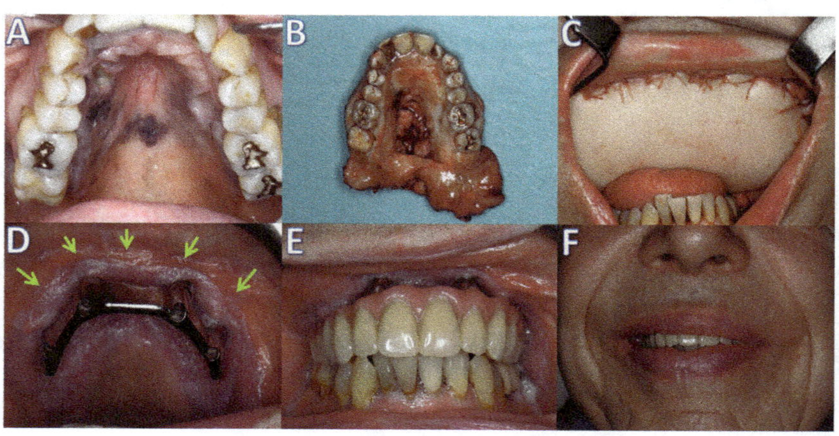

FIGURE 4 | Patient with a multilocular malignant mucosal melanoma of the upper jaw **(A)**, which was treated with extended maxillectomy **(B)** and a latissimus dorsi free flap **(C)**. After irradiation, reconstruction using a patient-specific implant (IPS Implants® Preprosthetic) and bar suprastructure; arrows: separation of anatomical units anterior to the implant posts **(D)**. Definitive palate-free prosthodontic restoration **(E)** and the clinical result **(F)**.

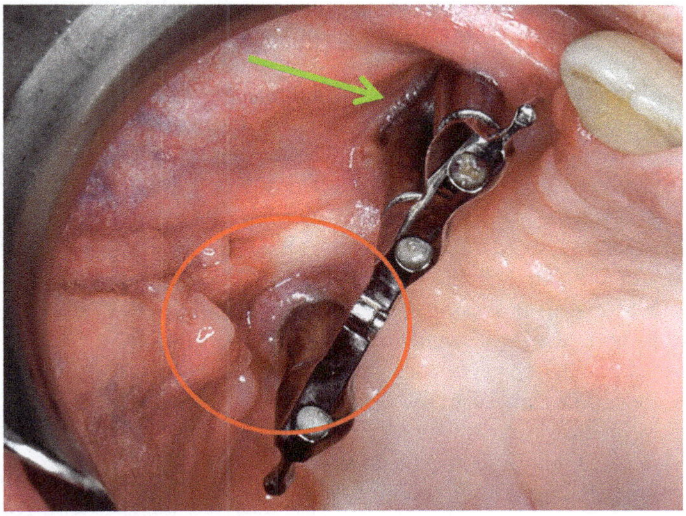

FIGURE 5 | Minor complications during follow-up. IPS Implants® preprosthetic with a bar-retained superstructure. The red circle shows mucositis of the soft tissue surrounding the dorsal post. The green arrow indicates an exposure of the underlying framework without any signs of inflammation.

post-radiation sequelae, the surgeon has to move up the soft tissue repair scale, from local flaps to microvascular soft tissue free flaps (fasciocutaneous or myocutaneous), in patients with extended maxillary defects. However, microvascular bone flaps donor sites when compared to microvascular soft tissue flaps are much fewer and donor-site morbidity is significantly higher (20, 21). In addition, after tumor resection, patients often shy away from complex reconstructions requiring tissue transplantation or augmentative procedures. Such patients require an alternative strategy similar to those with a history of failed reconstructions. Furthermore, many tumor patients are not eligible for major surgical interventions because of their reduced general condition. The excellent survival rates up to a follow-up period of up to 74 months indicate that this method is safe, with predictable results in terms of implant stability and definitive prosthodontic restoration. With regard to the quality of life, initial data show that restoration with patient-specific implants achieves outcomes that are comparable or even superior to those of conventional implants (22). This treatment option appears at first glance to be similar to the previously used subperiosteal implants, that were abandoned due to high complication rates (23). However, this is not true because the multivectorial and distant fixation of the implant using the midfacial buttresses or even the lateral skull base in selected cases fundamentally differs as an average of 22 screws achieves primary stability and allows full and immediate loading. Due to the possibilities of digital technologies, the abandoned idea of subperiosteally placed implants has been revisited and several approaches have been published (24–26), whereby individual designs and anchoring methods differ significantly. It is precisely this distant fixation as well as the multivectoral alignment of the comparatively large number of screws that distinguishes the implant system used from others that initially may appear similar. Particularly in compromised bone conditions, as in the patient group studied, anchoring with only a few screws appears dangerous, since patient-specific implants - unlike osteosynthesis plates, for example - cannot be repositioned due to their "one-fit-only" design if a screw fails to tighten.

Occasionally, signs of inflammation around the soft tissue surrounding the post were observed, but in contrast to conventional dental implants, where local infection may lead to implant loss *via* peri-implantitis, this does not seem to occur in IPS preprosthetic implants. The posts are not anchored directly in the bone and due to the distant fixation by screws, inflammation seems to remain limited to the soft tissue only. In contrast to osseointegrated conventional implants mucositis does not spread to the bone. This may be one reason that long-term stable conditions could be achieved even with recurrent episodes of mucosal inflammation and superficial exposure of framework structures. Severe postoperative complications, such as abscesses or dehiscence, requiring additional microvascular tissue transfer, only occurred in previously irradiated patients in whom the need for soft tissue was primarily underestimated. The principle of separating the anatomical units prior to IPS implant placement has to be strictly followed. As well as in alternative procedures, a history of irradiation leads to a higher rate of complications (27, 28).

Zygomatic implants used for implant-borne prosthodontic restoration are quite technology-dependent and often require an additional equipment, such as intraoperative real-time navigation (29). Furthermore, multiple complications such as sinusitis or incorrect positioning have been described (30, 31). This did not occur in the present study. Since the IPS preprosthetic implants are inserted under direct vision, there is no need for such technical prerequisites. The technical requirements for planning patient-specific implants are also shifted from the surgeon toward industrial partners. Furthermore, 3D features such as flanges toward the piriform aperture or around the transition zone between the malar prominence and zygomatic arch guarantee a one-fit-only position of IPS preprosthetic implants, in contrast to conventional dental or zygomatic implants. In addition, the possibility of positioning the implant shoulder of zygomatic implants is only possible up to the molar or premolar region and not in the esthetic zone. Zygomatic implants also do not offer a real solution to compensate for the severe postablative (pseudo-) skeletal class III relation. Owing to the patient-specific design of the IPS preprosthetic implant, a massive protrusion of the implant posts is feasible, especially in the anterior part of the (former) maxilla, enabling a functionally and esthetically satisfactory result. In contrast to restoration with conventional dental implants, the posts are aligned parallel from planning to implant insertion and final restoration. The noticeably shorter and less invasive surgical procedure compared to microvascular tissue transfer were noted, with an average duration of approximately 2 hours. Thus treatment as an outpatient is feasible.

Postablative maxillary defects often result in facial disfigurement and compromised function (6). Patients' desire for rapid functional and esthetic rehabilitation is often not possible with microvascular bone transplantation. After tumor resection or adjuvant therapy (in some cases), patients are often tired of treatment and shy away from complex reconstructions, especially after failure of tissue transfer or augmentation. Nevertheless, there is an understandable desire for dental rehabilitation with fixed palate-free dentures. The treatment algorithm presented here provides a predictable reconstruction, even after extended maxillary ablation, without time-consuming bone augmentation. With irradiated patients, the complication rate appears to increase, although all patients examined in this study were successfully rehabilitated. The patient cohort in this study is small, although the results are encouraging and the portfolio for the treatment of postablative maxillary defects is expanded. Especially if microvascular bone grafting seems not feasible or patients refuse such a procedure, secondary reconstruction using a patient-specific implant may be an alternative option.

AUTHOR CONTRIBUTIONS

PK and N-CG designed the study and drafted the manuscript. BR analysed the data and revised the manuscript. PJ and SS revised the article for important intellectual content. All authors contributed to the article and approved the submitted version.

ACKNOWLEDGMENTS

We would like to thank Editage (www.editage.com) for English language editing.

REFERENCES

1. Brown JS, Shaw RJ. Reconstruction of the Maxilla and Midface: Introducing a New Classification. *Lancet Oncol* (2010) 11:1001–8. doi: 10.1016/S1470-2045(10)70113-3
2. Andrades P, Militsakh O, Hanasono MM, Rieger J, Rosenthal EL. Current Strategies in Reconstruction of Maxillectomy Defects. *Arch Otolaryngol Head Neck Surg* (2011) 137:806–12. doi: 10.1001/archoto.2011.132
3. Jung S, Kook M-S, Park H-J, Oh H-K. Delayed Closure of the Palatal Defect Using Buccal Inversion and Palatal Rotation Flaps After Maxillectomy. *J Craniofac Surg* (2013) 24:660–4. doi: 10.1097/SCS.0b013e31827c8611
4. Vincent A, Burkes J, Williams F, Ducic Y. Free Flap Reconstruction of the Maxilla. *Semin Plast Surg* (2019) 33:30–7. doi: 10.1055/s-0039-1677701
5. Parr GR, Gardner LK. The Evolution of the Obturator Framework Design. *J Prosthet Dent* (2003) 89:608–10. doi: 10.1016/s0022-3913(03)00176-8
6. Lenox ND, Kim DD. Maxillary Reconstruction. *Oral Maxillofac Surg Clin North Am* (2013) 25:215–22. doi: 10.1016/j.coms.2013.01.004
7. Dahl G. Om MöJligheten FöR Inplantation I KäKen Avmetallskelett Som Bas Eller Retention FöR Fasta Eller Avtagbaraproteser. *Odontologisk Tidskrift* (1943) 51:440–9.
8. Goldberg NI, Gershkoff A. The Implant Lower Denture. *Dental Digest* (1949) 55:490–5.
9. Rohner D, Kunz C, Bucher P, Hammer B, Prein J. New Possibilities for Reconstructing Extensive Jaw Defects With Prefabricated Microvascular Fibula Transplants and ITI Implants. *Mund Kiefer Gesichtschir* (2000) 3:365–72. doi: 10.1007/s100060000228
10. Rohner D, Jaquiéry C, Kunz C, Bucher P, Maas H, Hammer B. Maxillofacial Reconstruction With Prefabricated Osseous Free Flaps: A 3-Year Experience With 24 Patients. *Plast Reconstr Surg* (2003) 112:748–57. doi: 10.1097/01.PRS.0000069709.89719.79
11. Rana M, Chin S-J, Muecke T, Kesting M, Groebe A, Riecke B, et al. Increasing the Accuracy of Mandibular Reconstruction With Free Fibula Flaps Using Functionalized Selective Laser-Melted Patient-Specific Implants: A Retrospective Multicenter Analysis. *J Craniomaxillofac Surg* (2017) 45:1212–9. doi: 10.1016/j.jcms.2017.04.003
12. Weitz J, Wolff K-D, Kesting MR, Nobis C-P. Development of a Novel Resection and Cutting Guide for Mandibular Reconstruction Using Free Fibula Flap. *J Craniomaxillofac Surg* (2018) 46:1975–8. doi: 10.1016/j.jcms.2018.09.007
13. Zavattero E, Bolzoni A, Dell'Aversana G, Santagata M, Massarelli O, Ferri A, et al. Accuracy of Fibula Reconstruction Using Patient-Specific Cad/Cam Plates: A Multicenter Study on 47 Patients. *Laryngoscope* (2021) 131:E2169–75. doi: 10.1002/lary.29379
14. Hackett S, El-Wazani B, Butterworth C. Zygomatic Implant-Based Rehabilitation for Patients With Maxillary and Mid-Facial Oncology Defects: A Review. *Oral Dis* (2021) 27:27–41. doi: 10.1111/odi.13305
15. Gellrich N-C, Zimmerer RM, Spalthoff S, Jehn P, Pott P-C, Rana M, et al. A Customised Digitally Engineered Solution for Fixed Dental Rehabilitation in Severe Bone Deficiency: A New Innovative Line Extension in Implant Dentistry. *J Craniomaxillofac Surg* (2017) 45:1632–8. doi: 10.1016/j.jcms.2017.07.022
16. Gellrich N-C, Rahlf B, Zimmerer R, Pott P-C, Rana M. A New Concept for Implant-Borne Dental Rehabilitation; How to Overcome the Biological Weak-Spot of Conventional Dental Implants? *Head Face Med* (2017) 13:17. doi: 10.1186/s13005-017-0151-3
17. Brown JS, Rogers SN, McNally DN, Boyle M. A Modified Classification for the Maxillectomy Defect. *Head Neck* (2000) 22:17–26. doi: 10.1002/(sici)1097-0347(200001)22:1<17::aid-hed4>3.0.co;2-2
18. Cao Y, Yu C, Liu W, Miao C, Han B, Yang J, et al. Obturators Versus Flaps After Maxillary Oncological Ablation: A Systematic Review and Best Evidence Synthesis. *Oral Oncol* (2018) 82:152–61. doi: 10.1016/j.oraloncology.2018.05.019
19. Buurman DJM, Speksnijder CM, de Groot RJ, Kessler P, Rieger JM. Mastication in Maxillectomy Patients: A Comparison Between Reconstructed Maxillae and Implant Supported Obturators: A Cross-Sectional Study. *J Oral Rehabil* (2020) 47:1171–7. doi: 10.1111/joor.13043
20. Ling XF, Peng X, Samman N. Donor-Site Morbidity of Free Fibula and DCIA

Flaps. *J Oral Maxillofac Surg* (2013) 71:1604–12. doi: 10.1016/j.joms.2013.03.006

21. Kansy K, Hoffmann J, Alhalabi O, Mistele N, Freier K, Shavlokhova V, et al. Long-Term Donor Site Morbidity in Head and Neck Cancer Patients and its Impact on Quality of Life: A Cross-Sectional Study. *Int J Oral Maxillofac Surg* (2019) 48:875–85. doi: 10.1016/j.ijom.2019.01.009
22. Jehn P, Spalthoff S, Korn P, Stoetzer M, Gercken M, Gellrich N-C, et al. Oral Health-Related Quality of Life in Tumour Patients Treated With Patient-Specific Dental Implants. *Int J Oral Maxillofac Surg* (2020) 49:1067–72. doi: 10.1016/j.ijom.2020.01.011
23. Schou S, Pallesen L, Hjørting-Hansen E, Pedersen CS, Fibaek B. A 41-Year History of a Mandibular Subperiosteal Implant. *Clin Oral Implants Res* (2000) 11:171–8. doi: 10.1034/j.1600-0501.2000.110210.x
24. Van den Borre C, Rinaldi M, De Neef B, Loomans NAJ, Nout E, Van Doorne L, et al. Radiographic Evaluation of Bone Remodeling After Additively Manufactured Subperiosteal Jaw Implantation (AMSJI) in the Maxilla: A One-Year Follow-Up Study. *J Clin Med* (2021) 10:3542. doi: 10.3390/jcm10163542
25. Cerea M, Dolcini GA. Custom-Made Direct Metal Laser Sintering Titanium Subperiosteal Implants: A Retrospective Clinical Study on 70 Patients. *BioMed Res Int* (2018) 2018:5420391. doi: 10.1155/2018/5420391
26. Mangano C, Bianchi A, Mangano FG, Dana J, Colombo M, Solop I, et al. Custom-Made 3D Printed Subperiosteal Titanium Implants for the Prosthetic Restoration of the Atrophic Posterior Mandible of Elderly Patients: A Case Series. *3D Print Med* (2020) 6:1. doi: 10.1186/s41205-019-0055-x
27. Schmidt BL, Pogrel MA, Young CW, Sharma A. Reconstruction of Extensive Maxillary Defects Using Zygomaticus Implants. *J Oral Maxillofac Surg* (2004) 62(9 Suppl 2):82–9. doi: 10.1016/j.joms.2004.06.027
28. Lodders JN, Leusink FKJ, Ridwan-Pramana A, Winters HAH, Karagozoglu KH, Dekker H, et al. Long-Term Outcomes of Implant-Based Dental Rehabilitation in Head and Neck Cancer Patients After Reconstruction With the Free Vascularized Fibula Flap. *J Craniomaxillofac Surg* (2021) 30: S1010–5182(21)00101-3. doi: 10.1016/j.jcms.2021.03.002
29. Schramm A, Gellrich NC, Schimming R, Schmelzeisen R. [Computer-Assisted Insertion of Zygomatic Implants (Brånemark System) After Extensive Tumor Surgery]. *Mund Kiefer Gesichtschir* (2000) 4:292–5. doi: 10.1007/s100060000211
30. Molinero-Mourelle P, Baca-Gonzalez L, Gao B, Saez-Alcaide L-M, Helm A, Lopez-Quiles J. Surgical Complications in Zygomatic Implants: A Systematic Review. *Med Oral Patol Oral Cir Bucal* (2016) 21:e751–7. doi: 10.4317/medoral.21357
31. D'Agostino A, Lombardo G, Favero V, Signoriello A, Bressan A, Lonardi F, et al. Complications Related to Zygomatic Implants Placement: A Retrospective Evaluation With 5 Years Follow-Up. *J Craniomaxillofac Surg* (2021) 5:S1010–5182(21)00033-0. doi: 10.1016/j.jcms.2021.01.020

14

Mandibular Reconstruction with Fibula Flap and Dental Implants through Virtual Surgical Planning and Three Different Techniques: Double-Barrel Flap, Implant Dynamic Navigation and CAD/CAM Mesh with Iliac Crest Graft

Raúl Antúnez-Conde, José Ignacio Salmerón, Alberto Díez-Montiel, Marc Agea, Dafne Gascón, Ángela Sada, Ignacio Navarro Cuéllar, Manuel Tousidonis, Santiago Ochandiano, Gema Arenas and Carlos Navarro Cuéllar*

Maxillofacial Surgery Department, Hospital General Universitario Gregorio Marañón, Madrid, Spain

***Correspondence:**
Raúl Antúnez-Conde
comunicacionrac@outlook.es

Introduction: Vertical discrepancy between the fibula flap and the native mandible results in difficult prosthetic rehabilitation. The aim of this study was to evaluate the outcomes of 3D reconstruction of the mandible in oncologic patients using three different techniques through virtual surgical planning (VSP), cutting guides, customized titanium mesh and plates with CAD/CAM technology, STL models and intraoperative dynamic navigation for implant placement. Material and methods

Material and Methods: Three different techniques for mandibular reconstruction and implant rehabilitation were performed in 14 oncologic patients. Five patients (36%) underwent VSP, cutting guides, STL models and a customized double-barrel titanium plate with a double-barrel flap and immediate implants. In six patients (43%), VSP, STL models and a custom-made titanium mesh (CAD/CAM) for 3D reconstruction with iliac crest graft over a fibula flap with deferred dental implants were performed. Three patients (21%) underwent VSP with cutting guides and customized titanium plates for mandibular reconstruction and implant rehabilitation using intraoperative dynamic navigation was accomplished. Vertical bone reconstruction, peri-implant bone resorption, implant success rate, effects of radiotherapy in vertical reconstruction, bone resorption and implant failure, mastication, aesthetic result and dysphagia were evaluated.

Results: Significant differences in bone growth between the double-barrel technique and iliac crest graft with titanium mesh technique were found ($p<0.002$). Regarding bone resorption, there were no significant differences between the techniques ($p=0.11$). 60 implants were placed with an osseointegration rate of 91.49%. Five implants were lost during the osseointegration period (8%). Peri-implant bone resorption was measured with a mean of 1.27 mm. There was no significant difference between the vertical gain technique used and implant survival (p>0.385). Implant survival rates were higher in non-irradiated patients (p<0.017). All patients were rehabilitated with a fixed implant-supported prosthesis reporting a regular diet (80%), normal swallowing (85.7%) and excellent aesthetic results.

Conclusions: Multi-stage implementation of VSP, STL models and cutting guides, CAD/CAM technology, customized plates and in-house dynamic implant navigation for mandibular defects increases bone-to-bone contact, resolves vertical discrepancy and improves operative efficiency with reduced complication rates and minimal bone resorption. It provides accurate reconstruction that optimizes implant placement, thereby improving facial symmetry, aesthetics and function.

Keywords: virtual surgical planning (VSP), 3D printing (3DP), CAD/CAM titanium mesh, mandibular reconstruction, STL models, implant dynamic navigation, double-barrel flap, iliac crest graft

INTRODUCTION

Mandibular defects in oncologic patients cause severe bone and soft tissue defects, with their consequent aesthetic and functional sequelae, and immediate mandibular reconstruction is mandatory. Mandibular segmental defects lead to malocclusion, mandibular deviation, TMJ alterations and soft tissue retraction (1). Retrusion of the lower third of the face occurs, especially in cases where the mandibulectomy includes the symphysis and mandibular body. In addition, there is significant lower lip ptosis and lip incompetence. When resection is located on the body of the mandible, facial asymmetry is evident, with soft tissue collapse on the affected side (2–4). If the tumor resection in the mandible includes the mandibular condyle, these sequelae are even more significant (1). In addition to lip incompetence, other disabling functional sequelae include salivary incontinence, difficulty in chewing, swallowing, and speech articulation. Patients undergoing mandibular resection who do not receive reconstruction present progressive deviation and retrusion towards the affected side, increasing the functional sequelae exposed (1, 2). In addition, vertical masticatory movements are replaced by oblique and diagonal movements directed by a single temporomandibular joint which, added to the limited lingual mobility in many cases, increases the patient's difficulties in social interaction.

Advances in reconstructive surgical techniques in the head and neck area have allowed a comprehensive treatment and a complete surgical approach with a significant improvement in the aesthetic and functional reconstruction of these patients. Microsurgical techniques, virtual surgical planning (VSP), CAD-CAM (computer-aided design/computer-aided manufacturing) technology, intraoperative dynamic navigation and advanced implantology have improved significantly the comprehensive reconstruction of the oncologic patients with segmental mandibular defects (5–8).

Free flaps are considered the main reconstructive technique for segmental defects of the mandible and adjacent soft tissues (9). Among them, the fibula free flap, the scapular flap, and the iliac crest flap stand out. The fibula flap has been the flap of choice since it was described for mandibular reconstruction due to several advantages: great length of bone which allows reconstructions of defects longer than 10 cm (10), medullary and periosteal vascular supply, a long and anatomically constant vascular pedicle (11), large skin paddle for soft tissue reconstruction, bicortical bone (10) and the feasibility for dental rehabilitation with implant-supported or implant-retained prostheses (12). The bicortical bone is ideal in order to achieve primary stability of dental implants, it provides the possibility of a two-team approach and the morbidity of the donor area is relatively low (2, 13). However, the fibula flap does not provide sufficient height of bone to restore the native height of the mandible (3). The vertical discrepancy between the remnant mandible and the fibula flap results in a reduction of the vertical dimension of the lower third of the face with the consequent aesthetic and functional sequelae and difficulty in implant placement and prosthetic rehabilitation that may cause implant overloading and endanger both the functional and aesthetic long-term results (9). There are several surgical techniques to solve this problem through virtual surgical planning: a double-barrel flap with a double-barrel customized titanium plate and immediate implant placement, a CAD/CAM titanium mesh filled with iliac crest onlay graft over the fibula flap in a second stage procedure, and a vertical distraction osteogenesis of the fibula flap. To complete the mandibular reconstruction and the aesthetic and functional oral rehabilitation of these patients, the placement of dental implants needs to be optimal. Therefore, intraoperative navigation allows highly accurate and predictable results necessary in cases with altered and complex mandibular anatomy.

The aim of this study was to evaluate the outcomes of three-dimensional aesthetic and functional reconstruction of the mandible in oncologic patients using three different techniques through virtual surgical planning: 1) VSP, STL models and cutting guides for mandibular resection and reconstruction with a double-barrel free flap and a customized double-barrel titanium plate with immediate implant placement; 2) VSP, STL models and a CAD/CAM titanium mesh with iliac crest graft in a second surgical procedure with delayed placement of dental implants; 3) VSP with cutting guides for mandibular reconstruction and intraoperative dynamic navigation for implant placement in a delayed surgical procedure. An additional aim of this study was to compare the success rate of the implants and the bone resorption between irradiated and non-irradiated patients. The specific aims were: a) to compare the vertical reconstruction of the mandible; b) to compare the peri-implant bone resorption; c) to compare the implant failure between the different techniques; d) to compare the effects of radiotherapy in vertical reconstruction and bone resorption; e) to stablish the association between radiotherapy and implant failure; f) to evaluate mastication; g) to evaluate the aesthetic result and h) to evaluate the presence or absence of dysphagia. The aesthetic result, the mastication and dysphagia were evaluated 1 year after prosthetic rehabilitation. The aesthetic and functional results with deglutition and speech articulation were evaluated 1 year after prosthetic rehabilitation. The review of medical records and data collection and the subsequent analysis of the data collected is endorsed by the Hospital Ethics Committee at Gregorio Marañón General Hospital, Madrid, Spain.

MATERIALS AND METHODS

To address the research purpose, the investigators designed and implemented a retrospective study during a 5-year period (2015–2020). Fourteen patients with segmental mandibular defect due to their oncologic process and mandibular segmental reconstruction with implant rehabilitation were included in this study at Hospital General Universitario Gregorio Marañón, Madrid, Spain. The inclusion criteria were: 1) oncologic patients with segmental mandibulectomy reconstructed through VSP with double-barrel fibula free flap, double-barrel customized plate and immediate implant placement with surgical guides; 2) oncologic patients with segmental mandibulectomy reconstructed with fibula flap and iliac crest graft with customized titanium mesh through VSP, CAD/CAM technology and dental implants in a second surgical stage; 3) oncologic patients with segmental mandibulectomy reconstructed with fibula flap and implant rehabilitation through VSP and "in house" dynamic navigation in a second surgical procedure. Patients with previous history of radiotherapy or chemotherapy were excluded from this study.

Eight oncologic patients were diagnosed with ameloblastoma and six patients were diagnosed with squamous cell carcinoma. In all cases, MRI was performed prior to surgical planning to ensure the viability of the patients' tibioperoneal vessels. In patients in which a skin paddle was necessary to reconstruct the soft tissue defect, the perforating vessels were marked on the skin, and the fibula flap was designed to include the perforators. Oncologic resection with clear margins was achieved in all patients through virtual surgical planning and cutting guides that improved the precision of the bone resection. Immediate reconstruction with fibula flap through VSP was performed in all patients. Patients were distributed into three groups according to the mandibular reconstruction and implant rehabilitation techniques employed.

In five patients (35%), the reconstruction technique used was the double-barrel fibula flap through virtual surgical planning, 3D printed models and a double-barrel customized titanium plate manufactured with a CNC milling machine (plate thickness: 2.0 mm with 1.5 mm in the upper extension and a 2.0 mm screw system) (KLS Martin). Immediate implant placement was accomplished through the 3D printed cutting guide This technique was performed in patients in which sufficient length of bone and length of vascular pedicle was available to allow an optimal reconstruction without compromise of microvascular anastomoses. The design of the peroneal cutting guide included the surgical guide for immediate implant placement (Ticare®, Valladolid, Spain).

In six patients (43%), a secondary 3D reconstruction of the mandible was accomplished through VSP, STL models and a custom-made titanium mesh (CAD/CAM) (Maffinter®, Madrid, Spain) with iliac crest graft and dental implants to enable both vertical and horizontal reconstruction of the fibula flap. This technique was performed in patients in which no sufficient length of bone was available to perform a double-barrel flap for complete reconstruction of the defect or in patients in which a previous single fibula flap was performed and a secondary 3D reconstruction of the fibula was needed prior to achieve an optimal prosthodontic rehabilitation with dental implants. In non-irradiated patients the second surgical stage was performed 4 months after initial surgery. In one irradiated patient the surgery was performed one year after the end of radiotherapy. A two-team approach was accomplished and a cortico-cancellous graft from the anterior superior iliac crest was harvested due to its thicker cortical layer. As it was a cortico-cancellous graft and not a microsurgical flap, no cutting guides were used, and the adaptation of the graft to the CAD/CAM titanium mesh was performed using a standard freehand procedure. A cervical approach was performed to expose the fibula flap and remove the osteosynthesis material. In this way, the cortico-cancellous graft was isolated from the oral cavity. In all patients cortico-cancellous graft was fixed using CAD/CAM titanium mesh, adapted and fixed to the remaining fibula. Six months later, the three dimensions of the mandible were evaluated by the Radiology Department through CT scan, providing relevant quantitative data regarding bone volume and bone resorption. The height of the graft was measured in both sagittal and coronal CT sequences, while the width of the graft was measured in the axial CT sequences. An intraoral approach was planned, the titanium mesh was removed and dental implants (Ticare®, Valladolid, Spain) were placed in all patients, who were subsequently rehabilitated with a fixed implant-supported prosthesis with the aim of achieving a comprehensive reconstruction, both aesthetic and functional.

Three patients (22%) underwent VSP with cutting guides and customized titanium plates with fibula flap with minimal vertical discrepancy that did not require complementary techniques. Rehabilitation with dental implants was performed using intraoperative dynamic navigation in a second surgical stage in patients previously reconstructed with fibula flap. The intraoperative dynamic navigation technique for implant placement is a recent technique in our department and, therefore, in patients in whom the vertical discrepancy between the fibula flap and the remnant mandible was not significant, implant placement was performed using an "in house" intraoperative dynamic navigation. Virtual 3D models of the jaw and surrounding tissues were generated from preoperative CT scan using 3D Slicer open-source software. The models were imported into a dental planning software and optimal position of the implants were determined. The virtual planning was transferred into the navigation software and a Polaris Spectra (NDI, Waterloo, Canada) optical tracking system was used to assess the real-time positioning of the surgical instruments. Tracked instruments included the drilling handpiece, and a pointer device in order to register the landmarks. The handpiece tracking was possible due to the attachment of a 3D printed adaptor specifically designed which included the optical markers. A 3D printed reference with optical markers was also designed in order to track the patients' position during surgery. This printed reference was attached to the jaw using a silicone jig fitted on the teeth. These references were manufactured with polylactic acid using a 3D printer at the hospital's FabLab. A software application was developed in 3D slicer showing the real-time position of the handpiece with respect to the preoperative images, 3D models and virtual planning. The handpiece tip position was recorded during drilling and the application enabled an accurate control of the drilling trajectory in order to achieve the virtual planning. Intraoperative measurements were performed to assess the position and angular deviation of the dental implants. Postoperative CT scan and panoramic radiographs were performed to evaluate the surgical outcomes.

The prosthetic rehabilitation of the oncologic patients was carried out in the Maxillofacial Surgery Department with fixed implant-supported prostheses with the aim of achieving the best aesthetic and functional reconstruction. During the follow-up period, the vertical gain obtained after surgery with each technique, the peri-implant bone resorption, the implant success rate and the effects of radiotherapy, were evaluated. Measurement of vertical bone gain was performed in all patients before implant placement. Esthetic assessment by the patients was performed in all groups to address scores in facial symmetry, facial scarring and facial projection, and the results were classified with scores 1 (poor), 2 (fair), and 3 (good). Functional outcomes such as mastication and deglutition were also evaluated. Dysphagia was reported as "yes" or "no", and mastication was assessed in all groups, and results were classified with scores 1 (liquid-soft diet), and 2 (regular/unrestricted diet).

Statistical analysis: qualitative variables were expressed as frequencies and percentages. Quantitative values were expressed as mean +/- standard error of mean. Mann-Whitney's tests were used to compare differences between groups of quantitative variables. Qualitative variables were compared using Chi-squared test. The statistical analysis was performed using the software SPSS 25.0. p value < 0.05 was considered statistically significant.

RESULTS

The mean follow-up time was 26 months (range 6-48 months) with no flap loss observed in any of the cases. The vertical discrepancy was solved, achieving in two patients a partial overcorrection of 112%. Fourteen patients with segmental mandibular defects were reconstructed with a free fibula flap. In all patients the origin of the defect was oncologic of which eight patients (57%) presented diagnosis of ameloblastoma and six patients (43%) of squamous cell carcinoma. In five patients (35%), mandibular reconstruction was performed in a single stage by means of VSP, double-barrel fibula flap, double-barrel customized titanium plate and immediate implant placement through surgical guides. Six patients (43%) underwent a second surgery with an iliac crest graft adapted according to the titanium meshes made specifically for each patient using CAD-CAM technology. Six months later, the titanium meshes were removed and dental implants were placed. In 3 patients (22%), the vertical dimension of a simple fibula flap was sufficient to provide a good aesthetic and functional result and implant placement was performed through VSP and dynamic navigation in a second surgical procedure. Therefore, 65% of patients required more than one surgical intervention for complete rehabilitation. The smallest mandibular segment was 6.3 cm and the largest was 16.4 cm, with a mean of 10.2 cm. In six patients, the fibula flap was exclusively a bone flap (43%) and in eight patients osseocutaneous flaps were harvested (57%). One flap required surgical revision due to partial thrombosis of one of the anastomosed veins in the immediate postoperative period.

VIRTUAL SURGICAL PLANNING FOR DOUBLE-BARREL FREE FLAP, CUTTING GUIDES, CUSTOMIZED DOUBLE-BARREL PLATE AND IMMEDIATE DENTAL IMPLANTS

Patients reconstructed with double-barrel fibula flap had a mean age of 46.4. Four patients were male (80%) and one patient was female (20%). Two patients were diagnosed with squamous cell carcinoma, 2 patients with multicystic ameloblastoma and 1 desmoplastic ameloblastoma. Three patients (60%) did not receive postoperative radiotherapy and two patients were irradiated (40%). Vertical reconstruction was 27.8+/-0.5mm and bone resorption was 1.23+/-0.09mm. A total of 20 implants were immediately placed with a mean of 3.8+/-0.26 implants per patient. There were no major complications. In one patient there was intraoral exposure of the osteosynthesis material, which was treated conservatively without incident. This technique allowed reconstruction of the natural mandibular height. Two patients (40%) with 8 implants were irradiated with 60Gy. Twelve implants (60%) were placed in the 3 non-irradiated patients. Of the implants placed in irradiated patients, one implant (12.5%) presented osseointegration failure. In non-irradiated patients there was loss of one implant (8.3%). The rest of the implants showed correct osseointegration (90%). All patients were rehabilitated with fixed implant-supported prostheses. One year after prosthetic rehabilitation, mesial and distal peri-implant bone resorption was evaluated. The mean bone resorption was 1.23 mm. In irradiated patients the resorption was slightly higher than in non-irradiated patients, where it was not relevant. (**Table 1A**).

Case Presentation

A 29-year-old male patient was diagnosed with mandibular desmoplastic ameloblastoma with involvement of the symphysis and right mandibular body and disruption of the lingual cortical bone. A virtual surgical planning was performed for resection with clear margins and reconstruction of a double-barrel fibula flap with four segments and immediate placement of five dental implants were performed (**Figure 1**). Cutting guides were designed for both resection and reconstruction, as well as a design for immediate implant placement (Osteoplac Innovations®, Madrid, Spain). For the reconstruction, a customized double-barrel titanium plate was designed and manufactured with a CNC milling machine (plate thickness: 2.0 mm with 1.5 mm in the upper extension and a 2.0 mm screw system) (KLS Martin) specifically so that the placement of the implants did not interfere with the osteosynthesis material (**Figure 2**). A two team approach was performed simultaneously and the cutting guides were used to perform the segmental mandibulectomy and to perform the osteotomies for a double-barrel fibula flap with four segments. The fibula cutting guide incorporated in its design the slots for the placement of the implants that were drilled during the harvesting of the flap. Once the mandible had been reconstructed and the microsurgical anastomoses had been performed, five dental implants were placed (Ticare®) (**Figures 3, 4**). Postoperative CT scan and panoramic radiograph demonstrated a correct union between the fibula flap and the remnant mandible and accurate implant placement as planned in the virtual surgical planning. Prosthetic rehabilitation was performed with an implant fixed prosthesis with an optimal aesthetic and functional result (**Figure 4**).

VIRTUAL SURGICAL PLANNING, STEREOLITOGRAPHIC MODELS AND CAD/CAM TITANIUM MESH FOR 3D RECONSTRUCTION OF FIBULA FLAP WITH ILIAC CREST GRAFT AND DENTAL IMPLANTS

The patients reconstructed with fibula flap and titanium mesh with iliac crest graft had a mean age of 52 years. Three patients were female (50%) and three patients were male (50%). Three patients were diagnosed with squamous cell carcinoma, 1 patient developed a recurrent ameloblastoma and 2 patients were diagnosed with multicystic ameloblastoma. One patient (17%) received postoperative radiotherapy while 5 patients (83%) were not irradiated. Mean vertical reconstruction was 12.1 mm (range 13.4 - 10.1 mm). Mean bone resorption was 1.48 mm. One patient received radiotherapy and iliac crest graft was delayed one year after the end of radiotherapy. In the remaining patients (83%), reconstruction of the vertical dimension with iliac crest graft and custom CAD-CAM titanium mesh was performed four months after initial surgery. In all cases a two-team approach was performed, at the cervical area and the anterosuperior iliac spine, respectively. The cervical approach allowed placement of the iliac crest graft without contamination of the oral cavity in all cases. Six months later, an intraoral approach was performed for mesh removal and implant placement. Twenty-eight implants were inserted in this group of patients with an average of 4.6 implants per patient. Osseointegration failure was evident in one implant (3.5%) in the irradiated patient. The osseointegration success rate was 92.86%. All patients were rehabilitated with an implant-supported fixed prosthesis (**Table 1B**).

Case Presentation

A 38-year-old patient was referred to our Department reporting progressive deformity of the mandibular symphysis. 3D CT scan showed a lytic lesion with destruction of the external mandibular cortex (**Figure 5A**). A multicystic ameloblastoma was diagnosed. Tumor resection with segmental mandibulectomy and clear margins, and immediate reconstruction with a two-segment fibula flap was performed (**Figure 5A**). A vertical discrepancy between the remnant mandible and the fibula flap was assessed and a virtual surgical planning (VSP) with a cortico-cancellous iliac crest graft was planned in a second surgical procedure. VSP was performed with the biomedical engineer (Maffinter®, Madrid, Spain) and a three-dimensional virtual reconstruction of the defect was performed with two titanium CAD/CAM meshes (**Figure 5B**). STL model and CAD/CAM titanium mesh were printed and checked before surgery (**Figure 6A**). Under general anesthesia, a cervical approach was performed to expose the fibula and remove the osteosynthesis material without communicating with the oral cavity (**Figure 6B**). Simultaneously, a cortico-cancellous graft of the left anterosuperior iliac crest was obtained. The graft was fixed to the fibula using the CAD/CAM titanium mesh and 1.5 mm screws (**Figure 6C**). There was no intraoral exposure of the graft and an increase in the vertical dimension of the fibula was achieved and demonstrated by panoramic radiograph and CT scan. Panoramic radiograph revealed a bone gap between the iliac crest graft and the remnant mandible mesial to the left first molar due to the angular shape of the titanium mesh at this level. Six months later, the ossification of the graft and volume of the soft tissue were verified. An intraoral approach was performed, the titanium mesh was removed and the increase in height and width achieved with the graft was verified, showing the space beneath the titanium mesh completely filled with new hard tissue (**Figure 7**). Seven dental implants were placed (Ticare®, Valladolid, Spain) and, four months later, the second surgical procedure of the implants was performed. Despite the gap between the iliac crest graft and the remnant mandible, the prosthetic rehabilitation was carried out by means of a fixed implant-supported prosthesis providing normal occlusion (**Figure 8**). Three years later, there was no evidence of significant peri-implant bone resorption. The prosthetic rehabilitation allowed a correct aesthetic and functional result with a regular diet and intelligible speech.

VIRTUAL SURGICAL PLANNING AND IN-HOUSE IMPLANT DYNAMIC NAVIGATION FOR MANDIBULAR RECONSTRUCTION AND DENTAL REHABILITATION

In three cases (21%), reconstruction with a free fibula flap was sufficient to obtain a vertical dimension of the segmental defect

TABLE 1 | Outcomes with three different techniques for mandible reconstruction and implant rehabilitation in oncologic patients.

A.- DOUBLE BARREL FIBULA FLAP WITH INMEDIATE DENTAL IMPLANTS

Gender/Age (Years)	Diagnosis	Length of Defect (cm)	Vertical Reconstruction (mm)	Vertical Fibula Height (mm)	Horizontal Dimension (mm)	Number ofImplants/ Failure	Bone resorption (mm)	Radiotherapy	Aesthetic Result	Mastication	Dysphagia
M/70	Squamous cell carcinoma	8.4	26.1	12.3	8.6	4/1	1.6	Yes	3	2	Yes
F/32	Ameloblastoma	7.8	24.5	12.0	8.0	3/1	1.5	No	3	2	No
M/29	Ameloblastoma	9.9	30.7	14.5	10.7	5	0.5	No	3	2	No
M/43	Ameloblastoma	9.3	28.2	13.7	9.5	4	1.2	No	2	2	No
M/58	Squamous cell carcinoma	10.6	29.4	14.2	10.9	4	1.4	Yes	3	1	No
Average		9.2	27.8	13.32	9.54	20/2 (90.0%)	1.23				

B.- FIBULA FLAP WITH ILIAC CREST GRAFT, TITANIUM MESH AND DENTAL IMPLANTS.

Gender/Age (Years)	Diagnosis	Length of Defect (cm)	Vertical Reconstruction (graft) (mm)	Vertical Fibula Height (mm)	Horizontal Dimension (mm)	Number of Implants/ Failure	Bone resorption (mm)	Radiotherapy	Aesthetic Result	Mastication	Dysphagia
M/42	Ameloblastoma	9.5	11.7	14.1	11.2	4	1.5	No	3	2	No
F/61	Squamous cell carcinoma	10.8	11.9	12.3	9.6	4	1.5	No	2	1	No
F/63	Squamous cell carcinoma	9.6	12.3	12.1	9.4	5/1	1.6	No	2	2	No
M/38	Ameloblastoma	12.6	13.2	14.4	11.7	7	0.5	No	3	2	No
F/35	Ameloblastoma	9.4	13.4	13.9	9.7	4	1.4	No	3	2	No
M/73	Squamous cell carcinoma	8.9	10.1	14.2	8.9	4/1	2.4	Yes	3	2	Yes
Average		10.05	12.22	13.55	10.1	28/2 (92.86%)	1.48				

C.- DYNAMIC NAVIGATION FOR IMPLANT REHABILITATION IN FIBULA FLAP

Gender/Age (Years)	Diagnosis	Length of Defect (cm)	Vertical Reconstruction (mm)	Vertical Fibula Height (mm)	Horizontal Dimension (mm)	Number of Implants/ Failure	Bone resorption (mm)	Radiotherapy	Aesthetic Result	Mastication	Dysphagia
M/18	Ameloblastoma	9.8	Not necessary	12.2	8.5	3	0.7	No	3	2	No
M/53	Ameloblastoma	8.8	Not necessary	13	9.2	4	0.8	No	3	2	No
M/61	Squamous cell carcinoma	8.2	Not necessary	11.8	9.8	5/1	1.8	Yes	2	2	No
Average		8.9		12.3	9.2	12/1 (91.6%)	1.1				

Esthetic result: 3=good; 2= fair; 1=poor. Mastication: 2= unrestricted diet; 1 = liquid and soft diet.

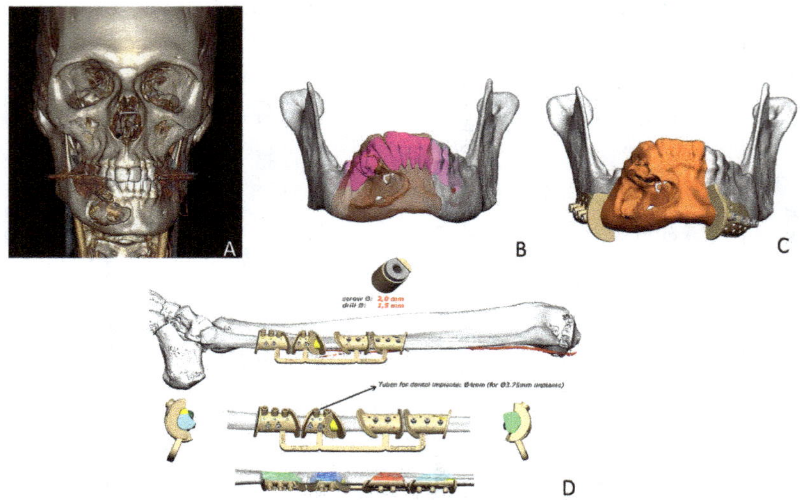

FIGURE 1 | **(A)** CT scan showing a right ameloblastoma. **(B)** Virtual planning of the mandibular resection. **(C)** Cutting guides designed for tumor resection with clear margins. **(D)** Fibula cutting guide designed for a double-barrel flap in 4 segments with the implant slots for implant placement.

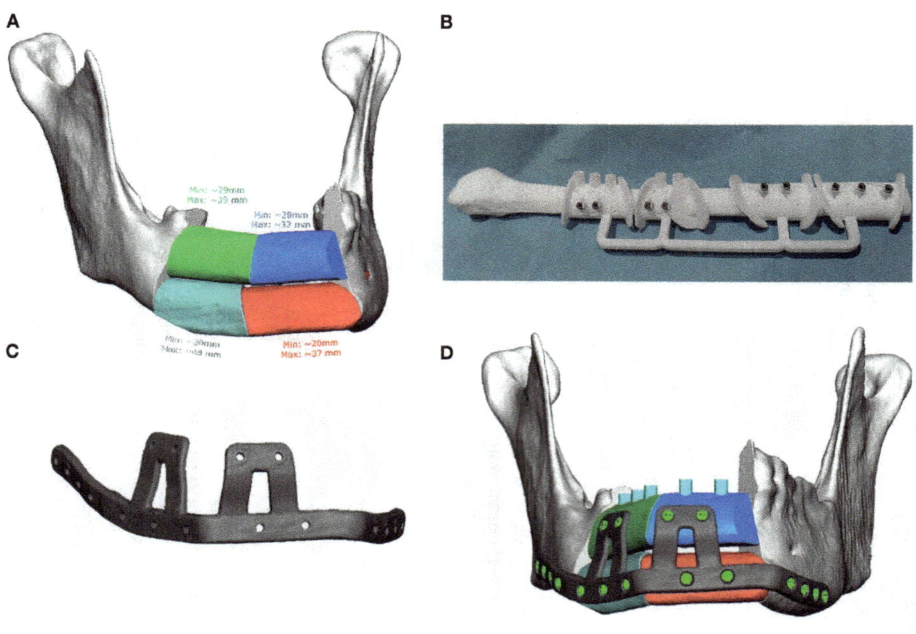

FIGURE 2 | **(A)** Double-barrel fibula flap designed in four segments for 3D reconstruction of the mandible. **(B)** Fibula cutting guide including the slots for implant placement. **(C)** Customized double-barrel titanium plate for rigid fixation. **(D)** Final design for mandibular reconstruction including the double-barrel flap, the double-barrel titanium plate and the position of dental implants.

similar to the remnant mandible, and no further techniques for vertical reconstruction were needed. In patients reconstructed with simple fibula flap, we usually deferred the placement of the implants because the possible interference of the osteosynthesis material could lead us to place the implants in a non-desirable position for future prosthetic rehabilitation. Therefore, implant dynamic navigation was performed to place dental implants in patients previously reconstructed with a simple fibula flap in whom implants had not been placed in the first surgical procedure. Implant rehabilitation of these patients was performed using 3D customized splint and intraoperative dynamic navigation. The mean age of these patients was 43 years. One patient was diagnosed with squamous cell carcinoma and 2 patients were diagnosed with ameloblastoma. Two patients (67%) did not receive radiotherapy, and implant surgery was performed four months after mandibular reconstruction. One patient (33%) was

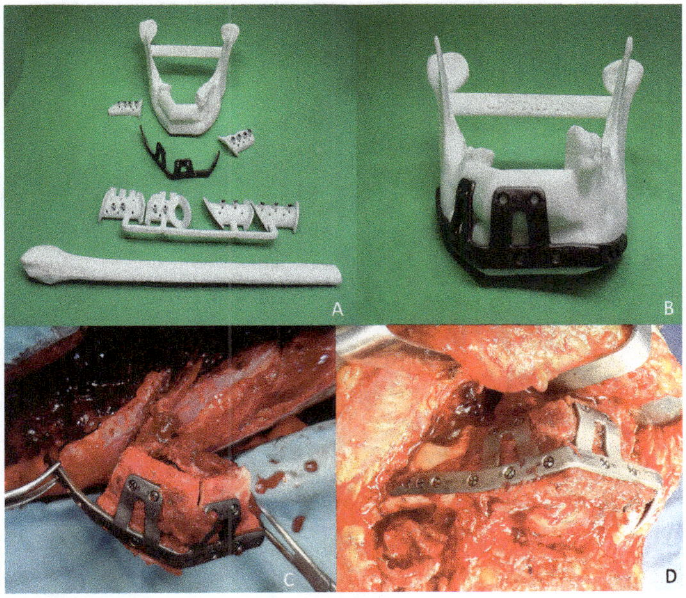

FIGURE 3 | **(A, B)** STL printed models with cutting guides and customized titanium plate. **(C)** Double-barrel fibula flap fixed to the titanium plate prior to vascular pedicle clamping. **(D)** Mandibular reconstruction after microvascular anastomoses.

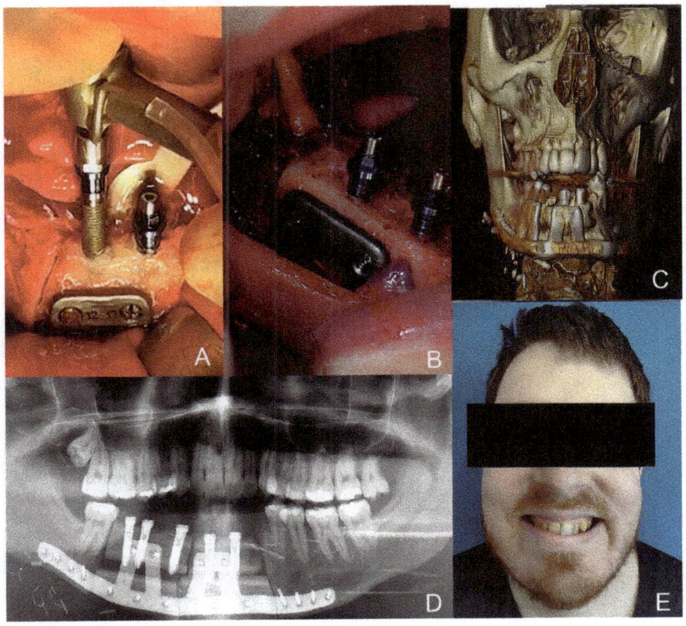

FIGURE 4 | **(A, B)** Immediate implant placement between the osteosynthesis material as previously planned in the VSP. **(C)** Postoperative CT scan demonstrating the 3D reconstruction with the double-barrel free flap, the double-barrel customized plate and the immediate implants. **(D)** Panoramic radiograph after surgery with 3D reconstruction of the mandible. **(E)** Final aesthetic and functional result.

irradiated after surgery and implant placement was performed one year after completion of radiotherapy. Twelve implants were placed assisted by this technology, of which seven (58.3%) were placed on non-irradiated peroneal flap and five (41.6%) on the irradiated patient. The average deviation in implant position was less than 1 mm and the average deviation in implant angulation was less than 5°. No major complications occurred. The mean peri-implant bone resorption measured in mesial and distal locations was 1.1 mm. One implant loss occurred in the irradiated patient, with a success rate of 91.6% (**Table 1C**).

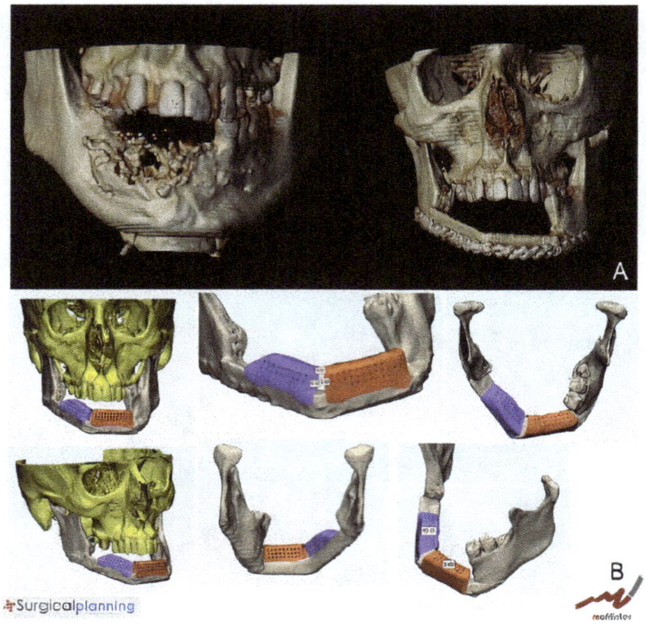

FIGURE 5 | **(A)** CT Scan showing destruction of the mandibular symphysis, segmental mandibulectomy from left mandibular body to right mandibular angle and immediate reconstruction with fibula free flap. **(B)** VSP for vertical reconstruction of the fibula with two CAD/CAM titanium meshes adapted to the two segments of the fibula flap.

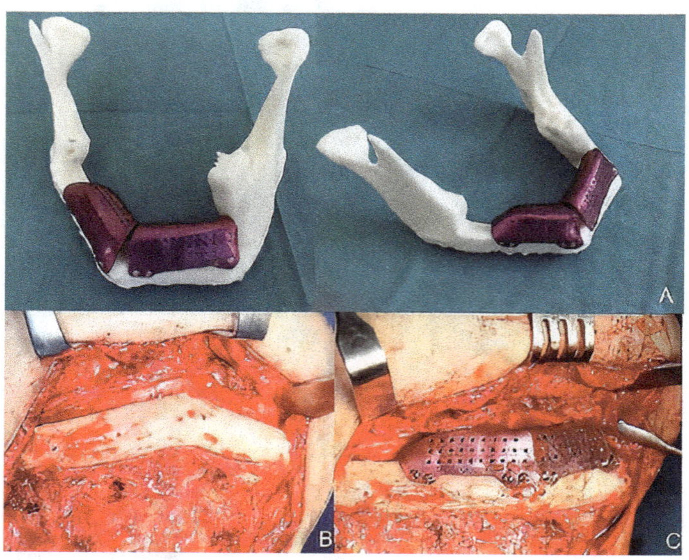

FIGURE 6 | **(A)** (STL) showing the vertical bone discrepancy and the adaptation of CAD/CAM titanium mesh to the fibula for three-dimensional bone reconstruction. **(B)** Cervical approach to avoid intraoral communication and exposure of the peroneal flap with good bone vascularization. **(C)** Iliac crest cortico-cancellous graft to reconstruct mandibular height and preserve the horizontal dimension of the fibula. Adjustment of the titanium mesh to the upper and lateral part of the two fibula segments.

Case Presentation

A 53-year-old patient was diagnosed with a recurrent left mandibular ameloblastoma. A virtual surgical planning of a segmental mandibulectomy from the parasymphysis to the left subcondylar area was performed, with the corresponding cutting guides designed. Virtual planning of mandibular reconstruction with fibula flap and customized titanium plate was designed simultaneously with the cutting guides for the fibula flap to

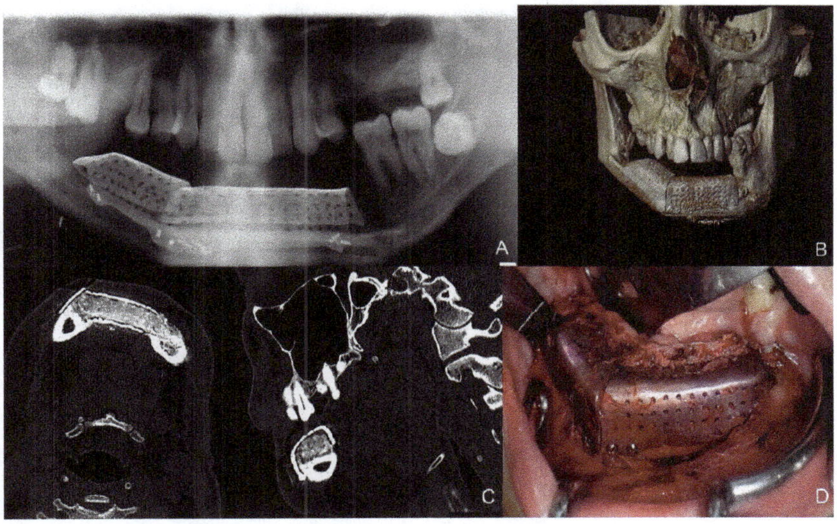

FIGURE 7 | **(A)** Panoramic radiograph showing a bone gap between the iliac crest graft and the remnant mandible mesially to the lower molar due to the angular shape of the titanium mesh at this level. CT Scan **(B)** with three-dimensional reconstruction of the mandible. CT Scan demonstrating the stability of the transverse dimension of the fibula with respect to the remnant mandible. **(C)** The three-dimensional preservation of the iliac crest graft with CAD/CAM mesh makes it possible to double the height of the fibula. **(D)** Intraoral approach showing the three-dimensional preservation of the customized mesh.

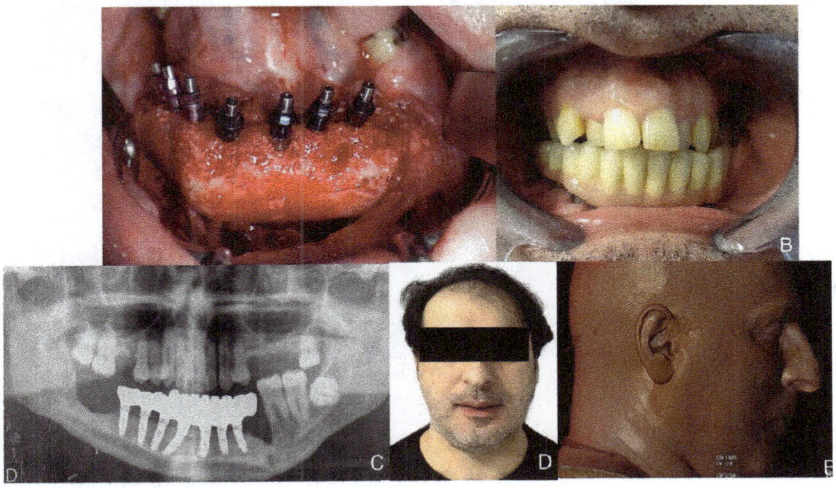

FIGURE 8 | **(A)** Placement of Ticare® dental implants. **(B)** Final dental restoration. **(C)** Panoramic radiograph demonstrating the reconstruction of the previous height of the mandible with a correct osseointegration of the implants. **(D)** Aesthetic result with mandibular symmetry. **(E)** Morphing performed after implant rehabilitation, demonstrating a significant aesthetic improvement after 3D reconstruction with iliac crest graft.

perform the osteotomies. The patient underwent segmental mandibulectomy with clear margins through the printed cutting guides and immediate reconstruction with a fibula free flap and a customized titanium plate. In the control panoramic radiograph, the mandibular reconstruction showed the mandibular reconstruction carried out by means of virtual surgical planning (**Figure 9**). Four months later, when planning the implant placement, it was decided to perform a dynamic intraoperative navigation. Splints were manufactured for CT scan and navigation planning of Ticare® implant placement. The placement of the implants was planned by means of in-house dynamic navigation using the 3D Slicer software (**Figure 10**). The "In House" navigation system uses an optical system with two infrared cameras and a free 3D Slicer software. The navigator detects the reflective spheres placed on the pointer, the handpiece adapter and the silicone key kit that is used as intraoral reference. This kit allows the navigator to compensate mandibular movements with submillimetric precision. The Ticare® implants were placed in the fibula flap using dynamic navigation with a mean deviation of less than 1 mm and an angular deviation of less than 5°. In the comparison between the

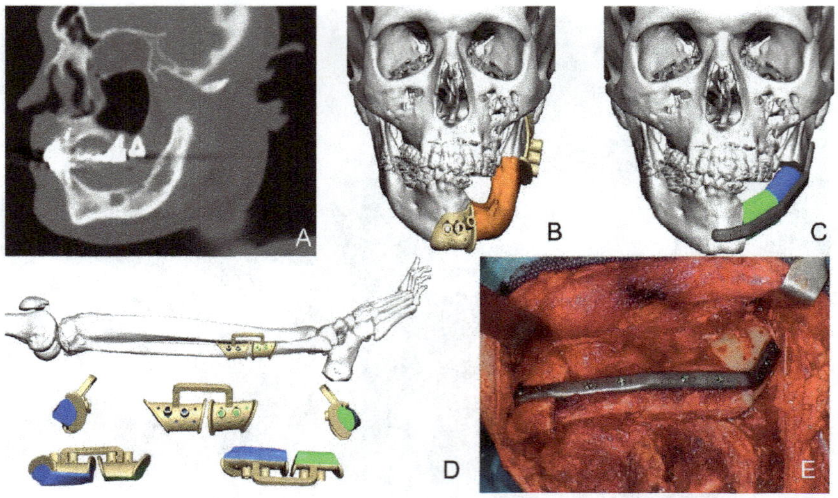

FIGURE 9 | **(A)** Recurrent ameloblastoma. **(B)** Virtual surgical planning of the oncologic resection with cutting guides. **(C)** Virtual reconstruction with fibula free flap and customized titanium plate. **(D)** Cutting guides for fibula flap. **(E)** Immediate reconstruction with fibula flap and customized titanium plate.

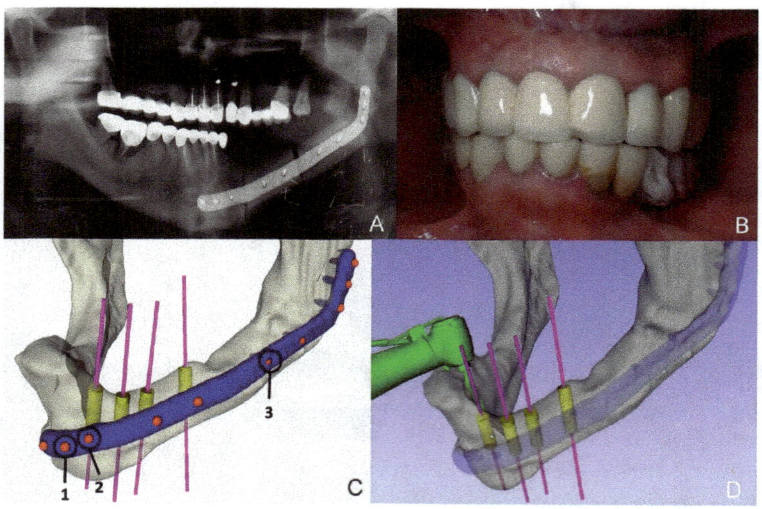

FIGURE 10 | **(A)** Panoramic radiograph after mandibular reconstruction. **(B)** Splint manufactured for dynamic navigation. **(C)** Virtual surgical planning of 4 Ticare® implants. **(D)** Intraoperative dynamic in-house navigation for implant placement.

preoperative planning of the implants and the postoperative panoramic radiograph after implant placement using "in house" navigation, it was observed that the accuracy achieved was submillimetric (**Figure 11**). Prosthetic rehabilitation was performed with an implant supported prosthesis and aesthetic and functional results were reported as excellent.

Vertical Mandible Reconstruction and Bone Resorption

Using Mann-Whitney test, the authors demonstrated significant differences in bone vertical gain in millimeters between the double barrel technique and iliac crest graft with titanium mesh technique ($p<0.002$). Regarding bone resorption in millimeters after implant placement and loading, the Mann-Whitney test determined that there were no significant differences between the double-barrel technique and the iliac crest graft technique ($p=0.11$).

Implant Success Rate

The overall implant success rate was 91.49%. By groups, the success rate of immediate implants on double-barrel fibula flap was 90%, 92.86% on iliac crest graft and 91.6% on peroneal flap with intraoperative navigation. Statistical analysis using the Chi-square table showed no statistically significant differences between the vertical gain (mm.) technique used and implant survival ($p>0.385$) (**Table 2**).

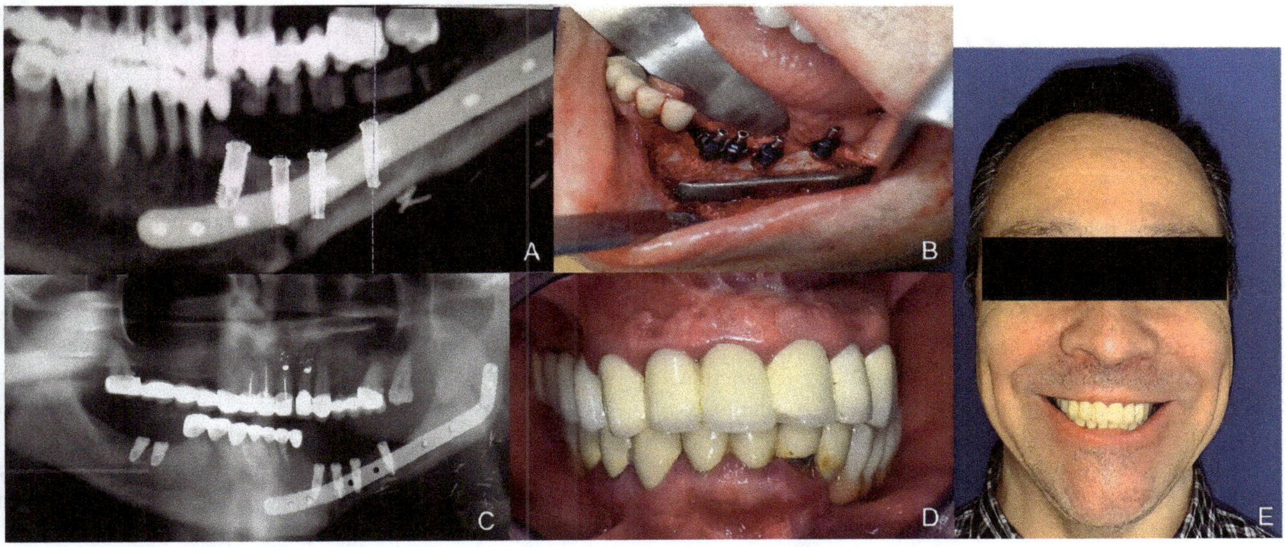

FIGURE 11 | **(A)** Virtual planning of dental implants. **(B)** Intraoperative implant placement through dynamic navigation. **(C)** Panoramic radiograph after surgery showing a high accuracy compared with the virtual planning. **(D)** Prosthetic rehabilitation with implant fixed prosthesis. **(E)** Aesthetic and functional result.

TABLE 2 | Implant failure between the different techniques.

			Implant Failure		*p* Value
			NO *n* (%)	YES *n* (%)	
TECHNIQUE	Double barrel fibula flap	Rate	18 (30%)	2 (3.3%)	0.385
	Iliac crest graft with titanium mesh over fibula flap	Rate	26 (43.3%)	2 (3.3%)	
	Dynamic navigation for implants in fibula flap	Rate	11 (18.3%)	1 (1.6%)	

Effect of Radiotherapy in Vertical Reconstruction and Bone Resorption

The Mann-Whitney test was applied to compare bone height and bone resorption in patients submitted to radiotherapy and showed no statistically significant difference, and radiotherapy was not associated with higher bone resorption (**Table 3**).

Association Between Radiotherapy and Implant Failure

Of the 60 implants, 43 implants were placed in non-irradiated bone with two losses (4.6%) and a success rate of 95.4%. Seventeen implants were inserted in irradiated bone, with two failures of osseointegration (11.7%) and a success rate of 88.3%. Chi-square analysis demonstrated significant results between both groups ($p<0.017$) (**Table 4**).

Mastication

Mastication was assessed in all groups, and results were classified with scores 1 (liquid-soft diet), and 2 (regular/unrestricted diet). Four patients reconstructed with a double-barrel flap and dental implants reported an unrestricted diet (80%), while 1 patient referred a soft diet (20%). Five patients reconstructed with a titanium mesh, iliac crest graft and implants reported a regular diet (83.3%), while 1 patient referred a liquid diet (16.7%). All patients in which oral rehabilitation was performed through dynamic navigation reported a regular diet (100%) (**Table 1**).

Aesthetics Outcomes

Esthetic assessment by the patients was performed in all groups to address scores in facial symmetry, facial scarring and facial projection. Ten patients (71.4%) reported a good aesthetic result while 4 patients referred a fair result (28.6%). A good aesthetic result was reported by 4 patients reconstructed with double-barrel flap, 4 patients reconstructed with CAD/CAM titanium mesh and 2 patients with dynamic navigation (**Table 1**).

TABLE 3 | Effects of radiotherapy in vertical reconstruction and bone resorption.

	Radiotherapy	No Radiotherapy	p
Vertical Reconstruction (mm)	16.5+/-1.25	16.21+/-0.74	0.22
Bone resorption (mm)	1.8+/-0.21	1.12+/-0.10	0.26

TABLE 4 | Association between radiotherapy and implant failure.

			Implant Failure		p Value
			NO *n* (%)	YES *n* (%)	
Radiotherapy	NO	Rate	41 (68.3%)	2 (3.33%)	0.017
	YES	Rate	14 (23.3%)	3 (5.0%)	

Dysphagia

Dysphagia was reported by the patients as "yes" or "no". Only 2 patients reported dysphagia, while 12 patients referred normal swallowing (85.7%) (**Table 1**).

All patients were rehabilitated with an implant-supported fixed prosthesis, obtaining excellent esthetic and functional results in terms of lip competence and speech articulation. No statistically significant differences were found in prosthetic rehabilitation between the three techniques and all patients reported an intelligible speech.

DISCUSSION

The use of computer-assisted surgery and navigation technology in head and neck oncology was described in the early 90's by A. Wagner (14). In recent years, the concept of "precision medicine" has become part of standard hospital practice, allowing different products to be adapted to each patient in a specific way (15). There has also been a significant development of this technology in the field of maxillofacial surgery: virtual surgical planning (VSP), CAD-CAM design and modeling and intraoperative navigation techniques have contributed, over the past few years, to simplify and improve the accuracy of surgeries. These techniques allow the pre-planning of the oncological resection, the dimensions of the neomandible and the precise location of the osteotomies in bone flaps (15, 16). CAD-CAM cutting guides help the surgical team to faithfully carry out the treatments devised, improving the precision, accuracy and reliability of the results in oncological resections and reconstructions. Intraoperative dynamic navigation systems allow immediate insertion of osseointegrated implants, contributing to faster dental rehabilitation (2, 17). Therefore, the combination of VSP and intraoperative navigation can guarantee the best possible postoperative results, especially in complex mandibular defects without occlusal stability. The main advantages of this technology are: 1) preoperative visualization of each patient's anatomy (18); 2) it enables oncologic resection with clear margins (19); 3) it improves the accuracy of the reconstruction by simplifying the osteosynthesis of the reconstruction increasing contact surfaces and achieving a better aesthetic contour (18, 19); 4) preoperative visualization of reconstruction limitations and preventing possible complications; 5) it decreases surgical time, especially ischemia time during the free flap harvest (19); 6) it provides more predictable results, increasing the stability of the results and patient outcomes (2, 18). On the other hand, the main disadvantages of virtual surgery planning are: 1) increased costs, often due to the need for an external digital laboratory (15, 18); 2) the surgical delay involved in surgical planning and obtaining the different models and cutting guides, which can delay the beginning of treatment in oncologic patients. Although a study of the economic costs using these techniques was not carried out as it was not an objective of this study, future studies are needed to evaluate the accuracy achieved compared with standard surgery and the total value added and the cost efficiency of VSP-CAD/CAM. Overall, the decreased patient morbidity and complications and the generalized improved outcomes may potentially offset the technological costs.

The fibula flap is the technique of choice for mandibular reconstruction. One of its main disadvantages is its low height of bone to be adapted to the remaining mandible in segmental defects, resulting in a reduction of the lower facial third with the consequent aesthetic and functional sequelae (2–4). In addition, this flap allows the implantological rehabilitation of oncologic patients, although it is necessary to perform a correct distribution of the masticatory dynamic loads to avoid overloading the implants in the flap bone and the remnant mandible (2, 3). The main disadvantage of this flap is the considerable vertical discrepancy between the remnant mandible and the fibula flap, which limits the prosthetic rehabilitation of the patients due to the unfavorable crown to implant ratio (4). To solve this problem, 3D mandibular reconstruction can be complemented by using the double-barrel technique and iliac crest grafts guided by titanium mesh over the fibula flap (3). The aim of this study was to describe three different options for mandibular reconstruction and rehabilitation with dental implants in oncologic patients with segmental defects, as well as to compare the different techniques in terms of vertical bone reconstruction, peri-implant bone resorption, implant success rate, the influence of radiotherapy and the aesthetic and functional outcomes such as deglutition and swallowing.

The study shows that vertical bone augmentation is higher in patients reconstructed with double-barrel fibula flap or with iliac crest graft over the fibula. The double-barrel flap will provide a vertical dimension dependent on the thickness of the fibula bone itself, so that the bone height to be achieved can be predicted intraoperatively. This gain is greater than the amount of the vertical dimension of each segment of the fibula, since there is usually a gap between them, secondary to their adaptation to achieve an adequate ridge and basal profile of the neomandible. Besides, the iliac crest graft over the fibula presents some bone resorption. Therefore, when performing the technique, the mandibular volume is usually overcorrected. In these cases, reconstruction is less predictable although the vertical gain is similar to that achieved with the double-barrel technique.

One of the limitations of this study is the sample size. Although implant survival is favorable in all three groups, larger studies are needed to highlight significant differences. Likewise, no differences were observed between vertical bone augmentation and bone resorption between patients treated with radiotherapy and non-irradiated patients. We consider important to emphasize that this is one of the few studies that demonstrates the stability of the reconstructive results achieved with VSP, double-barrel flap, STL models, titanium CAD-CAM meshes and implants placed with intraoperative navigation in any of the three variants presented. The stability of the implant rehabilitation of the oncologic patients submitted to these techniques is also shown, with very high functional and aesthetic results.

There are very few studies comparing vertical mandibular reconstruction techniques. Navarro-Cuéllar compared in his study a series of twenty-four patients submitted to vertical reconstruction of the fibula by means of double-barrel fibula, fibula with iliac crest onlay graft and distraction osteogenesis of the fibula. The good results mainly for the first two techniques stand out, in which a vertical bone augmentation of 18.5 mm and 17.75 mm is achieved, respectively, both in patients without adjuvant treatment and in irradiated patients. In addition, bone resorption was measured and compared, and no differences were observed between these two techniques or with respect to the group of irradiated patients, showing an average bone resorption of less than 1.5mm in both groups (2). Worse results were obtained in the group treated by distraction osteogenesis, in which the mean resorption was higher than 2 mm. Yue He reported the reconstruction of seven patients with the double-barrel fibula flap with a gain of more than 30 mm. Three patients had not been irradiated and one patient received radiotherapy. However, the author provides no data on bone resorption (4). Shen published a series of forty-five cases of double-barrel fibula with implant rehabilitation in eleven of them, with good esthetic and functional results (6); however, the author did not describe the implant success rate or the peri-implant bone resorption. Ferreti described the vertical reconstruction of mandibular atrophy by means of iliac crest grafts but did not show its application in cases of segmental defect or reconstruction with peroneal flap (20). None of the works consulted compared the ratio between the width of the flap and the remaining mandible. Given the small sample size of our study, this is another of its limitations. Further studies are needed to compare the values according to anatomical variations and patient-dependent factors. Very few studies have reported comparisons of techniques for mandibular reconstruction using peroneal flap with VSP and CAD-CAM technology. Navarro-Cuéllar reported a series of eight cases in which the author demonstrated an excellent result with this technique (3). Previously, Verhoeven had reported two-dimensional reconstructions with bone resorption of up to 25% of the height provided by the iliac crest graft (21). Vermeeren described a resorption close to 50%, results similar to those obtained by Johansson (22, 23). Casap reported a case of alveolar bone augmentation by impression of a titanium shell with BMP-2/allograft with excellent results in graft ossification but with a high rate of mesh exposure (24). Roser studies the accuracy of VSP in 11 patients comparing the distance between the real mandibular osteotomies and the virtual mandibular osteotomies with an accuracy rate of 2.0 ± 1.1 mm (25). Our study demonstrates that mandibular reconstruction can be achieved safely and effectively using an iliac crest graft adapted to preformed titanium mesh using VSP and CAD-CAM technology. This mesh is optimally adapted to the peroneal flap and the patient's anatomy. The stability of this reconstruction and the low bone resorption evaluated during the follow-up time by CBCT have also been demonstrated. The high rate of osseointegration of the implants on this bone regeneration has also been reported, providing a long-term stable occlusal rehabilitation with optimal aesthetic and functional outcomes.

The development of tissue engineering has provided the possibility to regenerate tissues from cells that develop on a matrix that guides their growth (26). Bone regeneration by means of iliac crest grafting is a form of autogenous regeneration considered to be of choice due to its osteogenic potential and its osteoinductive and osteoconductive properties (27). The success of bone grafts depends on the surfaces in contact with each other and their three-dimensional arrangement (3, 27). The design of the recipient site and its stability are also important. The fibula flap is a high quality recipient site due to its good vascularization and the provision of an extensive bone surface on which to place the graft and titanium mesh. The advantages of the iliac crest graft for 3D reconstruction of the mandible are (28): 1) high quality and quantity of cellular supply; 2) capacity for compacting the graft, which allows greater density of bone cells per unit of space; 3) good vascularization and the possibility of placing the graft in stable and well vascularized cavities. It also has certain disadvantages such as the need for a second surgical intervention, the morbidity secondary to iliac approach, the risk of exposure of the mesh containing the graft -which is higher in previously irradiated patients- and the deferred time of at least 6 months until implant surgery.

At this point and, considering the described techniques as good surgical options for vertical mandibular reconstruction, the choice of each technique will depend on the clinical status of each patient. An important point of discussion would be whether it is preferable to reconstruct the mandible in a single surgical time using a double barrel fibula flap or to delay the reconstructive process with two surgical procedures in patients in which bone regeneration is performed with titanium mesh-guided iliac crest grafting. Obviously, in patients in whom the height of the peroneal flap does not involve a high vertical discrepancy, implant rehabilitation will be faster and high accuracy can be achieved through dynamic navigation. The double-barrel fibula flap is the ideal technique for mandibular height reconstruction in order to solve the problem of bone discrepancy with the remaining mandible (2, 10). In addition, VSP, computer-aided design/computer-aided manufacturing (CAD/CAM), surgical navigation and advanced implantology complement this reconstructive technique with high precision. It has the following advantages: 1) great length of bone, allowing double-barrel reconstructions of 8-10 cm (10); 2) one surgical procedure, compared to iliac crest onlay grafts or techniques such as distraction osteogenesis (2); 3) it is a flap particularly suitable for dental implant rehabilitation and early implant placement due to the high primary stability provided by the cortical bone (12, 13); 4) this flap can be designed as an isolated bone flap or by providing a skin paddle to allow soft tissue reconstruction (2, 10); 5) it is a flap with low morbidity at the donor site; 6) it is the best surgical option for patients who will undergo radiotherapy due to the high vascularization and the minimal bone resorption of the flap (29); moreover, in cases of implant rehabilitation, low peri-implant resorption has been demonstrated. The major disadvantage of this technique is the limitation in patients with defects larger than 12-14 cm, which would require a flap length of almost 25 cm, which would increase the morbidity of the donor site (29) and decrease the length of the vascular pedicle for microvascular anastomosis. In these cases, an alternative surgical option is to reconstruct with the double-barrel only the mandibular region compromised with the occlusion in which the dental implants will be placed. Therefore, in oncologic patients, especially those receiving radiotherapy and, in patients with segmental defects smaller than 12-14 cm, this is the technique of choice. It allows early prosthetic rehabilitation and high success rate of the implants (2, 12, 13).

The cortico-cancellous iliac crest graft allows deferred mandibular reconstruction. It presents low bone resorption and high success rate of dental implants. It allows an adequate vertical reconstruction of the mandible, solving the problem of discrepancy with the remaining mandible and provides high volumes of autologous bone that supports well the treatment with radiotherapy (20). However, it has a number of disadvantages: it requires a second surgical procedure; it is essential to overcorrect the area to be treated by approximately 25% to compensate for the loss due to bone resorption, which entails the need for remodeling in some cases (30); the donor area implicates certain morbidity (6); it is necessary to wait at least six months for the ossification of the graft before placing dental implants, thus prolonging the prosthetic rehabilitation time (9). This technique is recommended mainly in patients who are not going to receive radiotherapy with extensive defects in the symphysis and mandibular body in which a double-barrel flap is not possible (2). When harvesting this technique, it is important to perform a cervical approach for the placement of the graft on the peroneal flap to avoid its contamination by flora of the oral cavity (1, 2). Implant success rates and peri-implant bone resorption are similar to those presented by the double bar fibula flap; however, the need for several surgical procedures and the impossibility of receiving radiation while the titanium mesh maintains the graft until ossification, limit the use of this technique, remaining as a second option in oncologic patients. Titanium mesh is ideal for the execution of this technique. It is a biocompatible material, with a high capacity to prevent deformation, and a 3D stability and adaptation that prevents the graft from collapsing. It is a non-absorbable material and protects the graft from invasion by adjacent soft tissue. It provides a smooth surface that isolates the graft from bacterial colonization and the elasticity of titanium prevents compression of the graft by intraoral tissues and mobile elements. In addition, the micropores on its surface maintain the vascular supply to the recipient area. Several studies have reported mesh exposure and bone resorption (31, 32); however, in our series we have demonstrated maintenance of the mesh without exposure in the oral cavity and minimal bone resorption due to the virtual surgical planning and the cervical approach performed to avoid contact between the graft and the oral cavity. Conventional surgery for titanium mesh with bone graft may show inadequate adaptation, irregular edges that may lead to exposure of the mesh and dead spaces that result in early bone resorption and the development of complications such as infection. Optimal mesh adaptation and proper design achieved by VSP and STL model production are critical for good aesthetic and functional results. Thus, it is possible to recreate and maintain the shape of the previous mandible, allowing a correct maxillo-mandibular position and a more predictable implant placement. The major limitation of VSP is the added cost of the surgical procedure; in any case, the notorious improvement of the results obtained needs to be valued with respect to the cost of the technology. Since this is one of the few works that report the experience with the use of this technology for mandibular reconstruction in oncologic patients, more studies are needed to evaluate and compare the results obtained with surgery performed using VSP, CAD-CAM technology, STL models and intraoperative navigation with respect to conventional surgery.

Although it is not the subject of this study, several authors advise against osteogenic distraction of the fibula in oncologic patients with a potential need for adjuvant radiotherapy treatment because of the 3-5 month period until stable vertical gain is achieved and, above all, because of the risk of exposure of the distractor and the bone during radiotherapy treatment. In addition, the technique requires three surgical procedures since the reconstruction until the distractor removal and implant placement (2).

In house navigation of dental implants allows real-time anatomical assessment of the patient's neo-mandible on which they are to be inserted. While VSP and CAD-CAM technology allow a more predictable flap design and mandibular reconstruction, it also provides the advantage of knowing the limitations of implant placement in an anatomically complex site (33). Thus, in patients rehabilitated with this technique, the VSP made possible to predict the exact position of the osteosynthesis material in the neomandible, proceeding to total or partial removal if it interfered with the correct position of the implant for a correct occlusal rehabilitation. The titanium plates with high adaptation to the anatomy of the flap used for the reconstruction may lead, in many cases, to place the implants to avoid interference with osteosynthesis screws. Intraoperative navigation allows in these cases to redirect the position of the implant and to achieve predictable, more accurate results with a reduction in surgical time. We used the in-house navigation technique for patients without dental implants in the previous fibula flap. Nowadays, and due to VSP, it is possible to perform mandibular reconstruction both in double-barrel or single fibula with immediate implant placement without the need of a second surgical time for implant placement through dynamic navigation. Therefore, we recommend this technique in patients in whom implant placement has not been performed previously.

From the aesthetic and functional point of view, mandibular reconstruction according to its original dimensions will provide a good projection of the lower third of the face. Otherwise, tissue collapse will occur, resulting in aesthetic and functional sequelae. Another point of discussion would be whether it is necessary to place the fibula at the inferior border of the mandible or in the midbody proximal to the alveolar ridge of the remnant mandible. Although the fibula positioned in the upper part of the defect is widely described in the literature, our recommendation would be to reconstruct the inferior border of the mandible to achieve optimal facial symmetry with a harmonious facial profile and to perform complementary techniques such as the double-barrel fibula flap to restore the previous height of the mandible and to place immediate implants. The reconstruction of the mandible by means of VSP, CAD-CAM and STL models makes possible to restore bone volumes similar to the previous dimensions, leading to a harmonious physical appearance of the patients. Mandibular profiles similar to the native mandible are achieved and osteosynthesis material arrangements that could compromise esthetics are avoided. In addition, functional results such as lip competence, deglutition and speech articulation are excellent in the patients of our study. In this study, the authors evaluated the functional outcomes according to patients' oral feeding ability. Patients were classified according to their ability to develop an unrestricted diet or a soft/liquid diet. Only 2 patients referred dysphagia and most of the patients reported a normal diet, and masticatory function was preserved after mandibular reconstruction with the described techniques. Similarly, 71.4% of the patients obtained good esthetic results both objectively and from the subjective evaluation of each patient.

It should be noted that segmental mandibular defects secondary to oncologic processes reconstructed with peroneal flap can solve the problem of vertical discrepancy and three-dimensional volume of the deficient mandible by means of double barrel techniques or by cortico-cancellous iliac crest grafting with titanium mesh developed by VSP, STL models and CAD-CAM technologies. In all cases the reconstruction can be completed by implant rehabilitation and intraoperative navigation. These techniques allow a precise 3D reconstruction and can be combined according to the needs of each patient, obtaining excellent esthetic and functional results.

Finally, it is important to emphasize that it is necessary to acknowledge all these surgical techniques, in order to individualize the mandibular reconstruction in oncologic patients. Multi-stage implementation of virtual surgical planning (VSP) with the use of stereolithographic models (STL), 3D printing of patient-specific surgical guides, CAD/CAM titanium mesh and intraoperative implant dynamic navigation for 3D mandibular defects offer a reconstructive accuracy improving the operative efficiency, reducing the complication rate and enabling the comprehensive rehabilitation of the patients, providing aesthetic and functional results that return quality of life to oncologic patients.

AUTHOR CONTRIBUTIONS

Conceptualization: RA-C and CN. Methodology: RA-C, MT, and JS. Software: AD-M and ÁS. Validation: RA-C, CN, and JS. Formal analysis: SO and DG. Investigation: RA-C and AD-M. Resources: IN, CN, MA, and GA. Data curation: JS and IN. Writing—original draft preparation: RA-C. Writing—review and editing: RA-C and CN. Visualization: SO. Supervision: RA-C. Project administration: RA-C and JS. All authors contributed to the article and approved the submitted version.

REFERENCES

1. Yu Y, Zhang WB, Liu XJ, Guo CB, Yu GY, Peng X. Three-Dimensional Accuracy of Virtual Planning and Surgical Navigation for Mandibular Reconstruction With Free Fibula Flap. *J Oral Maxillofac Surg* (2016) 74 (7):1503.e1–1503.e10.1. doi: 10.1016/j.joms.2016.02.020
2. Navarro Cuéllar C, Ochandiano Caicoya S, Navarro Cuéllar I, Valladares Pérez S, Fariña Sirandoni R, Antúnez-Conde R, et al. Vertical Ridge Augmentation of Fibula Flap in Mandibular Reconstruction: A Comparison Between Vertical Distraction, Double-Barrel Flap and Iliac Crest Graft. *J Clin Med* (2020) 10(1):101. doi: 10.3390/jcm10010101
3. Navarro Cuéllar C, Tousidonis Rial M, Antúnez-Conde R, Ochandiano Caicoya S, Navarro Cuéllar I, Arenas de Frutos G, et al. Virtual Surgical Planning, Stereolitographic Models and CAD/CAM Titanium Mesh for Three-Dimensional Reconstruction of Fibula Flap With Iliac Crest Graft and Dental Implants. *J Clin Med* (2021) 10(9):1922. doi: 10.3390/jcm10091922
4. He Y, Zhang ZY, Zhu HG, Wu YQ, Fu HH. Double-Barrel Fibula Vascularized Free Flap With Dental Rehabilitation for Mandibular Reconstruction. *J Oral Maxillofac Surg* (2011) 69(10):2663–9. doi: 10.1016/j.joms.2011.02.051
5. Cuéllar NC, Cuesta Gil M, Plasencia Delgado J, Guerra Martínez B, Acero Sanz J, López de Atalaya FJ, et al. Reconstrucción Oromandibular Con Colgajo Libre De Peroné E Implantes Osteointegrados [Oromandibular Reconstruction With Free Peroneal Flap and Osseointegrated Implants]. *Acta Otorrinolaringol Esp* (2003) 54(1):54–64. doi: 10.1016/s0001-6519(03)78384-8
6. Shen Y, Sun J, Li J, Li MM, Huang W, Ow A. Special Considerations in Virtual Surgical Planning for Secondary Accurate Maxillary Reconstruction With Vascularised Fibula Osteomyocutaneous Flap. *J Plast Reconstr Aesthet Surg* (2012) 65(7):893–902. doi: 10.1016/j.bjps.2011.12.035
7. Melville JC, Manis CS, Shum JW, Alsuwied D. Single-Unit 3d-Printed Titanium Reconstruction Plate for Maxillary Reconstruction: The Evolution of Surgical Reconstruction for Maxillary Defects-A Case Report and Review of Current Techniques. *J Oral Maxillofac Surg* (2019) 77(4):874.e1–874.e13. doi: 10.1016/j.joms.2018.11.030
8. Swendseid BP, Roden DF, Vimawala S, Richa T, Sweeny L, Goldman RA, et al. Virtual Surgical Planning in Subscapular System Free Flap Reconstruction of Midface Defects. *Oral Oncol* (2020) 101:104508. doi: 10.1016/j.oraloncology.2019.104508
9. Nocini PF, Wangerin K, Albanese M, Kretschmer W, Cortelazzi R. Vertical Distraction of a Free Vascularized Fibula Flap in a Reconstructed Hemimandible: Case Report. *J Craniomaxillofac Surg* (2000) 28(1):20–4. doi: 10.1054/jcms.2000.0106
10. Cuellar CN, de Atalaya Gutiérrez FJL, Vila CN, Sanz JA. Reconstrucción Mandibular Con El Colgajo Libre De Peroné. Tratado De Cirugía Oral Y

Maxilofacial. In: Navarro Vila C, Arán Ediciones SL, editors. Vol. 3. Madrid, Spain (2004). p. 1225–34.

11. Bähr W. Blood Supply of Small Fibula Segments: An Experimental Study on Human Cadavers. *J Craniomaxillofac Surg* (1998) 26(3):148–52. doi: 10.1016/s1010-5182(98)80004-8
12. Cuéllar CN, Caicoya SO, García FR, de Atalaya FJL, Sanz JA, Gil MC, et al. Rehabilitación Implantosoportada En El Colgajo Libre De Peroné. *Rev Esp Cir Oral Maxilofac* (2006) 28:263–75.
13. De Santis G, Chiarini L, Bedogni A, Nocini PF. Jaw Reconstruction by Free Fibular Transfer: Emphasis on Osseointegrated Implants, TMJ and Maxilla Reconstruction. *Eur J Plast Surg* (1999) 22:62–8. doi: 10.1007/s002380050149
14. Wagner A, Ploder O, Enislidis G, Truppe M, Ewers R. Virtual Image Guided Navigation in Tumor Surgery–Technical Innovation. *J Craniomaxillofac Surg* (1995) 23(5):217–3. doi: 10.1016/s1010-5182(05)80155-6
15. Huang MF, Alfi D, Alfi J, Huang AT. The Use of Patient-Specific Implants in Oral and Maxillofacial Surgery. *Oral Maxillofac Surg Clin North Am* (2019) 31 (4):593–600. doi: 10.1016/j.coms.2019.07.010
16. Naros A, Weise H, Tilsen F, Hoefert S, Naros G, Krimmel M, et al. Three-Dimensional Accuracy of Mandibular Reconstruction by Patient-Specific Pre-Bent Reconstruction Plates Using an "In-House" 3D-Printer. *J Craniomaxillofac Surg* (2018) 46(9):1645–51. doi: 10.1016/j.jcms.2018.05.047
17. Pietruski P, Majak M, Świątek-Najwer E, Popek M, Mazurek M, Świecka M, et al. Navigation-Guided Fibula Free Flap for Mandibular Reconstruction: A Proof of Concept Study. *J Plast Reconstr Aesthet Surg* (2019) 72(4):572–80. doi: 10.1016/j.bjps.2019.01.026
18. Yu Y, Zhang WB, Wang Y, Liu XJ, Guo CB, Peng X. A Revised Approach for Mandibular Reconstruction With the Vascularized Iliac Crest Flap Using Virtual Surgical Planning and Surgical Navigation. *J Oral Maxillofac Surg* (2016) 74(6):1285.e1–1285.e11. doi: 10.1016/j.joms.2016.02.021
19. Rodby KA, Turin S, Jacobs RJ, Cruz JF, Hassid VJ, Kolokythas A, et al. Advances in Oncologic Head and Neck Reconstruction: Systematic Review and Future Considerations of Virtual Surgical Planning and Computer Aided Design/Computer Aided Modeling. *J Plast Reconstr Aesthet Surg* (2014) 67 (9):1171–85. doi: 10.1016/j.bjps.2014.04.038
20. Ferretti C, Premviyasa V, Reyneke J, Ripamonti U. A Mass Guide for the Harvest of Cortico-Cancellous Bone From the Posterior Iliac Crest for Mandibular Reconstruction. *Br J Oral Maxillofac Surg* (2019) 57(7):627–31. doi: 10.1016/j.bjoms.2019.04.012
21. Verhoeven JW, Ruijter J, Cune MS, Terlou M, Zoon M. Onlay Grafts in Combination With Endosseous Implants in Severe Mandibular Atrophy: One Year Results of a Prospective, Quantitative Radiological Study. *Clin Oral Implants Res* (2000) 11(6):583–94. doi: 10.1034/j.1600-0501.2000.011006583.x
22. Vermeeren JI, Wismeijer D, van Waas MA. One-Step Reconstruction of the Severely Resorbed Mandible With Onlay Bone Grafts and Endosteal Implants. A 5-Year Follow-Up. *Int J Oral Maxillofac Surg* (1996) 25(2):112–5. doi: 10.1016/s0901-5027(96)80053-1
23. Johansson B, Grepe A, Wannfors K, Hirsch JM. A Clinical Study of Changes in the Volume of Bone Grafts in the Atrophic Maxilla. *Dentomaxillofac Radiol* (2001) 30(3):157–61. doi: 10.1038/sj/dmfr/4600601
24. Casap N, Rushinek H, Jensen OT. Vertical Alveolar Augmentation Using BMP-2/ACS/Allograft With Printed Titanium Shells to Establish an Early Vascular Scaffold. *Oral Maxillofac Surg Clin North Am* (2019) 31(3):473–87. doi: 10.1016/j.coms.2019.03.009
25. Roser SM, Ramachandra S, Blair H, Grist W, Carlson GW, Christensen AM, et al. The Accuracy of Virtual Surgical Planning in Free Fibula Mandibular Reconstruction: Comparison of Planned and Final Results. *J Oral Maxillofac Surg* (2010) 68(11):2824–32. doi: 10.1016/j.joms.2010.06.177
26. O'Brien F. Biomaterial and Scaffolds for Tissue Engineering. *Mater Today* (2011) 14:88–95. doi: 10.1016/S1369-7021(11)70058-X
27. Marx RE, Armentano L, Olavarria A, Samaniego J. rhBMP-2/ACS Grafts Versus Autogenous Cancellous Marrow Grafts in Large Vertical Defects of the Maxilla: An Unsponsored Randomized Open-Label Clinical Trial. *Int J Oral Maxillofac Implants* (2013) 28(5):e243–51. doi: 10.11607/jomi.te04
28. Iino M, Fukuda M, Nagai H, Hamada Y, Yamada H, Nakaoka K, et al. Evaluation of 15 Mandibular Reconstructions With Dumbach Titan Mesh-System and Particulate Cancellous Bone and Marrow Harvested From Bilateral Posterior Ilia. *Oral Surg Oral Med Oral Pathol Oral Radiol Endod* (2009) 107(4):e1–8. doi: 10.1016/j.tripleo.2008.12.018
29. Bähr W, Stoll P, Wächter R. Use of the "Double Barrel" Free Vascularized Fibula in Mandibular Reconstruction. *J Oral Maxillofac Surg* (1998) 56(1):38–44. doi: 10.1016/s0278-2391(98)90914-4
30. Sethi A, Kaus T, Cawood JI, Plaha H, Boscoe M, Sochor P. Onlay Bone Grafts From Iliac Crest: A Retrospective Analysis. *Int J Oral Maxillofac Surg* (2020) 49(2):264–71. doi: 10.1016/j.ijom.2019.07.001
31. Maiorana C, Santoro F, Rabagliati M, Salina S. Evaluation of the Use of Iliac Cancellous Bone and Anorganic Bovine Bone in the Reconstruction of the Atrophic Maxilla With Titanium Mesh: A Clinical and Histologic Investigation. *Int J Oral Maxillofac Implants* (2001) 16(3):427–32.
32. Proussaefs P, Lozada J, Kleinman A, Rohrer MD, McMillan PJ. The Use of Titanium Mesh in Conjunction With Autogenous Bone Graft and Inorganic Bovine Bone Mineral (Bio-Oss) for Localized Alveolar Ridge Augmentation: A Human Study. *Int J Periodontics Restorative Dent* (2003) 23(2):185–95.
33. Abbate V, Orabona GDA, Solari D, Bonavolontà P, Iaconetta G, Califano L. Mandibular Surgical Navigation: An Innovative Guiding Method. *J Craniofac Surg* (2017) 28(8):2122–6. doi: 10.1097/SCS.0000000000003816

15

Impact of Periosteal Branches and Septo-Cutaneous Perforators on Free Fibula Flap Outcome: A Retrospective Analysis of Computed Tomography Angiography Scans in Virtual Surgical Planning

Michael Knitschke [1], Anna Katrin Baumgart [1], Christina Bäcker [1], Christian Adelung [2], Fritz Roller [2], Daniel Schmermund [1], Sebastian Böttger [1], Philipp Streckbein [1], Hans-Peter Howaldt [1] and Sameh Attia [1]*

[1] *Department of Oral and Maxillofacial Surgery, Justus-Liebig-University, Giessen, Germany,* [2] *Department of Diagnostic and Interventional Radiology and Pediatric Radiology, Justus-Liebig-University, Giessen, Germany*

***Correspondence:**
Michael Knitschke
Michael.Knitschke@uniklinikum-giessen.de

Background: Virtual surgical planning (VSP) for jaw reconstruction with free fibula flap (FFF) became a routine procedure and requires computed tomography angiography (CTA) for preoperative evaluation of the lower limbs vascular system and the bone. The aim of the study was to assess whether the distribution and density of periosteal branches (PB) and septo-cutaneous perforators (SCP) of the fibular artery have an impact on flap success.

Method: This retrospective clinical study assessed preoperative CTA of the infra-popliteal vasculature and the small vessel system of 72 patients who underwent FFF surgery. Surgical outcome of flap transfer includes wound healing, subtotal, and total flap loss were matched with the segmental vascular supply.

Result: A total of 72 patients (28 females, 38.9 %; 44 males, 61.1 %) fulfilled the study inclusion criteria. The mean age was 58.5 (± 15.3 years). Stenoses of the lower limbs' vessel (n = 14) were mostly detected in the fibular artery (n = 11). Flap success was recorded in n = 59 (82.0%), partial flap failure in n = 4 (5.5%) and total flap loss in n = 9 (12.5%). The study found a mean number (± SD) of 2.53 ± 1.60 PBs and 1.39 ± 1.03 SCPs of the FA at the donor-site. The proximal FFF segment of poly-segmental jaw reconstruction showed a higher rate of PB per flap segment than in the distal segments. Based on the total number of prepared segments (n = 121), 46.7% (n = 7) of mono-, 40.4% (n = 21) of bi-, and 31.5 % (n = 17) of tri-segmental fibula flaps were at least supplied by one PB in the success group. Overall, this corresponds to 37.2% (45 out of 121) of all successful FFF. For total flap loss (n = 14), a relative number of 42.9% (n = 6) of distinct supplied segments was recorded. Wound healing disorder of the donor site was not statistically significant influenced by the detected rate of SCP.

Conclusion: In general, a correlation between higher rates of PB and SCP and the flap success could not be statistically proved by the study sample. We conclude, that preoperative PB and SCP mapping based on routine CTA imaging is not suitable for prediction of flap outcome.

Keywords: virtual surgical planning, jaw reconstruction, CTA, flap failure, head and neck tumor, fibula free flap

INTRODUCTION

Taylor presented the free fibula flap (FFF) for the first time in 1975 (1), and Hidalgo employed it for mandible reconstruction 14 years later (2). This flap has a high success rate and is commonly used in reconstructive surgery (3). It allows the treatment of both bone and soft tissue defects with a single free flap from a single donor site (4). The FFF is the gold standard in mandibular reconstruction as it may be molded to a nearly ideal form of the missing jaw sections (5). Sufficient jaw reconstruction improves the quality of life (QoL) after ablative cancer surgery. After successful treatment, the overall QoL is comparable to that of the general population (6, 7). The osseous FFF permits for stable long-term prosthetic rehabilitation with dental implants with manageable donor-site complications (8–11). Computed tomography (CT) scans and DICOM data sets of the donor and recipient sites are required for virtual surgical planning (VSP) and the facilitation of custom-made, laser-melted, patient-specific titanium osteosynthesis plates (12, 13), which becomes widespread routine in many reconstructive centers (14). MRA was found as a reliable and non-invasive technique to identify anatomical variants and arterial stenoses (15, 16) without radiation in preoperative FFF planning (17). But CTA has been shown to be better than MRA for perforator mapping (18), as well as being more widely available, adequately accurate, and economic (19–21). The method of VSP was described by Eckardt and Swennen in 2005 for mandible reconstruction (22) and becomes more popular since than (23–27). The transfer from virtual planning to operating fields became accurate due to the possible because of the three-dimensionally designed and configured plate (28). Thank this planning method an exact and predictable uni- and poly-segmental bone restorations are possible (14, 29, 30). Success rates of the FFF ranging between 90% to 95% have been reported in the literature (31–34). Despite these significant benefits, surgery remains challenging in terms of insufficient perforator vessels, vascular bundle complications, or inadequate resections margins (35, 36). A thorough preoperative examination of the vascular system using a computed tomography angiography scan (CTA) to reduce those risks is required, as CTA scans allow for simultaneous evaluation of bony and vascularly structures (37).

The descriptive term periosteal branch (PB) is very general and has to be precise. Studies showed that bone perfusion of the skeleton is maintained by a system of three types of vessels (38, 39): endosteal nutrient vessels, penetrating periosteal vessels, and non-penetrating periosteal vessels. There are crosslinks between periosteal and endosteal vessels but without clear borders of perfusion. Experimental studies show that the inner two-thirds of the cortical bone is supplied by the endosteal system and the outer third by the periosteal system (40). Age seems to play a vital role, as the endosteal supply dominates the perfusion of cortical bone in youth, while in advanced age, a greater cortical thickness can be supplied by periosteum (41). While the nutrient vessels contribute to periosteal and endosteal blood supply (41), the non-penetrating branches do not appear to have a contribution to the endosteal perfusion (39, 42). The FFF is supplied by the non-penetrating perforator vessel subtypes direct periosteal and musculo-periosteal and nutrient vessels (1, 43). Several studies supported the thesis that non-penetrating branches only perfuse the outer section of the cortical bone (42, 44).

An anatomical examination of 30 formalin-fixed legs revealed that 27 legs (90%) had a singular nutrient vessel, and two (6.6 %) had a double nutrient vessel. In one leg, no nutrient vessel was observed. These vessels enter the fibula predominantly in the middle third, at its medial crest. In contrast, only one entered from the posterior surface and showed, on average, a diameter of 0.9 mm – 1.5 mm (45). Based on 54 cadaveric legs, it was found that the fibular nutrient artery, which arose from the fibular artery as a short descending branch, penetrated the M. flexor hallucis longus to enter the fibular nutrient foramen (46). Between the distal half of the first-quarter and second-quarter segments of the fibula, the fibular nutrient artery, and up to three arcuate arteries were located constantly (47). The term periosteal branch summarizes, therefore, nutrient and non-penetrating vessels.

Previous radiological analyzes of our research group on the same study sample revealed different distribution patterns and frequencies for PB and SCP based on CTA scans of both legs. A bimodal distribution pattern for PB and three peaks for SCP in performed CTA for VSP were recorded (48). Further, significant differences concerning the number of periosteal branches in the bone segment of different sizes were found compared to cadaver studies (49). The more proximal the FFF segment, the more frequently a potential PB was observed in the CTA scans. So that a comparison of the previous published radiological findings to the clinical data of the same patient's collection is of great interest, which is the topic of this paper.

This investigation aimed to evaluate the impact of detected small vessels (PB and SCP) on the surgical outcome after VSP of uni- and poly-segmental mandible reconstruction with FFF. Additionally, the following questions were evaluated in the study.

1. How do infra-popliteal branching pattern and fibular artery vascular anomalies (stenoses) affect the outcome of flap surgery?
2. How does the distribution of CTA-based detected PB and SCP influence the surgical result of mono- and poly-segmental jaw reconstructions with partial or total flap loss?

3. Does the observed distribution of PB and SCP impact wound healing of the donor site?

MATERIAL AND METHODS

Patient Collection, Ethical Consideration and Inclusion Criteria

The ethics committee of the Justus-Liebig-University Giessen approved the study (approval number: AZ33/20, approval date: 25.5.2020). No written obtained consent was required from the considered patients. Individuals meeting the following criteria were included: Immediate or delayed mandible reconstruction using FFF planned virtually, availability of preoperative CTA scans with a maximum slice thickness of 1.5 mm, treatment performed between January 2015 and December 2020.

A total number of 77 patients fulfilled the inclusion criteria. Five could not be included because of one fibula CTA after reconstruction with contralateral fibula after flap loss (n = 4) and after tumor recurrence (n = 1). Finally, 72 patients with CTA scans of 144 legs were available for the analyzis (**Figure 1**).

Dissection of the fibula flap was conducted using Gilbert's lateral approach (50). A segment of 8cm at the proximal end and the distal end, a 6-8cm length, was left in place to preserve knee and ankle stability. When a composite flap was harvested, the perforators were protected with a muscle cuff of M. soleus and M. flexor hallucis longus. A summarized clinical example is given in **Figures 2–4**. Wound closure of the donor site was done primarily in cases of non-composite FFF. When composite FFF were harvested, all donor site defects were covered with meshed split thickness skin graft.

All CTA scans were done at the University Hospital Giessen's Departments of Diagnostic and Interventional Radiology and Pediatric Radiology. The CT scans were done using a first-generation dual-energy CT scanner and a third-generation dual-energy CT scanner (SOMATOM Definition AS & Force, Siemens Healthineers, Forchheim, Germany). Above the aortic bifurcation to the feet, scans of both legs were performed with a slice thickness of 1.5 mm (70 kV, 300 mA max, pitch 0.5, collimation 0.6 mm, matrix size 512 x 512). Intravenously, non-ionic contrast fluids containing 350 mg of iodine per milliliter (Ultravist 370, Bayer, Leverkusen, Germany) were given. The amount of contrast media used is determined on the patient's weight.

CTA DICOM data sets were analyzed in HOROS-Software for Mac (Version 4.0.0 RC5, Horosproject). Horos is a free and open-source code software (FOSS) program distributed free of charge under the LGPL license at Horosproject.org and sponsored by Nimble Co LLC d/b/a Purview in Annapolis, MD, USA. The CTA quality was assessed by side-by-side comparison with an ROI in the center of the popliteal artery and dorsal vessels of the dorsum of the foot. For every CTA, the measurements were performed on both patients' legs.

Study Parameters

The following parameters were collected in a previous investigation on the study sample: Length of the fibula, bone and

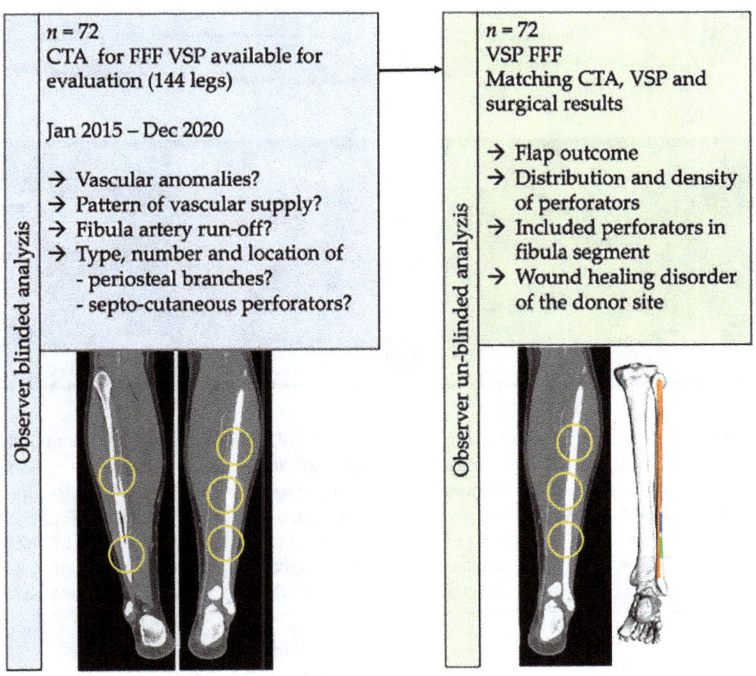

FIGURE 1 | Workflow of the present study. A total number of n = 72 computed tomography angiography (CTA) DICOM-datasets of virtual planned jaw reconstructions with a free fibula flap were included in the investigation. Findings on the vascular infra-popliteal branching pattern, stenoses, and distribution and density of periosteal branches and septo-cutaneous perforators of the fibular artery were matched with flap surgery outcome.

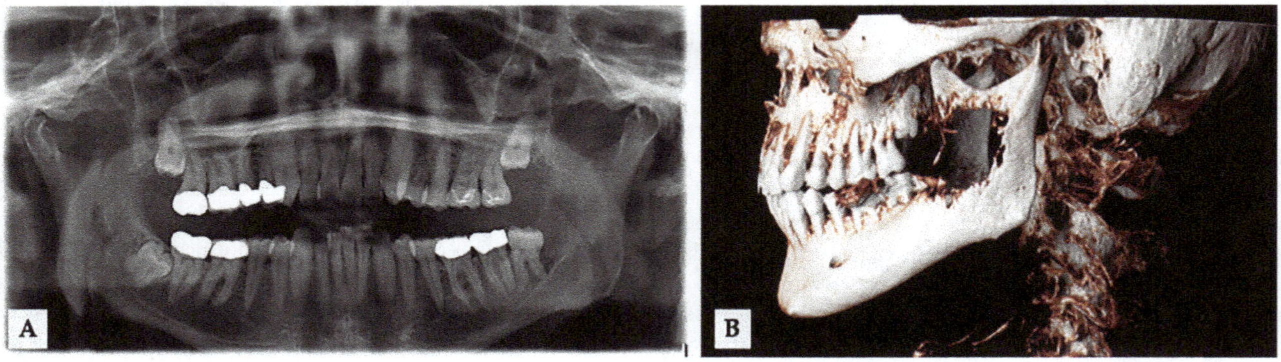

FIGURE 2 | 56 years old male with an infiltrative growth of oral squamous cell carcinoma (T4) in regio 38 (ID 18 in **Figure 5**). **(A)** Extension of osseous destruction in OPT and **(B)** cinematic volume rendering CT reconstruction.

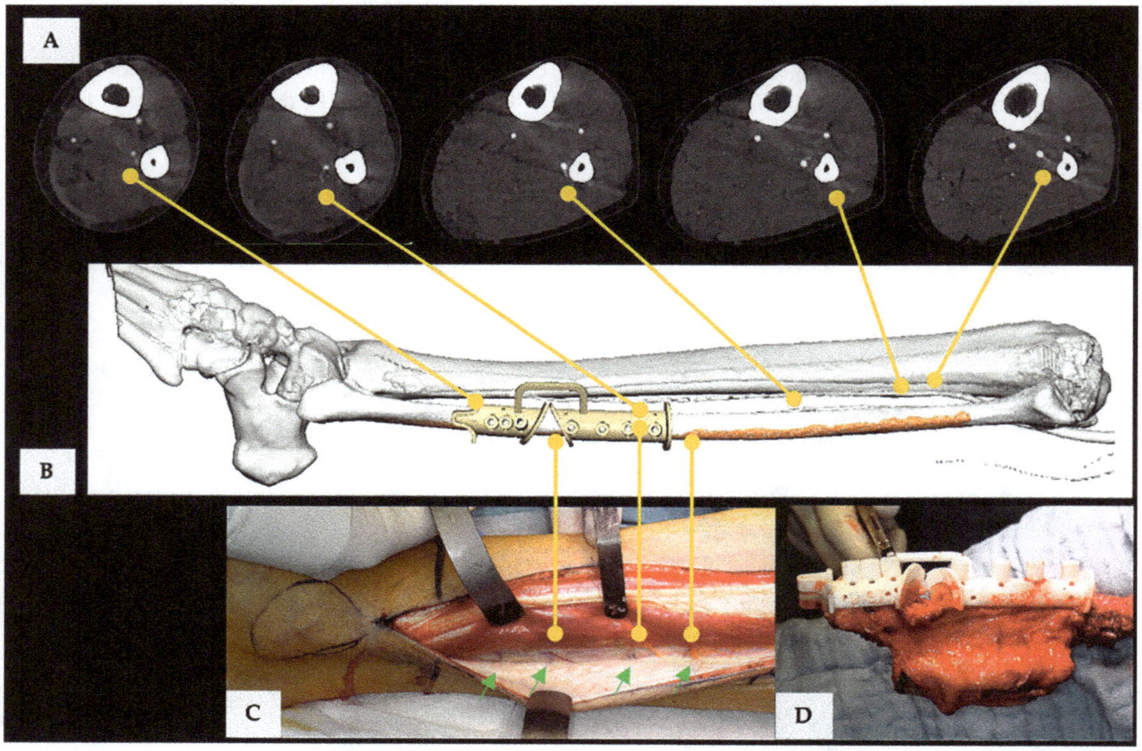

FIGURE 3 | **(A)** CTA scan (axial plane) of the donor site. Yellow lines connect found PB and SCP with virtual surgical planning. **(B)** Final virtual surgical planning for bi-segmental mandible reconstruction with free fibula flap. **(C)** Yellow lines connect corresponding vessels with the operating field. **(D)** Applied cutting guide, performed osteotomies, and shaped neo-condyle. Case is ID 18 in **Figure 5**. In CTA assessment were 5 PB and one SCP of the FA at donor site recorded. Each fibula flap segment was supplied by one PB, while three were located proximal to the designed flap. The CTA-based SCP position was in the middle of the skin paddle in the proximal fibula flap segment. The radiological examination of the FA was without pathological findings (type I-B: infra-popliteal branching pattern, which means trifurcation of the popliteal artery in ATA, PTA, and FA). Overall, there were no radiological reservations or restrictions to surgery. **Figure 3A, C** shows that there was a discrepancy between the radiological and the operative findings. The number of SCP was at least 4 (green arrows).

vascular anomalies, vascular anatomy and branching pattern of the infra-popliteal vessels will the classified concerning Kim et al. (51), length of TTF, number and localization of SCPs and PBs from the distal tip of the fibula bone to branching and between the branches.

These findings were matched with the surgical outcome including: Patient's age (at CT scan), gender, body height, and weight, BMI, flap-type (composite or non-composite flap), site of flap harvesting, distance to the distal tip of the fibula (ankle), as well

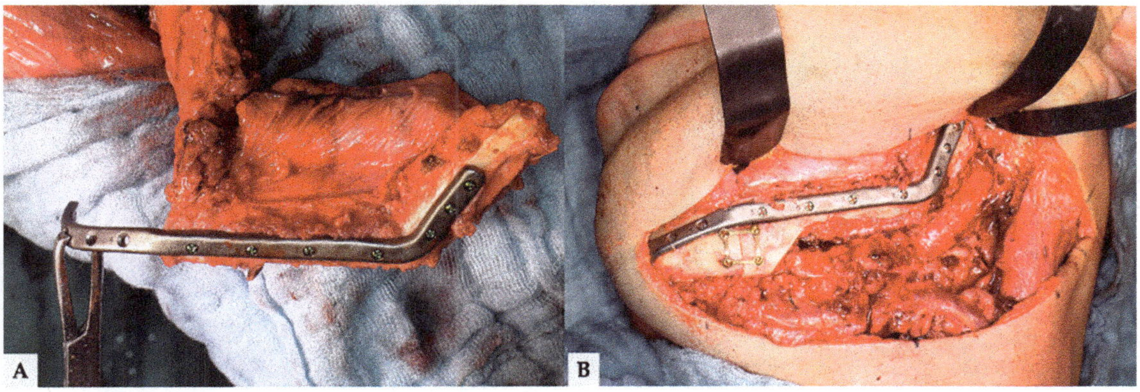

FIGURE 4 | **(A)** Final molded bi-segmental composite fibula flap and **(B)** neo-mandible. Additional triangular free bone transplant to smooth the contour of neo-mandible's jawline. Finally, total flap loss occurred in this case. The surgical revision revealed a combined arterial and venous thrombosis.

as the number, length, and position of fibula segments. Additionally, total transplant length, which were taken out of the virtual planning report was recorded. Information about flap status (complete flap success, partial (bone or skin paddle), or total flap loss) was extracted from the medical records. PFF was defined as any loss of parts of the skin paddle (skin), parts or segments (poly-segmental reconstruction) of bone grafts (bone), or a combination of both (52). The donor site's wound healing disorder (WHD) was classified as minor WHD when only a conservative wound had been performed. Major WHD implicates large wounds with exposed tendons and surgical treatment by applying split-thickness skin graft after wound debridement.

Statistical Analysis

Pearson's $\chi 2$ test, Fisher's exact test, and the Freeman–Halton extension (53) were conducted on the categorical variables used to analyze flap outcome concerning: gender, flap-type (composite or non-composite flap), donor site, number of bone segments, and number and type of included perforators and ASA-score. Kruskal-Wallis test was performed to analyze defined flap outcome groups concerning metric parameters. The continuous parameters: age, body height, and weight, body-mass-index (BMI), the total length of the fibula, the length of the fibular artery (FA) from origin to the distal tip of the fibula bone, the diameter of the fibular artery, the length and the diameter of the truncus tibiofibularis (TTF), the number and the distance of septo-cutaneous perforators (SCP), the periosteal branches (PB), overall reconstruction length, and the segment length were verified for normality. The distribution was presented as a mean (standard deviation), and Student's t-test was performed. $p < 0.05$ was defined as statistically significant. The statistical analyzes were carried out with SPSS (IBM SPSS Statistics, v28.0, Armonk, NY, USA).

RESULTS

A total of 72 patients (28 women, 38.9 %; 44 men, 61.1 %) fulfilled the inclusion criteria. The mean age was 58.5 ± 15.3 years (range: 14.8 – 82.6 years). Firstly, the vascular system of the study sample was assessed and the sample was categorized into donor and non-donor site for further analyzis.

In the gender-mixed sample, no significant difference in fibular bone length was found. Concerning the infra-popliteal branching pattern type as classified by Kim et al., all donor fibulae had a regular vascular supply equivalent to types I-A through II-C. In contrast, at the non-donor site, two cases of type III-A and two cases of type III-B were found (51). Out of 144 legs, 88.9 % (n = 128) were assigned as type I-A. Detailed evaluation of the donor site vascular architecture revealed that type I-A was found in 93.1 % (non-donor site: 84.7 %). Two donor site vascular systems were classified as type I-B, and one case was assigned to categories I-C to II-B. Four legs of the non-donor site showed dominant fibular artery (FA) variants (III-A: n = 2; III-B: n = 2). No type III-C branching pattern was observed, defined as a dominant fibular artery, that can lead to critical perfusion (**Tables 1** and **2**).

At all, 14 stenoses of the lower limbs' vessels were recognized. Five stenoses of the FA were detected at the donor site, while in the non-donor site, stenoses in all three vessels had been found (FA: n = 6; ATA: n = 1; PTA: n = 2). In donor vs. non-donor site comparison, no significant differences for the total length of the TTF and FA and the diameters were found. PB and SCP were located in equal parts at donor- vs. non-donor sites. The study detected a mean number (± SD) of 2.53 ± 1.60 PB and 1.39 ± 1.03 SCP of the FA at the donor-site in the region of interest between the exit of FA from the TTF and 5.0 cm above the distal tip of the fibula bone. Compared to the non-donor site, a non-significant difference in the mean number of recorded PB and SCP was found.

The findings were matched with virtual surgical planning (VSP) and surgery results, and flap outcome was categorized concerning complete flap success (FS), partial (PFF), and total flap failure (TFF). Partial flap failure was defined as (sub-)total loss of the skin paddle and/or parts or segments of poly-segmental reconstructions. The detailed results are summarized in **Table 3** and **Figure 5**. Total flap loss was recorded in n = 9 cases (12.5%). The highest average age with 64.9 ± 8.0 years was found in the TFF-group, while the lowest

TABLE 1 | CTA assessment for fibular bone and vascular system parameters of the study sample.

n = 144	Donor site (*n* = 72)	Non-donor site (*n* = 72)	Total	*p*-value
Fibula length, mean (mm) ± SD	373.9 ± 30.2	372.8 ± 30.9	142	0.829
Fibula bone anomalies				
Fracture	0	1	1	–
Branching pattern of the calf (51)				
Regular (I-A to II-C)	72	68	140	
Absent ATA (III-A)	0	2	2	
Absent PTA (III-B)	0	2	2	0.119
Stenoses				
ATA	0	1	1	
PTA	0	2	2	
FA	5	6	11	0.670
Length of TTF, mean (mm) ± SD	32.6 ± 12.9 (*n* = 67)	32.5 ± 14.6 (*n* = 61)	128	0.965
Diameter of TTF, mean (mm) ± SD	4.13 ± 0.95 (*n* = 67)	4.16 ± 1.0 (*n* = 61)	128	0.862
Length of FA, mean (mm) ± SD	244.9 ± 36.9	243.0 ± 43.3	142	0.777
Diameter of FA, mean (mm) ± SD	3.12 ± 0.79	3.21 ± 0.78	142	0.493
Overall found SCP, *n* (%)	101 (47.4%)	112 (52.6%)	213	
Diameter SCP, mean (mm) ± SD	0.93 ± 0.28	0.93 ± 0.32	0.93 ± 0.30	1.0
Mean SCP per fibula (mm) ± SD	1.39 ± 1.03	1.52 ± 1.23	1.40 ± 1.01	0.407
Overall found PB, *n* (%)	185 (51.2%)	176 (48.8%)	361	
Diameter PB, mean (mm) ± SD	0.87 ± 0.24	0.87 ± 0.26	0.87 ± 0.56	1.0
Mean PB per fibula (mm) ± SD	2.53 ± 1.60	2.42 ± 1.60	2.47 ± 1.54	0.514

SD, standard deviation; ATA, anterior tibial artery; FA, fibular artery; PB, periosteal branch; PTA, posterior tibial artery; SCP, septo-cutaneous perforator; TTF, truncus tibiofibularis.

mean age with 49.8 ± 20.6 years was estimated in the PFF group. The finding was without statistical significance. Differences concerning body weight were found significant for PFF in comparison to FS (PFF: 92.3 ± 10.6 kg vs. TFF: 64.9 ± 8.0 kg; p = 0.012) and a trend towards significance concerning the TFF (PFF: 92.3 ± 10.6 kg vs. FS: 58.4 ± 15.6 kg; p = 0.061). About 43.1 % of the study sample were classified at least ASA-score 3. PFF and TFF were found only for ASA-score 2 and 3 and within each class in equal proportions. All registered PFFs and TFFs (except for one type, I-B) occurred in a I-A branching pattern.

The donor site was in nearly two-thirds of the cases (63.9 %) the right leg, and a minimal distance to the distal tip of the fibular of more than 70 mm was planned in 91.7 % of our cases to preserve ankle stability. TFF has not been observed when tri-segmental jaw reconstruction has been performed.

No significant difference (p = 0.431) was found for the length of TTF concerning flap outcome (FS: 31.3 ± 12.2 mm vs. TFF: 40.1 ± 14.9 mm).

Only when composite flaps were used, wound healing disorders of the donor site were registered. Harvesting defects were standardized covered with a meshed split-thickness skin graft (0.4 mm). The proportion of significant wound healing disorders (WHD) was almost twice as high as that of minor WHD in the FS-group (33.9 % vs. 18.6 %). In the TFF-group, this proportion quadrupled and must be viewed critically due to the small number of cases. No WHD was observed summarized in half of the patients in all groups (**Table 4**).

The total number of in FFF included SCP and PB of the FA were analyzed in relation to the found vessels beyond the flap and classified concerning flap outcome (**Figure 6**). No significant differences were observed for different flap outcomes and the number of included SCP (CS 46.3 % vs. PFF 50.0 %, TFF 45.4 %) and PB (CS 37.7 % vs. PFF 38.5 %, TFF 28.6 %).

Further, the number of every single segment of a mono- and poly-segmental reconstruction which was supplied by at least one PB (**Table 5**), and analog for SCP (only for composite flaps, n = 61) (**Table 6**) was assessed. Based on the number of prepared segments, at least one PB supplied 46.7% in the mono-, 40.4% in the bi-, and 31.5 % in the tri-segmental group. Overall, this corresponds to 37.2% (45 out of 121) of all successful FFF. For TFF, a relative number of 42.9% of single addressed segments was calculated. The findings were non-significant. In summary, the number of SCP per segment were lower in poly-segmental composite FFF than in mono-segmental composite reconstruction (**Table 6**). These results are without significance.

Minimal and maximal segment length of each virtually shaped FFF segment was assessed and categorized concerning flap outcome. With an increasing number of used FFF segments for reconstruction, the mean segment length decreases (**Table 3**). With the same number of used segments, no statistically significant differences could be found. In detail, the shortest segment length was found in mean with ≥ 34.5 ± 14.2 mm for successful tri-segmental reconstructions, with ≥ 27.1 ± 6.4 mm for partial flap failure in tri-segmental reconstructions, and with ≥ 40.3 ± 16.8 mm

TABLE 2 | Infrapopliteal arterial branching variations were classified by Kim (51) of the investigated sample (n = 144).

Type	Donor site (*n* = 72) *n* (%)	Non-donor site (*n* = 72) *n* (%)	Total (*n* = 144) *n* (%)
I-A	67 (93.1)	61 (84.7)	128 (88.9)
I-B	2 (2.8)	1 (1.4)	3 (2.1)
I-C	1 (1.4)	–	1 (0.7)
II-A	1 (1.4)	2 (2.8)	3 (2.1)
II-B	1 (1.4)	4 (5.6)	5 (3.6)
II-C	–	–	–
III-A	–	2 (2.8)	2 (1.4)
III-B	–	2 (2.8)	2 (1.4)
III-C	–	–	–

TABLE 3 | Demographic and surgery-associated parameters.

n = 72	**Flap success 59 (82.0%)**	**Partial flap failure 4 (5.5%)**	**Total flap failure 9 (12.5%)**	***p*-value**
Age (years), mean ± SD	58.4 ± 15.6	49.8 ± 20.6	64.9 ± 8.0	0.338
Gender, n (%)				
Male	33 (44.1)	4 (100.0)	7 (77.8)	
Female	26 (55.9)	0	2 (22.2)	0.150
Body weight (kg), mean ± SD	71.7 ± 15.7	92.3 ± 10.6	74.6 ± 15.2	*0.012
Body height (cm), mean ± SD	169.9 ± 10.0	179.3 ± 3.9	176.8 ± 11.3	0.067
BMI (kg/m^2), mean ± SD	24.7 ± 5.2	28.8 ± 3.6	23.6 ± 4.8	0.189
ASA-score, n (%)				
1	3 (5.1)	0	0	
2	31 (52.5)	2 (50.0)	5 (55.6)	
3	23 (39.0)	2 (50.0)	4 (44.4)	
4	2 (3.4)	0	0	0.973
Reconstruction site				
Maxilla	15 (25.4)	1 (25.0)	2 (22.2)	
Mandibula	44 (74.6)	3 (75.0)	7 (77.8)	1.0
FFF type, n (%)				
Composite flap	51 (86.5)	3 (75.0)	7 (77.8)	
Non-composite flap	8 (13.5)	1 (25.0)	2 (22.2)	0.573
Donor site, n (%)				
Left	22 (37.3)	0	4 (44.4)	
Right	37 (62.7)	4 (100.0)	5 (55.6)	0.384
Distance to the tip of the fibula (ankle), mean ± SD				
60 mm	6 (10.2)	0	0	
70 mm	31 (52.5)	4 (100.0)	5 (55.6)	
80 mm	17 (28.8)	0	2 (22.2)	
90 mm	5 (8.5)	0	1 (11.1)	
118.9 mm	0	0	1 (11.1)	0.175
Number of segments, n (%)				
1	15 (25.4)	1 (25.0)	4 (44.4)	
2	26 (44.1)	2 (50.0)	5 (55.6)	
3	18 (30.5)	1 (25.0)	0	0.351
Total transplant length (mm), mean ± SD (range)				
1	56.1 ± 15.3 (35.0 – 94.9)	55.0	68.1 ± 17.8 (47.3 – 90.2)	0.458
2	106.6 ± 21.5 (71.0 – 143.6)	99.8 ± 18.2 (86.9 – 112.6)	109.9 ± 18.7 (90.5 – 133.1)	0.804
3	142.3 ± 21.2 (103.7 – 176.3)	126.7	–	0.361
Minimal segment length (mm), mean ± SD (range)				
1	45.3 ± 16.8 (17.0 – 84.7)	32.0	52.6 ± 12.5 (34.0 – 60.2)	0.261
2	36.7 ± 14.3 (16.0 – 64.8)	37.0 ± 14.7 (28.4 – 59.0)	40.3 ± 16.8 (22.7 ± 73.0)	0.926
3	34.5 ± 14.2 (16.7 – 71.3)	27.1 ± 6.4 (25.8 – 29.5)	–	0.650
Maximal segment length (mm), mean ± SD (range)				
1	53.7 ± 16.4 (29.0 – 91.5)	52	62.2 ± 12.1 (45.0 – 71.5)	0.464
2	49.4 ± 16.1 (20.0 – 80.2)	45.1 ± 14.7 (32.9 – 64.5)	47.2 ± 16.1 (32.3 ± 79.3)	0.809
3	43.1 ± 13.5 (27.4 – 89.5)	36.8 ± 2.1 (29.9 – 42.4)	–	0.508
Length of TTF, mean ± SD (n‡)	31.3 ± 12.2 (55)	32.3 ± 11.7 (4)	40.1 ± 14.9 (8)	‡0.034

*BMI, body mass index; FFF, free fibula flap; PB, periosteal branch; SCP, septo-cutaneous perforator; SD, standard deviation; TTF, truncus tibiofibularis; WHD, wound healing disorder. *Significant difference was only found between flap success and partial flap failure group. ‡TTF was only assessed in type I-A branching pattern.*

for total flap failure in bi-segmental reconstructions. The length of each fibula flap segment was non-significant different in mono- (p = 0.194) and bi-segmental (p = 0.752) reconstructions concerning flap success. In poly-segmental jaw reconstructions, the proximal FFF segments (proximal in bi- and proximal > medial in tri-segmental reconstruction), a higher rate of PB per flap segment was assessed than in the distal segments (**Figure** 7).

DISCUSSION

Despite advances in the planning of free flaps, improvements of microsurgical techniques (54), and flap monitoring (55–57), the result of surgical reconstruction is still threatened by perfusion disorders of macro- and microcirculation. Flap loss severely disturbs patients' quality of life and increases the risk of further surgical procedures. Intensive preoperative assessment and imaging evaluation are necessary to decrease peri- and postoperative complications and increase flap success (58–63). CTA has been shown as a sensitive and specific method for microsurgical free flap (21, 64–66) and perforator flap harvesting in reconstructive surgery (67–75).

Over 43 % (n = 31) of the included study subjects were classified at least ASA-score 3. PFF occurred in 2 cases (6.5 %) and TFF in 4 cases (12.9 %). On the other hand, in the ASA-score 1 and 2 groups (n = 41), we documented n = 2 PFF (4.9 %) and n

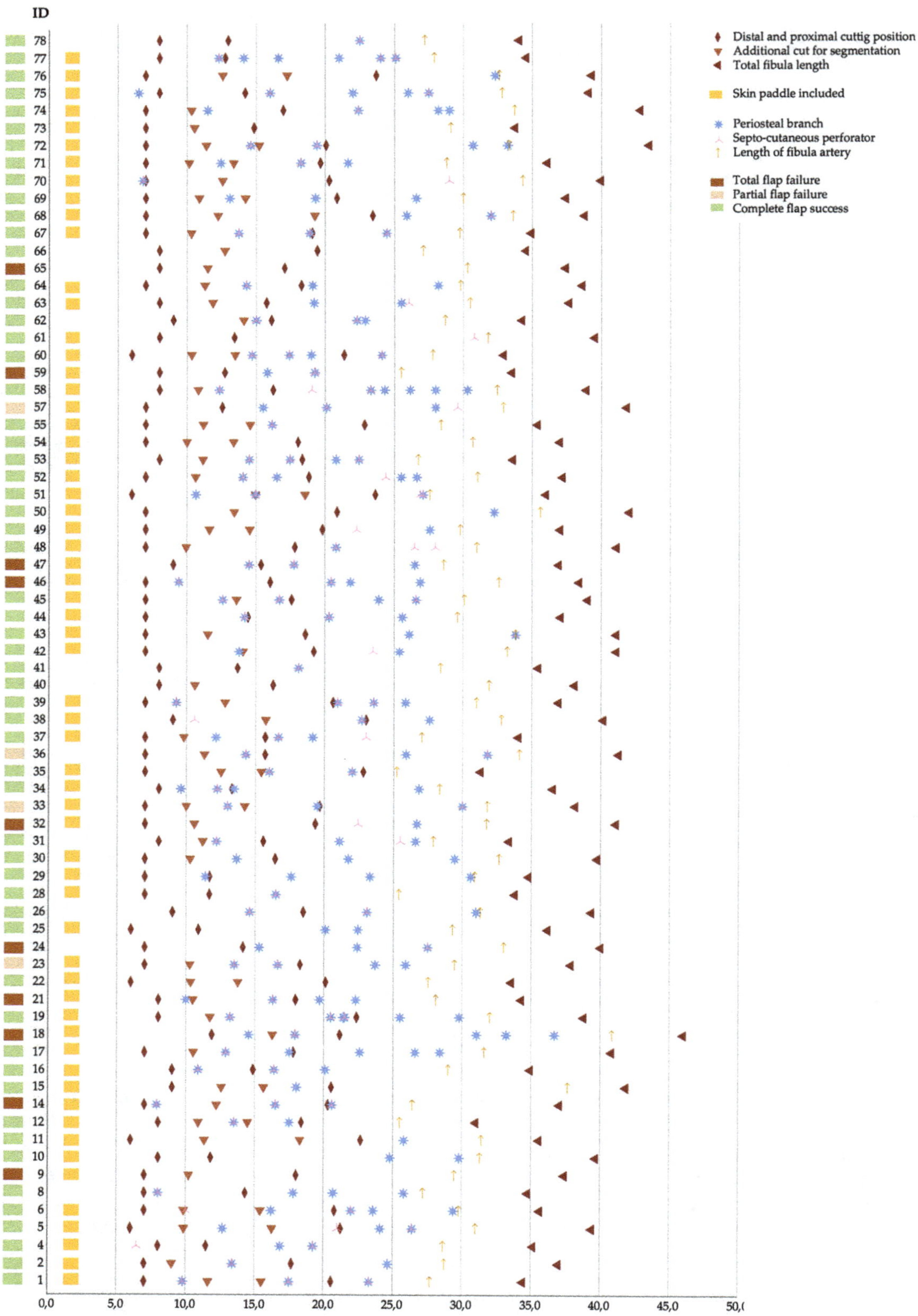

FIGURE 5 | Sample of n = 72 virtual planned jaw reconstructions. Matching virtually planned parameters, CTA detected vessels (PB and SCP), and surgical outcome. All position marks (x-axis) are given in centimeters.

TABLE 4 | Wound healing disorders of the donor site.

n = 72	Flap success 59 (82.0%)	Partial flap failure 4 (5.5%)	Total flap failure 9 (12.5%)	*p*-value
Composite flap, n (%)				
None	20 (33.9)	1 (25.0)	2 (22.2)	
Minor WHD	11 (18.6)	0	1 (11.1)	
Major WHD	20 (33.9)	2 (50.0)	4 (44.4)	
Non-composite flap				
None	8 (13.6)	1 (25.0)	2 (22.2)	0.523

= 5 (12.2 %) TFF. Despite the presence of comorbidities, we did not observe an increase in complications and flap loss. These results are comparable to the literature reported by other study groups (76–78).

How do Infra-Popliteal Branching Pattern and Fibular Artery Vascular Anomalies (Stenoses) Affect the Outcome of Flap Surgery?

Evaluation of the donor site vascular architecture revealed that type I-A was found in 93.1 % (non-donor site: 84.7 %) according to the classification by Kim et al. (51). Two donor site vascular systems were classified as type I-B, and one case was assigned to categories I-C to II-B. Four legs of the non-donor site showed dominant FA variants (III-A: n = 2; III-B: n = 2). The foot's blood supply is then shared between FA and non-hypoplastic ATA or PTA in type III-A and B, and FA is enlarged as a result (79–81). It was previously estimated that 5.2 % of limbs have dominant FAs (66). The study sample presented either on the donor or non-donor site none peroneal artery magna (type III-C), in which FA supplies blood to the lower leg and foot.

Overall, the distribution of the recorded branching variants of the popliteal artery is comparable to previous published data (82). However, it is imperative to identify this particular singular vasculature before FFF harvesting to prevent critical limb and foot ischemia (63, 83, 84). The investigation revealed that all but one of the PFF and TFF cases could be assigned to type I-A and I-B branching patterns. In accordance with the literature, type I-A is the most common branching pattern. Successful flap transfers occurred in types I-B, I-C, II-A, and II-B (each n = 1).

9.7 % of cases with vascular stenoses (n = 14) were identified in the sample, and from these, 11 were localized in the FA. There were five stenoses in the distal course of the FA run-off at the donor site, and two of these were associated with TFF. On the other hand, three cases of FA stenoses did not impact flap success. Remarkably, the majority of the recorded stenoses were located in FA. Other studies suggest the FA is not as severely affected by the peripheral arterial occlusive disease (PAOD) as the tibial arteries (60, 85, 86). Despite vascular calcifications impacting the flap vascular pedicle, successful microvascular FFF has been described, with a 0 % complete flap failure rate and a 7 % partial flap failure rate (87). Preoperative optimizing of leg perfusion by endovascular interventions has also been reported as a therapeutic option in possible critical limb perfusion (88).

Further study findings revealed significant differences concerning the length of TTF in the flap failure group compared to flap success and were assessed with an extended length of 40.1 ± 14.9 mm (p = 0.034). A more prolonged TTF implicates a decreasing length of the FA and, therefore, the entire vascular pedicle of the FFF. While short pedicle length can aggravate microsurgical anastomosis (89), a long pedicle is

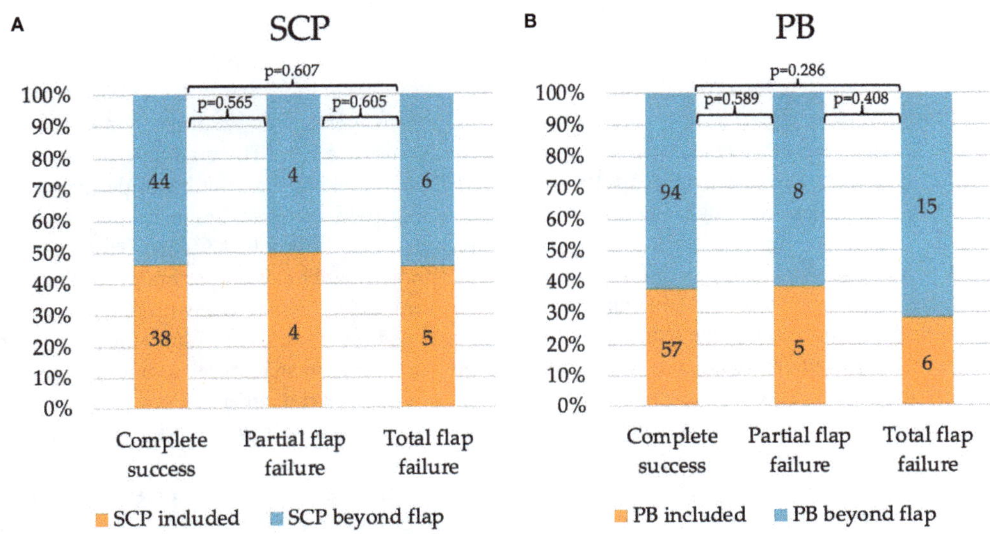

FIGURE 6 | Impact of relative distribution of **(A)** SCP and **(B)** PB concerning FFF outcome: Complete success, *n* = 59; Partial flap failure, *n* = 4; Total flap failure, *n* = 9. An absolute number of recorded vessel types are noted in the bars. Annotation: All possible SCP were recorded without consideration of including a skin paddle (composite FFF type). FFF, free fibula flap; PB, periosteal branch; SCP, septo-cutaneous perforator.

TABLE 5 | Absolute (n) and relative (%) number of fibular segments were addressed by at least one periosteal branch (PB) based on preoperative CTA for VSP.

PB ≥1 per segment (total segments *n* = 143)	Flap success 121 (= 59 FFF)	Partial flap failure 8 (= 4 FFF)	Total flap failure 14 (= 9 FFF)
1 SFFF, n (%)	7 (46.7)	0	2 (50.0)
2 SFFF, n (%)	21 (40.4)	2 (50.0)	4 (40.0)
3 SFFF, n (%)	17 (31.5)	2 (66.7)	–
All, n (%)	45 (37.2)	4 (50.0)	6 (42.9)

TABLE 6 | Absolute (n) and relative (%) number of fibula segments of composite FFF, which were addressed by at least one septo-cutaneous perforator (SCP) based on preoperative CTA for VSP.

SCP ≥1 per segment (total segments *n* = 126)	Flap success 109 (= 51 FFF)	Partial flap failure 6 (= 3 FFF)	Total flap failure 11 (= 7 FFF)
1 SFFF, n (%)	4 (36.4)	0	2 (66.7)
2 SFFF, n (%)	13 (29.5)	1 (50.0)	3 (37.5)
3 SFFF, n (%)	12 (22.2)	1 (33.3)	–
All, n (%)	29 (26.6)	2 (33.3)	5 (45.4)

endangered for kinking and twisting with critical blood flow of the vascular axis (90). Published literature hypothesizes a relation between length and course of TTF and high body mass. This condition may contribute to enlarged and curved/twisted TTF, promoting local atherosclerosis and impeding microsurgery (91).

Summarized, the infra-popliteal branching pattern types I-A to II-B did not affect the flap surgery outcome in the present study. Furthermore, despite recorded vascular stenoses of the FA, flap success was observed in more than the half of those cases.

How Does the Distribution of CTA-Based Detected PB and SCP Influence the Surgical Result of Mono- and Poly-Segmental Jaw Reconstructions With Partial or Total Flap Loss?

The results of this study show that a PB and SCP (musculo-fascio-periosteal perforators) could not be visualized in every virtually planned and transplanted segment in the preoperatively performed lower limb CTA scan. Nevertheless, mono- and poly-segmental reconstructions were successful when no PB was found in CTA evaluation and failed, although PB (and SCP) were verifiable.

When matching harvested segments with detected PB, 38.5 % of all virtual planned segments (n = 143 in 72 patients) were congruent to one or more PB localization. If the segments which at least one PB distinctively supplied are assigned to the defined flap outcome groups, it was found that the FS group has the lowest rate with 37.2 %, the PFF group has the highest rate with 50.0 %, and the TFF group is between both with 42.9 % (**Table 5**). Therefore, the rate of in CTA detected PB found per segment did not provide information concerning expected flap success. The explored distribution patterns reflect PB and SCP clustering and confirm the high variability of the localization and course. It is noticeable that in poly-segmental reconstructions, the probability of observing a PB in the CTA increases in the more proximal segment. Previous investigations on the study sample revealed a bimodal distribution pattern for PB and three peaks for SCP in performed CTA for VSP (48). These patterns of distribution are similar to the results of other studies (17, 20, 92).

Investigations of CT-scans in fresh frozen cadaver lower limbs showed in mean 12.8 periosteal branches of the fibular artery with a mean intersegmental distance of 1.36 cm between them, and at least one branch in 65.1% in 1.0 cm segments, and up to 94% of the 2.0 cm segments (49). Their radiological findings of the detected periosteal branches (49) support the measurements of fibular segments perfusion in cadavers (93), but differ from our conclusions presented. The previous analysis of the study sample has shown that in 10.8 %, one PB was found in a 1.0 cm fibula section in our defined region of interest between the origin of the FA and a plane 5 cm above the distal tip of the fibula section. The likelihood increases in 2.0 cm segment up to 21.1 % and in 3.0 cm segment length to 29.2 %, having included at least one PB (48). Further, there is no difference regarding the density of periosteal and musculo-periosteal vessels in the long and short fibula segments. Existing collaterals between the superficial, periosteal, and the internal endoperiosteal system, were not able to compensate for the work of the non-functional vessels if the segment length was too short. However, this is more likely to occur if the segments are longer (93). Larger segments and fewer osteotomies were associated with higher perfusion (94). Battaglia et al. reported a series of 20 patients in matching in CTA images identified perforators with the intraoperative perforator location while FFF harvesting (65). An average distance between CTA perforator positions and intraoperative perforator positions of 1 mm (range 0 to 2 mm) was assessed. They concluded that preoperative CTA evaluation to investigate lower-extremity vascular patterns for patients undergoing composite FFF is a valuable approach for reducing VSP complications due to variable vascular anatomy. Still, more follow-up studies are needed to assess this modern technique's long-term outcomes and benefits (65). Ettinger et al. report that further development of CTA imaging protocols and existing VSP workflows is necessary to be optimized to allow faster and more accurate preoperative modeling of cutaneous perforator anatomy for consideration in VSP of reconstructions (64). These authors point out also, that CTA for VSP allows taking the position of perforators into account when planning poly-segmental reconstruction and skin paddle (64). A previous study found that CTA could detect the size, course, and penetration pattern of all perforators with a diameter more than 0.3 mm (21). Recent investigation on the study population confirmed these statements (48). However, it can be assumed that the discrepancy in anatomical findings is based on the quality of the CTA scans. Several other factors influence CTA scan accuracy, including the timing, dosage, and coordination of the contrast bolus with the sequence of images (95).

Overall, the rate of CTA detected PB per segment did not indicate flap success. Mono- and poly-segmental reconstructions were successful when no PB (and SCP) were found in the CTA evaluation and even were unsuccessful when PB (and SCP) were recorded.

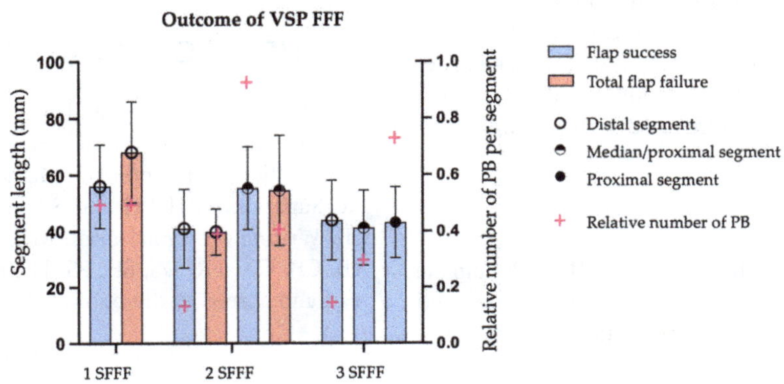

FIGURE 7 | Impact of FFF outcome concerning length of fibular bone segments of mono- (1 SFFF), bi- (2 SFFF) or tri-segmental (3 SFFF) flap for achieving jaw reconstruction (left y-axis). The relative number of periosteal branches (PB) per segment (right y-axis) was calculated and superimposed (magenta cross). 1 SFFF flap success: $n = 16$ vs. total flap failure: $n = 4$; 2 SFFF flap success: $n = 28$ vs. $n = 5$; 3 SFFF flap success: $n = 19$ vs. $n = 0$; Amount of observed PB in region of transplanted fibular bone segments $n = 66$ based on the preoperative CTA.

Does the Observed Distribution of PB and SCP Impact Wound Healing of the Donor Site?

WHD of the donor site were recorded only in the composite flap group, and the proportion of WHD was less high in the TFF-group (55.5 %) than in the FS-group (52.5 %). The differences should be viewed critically according to the small number of cases. A separation between minor WHD (small wound area and local therapy) and major WHD (large wound, exposed tendon, and need of surgical therapy with debridement, new skin grafting) had been done and showed, that major WHD (33.9%) had been recorded near to twice than minor WHD (18.6%) in the FS-group. In summary, more than 52.8 % of the entire study sample WHD were found. Published literature shows complication rates from 0% to 33% (62, 96, 97). In the present study, donor site defect of composite FFF were covered in all cases with a meshed split-thickness skin graft, and every (sub-)total graft loss was counted and defined as WHD. Primarily wound closure was only performed after non-composite FFF harvesting, and wound healing disorder was not found in this group.

According to SCP per segment matching rate, only composite flaps were evaluated. A total number of n = 126 segments in 64 patients has shown that overall, 28.6 % of all virtual planned segments were congruent to one or more SCP localization. However, this finding does not allow providing information concerning wound healing disorder. On the one hand, the authors believe that the size of the skin paddle and the donor site defect, and the patient's general condition with comorbidities play a decisive role in wound healing. Heavy tobacco use was found to have as a risk factor for wound impairment (97).

The problem of WHD as a donor site morbidity has been known in the literature for a long time. Up to now, closure of the donor site is controversial and ranges from primarily closure, open wound healing, split-thickness skin graft, full skin graft, free flap (96, 98). Open healing of the fibular donor site and meshing of the surrounded tissue has been reported as a modification to decrease the wound area and avoid the morbidity associated with graft and resulted in a good cosmetic outcome (99). The use of vacuum-assisted closure allows patients to be mobilized sooner, assures greater graft acceptance, and reduces healing time up to 50% (100).

Up to now, information about the number and course of PB and SCP has not been of interest in our entire virtual planning process. Designing the composite flap and especially the skin paddle's dimension depends on the defect size and visible SCP in the posterior intermuscular septum. From our clinical experience, we agree with others that handheld Doppler sonography examination is often unsuitable in general anesthesia to identify SCP reliably. Identifying tiny perforators and distinguishing between superficial muscular perforators and cutaneous perforators is difficult (101). Islam et al. discovered that real-time, color-flow Doppler ultrasonography was beneficial in the planning and harvesting free perforator flaps and suggested that it be used more widely than traditional hand-held Doppler equipment (102). We prefer the direct assessment and visualization of the SCP during dissection (**Figure 3**).

The distribution of in preoperative CTA detected PB and SCP per segment was not associated with the rate of wound healing disorders of the donor site after composite flap harvesting.

Limitations of the Study

There are some limitations in this retrospective study. Only patients who underwent the following FFF procedure were included in the investigation. Patients who were not suitable for FFF after CTA scan were not included, and the number of cases remains unclear. The investigated study population consisted a mixture of malignant and benign diseases which give an inhomogeneity to the study subjects. Another limitation is that multiple surgeons were involved in the treatment of the study population. Three different surgeons were involved in FFF harvesting over the entire study period. Evaluated CTA scans were not performed under experimental, controlled conditions. Instead, they were run as routine clinical imaging which reported by different radiologists.

Furthermore, as concluded in a previous study, the in CTA observed number of PBs and SCPs is substantially less than accurate as the anatomical findings (48). Therefore, the number of small vessels could be underestimated. Further studies using better developed volume visualization software to improve the illustration of small vessels are necessary as a future research step in this topic.

CONCLUSION

Preoperatively CTA for VSP of free fibula flap (FFF) is suitable for vascular mapping of the infra-popliteal vascular system and smaller vessels. Despite recorded stenoses of fibular artery in five cases, FFF was in 60% successful.

Correlation between higher rates of PB, SCP and the flap success could not be statistically proved in study sample. We conclude, that preoperative PB and SCP mapping based on routine CTA imaging is not suitable for prediction of flap outcome.

AUTHOR CONTRIBUTIONS

Conceptualization, MK and SA. Data curation, DS and SB. Formal analysis, MK and PS. Funding acquisition, H-PH. Investigation, MK and AB. Methodology, MK, AB, CA, and FR. Supervision, H-PH and SA. Validation, SA. Visualization, CB. Writing - original draft, MK. Writing - review & editing, AB, CB, CA, FR, DS, SB, PS, H-PH, and SA. All authors have read and agreed to the published version of the manuscript.

ACKNOWLEDGMENTS

This publication is part of the dental doctoral thesis of AB.

REFERENCES

1. Taylor GI, Miller GD, Ham FJ. The Free Vascularized Bone Graft. A Clinical Extension of Microvascular Techniques. *Plast Reconstr Surg* (1975) 55 (5):533–44. doi: 10.1097/00006534-197505000-00002
2. Hidalgo DA. Fibula Free Flap: A New Method of Mandible Reconstruction. *Plast Reconstr Surg* (1989) 84(1):71–9. doi: 10.1097/00006534-198907000-00014
3. Cordeiro PG, Disa JJ, Hidalgo DA, Hu QY. Reconstruction of the Mandible With Osseous Free Flaps: A 10-Year Experience With 150 Consecutive Patients. *Plast Reconstr Surg* (1999) 104(5):1314–20. doi: 10.1097/00006534-199910000-00011
4. Wei FC, Chen HC, Chuang CC, Noordhoff MS. Fibular Osteoseptocutaneous Flap: Anatomic Study and Clinical Application. *Plast Reconstr Surg* (1986) 78 (2):191–200. doi: 10.1097/00006534-198608000-00008
5. Kumar BP, Venkatesh V, Kumar KA, Yadav BY, Mohan SR. Mandibular Reconstruction: Overview. *J Maxillofac Oral Surg* (2016) 15(4):425–41. doi: 10.1007/s12663-015-0766-5
6. Löfstrand J, Nyberg M, Karlsson T, Thórarinsson A, Kjeller G, Lidén M, et al. Quality of Life After Free Fibula Flap Reconstruction of Segmental Mandibular Defects. *J Reconstr Microsurg* (2018) 34(2):108–20.
7. Tarsitano A, Ciocca L, Cipriani R, Scotti R, Marchetti C. Mandibular Reconstruction Using Fibula Free Flap Harvested Using a Customised Cutting Guide: How We do it. *Acta Otorhinolaryngol Ital* (2015) 35 (3):198–201.
8. Attia S, Wiltfang J, Streckbein P, Wilbrand JF, El Khassawna T, Mausbach K, et al. Functional and Aesthetic Treatment Outcomes After Immediate Jaw Reconstruction Using a Fibula Flap and Dental Implants. *J Craniomaxillofac Surg* (2019) 47(5):786–91. doi: 10.1016/j.jcms.2018.12.017
9. Attia S, Diefenbach J, Schmermund D, Bottger S, Pons-Kuhnemann J, Scheibelhut C, et al. Donor-Site Morbidity After Fibula Transplantation in Head and Neck Tumor Patients: A Split-Leg Retrospective Study With Focus on Leg Stability and Quality of Life. *Cancers (Basel)* (2020) 12(8). doi: 10.3390/cancers12082217
10. Attia S, Wiltfang J, Pons-Kühnemann J, Wilbrand JF, Streckbein P, Kähling C, et al. Survival of Dental Implants Placed in Vascularised Fibula Free Flaps After Jaw Reconstruction. *J Craniomaxillofac Surg* (2018) 46(8):1205–10. doi: 10.1016/j.jcms.2018.05.008
11. Petrovic I, Baser R, Blackwell T, McCarthy C, Ganly I, Patel S, et al. Long-Term Functional and Esthetic Outcomes After Fibula Free Flap Reconstruction of the Mandible. *Head Neck* (2019) 41(7):2123–32. doi: 10.1002/hed.25666
12. Wilde F, Winter K, Kletsch K, Lorenz K, Schramm A. Mandible Reconstruction Using Patient-Specific Pre-Bent Reconstruction Plates: Comparison of Standard and Transfer Key Methods. *Int J Comput Assist Radiol Surg* (2015) 10(2):129–40. doi: 10.1007/s11548-014-1065-1
13. Wilde F, Schramm A. [Computer-Aided Reconstruction of the Facial Skeleton : Planning and Implementation in Clinical Routine]. *HNO* (2016) 64(9):641–9. doi: 10.1007/s00106-016-0220-0
14. Wilde F, Hanken H, Probst F, Schramm A, Heiland M, Cornelius CP. Multicenter Study on the Use of Patient-Specific CAD/CAM Reconstruction Plates for Mandibular Reconstruction. *Int J Comput Assist Radiol Surg* (2015) 10(12):2035–51. doi: 10.1007/s11548-015-1193-2
15. Ersoy H, Rybicki FJ. MR Angiography of the Lower Extremities. *AJR Am J Roentgenol* (2008) 190(6):1675–84. doi: 10.2214/AJR.07.2223
16. Lorbeer R, Grotz A, Dörr M, Völzke H, Lieb W, Kühn JP, et al. Reference Values of Vessel Diameters, Stenosis Prevalence, and Arterial Variations of the Lower Limb Arteries in a Male Population Sample Using Contrast-Enhanced MR Angiography. *PLoS One* (2018) 13(6):e0197559. doi: 10.1371/journal.pone.0197559
17. Schuderer JG, Meier JK, Klingelhöffer C, Gottsauner M, Reichert TE, Wendl CM, et al. Magnetic Resonance Angiography for Free Fibula Harvest: Anatomy and Perforator Mapping. *Int J Oral Maxillofac Surg* (2020) 49 (2):176–82. doi: 10.1016/j.ijom.2019.09.005
18. Rozen WM, Phillips TJ, Ashton MW, Stella DL, Gibson RN, Taylor GI. Preoperative Imaging for DIEA Perforator Flaps: A Comparative Study of Computed Tomographic Angiography and Doppler Ultrasound. *Plast Reconstr Surg* (2008) 121(1 Suppl):1–8. doi: 10.1097/01.prs.0000293874.71269.c9
19. Abdel Razek AA, Denewer AT, Hegazy MA, Hafez MT. Role of Computed Tomography Angiography in the Diagnosis of Vascular Stenosis in Head and Neck Microvascular Free Flap Reconstruction. *Int J Oral Maxillofac Surg* (2014) 43(7):811–5. doi: 10.1016/j.ijom.2014.03.014
20. Garvey PB, Chang EI, Selber JC, Skoracki RJ, Madewell JE, Liu J, et al. A Prospective Study of Preoperative Computed Tomographic Angiographic Mapping of Free Fibula Osteocutaneous Flaps for Head and Neck Reconstruction. *Plast Reconstr Surg* (2012) 130(4):541e–9e. doi: 10.1097/PRS.0b013e318262f115
21. Ribuffo D, Atzeni M, Saba L, Guerra M, Mallarini G, Proto EB, et al. Clinical Study of Peroneal Artery Perforators With Computed Tomographic Angiography: Implications for Fibular Flap Harvest. *Surg Radiol Anat* (2010) 32(4):329–34. doi: 10.1007/s00276-009-0559-y
22. Eckardt A, Swennen GR. Virtual Planning of Composite Mandibular Reconstruction With Free Fibula Bone Graft. *J Craniofac Surg* (2005) 16 (6):1137–40. doi: 10.1097/01.scs.0000186306.32042.96
23. Seruya M, Fisher M, Rodriguez ED. Computer-Assisted Versus Conventional Free Fibula Flap Technique for Craniofacial Reconstruction: An Outcomes Comparison. *Plast Reconstr Surg* (2013) 132(5):1219–28. doi: 10.1097/PRS.0b013e3182a3c0b1
24. Han HH, Kim HY, Lee JY. The Pros and Cons of Computer-Aided Surgery

for Segmental Mandibular Reconstruction After Oncological Surgery. *Arch Craniofac Surg* (2017) 18(3):149–54. doi: 10.7181/acfs.2017.18.3.149
25. Saini V, Gaba S, Sharma S, Kalra P, Sharma RK. Assessing the Role of Virtual Surgical Planning in Mandibular Reconstruction With Free Fibula Osteocutaneous Graft. *J Craniofac Surg* (2019) 30(6):e563–6. doi: 10.1097/SCS.0000000000005538
26. Tang NSJ, Ahmadi I, Ramakrishnan A. Virtual Surgical Planning in Fibula Free Flap Head and Neck Reconstruction: A Systematic Review and Meta-Analysis. *J Plast Reconstr Aesthet Surg* (2019) 72(9):1465–77. doi: 10.1016/j.bjps.2019.06.013
27. Barr ML, Barr ML, Haveles CS, Rezzadeh KS, Nolan IT, Castro R, Lee JC, et al. Virtual Surgical Planning for Mandibular Reconstruction With the Fibula Free Flap: A Systematic Review and Meta-Analysis. *Ann Plast Surg* (2020) 84(1):117–22. doi: 10.1097/SAP.0000000000002006
28. Cornelius CP, Smolka W, Giessler GA, Wilde F, Probst FA. Patient-Specific Reconstruction Plates are the Missing Link in Computer-Assisted Mandibular Reconstruction: A Showcase for Technical Description. *J Craniomaxillofac Surg* (2015) 43(5):624–9. doi: 10.1016/j.jcms.2015.02.016
29. Wilde F, Cornelius CP, Schramm A. Computer-Assisted Mandibular Reconstruction Using a Patient-Specific Reconstruction Plate Fabricated With Computer-Aided Design and Manufacturing Techniques. *Craniomaxillofac Trauma Reconstr* (2014) 7(2):158–66. doi: 10.1055/s-0034-1371356
30. Geusens J, Sun Y, Luebbers HT, Bila M, Darche V, Politis C. Accuracy of Computer-Aided Design/Computer-Aided Manufacturing-Assisted Mandibular Reconstruction With a Fibula Free Flap. *J Craniofac Surg* (2019) 30(8):2319–23. doi: 10.1097/SCS.0000000000005704
31. Kansy K, Mueller AA, Mücke T, Kopp JB, Koersgen F, Wolff KD, et al. Microsurgical Reconstruction of the Head and Neck-Current Concepts of Maxillofacial Surgery in Europe. *J Craniomaxillofac Surg* (2014) 42(8):1610–3. doi: 10.1016/j.jcms.2014.04.030
32. Shroff SS, Nair SC, Shah A, Kumar B. Versatility of Fibula Free Flap in Reconstruction of Facial Defects: A Center Study. *J Maxillofac Oral Surg* (2017) 16(1):101–7. doi: 10.1007/s12663-016-0930-6
33. Hölzle F, Kesting MR, Hölzle G, Watola A, Loeffelbein DJ, Ervens J, et al. Clinical Outcome and Patient Satisfaction After Mandibular Reconstruction With Free Fibula Flaps. *Int J Oral Maxillofac Surg* (2007) 36(9):802–6. doi: 10.1016/j.ijom.2007.04.013
34. Colletti G, Autelitano L, Rabbiosi D, Biglioli F, Chiapasco M, Mandala M, et al. Technical Refinements in Mandibular Reconstruction With Free Fibula Flaps: Outcome-Oriented Retrospective Review of 99 Cases. *Acta Otorhinolaryngol Ital* (2014) 34(5):342–8.
35. Barry CP, MacDhabheid C, Tobin K, Stassen LF, Lennon P, Toner M, et al. 'Out of House' Virtual Surgical Planning for Mandible Reconstruction After Cancer Resection: Is it Oncologically Safe? *Int J Oral Maxillofac Surg* (2020). doi: 10.1016/j.ijom.2020.11.008
36. Knitschke M, Bäcker C, Schmermund D, Böttger S, Streckbein P, Howaldt HP, et al. Impact of Planning Method (Conventional Versus Virtual) on Time to Therapy Initiation and Resection Margins: A Retrospective Analysis of 104 Immediate Jaw Reconstructions. *Cancers (Basel)* (2021) 13(12). doi: 10.3390/cancers13123013
37. Ma C, Wang L, Tian Z, Qin X, Zhu D, Qin J, et al. Standardize Routine Angiography Assessment of Leg Vasculatures Before Fibular Flap Harvest: Lessons of Congenital and Acquired Vascular Anomalies Undetected by Color Doppler and Physical Examinations. *Acta Radiol* (2021) p:284185120980001. doi: 10.1177/0284185120980001
38. Panje W, Cutting C. Trapezius Osteomyocutaneous Island Flap for Reconstruction of the Anterior Floor of the Mouth and the Mandible. *Head Neck Surg* (1980) 3(1):66–71. doi: 10.1002/hed.2890030112
39. Sparks DS, Saleh DB, Rozen WM, Hutmacher DW, Schuetz MA, Wagels M. Vascularised Bone Transfer: History, Blood Supply and Contemporary Problems. *J Plast Reconstr Aesthet Surg* (2017) 70(1):1–11. doi: 10.1016/j.bjps.2016.07.012
40. Menck J, Sander A. [Periosteal and Endosteal Blood Supply of the Human Fibula and its Clinical Importance]. *Acta Anat (Basel)* (1992) 145(4):400–5. doi: 10.1159/000147397
41. Simpson AH. The Blood Supply of the Periosteum. *J Anat* (1985) 140(Pt 4):697–704.
42. Rhinelander FW. Tibial Blood Supply in Relation to Fracture Healing. *Clin Orthop Relat Res* (1974) 105):34–81. doi: 10.1097/00003086-197411000-00005
43. Schmidt AB, Giessler GA. The Muscular and the New Osteomuscular Composite Peroneus Brevis Flap: Experiences From 109 Cases. *Plast Reconstr Surg* (2010) 126(3):924–32. doi: 10.1097/PRS.0b013e3181e3b74d
44. Kofoed H, Sjontoft E, Siemssen SO, Olesen HP. Bone Marrow Circulation After Osteotomy. Blood Flow, Po2, Pco2, and Pressure Studied in Dogs. *Acta Orthop Scand* (1985) 56(5):400–3. doi: 10.3109/17453678508994357
45. Kocabiyik N, Yalcin B, Ozan H. Variations of the Nutrient Artery of the Fibula. *Clin Anat* (2007) 20(4):440–3. doi: 10.1002/ca.20442
46. Anetai H, Kinose S, Sakamoto R, Onodera R, Kato K, Kawasaki Y, et al. Anatomic Characterization of the Tibial and Fibular Nutrient Arteries in Humans. *Anat Sci Int* (2021) 96(3):378–85. doi: 10.1007/s12565-020-00600-9
47. Zhu YL, Xu YQ, Yang J, Li J, Lan XF. An Anatomic Study of Vascularized Fibular Grafts. *Chin J Traumatol* (2008) 11(5):279–82. doi: 10.1016/S1008-1275(08)60056-5
48. Knitschke M, Baumgart AK, Bäcker C, Adelung C, Roller F, Schmermund D, et al. Computed Tomography Angiography (CTA) Before Reconstructive Jaw Surgery Using Fibula Free Flap: Retrospective Analysis of Vascular Architecture. *Diagnostics (Basel)* (2021) 11(10). doi: 10.3390/diagnostics11101865
49. Fry AM, Laugharne D, Jones K. Osteotomising the Fibular Free Flap: An Anatomical Perspective. *Br J Oral Maxillofac Surg* (2016) 54(6):692–3. doi: 10.1016/j.bjoms.2015.11.009
50. Gilbert A. Vascularised Transfer of the Fibula Shaft. *Int J Microsurg* (1979) 1:100.
51. Kim D, Orron DE, Skillman JJ. Surgical Significance of Popliteal Arterial Variants. A Unified Angiographic Classification. *Ann Surg* (1989) 210 (6):776–81. doi: 10.1097/00000658-198912000-00014
52. Knitschke M, Sonnabend S, Bäcker C, Schmermund D, Böttger S, Howaldt HP, et al. Partial and Total Flap Failure After Fibula Free Flap in Head and Neck Reconstructive Surgery: Retrospective Analysis of 180 Flaps Over 19 Years. *Cancers (Basel)* (2021) 13(4). doi: 10.3390/cancers13040865
53. Freeman GH, Halton JH. Note on an Exact Treatment of Contingency, Goodness of Fit and Other Problems of Significance. *Biometrika* (1951) 38 (1-2):141–9. doi: 10.1093/biomet/38.1-2.141
54. Wieker H, Fritz Schomaker MC, Florke C, Karayurek F, Naujokat H, Acil Y, et al. A Retrospective Analysis of the Surgical Outcomes of Different Free Vascularized Flaps Used for the Reconstruction of the Maxillofacial Region: Hand-Sewn Microvascular Anastomosis vs Anastomotic Coupler Device. *J Craniomaxillofac Surg* (2021) 49(3):191–5. doi: 10.1016/j.jcms.2020.12.015
55. Thiem DGE, Frick RW, Goetze E, Gielisch M, Al-Nawas B, Kämmerer PW. Hyperspectral Analysis for Perioperative Perfusion Monitoring-a Clinical Feasibility Study on Free and Pedicled Flaps. *Clin Oral Investig* (2021) 25 (3):933–45. doi: 10.1007/s00784-020-03382-6
56. Salgado CJ, Moran SL, Mardini S. Flap Monitoring and Patient Management. *Plast Reconstr Surg* (2009) 124(6 Suppl):e295–302. doi: 10.1097/PRS.0b013e3181bcf07b
57. Ludolph I, Lehnhardt M, Arkudas A, Kneser U, Pierer G, Harder Y, et al. [Plastic Reconstructive Microsurgery in the Elderly Patient - Consensus Statement of the German Speaking Working Group for Microsurgery of the Peripheral Nerves and Vessels]. *Handchir Mikrochir Plast Chir* (2018) 50 (2):118–25. doi: 10.1055/s-0043-115730
58. Akashi M, Nomura T, Sakakibara S, Sakakibara A, Hashikawa K. Preoperative MR Angiography for Free Fibula Osteocutaneous Flap Transfer. *Microsurgery* (2013) 33(6):454–9. doi: 10.1002/micr.22128
59. Bretzman PA, Manaster BJ, Davis WL, Coleman DA. MR Angiography for Preoperative Evaluation of Vascularized Fibular Grafts. *J Vasc Interv Radiol* (1994) 5(4):603–10. doi: 10.1016/S1051-0443(94)71561-X
60. Kelly AM, Cronin P, Hussain HK, Londy FJ, Chepeha DB, Carlos RC. Preoperative MR Angiography in Free Fibula Flap Transfer for Head and Neck Cancer: Clinical Application and Influence on Surgical Decision Making. *AJR Am J Roentgenol* (2007) 188(1):268–74. doi: 10.2214/AJR.04.1950

61. Kessler P, Wiltfang J, Schultze-Mosgau S, Lethaus B, Greess H, Neukam FW. The Role of Angiography in the Lower Extremity Using Free Vascularized Fibular Transplants for Mandibular Reconstruction. *J Craniomaxillofac Surg* (2001) 29(6):332–6. doi: 10.1054/jcms.2001.0251
62. Ling XF, Peng X. What is the Price to Pay for a Free Fibula Flap? A Systematic Review of Donor-Site Morbidity Following Free Fibula Flap Surgery. *Plast Reconstr Surg* (2012) 129(3):657–74. doi: 10.1097/PRS.0b013e3182402d9a
63. Rosson GD, Singh NK. Devascularizing Complications of Free Fibula Harvest: Peronea Arteria Magna. *J Reconstr Microsurg* (2005) 21(8):533–8. doi: 10.1055/s-2005-922432
64. Ettinger KS, Alexander AE, Arce K. Computed Tomographic Angiography Perforator Localization for Virtual Surgical Planning of Osteocutaneous Fibular Free Flaps in Head and Neck Reconstruction. *J Oral Maxillofac Surg* (2018) 76(10):2220–30. doi: 10.1016/j.joms.2018.04.002
65. Battaglia S, Maiolo V, Savastio G, Zompatori M, Contedini F, Antoniazzi E, et al. Osteomyocutaneous Fibular Flap Harvesting: Computer-Assisted Planning of Perforator Vessels Using Computed Tomographic Angiography Scan and Cutting Guide. *J Craniomaxillofac Surg* (2017) 45 (10):1681–6. doi: 10.1016/j.jcms.2017.07.017
66. Abou-Foul AK, Borumandi F. Anatomical Variants of Lower Limb Vasculature and Implications for Free Fibula Flap: Systematic Review and Critical Analysis. *Microsurgery* (2016) 36(2):165–72. doi: 10.1002/micr.30016
67. Alonso-Burgos A, Garcia-Tutor E, Bastarrika G, Cano D, Martinez-Cuesta A, Pina LJ. Preoperative Planning of Deep Inferior Epigastric Artery Perforator Flap Reconstruction With Multislice-CT Angiography: Imaging Findings and Initial Experience. *J Plast Reconstr Aesthet Surg* (2006) 59 (6):585–93. doi: 10.1016/j.bjps.2005.12.011
68. Chiu WK, Lin WC, Chen SY, Tzeng WD, Liu SC, Lee TP, et al. Computed Tomography Angiography Imaging for the Chimeric Anterolateral Thigh Flap in Reconstruction of Full Thickness Buccal Defect. *ANZ J Surg* (2011) 81(3):142–7. doi: 10.1111/j.1445-2197.2010.05483.x
69. Duymaz A, Karabekmez FE, Vrtiska TJ, Mardini S, Moran SL. Free Tissue Transfer for Lower Extremity Reconstruction: A Study of the Role of Computed Angiography in the Planning of Free Tissue Transfer in the Posttraumatic Setting. *Plast Reconstr Surg* (2009) 124(2):523–9. doi: 10.1097/PRS.0b013e3181addafa
70. Gelati C, Lozano Miralles ME, Morselli PG, Fabbri E, Cipriani R. Deep Inferior Epigastric Perforator Breast Reconstruction With Computer-Aided Design/Computer-Aided Manufacturing Sizers. *Ann Plast Surg* (2020) 84 (1):24–9. doi: 10.1097/SAP.0000000000002020
71. Higueras Sune MC, Lopez Ojeda A, Narvaez Garcia JA, De Albert De Las Vigo M, Roca Mas O, Perez Sidelnikova D, et al. Use of Angioscanning in the Surgical Planning of Perforator Flaps in the Lower Extremities. *J Plast Reconstr Aesthet Surg* (2011) 64(9):1207–13. doi: 10.1016/j.bjps.2011.03.015
72. Masia J, Clavero JA, Larranaga JR, Alomar X, Pons G, Serret P. Multidetector-Row Computed Tomography in the Planning of Abdominal Perforator Flaps. *J Plast Reconstr Aesthet Surg* (2006) 59(6):594–9. doi: 10.1016/j.bjps.2005.10.024
73. Ngaage LM, Hamed R, Oni G, Di Pace B, Ghorra DT, Koo BBC, et al. The Role of CT Angiography in Assessing Deep Inferior Epigastric Perforator Flap Patency in Patients With Pre-Existing Abdominal Scars. *J Surg Res* (2019) 235:58–65. doi: 10.1016/j.jss.2018.09.059
74. Prokop M. Multislice CT Angiography. *Eur J Radiol* (2000) 36(2):86–96. doi: 10.1016/S0720-048X(00)00271-0
75. Zhang Y, Pan X, Yang H, Yang Y, Huang H, Rui Y. Computed Tomography Angiography for the Chimeric Anterolateral Thigh Flap in the Reconstruction of the Upper Extremity. *J Reconstr Microsurg* (2017) 33 (3):211–7. doi: 10.1055/s-0036-1597587
76. Piazza C, Grammatica A, Paderno A, Taglietti V, Del Bon F, Marengoni A, et al. Microvascular Head and Neck Reconstruction in the Elderly: The University of Brescia Experience. *Head Neck* (2016) 38 Suppl 1:E1488–92. doi: 10.1002/hed.24264
77. van Gemert JTM, Abbink JH, van Es RJJ, Rosenberg A, Koole R, Van Cann EM. Early and Late Complications in the Reconstructed Mandible With Free Fibula Flaps. *J Surg Oncol* (2018) 117(4):773–80. doi: 10.1002/jso.24976
78. Lodders JN, Schulten EA, de Visscher JG, Forouzanfar T, Karagozoglu KH. Complications and Risk After Mandibular Reconstruction With Fibular Free Flaps in Patients With Oral Squamous Cell Carcinoma: A Retrospective Cohort Study. *J Reconstr Microsurg* (2016) 32(6):455–63. doi: 10.1055/s-0036-1571794
79. Abou-Foul AK, Fasanmade A, Prabhu S, Borumandi F. Anatomy of the Vasculature of the Lower Leg and Harvest of a Fibular Flap: A Systematic Review. *Br J Oral Maxillofac Surg* (2017) 55(9):904–10. doi: 10.1016/j.bjoms.2017.08.363
80. Carroll WR, Esclamado R. Preoperative Vascular Imaging for the Fibular Osteocutaneous Flap. *Arch Otolaryngol Head Neck Surg* (1996) 122(7):708–12. doi: 10.1001/archotol.1996.01890190006003
81. Seres L, Csaszar J, Borbely L, Voros E. [Donor Site Digital Subtraction Angiography Before Mandible Reconstruction With Free Fibula Transplantation]. *Fogorv Sz* (2001) 94(1):15–20.
82. Yanik B, Bulbul E, Demirpolat G. Variations of the Popliteal Artery Branching With Multidetector CT Angiography. *Surg Radiol Anat* (2015) 37(3):223–30. doi: 10.1007/s00276-014-1346-y
83. Futran ND, Stack BC Jr, Zachariah AP. Ankle-Arm Index as a Screening Examination for Fibula Free Tissue Transfer. *Ann Otol Rhinol Laryngol* (1999) 108(8):777–80. doi: 10.1177/000348949910800811
84. Astarci P, Siciliano S, Verhelst R, Lacroix V, Noirhomme P, Rubay J, et al. Intra-Operative Acute Leg Ischaemia After Free Fibula Flap Harvest for Mandible Reconstruction. *Acta Chir Belg* (2006) 106(4):423–6. doi: 10.1080/00015458.2006.11679921
85. Young DM, Trabulsy PP, Anthony JP. The Need for Preoperative Leg Angiography in Fibula Free Flaps. *J Reconstr Microsurg* (1994) 10(5):283–7; discussion 287-9. doi: 10.1055/s-2007-1006596
86. Oxford L, Ducic Y. Use of Fibula-Free Tissue Transfer With Preoperative 2-Vessel Runoff to the Lower Extremity. *Arch Facial Plast Surg* (2005) 7 (4):261–4; discussion 265. doi: 10.1001/archfaci.7.4.261
87. Lee MK, Blackwell KE, Kim B, Nabili V. Feasibility of Microvascular Head and Neck Reconstruction in the Setting of Calcified Arteriosclerosis of the Vascular Pedicle. *JAMA Facial Plast Surg* (2013) 15(2):135–40. doi: 10.1001/2013.jamafacial.208
88. Kim RY, Burkes JN, Broker HS, Williams FC. Preoperative Vascular Interventions to Improve Donor Leg Perfusion: A Report of Two Fibula Free Flaps Used in Head and Neck Reconstruction. *J Oral Maxillofac Surg* (2019) 77(3):658–63. doi: 10.1016/j.joms.2018.10.017
89. Lorenz RR, Esclamado R. Preoperative Magnetic Resonance Angiography in Fibular-Free Flap Reconstruction of Head and Neck Defects. *Head Neck* (2001) 23(10):844–50. doi: 10.1002/hed.1123
90. Bui DT, Cordeiro PG, Hu QY, Disa JJ, Pusic A, Mehrara BJ. Free Flap Reexploration: Indications, Treatment, and Outcomes in 1193 Free Flaps. *Plast Reconstr Surg* (2007) 119(7):2092–100. doi: 10.1097/01.prs.0000260598.24376.e1
91. Wood NB, Zhao SZ, Zambanini A, Jackson M, Gedroyc W, Thom SA, et al. Curvature and Tortuosity of the Superficial Femoral Artery: A Possible Risk Factor for Peripheral Arterial Disease2006. *J Appl Physiol (1985)* (2006) 101 (5):1412–8. doi: 10.1152/japplphysiol.00051.2006
92. Jones NF, Monstrey S, Gambier BA. Reliability of the Fibular Osteocutaneous Flap for Mandibular Reconstruction: Anatomical and Surgical Confirmation. *Plast Reconstr Surg* (1996) 97(4):707–16; discussion 717-8. doi: 10.1097/00006534-199604000-00003
93. Bähr W. Blood Supply of Small Fibula Segments: An Experimental Study on Human Cadavers. *J Craniomaxillofac Surg* (1998) 26(3):148–52. doi: 10.1016/S1010-5182(98)80004-8
94. Fichter AM, Ritschl LM, Georg R, Kolk A, Kesting MR, Wolff KD, et al. Effect of Segment Length and Number of Osteotomy Sites on Cancellous Bone Perfusion in Free Fibula Flaps. *J Reconstr Microsurg* (2018).
95. Chang EI, Chu CK, Chang EI. Advancements in Imaging Technology for Microvascular Free Tissue Transfer. *J Surg Oncol* (2018) 118(5):729–35. doi: 10.1002/jso.25194
96. Momoh AO, Yu P, Skoracki RJ, Liu S, Feng L, Hanasono MM. A Prospective Cohort Study of Fibula Free Flap Donor-Site Morbidity in 157 Consecutive Patients. *Plast Reconstr Surg* (2011) 128(3):714–20. doi: 10.1097/PRS.0b013e318221dc2a
97. Shindo M, Fong BP, Funk GF, Karnell LH. The Fibula Osteocutaneous Flap in Head and Neck Reconstruction: A Critical Evaluation of Donor Site Morbidity. *Arch Otolaryngol Head Neck Surg* (2000) 126(12):1467–72. doi: 10.1001/archotol.126.12.1467
98. Fang H, Liu F, Sun C, Pang P. Impact of Wound Closure on Fibular Donor-Site Morbidity: A Meta-Analysis. *BMC Surg* (2019) 19(1):81. doi: 10.1186/s12893-019-0545-1
99. Fry AM, Patterson A, Orr RL, Colver GB. Open Wound Healing of the

Osseocutaneous Fibula Flap Donor Site. *Br J Oral Maxillofac Surg* (2014) 52 (9):861–3. doi: 10.1016/j.bjoms.2014.05.003

100. Bach CA, Guillere L, Yildiz S, Wagner I, Darmon S, Chabolle F. Comparison of Negative Pressure Wound Therapy and Conventional Dressing Methods for Fibula Free Flap Donor Site Management in Patients With Head and Neck Cancer. *Head Neck* (2016) 38(5):696–9. doi: 10.1002/hed.23952

101. Yu P, Youssef A. Efficacy of the Handheld Doppler in Preoperative Identification of the Cutaneous Perforators in the Anterolateral Thigh Flap. *Plast Reconstr Surg* (2006) 118(4):928–33. doi: 10.1097/01.prs.0000232216.34854.63

102. Islam S, Ansari U, Walton GM. Role of Real-Time Colour-Flow Doppler in Perforator Free Flap Head and Neck Reconstruction. *Br J Oral Maxillofac Surg* (2021) 59(1):111–3. doi: 10.1016/j.bjoms.2020.08.008

16

Deviation Analyses of Computer-Assisted, Template-Guided Mandibular Reconstruction with Combined Osteotomy and Reconstruction Pre-Shaped Plate Position Technology

*Jie Chen[1,2,3], Ruipu Zhang[1,2,3], Ye Liang[1,2,3], Yujie Ma[1,2,3], Saiwen Song[1,2,3] and Canhua Jiang[1,2,3]**

[1] Department of Oral and Maxillofacial Surgery, Center of Stomatology, Xiangya Hospital, Central South University, Changsha, China, [2] Research Center of Oral and Maxillofacial Tumor, Xiangya Hospital, Central South University, Changsha, China, [3] Institute of Oral Cancer and Precancerous Lesions, Central South University, Changsha, China

***Correspondence:**
Canhua Jiang
canhuaj@csu.edu.cn

Background: Computer-assisted and template-guided mandibular reconstruction provides higher accuracy and less variation than conventional freehand surgeries. The combined osteotomy and reconstruction pre-shaped plate position (CORPPP) technique is a reliable choice for mandibular reconstruction. This study aimed to evaluate the accuracy of CORPPP-guided fibular flap mandibular reconstruction and analyze the possible causes of the deviations.

Patients and Methods: From June 2015 to December 2016, 28 patients underwent fibular flap mandibular reconstruction. Virtual planning and personalized CORPPP-guided templates were applied in 15 patients while 13 patients received conventional freehand surgeries. Deviations during mandibulectomy and fibular osteotomy, and overall and triaxial deviation of the corresponding mandibular anatomical landmarks were measured by superimposing the pre- and postoperative virtual models.

Results: The deviation of the resection line and resection angle was 1.23 ± 0.98 mm and 4.11° ± 2.60°. The actual length of fibula segments was longer than the designed length in 7 cases (mean: 0.35 ± 0.32 mm) and shorter in 22 cases (mean: 1.53 ± 1.19 mm). In patients without ramus reconstruction, deviations of the ipsilateral condylar head point (Co.), gonion point (Go.), and coracoid process point (Cor.) were 6.71 ± 3.42 mm, 5.38 ± 1.71 mm, and 11.05 ± 3.24 mm in the freehand group and 1.73 ± 1.13 mm, 1.86 ± 0.96 mm, and 2.54 ± 0.50 mm in the CORPPP group, respectively, with significant statistical differences ($p < 0.05$). In patients with ramus reconstruction, deviations of ipsilateral Co. and Go. were 9.79 ± 4.74 mm *vs*. 3.57 ± 1.62 mm ($p < 0.05$), and 15.17 ± 6.53 mm *vs*. 4.36 ± 1.68 mm ($p < 0.05$) in the freehand group and CORPPP group, respectively.

Conclusion: Mandibular reconstructions employing virtual planning and personalized CORPPP-guided templates show significantly higher predictability, convenience, and accuracy of mandibular reconstruction compared with conventional freehand surgeries. However, more clinical cases were required for further dimensional deviation analysis. The application and exploration of clinical practice would also continuously improve the design of templates.

Keywords: mandibular reconstruction, virtual surgical planning, template-guided surgery, 3D printing, deviation analyses

1 INTRODUCTION

Mandibular defects can be caused by radical surgery of oral and maxillofacial tumors, osteomyelitis, or trauma of the jaw, and can lead to severe functional and aesthetic deficits, negatively affecting quality of life. Vascularized autologous bone grafting, especially the fibular free flap, serves as the workhorse for segmental mandibular defect reconstruction (1–4). Successful reconstruction includes restoration of symmetrical appearance, sufficient chewing space, and correct joint position, signifying its great demand for accurate position of both the fibula and the remaining mandible (5, 6). However, due to the interruption of the mandibular continuity, even a small displacement may cause the entire jaw to be deflected.

With the aid of computer-assisted surgery (CAS) and three-dimensional (3D) printing technology, template-guided surgeries are gaining increasing popularity (7). Personalized guiding templates can be fabricated, and the titanium plates can be pre-shaped in advance to shorten the operation duration. Template-guided mandibular reconstruction provides higher accuracy, acceptability, and less variation than the conventional free-hand surgeries (8–12).

The combined osteotomy and reconstruction pre-shaped plate position (CORPPP) technique, as previously described, is a reliable choice for mandibular reconstruction (13). In this study, we evaluated the accuracy of CORPPP-guided mandibular reconstruction with fibula free flaps and analyzed the possible causes of the deviations. Furthermore, we applied coordinate conversion to analyze the deviations between the designed model and the actual model in triaxial directions. Results were analyzed to provide suggestions for further accuracy improvement of mandibular reconstruction.

2 PATIENTS AND METHODS

2.1 Clinical Characteristics of Patients

This study was approved by the Center of Medical Ethics of Central South University (Changsha, China; serial number 201512515). Written informed consents were obtained from the patients in accordance with the Declaration of Helsinki. All methods were performed in accordance with the relevant guidelines and regulations approved by the institutional review board of the Center of Medical Ethics of Central South University.

From June 2015 to December 2016, 28 patients were recruited in this study and underwent segmental mandibulectomy. Clinical characteristics of all the patients are presented in **Table 1**. Reconstruction with fibula free flaps were conducted either by the conventional freehand procedure (freehand group, 15 patients) or the CORPPP-guided surgical templates (CORPPP group, 13 patients) based on their personal preference. The mandible defects after surgical resection were classified by the Urken's CRBS (Condyle, Ramus, Body, Symphysis) classification criteria (14).

2.2 Surgical Simulation and Design of the CORPPP Guiding Template

Preoperative virtual surgical simulation and design of the CORPPP guiding template were conducted as previously described (13). First, imaging data were obtained from the patients' maxillofacial region by large-field cone-beam computed tomography (CBCT; 0.25-mm slice interval; Imaging Sciences International 17-19 System, KaVo, USA) at intercuspal position, and from the fibular donor sites by Spiral CT (0.5-mm slice interval; SOMATOM Definition AS, SIEMENS, Germany). Then imaging data were loaded into the E3D CMF software (Digital Medicine and Virtual Reality Research Center, Central South University, China) for surgical simulations. Based on the mandibular lesion, the resection range was determined (**Figure 1A**), and simulated fibula segments were arranged into mandibular defects to fit the curved contour of the mandible (**Figure 1B**), generating the expected reconstructed mandibular model (**Figure 1C**). The fibular osteotomy was designed accordingly with consideration of proper length of the distal end of the fibula as well as the peroneal artery (**Figures 2A, B**).

The titanium template was shaped and fixed to the ideal position with plastic ligatures on a 3D printout of the expected reconstructed mandibular model, and proper fixing holes were chosen from the titanium template. Then, the model was scanned again together with the titanium template by CBCT to generate the composite model. By overlapping the composite model and the expected model in the software, location of the

TABLE 1 | Clinical characteristics of the patients.

	Freehand group	CORPPP group
Number of cases	15	13
Gender		
Male	10	8
Female	5	5
Age		
Range	29–67	21–64
Mean ± SD	43.4 ± 13.1	38.9 ± 14.4
Mandibular lesions	Ameloblastoma/9 Ossifying fibroma/1 Oral malignancies/5	Ameloblastoma/9 Gingival cancer/1 Osteoradionecrosis/1 Other benign tumors/2
Whether the ramus was reconstructed		
Yes	8	7
No	7	6
Number of cases by Urken's classification		
BR	7	6
S^HBR	1	1
B	2	1
S^HB	4	3
BS	1	1
BSB	0	1
Number of fibula segments		
1	2	1
2	12	9
3	1	2
4	0	1

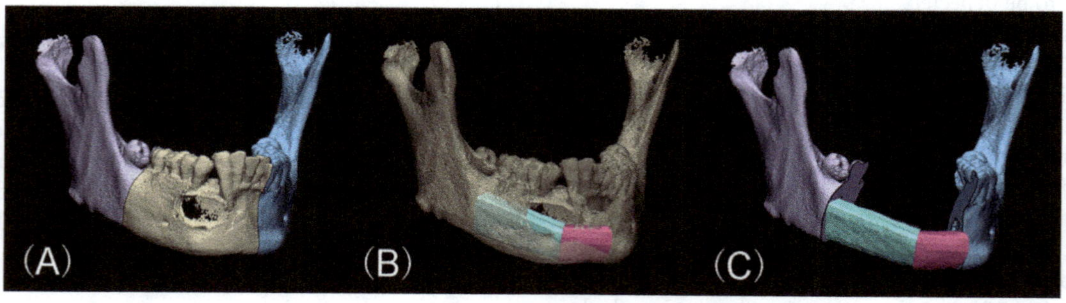

FIGURE 1 | Virtual surgery simulation of mandibular lesion resection and fibular reconstruction. **(A)** Determination of the range of the mandibulectomy. **(B)** Arrangement of the fibula segments into the defect region according to the contour of the original mandible. **(C)** Expected virtual mandibular model after fibular reconstruction.

fixing holes can simply be transferred onto both the remaining mandible as well as each fibula segment in expected model. Resection guiding templates (**Figures 3A–C**) and fibular osteotomy templates (**Figures 3D, E**) were then designed to include the designed fixing holes, and the guide wings (or grooves) of the templates were consistent with the expected osteotomy template. In this way, the fixing holes were unified, which play the dual role of fixing the guiding template to the bone surface and determine the position for the subsequent fixation of the titanium template.

All the designed guiding templates are stored in Stereolithography (STL) documents and the 3D printout templates and models were fabricated using polymer nylon materials by Hunan Huaxiang Incremental Manufacturing Co. Ltd (**Figure 4**). The templates and the pre-shaped titanium template were then sterilized and prepared for further use.

2.3 Surgical Procedures and Postoperative Data Collection

The mandibular reconstruction with fibular flaps were conducted as previously described (6, 13). For the patients in the CORPPP-guided group, segmental mandibulectomy was performed with the assistance of the resection guiding template (**Figures 5A, B**). Through the fixing holes, the mandible was drilled, and the fixing holes were used for fixation of the titanium plate to restore the correct occlusal relation and the position of the

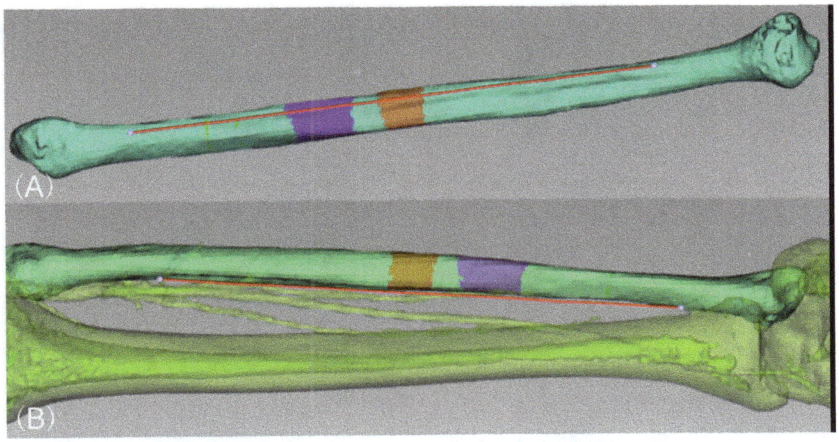

FIGURE 2 | Virtual surgery simulation of designing the location fibular flap osteotomy. **(A)** Determination of proper osteotomy location and arrangement of all segments on the virtual fibula model (purple and orange). **(B)** The fibular flap was designed in consideration of preserving proper length at the distal end of the fibula as well as the location of proximal end of the peroneal artery.

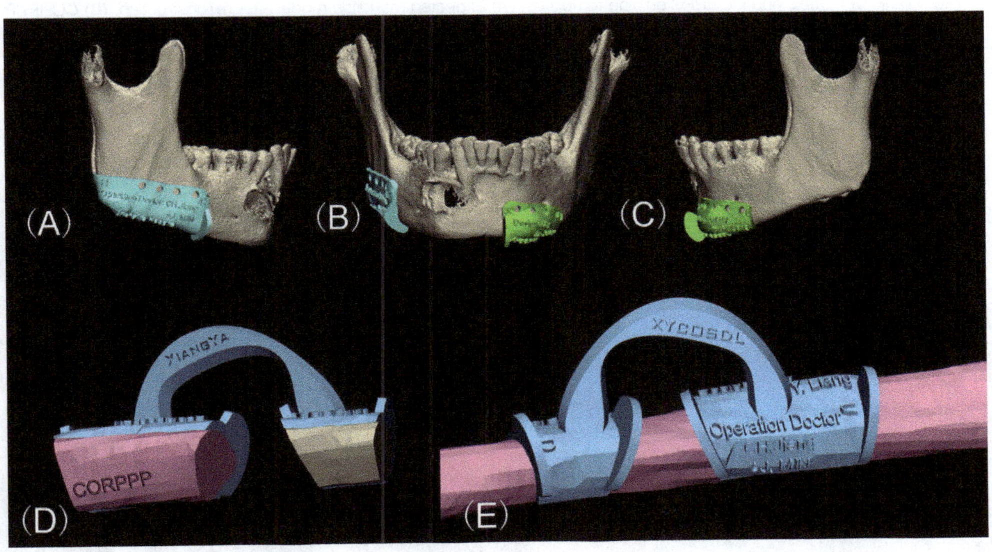

FIGURE 3 | Virtual design of the CORPPP guiding template. **(A–C)** Lateral and frontal view of placement of CORPPP mandibulectomy guiding templates with guiding wings and designed fixing holes. **(D, E)** Medial and external view of the placement of CORPPP fibular osteotomy templates.

condyles (**Figure 5C**). At the same time, fibular flaps were harvested with the osteotomy template (**Figure 5D**). With the assistance of the positioning templates, the fibula segments were arranged and fixed as designed (**Figure 5E**). For patients in the freehand group, conventional procedures were performed without guiding templates. Vascular anastomosis was then processed, and the skin paddle was used to repair the defect as well as monitoring the circulation of the flap if needed (**Figure 5F**).

All patients received conventional free flap post-operative care and medication. During the routine follow-up visit at the 6th month after operation, CBCT scan was performed to obtain the post-operative data for deviation evaluation.

2.4 Virtual Model Superimposing and Deviation Evaluation

Post-operative image data were used to reconstruct the actual 3D model in the software. Superimposing of the actual model and the expected model was conducted using the model superimpose tracing function in 3D analysis module of the InVivoDental software (Version 5.2.4, Anatomage, USA).

2.4.1 Deviation Measurement in CORPPP-Guided Mandibular Lesion Resection

To measure the deviation during mandibulectomy, both (1) the deviation of osteotomy angle and (2) the deviation of lesion

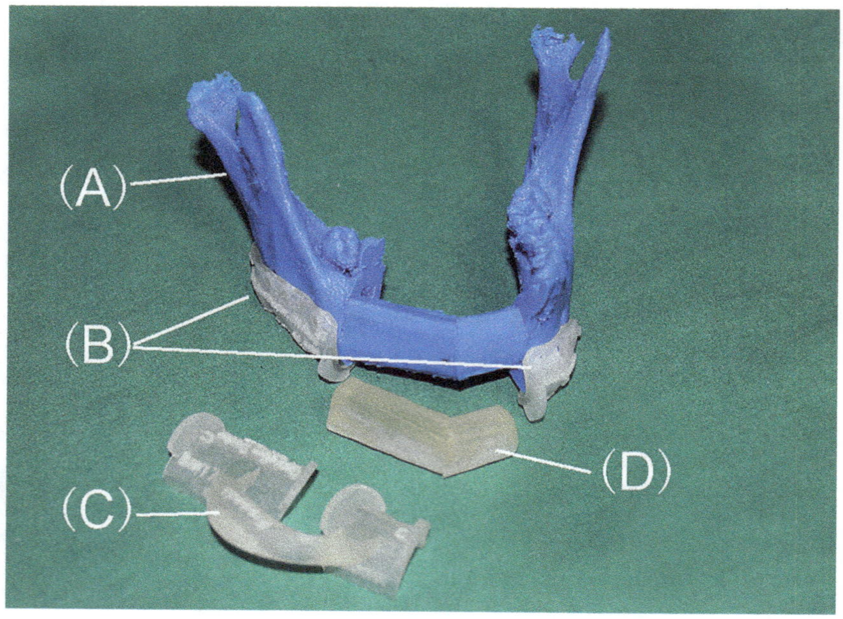

FIGURE 4 | 3D printout templates of models and CORPPP guiding templates. **(A)** Expected mandible model after reconstruction. **(B)** CORPPP mandibulectomy guiding templates with fixing holes. **(C)** CORPPP fibular osteotomy template. **(D)** CORPPP positioning template.

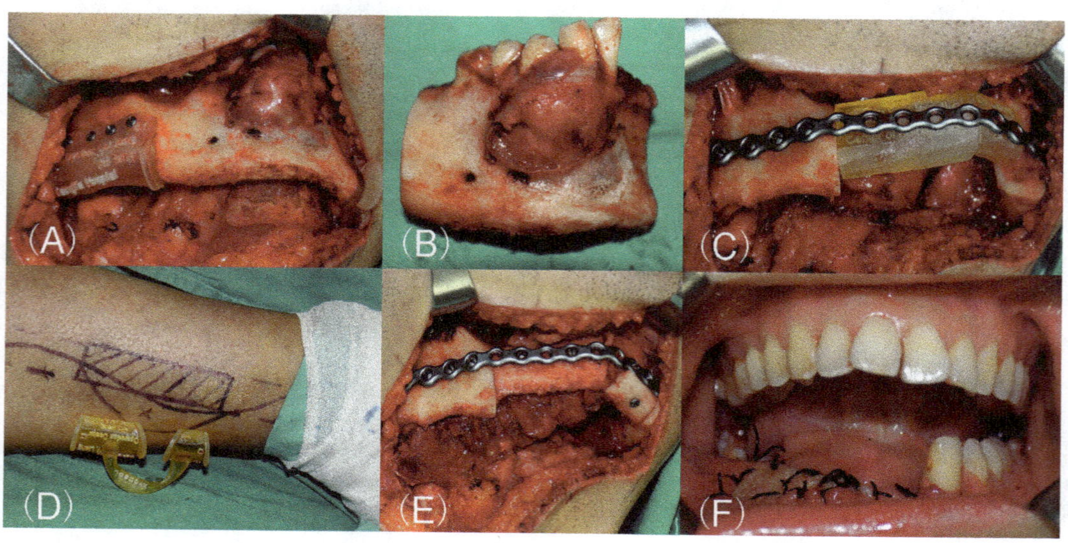

FIGURE 5 | Surgical procedure of CORPPP-guided mandibular reconstruction. **(A)** Placement of the resection guiding templates with the designed fixing holes and screws. **(B)** Mandibular lesion specimen after segmental resection. **(C)** Placement of the pre-shaped titanium plate with the designed fixing holes. **(D)** Design of the fibular flap. **(E)** Fixation of fibula segments into the defect.

resection line were measured. Three points were selected on the expected mandibular model in the software to form the designed osteotomy plane, and the actual osteotomy plane was formed on the post-operative model with the same method. The acute angle formed by the two planes was defined as the resection angle deviation. The inferior mandibular margin points were marked in both the actual model and the expected model, and the distance between them was defined as the deviation of the lesion resection line.

2.4.2 Deviation Measurement in CORPPP-Guided Fibular Osteotomy

The length of all fibula segments was measured in both the expected mandibular model and the actual model in CORPPP-guided patients. The absolute value of the actual length minus the designed length was recorded as the deviations in CORPPP-guided fibular osteotomy.

2.4.3 Overall Deviation Measurement of the Mandibular Anatomical Landmarks

Patients were divided into two groups based on whether the ramus was reconstructed. To evaluate the displacement and rotation of the remaining mandible, the maxillary was used for superimposing the pre- and postoperative virtual models. Mandibular anatomical landmarks including the condylar head point (Co.), gonion point (Go.), and coracoid process point (Cor.) on the ipsilateral side were chosen for measurement. Those points were marked on both the postoperative actual model and the preoperative expected model, and the distance was recorded as the overall deviation.

2.4.4 Establishment of Coordinate System and Triaxial Deviation Measurement of the Mandibular Anatomical Landmarks

We applied coordinate conversion to analyze the deviations between the designed model and the actual model in triaxial directions. A coordinate system was established as follows. Plane A, an imaginary plane that was parallel to the Frankfort plane, was established at the level of the mandibular incisal notch. The midpoint of the line segment connecting the central fossa points of the bilateral mandibular first molars was projected to Plane A, forming the origin of the coordinate axis. In the first molar missing situation, the bilateral central fossa points were substituted in the order of bilateral outermost points of the condyle, bilateral points of the mandibular angle, or bilateral points of the sigmoid notch. The x-axis was defined as the horizontal axis passing through the origin and Plane A, and the positive direction was defined from the contralateral side to the ipsilateral side, and from right to left in patients with bilateral lesions by default. The y-axis was formed by connecting the origin and the aforementioned midpoint, and the positive direction was defined posteriorly. The z-axis was formed vertical to Plane A, defining the positive direction superiorly.

We further analyzed the overall deviations of each mandibular anatomical landmarks in three-dimensional directions. Matrix Laboratory (R2014B version, MathWorks, USA) was used to complete the coordinate conversion of the landmarks from the actual model and the expected model into the same coordinate system. Vectors of each point (from the actual model towards the expected model) were calculated respectively, generating the triaxial deviation, and the signs (positive or negative) of the coordinates represent the direction.

2.5 Statistical Analyses

Deviations were measured and presented as mean ± SD. Homogeneity of variance was evaluated by Levene Variance Equality Test first, and t test or Mann–Whitney test was performed accordingly. Statistical significance was reached for $p < 0.05$. All statistical analyses were performed using SPSS Version 19.0.

3 RESULTS

All patients in both the CORPPP group and the freehand group underwent successful mandibular reconstruction. All flaps survived and postoperative recovery was uneventful. The design and preparation of the CORPPP guiding templates for all 13 cases were successful. In the CORPPP group, the lesions were resected in accordance with the preoperative designs, the pre-shaped titanium plates and titanium screws were placed smoothly, and the occlusal relation was well recovered. All patients came for follow-up visits as expected.

Deviations were inevitable despite the assistance of the guiding templates. The deviation of the resection line was 1.23 ± 0.98 mm with a maximum of 2.54 mm, while the deviation of the mandibular resection angle was 4.11° ± 2.60° and the maximum was 9.53°. The actual length of fibula segments was longer than the designed length in 7 cases (mean: 0.35 ± 0.32 mm, maximum: 1.12 mm), and shorter in 22 cases (mean: 1.53 ± 1.19 mm, maximum: 4.61 mm).

The overall deviation of the mandibular anatomical landmarks in cases without ramus reconstruction was measured and presented in **Table 2**. The deviations of all anatomical landmarks (Co., Go., and Cor.) in the CORPPP group (1.73 ± 1.13 mm, 1.86 ± 0.96 mm, and 2.54 ± 0.50 mm, respectively) were significantly smaller than that in the freehand group (6.71 ± 3.42 mm, 5.38 ± 1.71 mm, and 11.05 ± 3.24 mm, respectively). Similarly, the overall deviations of Co. and Go. in cases with ramus reconstruction were also compared. In the CORPPP group, among seven cases, the deviation of Co. was 3.57 ± 1.62 mm, and the deviation of Go. was 4.36 ± 1.68 mm. In the freehand group, the deviation of condylar head was 9.79 ± 4.74 mm, and the deviation of gonion was 15.17 ± 6.53 mm in eight cases (**Table 3**).

The triaxial deviations of all mandibular anatomical landmarks of the ipsilateral side of the mandible in the CORPPP-guided patients were measured. Patients without ramus reconstruction (**Table 4**) and with ramus reconstruction (**Table 5**) were calculated separately. However, statistical analysis could not perform due to the limited case numbers.

TABLE 2 | Deviation comparison between CORPPP group and freehand group in patients without ramus reconstruction.

Group	Number of cases	Deviation of Co. (mm)	Deviation of Go. (mm)	Deviation of Cor. (mm)
Freehand	7	6.71 ± 3.42	5.38 ± 1.71	11.05 ± 3.24
CORPPP	6	1.73 ± 1.13*	1.86 ± 0.96*	2.54 ± 0.50*

*$p < 0.05$.

TABLE 3 | Deviation comparison between CORPPP group and freehand group in patients with ramus reconstruction.

Group	Number of cases	Deviation of Co. (mm)	Deviation of Go. (mm)
Freehand	8	9.79 ± 4.74	15.17 ± 6.53
CORPPP	7	3.57 ± 1.62*	4.36 ± 1.68*

*$p < 0.05$.

4 DISCUSSION

4.1 Advantages and Limitations of the Template-Guided Mandibular Reconstruction

Digital surgical technology has yielded excellent clinical results in personalized functional mandibular reconstruction. Although surgical navigation is currently considered one of the best solutions for real-time confirmation in mandibular reconstruction, it can hardly be widely promoted due to the expensive equipment and time-consuming matching procedure (15).

Virtual surgery allows simulation of all the critical steps before the actual operation, including determination of the range for lesion resection, design of the fibula osteotomy, and the positioning and contouring of the fibular segments. By combining with the 3D printing technology, models and surgical guiding templates are designed and fabricated. In addition, it facilitates young surgeon training, and enhances the predictability and streamlining of surgery (7, 16, 17).

CORPPP technique, as previously designed and applied by our group, were specially designed for better positioning of the titanium plate and the seating of the bone grafts (13). The titanium plates were pre-shaped according to the 3D-printed mandible model preoperatively. Templates referring to each specific step are "printed-out" in advance, and the operation was processed step by step under the guidance. This advantage was also shared by other similar 3D-printed patient-specific surgeries. Gupta et al. reported that the total operation time was significantly reduced by nearly 1/3 in 3D-guided surgeries, which was 83.9 min in the 3D group and 124 min in the freehand group (18). Another study reported by Weitz et al. showed that the operations were 34 min shorter in virtually planned cases with optimizing accuracy (19). With the help of the models and templates, the intraoperative time was significantly reduced, improving the efficiency of the surgery and contributing to rapid recovery of patients.

The cost of the guiding template was mainly dependent on the type and the dosage of the material for 3D printing. Compared to other 3D-printed guiding templates, CORPPP neither changed the type nor increased the dosage of the material, and the manufacturing cost was generally the same as other guiding templates. In addition, the special fixing holes of CORPPP were designed to stabilize the guiding template to the bone surface as well as determine the position for the subsequent fixation of the titanium template. This special design can also be applied in combination with other similar 3D-printed guiding templates to reduce the skewing of the titanium plates, improve accuracy, and facilitate the reconstruction process. However, even under the guidance of the CORPPP guiding template, there were still inevitable deviations when each step was performed.

4.2 Deviation Analyses in CORPPP-Guided Mandibular Lesion Resection

By comparing the postoperative measurement with the preoperative virtual design, the average deviation of mandibulectomy line was 1.23 ± 0.98 mm, and the average

TABLE 4 | Triaxial deviation of mandibular anatomical landmarks in CORPPP-guided patients without ramus reconstruction.

Landmark	Triaxial deviation	Positive direction (mm)	Number of cases	Negative direction (mm)	Number of cases
Co.	*x*	0.76 ± 0.57	5	−0.35	1
	y	1.39 ± 1.47	4	−1.28 ± 1.50	2
	z	0.20 ± 0.18	4	−0.19 ± 0.11	2
Go.	*x*	0.77 ± 0.53	5	−0.18	1
	y	0.11 ± 0.14	2	−0.91 ± 1.04	4
	z	0.59 ± 0.49	5	−0.16	1
Cor.	*x*	1.67 ± 1.21	6	/	0
	y	0.86 ± 0.45	6	/	0
	z	1.27 ± 0.99	5	−0.52	1

TABLE 5 | Triaxial deviation of mandibular anatomical landmarks in CORPPP-guided patients with ramus reconstruction.

Landmark	Triaxial deviation	Positive direction (mm)	Number of cases	Negative direction (mm)	Number of cases
Co.	*x*	1.72 ± 1.48	4	2.26 ± 2.15	3
	y	0.83 ± 0.63	4	1.21 ± 0.94	3
	z	1.11 ± 0.55	4	3.17 ± 3.00	3
Go.	*x*	2.78 ± 1.47	3	2.27 ± 2.14	4
	y	1.77 ± 0.95	3	1.30 ± 1.22	4
	z	2.60 ± 0.50	4	−0.69 ± 0.49	3

deviation of osteotomy angle was 4.11° ± 2.60°. We believed that these deviations were produced by a tiny shift of the templates and the saw blades. The setting of the resection guiding template was designed by matching its inner surface with the specific structures on the external surface of the mandible. However, the chosen surface structures on the mandible were not so prominent that a tiny slippage of the template happens during positioning, which would lead to deviation of the mandibulectomy line. The simple solution was to increase the contact area between the template and the mandible surface, but expansion of the template would increase the stripping range of the remaining healthy mandible, resulting in loss of muscle attachment and periosteal blood supply, which might aggravate the mandibular ischemia, especially in patients with osteoradionecrosis.

As for the deviation of mandibulectomy angle, when performing mandibular resection, it was important to ensure that the saw blade travels along the guiding wings of the template to ensure accurate angulation of the osteotomy plane. However, during actual operation, the saw blade might tilt away from the wings when working in the blind field of the vision such as the lingual side of the mandible, thus causing a certain rotation of the mandibular osteotomy plane. Increased restriction and directional guidance of the saw blade path to ensure that the blade did not drift during osteotomy would reduce the deviation.

Integrating the above solutions, another template with guiding wing was added on the lesion side of the mandible, covering the mandibular lesion, and changing the design of the unilateral guiding wing to a guiding groove (17, 20). The contact area between the template and the mandible surface was greatly increased without extra stripping of the muscle attachment and periosteum. At the same time, the slot generated a stronger guiding effect on the saw blade, which effectively reduced the osteotomy angle deviation. Therefore, in our later recruited CORPPP cases, guiding grooves were used instead of wings, as shown in **Supplementary Figure 1**.

4.3 Deviation Analyses in CORPPP-Guided Fibular Osteotomy

In total, 28 fibular segments were measured, and the average length deviation was only 1.24 ± 1.17 mm, confirming the reliability and repeatability of CORPPP techniques. Interestingly, we found that most (22/28, 78.6%) of the fibular segments were shorter than the original design. The main reason was considered to be the excessive trimming during the fibula positioning. Similar to the mandibular resection step, deviations happened during fibular osteotomy, resulting in increased fibular length.

However, the positioning templates and the pre-shaped titanium plate were made strictly according to the design. Thus, the extra intercepted part of the fibula formed early contact points, resulting in changes in the overall length and the angles of the fibular segments, and the fixing holes on the fibula could not be matched with the corresponding holes on the pre-shaped titanium plate, so repeated trimming and grinding was frequently required. The fibula was stiff in texture and hard for trimming after osteotomizing into small segments. Ultimately, the grafted fibula segment would be shorter than designed. That was also the reason for the gaps between fibular segments found on review of the postoperative CBCT images.

4.4 Overall and Triaxial Deviation Analyses of Mandibular Anatomical Landmarks in CORPPP-Guided Mandibular Reconstruction

Conventional absolute deviations were measured by superimposing the reconstructed mandibles onto the preoperative virtual models based on the healthy side of the mandible. However, in the physiological state, the reconstructed mandible was distracted by muscles and adapted to occlusion, leading to physiological deviations on both the lesion side and the healthy side. Yang et al. discussed the novel algorithm for physiological deviation assessment. In the 3D-printed plate group, greater impact of temporomandibular joint (TMJ) deviations were found on the lesion side than the healthy side. Moreover, patients without preservation of both the condyle and ramus had significantly higher deviations of the condyle and joint space (21). This result was consistent with our study. We evaluated the physiological deviation on the ipsilateral side, and the CORPPP group showed significantly lower deviations of the mandibular anatomical landmarks on the ipsilateral side than the freehand group, suggesting that CORPPP technique improved the physiological position of reconstructed mandible.

The recruited 13 patients were divided into two groups according to whether the ramus was restored. There were two main reasons for grouping. Firstly, for measurement reason, due to the great difference in shape between mandible and fibula, anatomical landmarks on the residual mandible should be priorly selected for measurement to reduce the selection error, so the presence or absence of the ramus on ipsilateral side might affect the deviation (22, 23). Secondly, the deviations of the reconstructed mandible were assumed to be affected by the resection range, especially the posterior part of the mandible (24). The anatomical anchor of the fossa-condyle structure and the intact joint capsule stabilized the TMJ, and the masticatory muscles were mainly attached to the posterior mandible (21). Therefore, when the ramus was involved in the defect, the stability from the TMJ and the muscles greatly decreased, and reconstruction procedures became more complex at the same time, leading to increasing deviation.

It was generally accepted that the overall deviation was directly related to the final reconstruction outcome. Our result showed that among all the patients, no matter with or without ramus reconstruction, there were significantly smaller overall deviations of Co., Go., and Cor. in the CORPPP-guided group than the conventional free-hand group. Several studies have also reported less overall deviation of length and angles in the computer-aided group *versus* the conventional freehand group, when superimposing the virtual planning on post-operative mandible. Foley et al. reported the average deviation for free fibula flap 0.9 mm in the A–P dimension, 2.7 mm from condyle to condyle, and 2.5 mm from gonial angle to gonial angle in the transverse dimension (25). In a retropective study conducted by Zhang et al., the deviation in fibula segment length was 1.34 ± 1.09 mm, the angular deviation was 2.29° ± 1.19°, and the mean 3-D deviation was

0.53 ± 0.06 mm in the computer-aided group, indicating high accuracy in templated guided fibular flap mandibular reconstruction (26). Those findings were consistent and comparable with our results. As for esthetic evaluation, Bartier et al., in a CT symmetry study of 25 patients in the 3D group and 8 in the freehand group, found that deviations in the 3D group of the coronal mandibular angle, mandibular body height, and ramus length on the affected side were significantly lower, and the sagittal mandibular angle symmetry was better, indicating that 3D-guided mandibular reconstruction with fibula free flaps helped to restore a greater symmetry and improved esthetic outcome (27).

To find other potential causes for the offset of CORPPP-guided mandibular reconstruction, we further analyze the deviations of each mandibular anatomical landmarks in three-dimensional directions. Our results revealed that in almost all the CORPPP-guided cases with preserved ramus, deviations of the Cor. happened towards the medial, superior, and posterior directions, with the most pronounced displacement in the medial direction, averaging 1.26 mm. Unfortunately, the results of Co. and Go. could not be statistically analyzed due to the limited cases.

The reasons for the deviation of Cor. in CORPPP-guided cases were considered as follows. Firstly, intraoperative stripping of the muscles attached to the surface of the mandible affected the force balance of masticatory muscle groups. Therefore, under the traction of the temporalis muscle, posterior–superior displacement of the coracoid process happened. Secondly, after detailed observation of the overlapping images in the InVivoDental software, it was found that the inward migration was not only present at the coracoid process, but the entire anterior edge of the ramus had the tendency to rotate inward in some cases. The inward rotation also led to an inadequate fit of the ramus to the titanium plate, indicating that the ramus was not sufficiently stable during fixation.

The commercialized mandibular reconstruction plate that is commonly used consisted of two parts: the horizontal part and the ascending part, which were connected by an arched turn of nearly 130°. Usually, the screws on the ascending part were arranged in a linear pattern after ramus fixation, which was not stable enough. In addition, the pre-shaped titanium plate did not fit perfectly to the surface of the mandible, so rotation might occur during fixation. Since the rotation towards the lateral side was blocked by the titanium plate, the anterior edge of the ramus could only rotate towards internally.

Therefore, when designing the fixation position of the titanium plate, we should consider appropriate posterior displacement and try to use a few nail holes on the horizontal part of the titanium plate to increase the stability of ramus fixation. It was also possible to increase the fitting of the titanium plate to the surface of the mandible and to reduce the forces exerted on the mandible by the titanium plate and screws in additional directions during fixation.

With further advances in 3D printing technology, personalized mandibular titanium plates can also be printed for better fitting, higher reconstruction accuracy (28). Based on preoperative CT-scan data, personalized titanium plate can be precisely preformed. Even for patients who underwent double-barrel fibular flap reconstruction, a special "one-piece" reconstruction plate has been reported to fix both barrels simultaneously, achieving satisfactory outcomes (29). After being sterilized, those personalized plates can be used directly without the need for bending. Moreover, it provides stronger guiding for the alignment and fixation of bone segments that may help reduce the deviations.

This study suggested that the CORPPP technique significantly improved the predictability, convenience, and accuracy of mandibular reconstruction. However, more clinical cases were required for further dimensional deviation analysis. The application and exploration of clinical practice would also continuously improve the design of templates.

AUTHOR CONTRIBUTIONS

JC: Writing—original draft preparation, writing—review and editing. RZ: Data curation, formal analysis, resources, and software. YL: Conceptualization, visualization, software, and methodology. YM: Writing—original draft and writing—review and editing. SS: Writing—original draft and writing—review and editing. CJ: Conceptualization, funding acquisition, surgical operator supervision, methodology, and validation. All authors contributed to the article and approved the submitted version.

REFERENCES

1. Kakarala K, Shnayder Y, Tsue TT, Girod DA. Mandibular Reconstruction. *Oral Oncol* (2018) 77:111–117. doi: 10.1016/j.oraloncology.2017.12.020
2. Brown JS, Lowe D, Kanatas A, Schache A. Mandibular Reconstruction With Vascularised Bone Flaps: A Systematic Review Over 25 Years. *Br J Oral Maxillofac Surg* (2017) 55(2):113–26. doi: 10.1016/j.bjoms.2016.12.010
3. Dupret-Bories A, Vergez S, Meresse T, Brouillet F, Bertrand G. Contribution of 3D Printing to Mandibular Reconstruction After Cancer. *Eur Ann Otorhinolaryngol Head Neck Dis* (2018) 135(2):133–6. doi: 10.1016/j.anorl.2017.09.007
4. Hou JS, Chen M, Pan CB, Tao Q, Wang JG, Wang C, et al. Immediate Reconstruction of Bilateral Mandible Defects: Management Based on Computer-Aided Design/Computer-Aided Manufacturing Rapid Prototyping Technology in Combination With Vascularized Fibular Osteomyocutaneous Flap. *J Oral Maxillofac Surg* (2011) 69(6):1792–7. doi: 10.1016/j.joms.2010.07.047
5. Bak M, Jacobson AS, Buchbinder D, Urken ML. Contemporary Reconstruction of the Mandible. *Oral Oncol* (2010) 46(2):71–6. doi: 10.1016/j.oraloncology.2009.11.006
6. Chen J, Yin P, Li N, Wu L, Jian X, Jiang C. Functional Mandibular Reconstruction With Double-Barrel Fibular Flap and Primary Osseointegrated Dental Implants Improve Facial Esthetic Outcome. *J Oral Maxillofac Surg* (2019) 77(1):218–25. doi: 10.1016/j.joms.2018.08.008
7. Louvrier A, Marty P, Barrabe A, Euvrard E, Chatelain B, Weber E, et al. How Useful Is 3D Printing in Maxillofacial Surgery? *J Stomatol Oral Maxillofac Surg* (2017) 118(4):206–12. doi: 10.1016/j.jormas.2017.07.002
8. Ince B, Ismayilzade M, Dadaci M, Zuhal E. Computer-Assisted *Versus* Conventional Freehand Mandibular Reconstruction With Fibula Free Flap: A Systematic Review and Meta-Analysis. *Plast Reconstr Surg* (2020) 146 (5):686e–7e. doi: 10.1097/PRS.0000000000007295
9. Nobis CP, Kesting MR, Wolff KD, Frohwitter G, Rau A, Weitz J. Development of a Template Tool for Facilitating Fibula Osteotomy in Reconstruction of Mandibular Defects by Digital Analysis of the Human Mandible. *Clin Oral Investig* (2020) 24(9):3077–83. doi: 10.1007/s00784-019-03177-4

10. Ren W, Gao L, Li S, Chen C, Li F, Wang Q, et al. Virtual Planning and 3D Printing Modeling for Mandibular Reconstruction With Fibula Free Flap. *Med Oral Patol Oral Cir Bucal* (2018) 23(3):e359–66. doi: 10.4317/medoral.22295
11. Powcharoen W, Yang WF, Yan Li K, Zhu W, Su YX. Computer-Assisted *Versus* Conventional Freehand Mandibular Reconstruction With Fibula Free Flap: A Systematic Review and Meta-Analysis. *Plast Reconstr Surg* (2019) 144 (6):1417–28. doi: 10.1097/PRS.0000000000006261
12. Yang WF, Powcharoen W, Su YX. Computer-Assisted Surgery Increases Efficiency of Mandibular Reconstruction With Fibula Free Flap. *Plast Reconstr Surg* (2020) 146(5):687e–8e. doi: 10.1097/PRS.0000000000007296
13. Liang Y, Jiang C, Wu L, Wang W, Liu Y, Jian X. Application of Combined Osteotomy and Reconstruction Pre-Bent Plate Position (CORPPP) Technology to Assist in the Precise Reconstruction of Segmental Mandibular Defects. *J Oral Maxillofac Surg* (2017) 75(9):2026.e1–10. doi: 10.1016/j.joms.2017.04.046
14. Urken ML, Weinberg H, Vickery C, Buchbinder D, Lawson W, Biller HF. Oromandibular Reconstruction Using Microvascular Composite Free Flaps. Report of 71 Cases and a New Classification Scheme for Bony, Soft-Tissue, and Neurologic Defects. *Arch Otolaryngol Head Neck Surg* (1991) 117(7):733–44. doi: 10.1001/archotol.1991.01870190045010
15. Abbate V, Orabona GDA, Solari D, Bonavolonta P, Iaconetta G, Califano L. Mandibular Surgical Navigation: An Innovative Guiding Method. *J Craniofac Surg* (2017) 28(8):2122–6. doi: 10.1097/SCS.0000000000003816
16. Wilde F, Cornelius CP, Schramm A. Computer-Assisted Mandibular Reconstruction Using a Patient-Specific Reconstruction Plate Fabricated With Computer-Aided Design and Manufacturing Techniques. *Craniomaxillofac Trauma Reconstr* (2014) 7(2):158–66. doi: 10.1055/s-0034-1371356
17. Lu T, Shao Z, Liu B, Wu T. Recent Advance in Patient-Specific 3D Printing Templates in Mandibular Reconstruction. *J Mech Behav BioMed Mater* (2020) 106:103725. doi: 10.1016/j.jmbbm.2020.103725
18. Gupta S, Goil P. Formulating an Easy, Affordable, and Reproducible Method for Virtual Planning and 3D Reconstruction: A State Institution's Approach for Mandibular Reconstruction. *Ann Plast Surg* (2021) 87(1):65–72. doi: 10.1097/SAP.0000000000002832
19. Weitz J, Bauer FJ, Hapfelmeier A, Rohleder NH, Wolff KD, Kesting MR. Accuracy of Mandibular Reconstruction by Three-Dimensional Guided Vascularised Fibular Free Flap After Segmental Mandibulectomy. *Br J Oral Maxillofac Surg* (2016) 54(5):506–10. doi: 10.1016/j.bjoms.2016.01.029
20. Ganry L, Quilichini J, Bandini CM, Leyder P, Hersant B, Meningaud JP. Three-Dimensional Surgical Modelling With an Open-Source Software Protocol: Study of Precision and Reproducibility in Mandibular Reconstruction With the Fibula Free Flap. *Int J Oral Maxillofac Surg* (2017) 46(8):946–57. doi: 10.1016/j.ijom.2017.02.1276
21. Yang WF, Choi WS, Zhu WY, Zhang CY, Li DTS, Tsoi JK, et al. Spatial Deviations of the Temporomandibular Joint After Oncological Mandibular Reconstruction. *Int J Oral Maxillofac Surg* (2021) S0901-5027(21)00129-6. doi: 10.1016/j.ijom.2021.02.033
22. Sawh-Martinez R, Parsaei Y, Wu R, Lin A, Metzler P, DeSesa C, et al. Improved Temporomandibular Joint Position After 3-Dimensional Planned Mandibular Reconstruction. *J Oral Maxillofac Surg* (2017) 75(1):197–206. doi: 10.1016/j.joms.2016.07.032
23. Shiozaki M, Terao Y, Taniguchi K. Evaluation of Temporomandibular Joint Movement After Mandibular Reconstruction. *J Craniofac Surg* (2019) 30 (1):154–7. doi: 10.1097/SCS.0000000000005046
24. Wang L, Liu K, Shao Z, Shang ZJ. Management of the Condyle Following the Resection of Tumours of the Mandible. *Int J Oral Maxillofac Surg* (2017) 46 (10):1252–6. doi: 10.1016/j.ijom.2017.04.029
25. Foley BD, Thayer WP, Honeybrook A, McKenna S, Press S. Mandibular Reconstruction Using Computer-Aided Design and Computer-Aided Manufacturing: An Analysis of Surgical Results. *J Oral Maxillofac Surg* (2013) 71(2):e111–9. doi: 10.1016/j.joms.2012.08.022
26. Zhang L, Liu Z, Li B, Yu H, Shen SG, Wang X. Evaluation of Computer-Assisted Mandibular Reconstruction With Vascularized Fibular Flap Compared to Conventional Surgery. *Oral Surg Oral Med Oral Pathol Oral Radiol* (2016) 121(2):139–48. doi: 10.1016/j.oooo.2015.10.005
27. Bartier S, Mazzaschi O, Benichou L, Sauvaget E. Computer-Assisted *Versus* Traditional Technique in Fibular Free-Flap Mandibular Reconstruction: A CT Symmetry Study. *Eur Ann Otorhinolaryngol Head Neck Dis* (2021) 138(1):23–7. doi: 10.1016/j.anorl.2020.06.011
28. Yang WF, Choi WS, Wong MC, Powcharoen W, Zhu WY, Tsoi JK, et al. Three-Dimensionally Printed Patient-Specific Surgical Plates Increase Accuracy of Oncologic Head and Neck Reconstruction *Versus* Conventional Surgical Plates: A Comparative Study. *Ann Surg Oncol* (2021) 28(1):363–75. doi: 10.1245/s10434-020-08732-y
29. Yang WF, Choi WS, Zhu WY, Su YX. One-Piece" Patient-Specific Reconstruction Plate for Double-Barrel Fibula-Based Mandibular Reconstruction. *Int J Oral Maxillofac Surg* (2020) 49(8):1016–9. doi: 10.1016/j.ijom.2019.12.006

17

In-House, Open-Source 3D-Software-Based, CAD/CAM-Planned Mandibular Reconstructions in 20 Consecutive Free Fibula Flap Cases: An Explorative Cross-Sectional Study with Three-Dimensional Performance Analysis

Lucas M. Ritschl[1], Paul Kilbertus[1], Florian D. Grill[1], Matthias Schwarz[1], Jochen Weitz[1,2], Markus Nieberler[1], Klaus-Dietrich Wolff[1] and Andreas M. Fichter[1]*

[1] *Department of Oral and Maxillofacial Surgery, School of Medicine, Technical University of Munich, Klinikum rechts der Isar, Munich, Germany,* [2] *Department of Oral and Maxillofacial Surgery, Josefinum, Augsburg and Private Practice Oral and Maxillofacial Surgery im Pferseepark, Augsburg, Germany*

Correspondence:
Lucas M. Ritschl
lucas.ritschl@tum.de

Background: Mandibular reconstruction is conventionally performed freehand, CAD/CAM-assisted, or by using partially adjustable resection aids. CAD/CAM-assisted reconstructions are usually done in cooperation with osteosynthesis manufacturers, which entails additional costs and longer lead time. The purpose of this study is to analyze an in-house, open-source software-based solution for virtual planning.

Methods and Materials: All consecutive cases between January 2019 and April 2021 that underwent in-house, software-based (Blender) mandibular reconstruction with a free fibula flap (FFF) were included in this cross-sectional study. The pre- and postoperative Digital Imaging and Com munications in Medicine (DICOM) data were converted to standard tessellation language (STL) files. In addition to documenting general information (sex, age, indication for surgery, extent of resection, number of segments, duration of surgery, and ischemia time), conventional measurements and three-dimensional analysis methods (root mean square error [RMSE], mean surface distance [MSD], and Hausdorff distance [HD]) were used.

Results: Twenty consecutive cases were enrolled. Three-dimensional analysis of preoperative and virtually planned neomandibula models was associated with a median RMSE of 1.4 (0.4–7.2), MSD of 0.3 (-0.1–2.9), and HD of 0.7 (0.1–3.1). Three-dimensional comparison of preoperative and postoperative models showed a median RMSE of 2.2 (1.5–11.1), MSD of 0.5 (-0.6–6.1), and HD of 1.5 (1.1–6.5) and the differences were significantly different for RMSE ($p < 0.001$) and HD ($p < 0.001$). The difference was not significantly different for MSD ($p = 0.554$). Three-dimensional analysis of virtual and postoperative models had a median RMSE of 2.3 (1.3–10.7), MSD of -0.1 (-1.0–5.6), and HD of 1.7 (0.1–5.9).

Conclusions: Open-source software-based in-house planning is a feasible, inexpensive, and fast method that enables accurate reconstructions. Additionally, it is excellent for teaching purposes.

Keywords: in-house CAD/CAM planning, 3D printing, mandibular reconstruction, free fibula flap, open-source software

INTRODUCTION

The application of computer-aided design and computer-aided manufacturing (CAD/CAM) technology in primary and secondary mandibular reconstruction with the free fibula flap (FFF) following ablative surgery is considered to be state of the art nowadays. Several studies have proven its benefits and superiority in terms of operating time, ischemic time, symmetry, bony consolidation, and function (1–4), which may result in a positive cost–benefit balance sheet (5, 6) as well as better functional and aesthetic results (7–9).

After increasing standardization of the surgical processes and the integration of virtual planning processes in the last decade, the trend continues toward cost reduction, as patient-specific cutting guides and osteosynthesis plates are usually offered and produced by various osteosynthesis manufacturers and may even not have led to overall cost reduction (10). On the one hand, this necessitates a functioning infrastructure with nationwide coverage by these companies, and on the other hand, the effort expended entails additional costs for the surgical department and ultimately the healthcare system (10). In addition, the dependence on the industry reduces flexibility of planning timing and, depending on the complexity of the case, requires a lead time of at least seven to ten working days, during which one to three web meetings are held to discuss the planning and its implementation. In this context, two developments can be observed in the daily routine and more recent literature: first, the establishment of low-cost solutions for the in-house production of cutting guides using open-source software and in-house printers (11–14) and, second, the use of partially adjustable resection aids such as the ReconGuide (KLS Martin Group; Gebrüder Martin GmbH & Co. KG; Tuttlingen, Germany) and the MUC-Jig (15, 16).

The purpose of this study was to evaluate our workflow and results of in-house-planned mandibular reconstructions with the FFF and to describe potential pitfalls and solutions for a wider application of this versatile opportunity.

MATERIALS AND METHODS

Ethical Statement and Enrolled Patients

All clinical investigations were conducted according to the principles expressed in the Declaration of Helsinki. The exploratory cross-sectional study of a historical cohort was approved by the institutional ethics committee of the Technical University of Munich, Klinikum rechts der Isar (Approval number: 326/21 S-EB).

All patients who underwent mandibular resection and a reconstruction with an in-house-planned CAD/CAM FFF in our department for a benign or malignant disease between January 2019 and May 2021 were included. Patients without a postoperative computed tomography (CT) scan or with any otherwise planned and performed mandibular reconstruction (for example the use of partially adjustable resection aids or other microvascular bone flap) within this observation period were excluded (**Figure 1**). Data collection included: gender, age, indication for mandibular reconstruction, extent of resection according to Brown et al. (I–IV) (17), number of fibular segments, duration of surgery [min], ischemia time [min], and estimated resin volume and printing duration per case. Ischemia time was defined as the interval between ligation of the pedicle, mandibular reconstruction with completed osteosynthesis and opening of the vessel clamp following microvascular anastomoses.

All enrolled FFF cases were preoperatively planned and flaps were harvested by either the first- or last-named author (LMR, AMF), using the lateral approach (18) and using templates printed in-house (cutting guides and repositioning aids).

Blender-Based In-House CAD/CAM Planning

The digital workflow for the production of the in-house-planned and printed cutting and reconstruction guides complies with the general principles of CAD/CAM-assisted techniques as described elsewhere in detail (1, 19–21).

Available pre- and postoperative CT scans of enrolled patients were collected. Corresponding Digital Imaging and Communications in Medicine (DICOM) data sets of the CT scans were anonymized and converted to corresponding standard tessellation language (STL) files using Mimics® software (Mimics® 17.0, Materialise; Leuven, Belgium). The open-source software solution Blender (Blender® Version 2.79; Blender Foundation and Institute; Amsterdam, Netherlands) was used for the in-house computer planning and design of corresponding mandibular and fibular cutting guides and repositioning aids (**Figure 2**). No validation or comparison of the Blender-based planning with another software was performed.

The purely Blender-based planning procedure contained following key steps (**Supplementary Data**): First, the preoperative STL file of the mandible was imported to the Blender software and positioned in three-dimensional space ("*Object_Transform_Geometry to Origin*"). Then the necessary cutting planes were set and aligned as surgically required (paramedian, corpus, ramus, etc.)

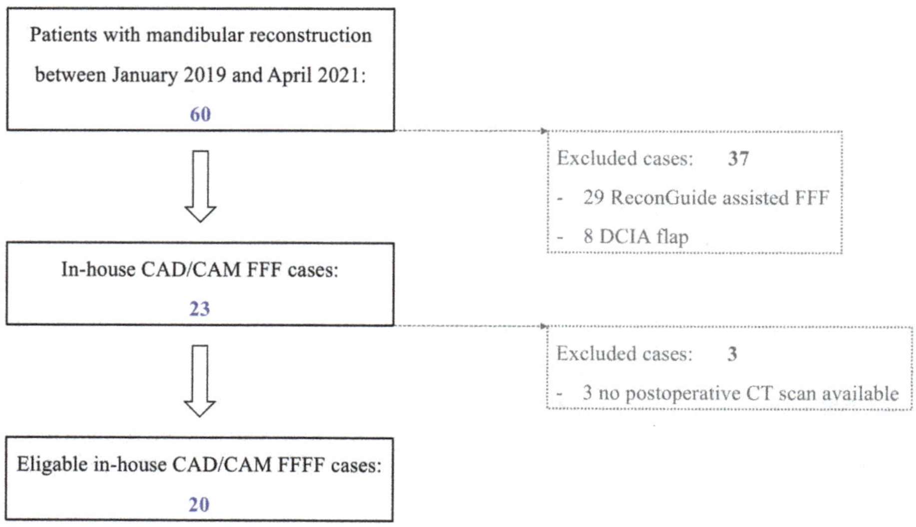

FIGURE 1 | Patient enrollment protocol of this exploratory cross-sectional study of a historical cohort. (FFF, free fibula flap; DCIA, microvascular iliac crest flap, deep circumflex iliac artery).

("*Create_Cube*" → transform and manipulate in *object* and *edit mode*). Now, depending on the number of necessary fibula segments, the STL file of the fibula was imported and superimposed onto the expected mandibular defect according to the functional and reconstructive requirements. After simulation of the reconstructive result (= neomandibula) and final adjustment of the fibula segment positions, the corresponding cutting guides for the mandible and the fibula, as well as the repositioning aids for the final neomandibula, were designed ("*Create_Cube*" → transformation and manipulation in *object* and *edit mode*, and "*Add Modifier_Boolean_Difference*"). Repositioning aids were only created for the junction between neomandibula body and original mandibular as well as for the neomandibular angle. No repositioning aids were designed for the ramus/condylar junction due to lack of space. In this region, pre-bent miniplates were the only aid to transfer the virtual plan.

In addition, holes with a diameter of 4.2 mm were integrated to incorporate drill sleeves for safe intraoperative temporary fixation (KLS Martin Group; Gebrüder Martin GmbH & Co. KG; Tuttlingen, Germany).

The cutting guides and repositioning aids were printed in-house with a Form 2 stereolithographic printer (Form 2, Formlabs; USA) using a Class 1 autoclavable, biocompatible photopolymer resin (Dental SG, FLDGOR01; Formlabs; USA) with a layer thickness of 50 μm. The post-processing of the printed geometries was carried out according to the manufacturer's instructions.

Conventional Measurements and Three-Dimensional Analysis of Postoperative Results

Postoperative analysis of the surgical results included conventional measurements and three-dimensional surface matching methods. The conventional measurements included the following distances: horizontal distance condylar head–condylar head (head–head) medial (1), lateral (2), and the condylar angles left (3) and right (4) according to Ueki et al. (22).

After the segmented pre- and postoperative mandibles and the virtual model were six-point-aligned, the following three three-dimensional parameters were determined for the comparison of three possible constellations [preoperative *vs.* virtual model (pre-virt); preoperative *vs.* postoperative model (pre-post); virtual model *vs.* postoperative (virt-post)]: root mean square error [RMSE, [mm)], mean surface distance [MSD, (mm)], and Hausdorff distance [HD, (voxel)] (23–25) (**Figure 3**). All conventional and three-dimensional analyses were performed using the open-source software MeshLab (MeshLab_64bit_fp v2020.12) and Blender.

All measurements were performed independently by two investigators (PK and FDG). All analyses were performed twice; the second round of analysis was performed at least seven to fourteen days later to minimize a habitual landmark setting and six-point alignment (26).

Statistical Analysis

The intraclass correlation (ICC) coefficient (Cohen's kappa = κ) was calculated to determine the intra- and interrater reliability and consistency of measurements performed by two raters applying a two-way mixed model. For the analysis of pre- and postoperative differences of the conventional parameters the Wilcoxon signed-rank test was used. For the differences of RMSE, MSD, and HD between pre-virt *vs.* pre-post models uni- and multivariate regression analyses were performed.

All statistical tests were performed on an exploratory two-sided 5% significance level. No adjustments were made for multiple testing. Analysis was done with IBM SPSS 24 for Mac software (IBM Corp, Armonk; New York, United States).

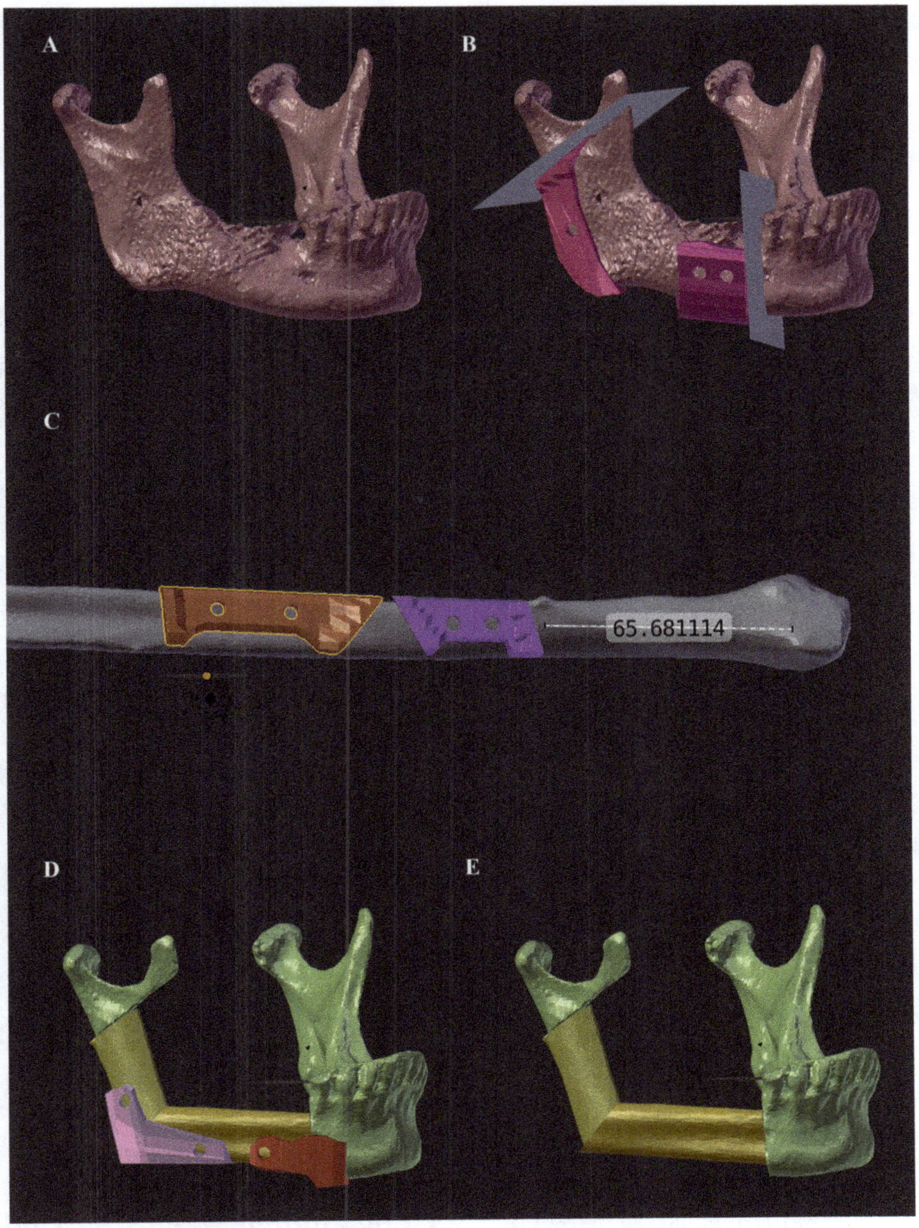

FIGURE 2 | Workflow for in-house Blender-based (Blender® Version 2.79; Blender Foundation and Institute; Amsterdam, Netherlands) planning and design of corresponding mandibular and fibular cutting guides and repositioning aids for mandibular reconstruction with the free fibula flap. **(A)** preoperative mandibular situation, **(B)** simulated resection planes and designed mandibular cutting guides, **(C)** corresponding fibular cutting guides, **(D)** repositioning aids (at angle and neomandibular/mandibula body junction), and **(E)** final virtually reconstructed mandible.

RESULTS

General Information and Descriptive Statistics

Twenty patients (9 female, 11 male) met the inclusion criteria (**Figure 1**). Age, indication for surgery, distribution of mandibular defect class according to Brown et al. (17), and the distribution of corresponding number of segments are shown in **Table 1**.

The overall median estimated resin volume and printing duration per case were 43.6 ml (13.8–77.4) and 180 minutes (120–255). Median costs per case were EUR 14.30 (4.50–25.30). The median overall operation duration was 650 minutes (480–840) and ischemic time was 165 minutes (90–240). In the class II mandibular defect constellation the operation duration was 630 minutes (480–840) and ischemic time was 150 minutes (90–240). In the class IV mandibular defect constellation the operation duration was 660 minutes

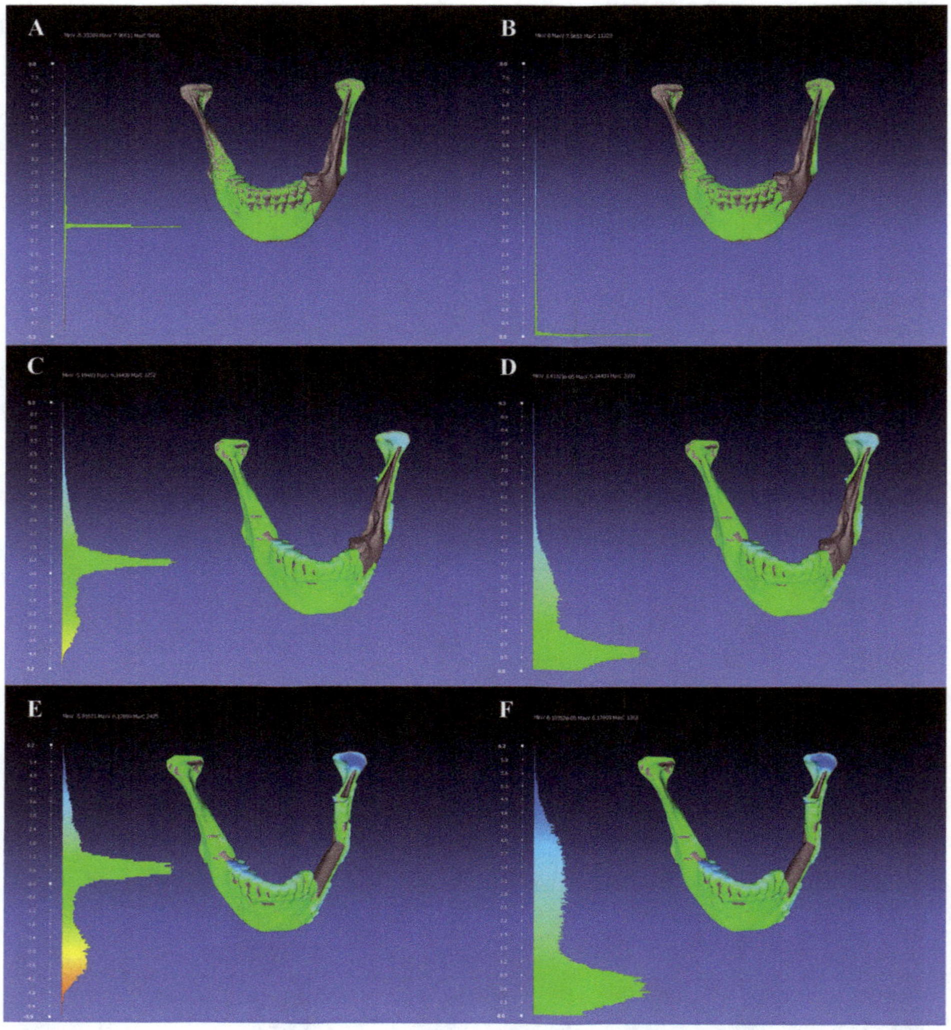

FIGURE 3 | Three-dimensional analyses were done with the open-source software MeshLab (MeshLab_64bit_fp v2020.12) showing root mean square error [RMSE, (mm)] in the left column and Hausdorff distance [HD, (voxel)] in the right column: **(A, B)** preoperative *vs.* virtual (pre-virt) model, **(C, D)** preoperative *vs.* postoperative (pre-post), and **(E, F)** virtual model *vs.* postoperative (virt-post).

(600–750) and ischemic time was 180 minutes (120–185) (p = 0.180; p = 0.928, respectively).

The Intraclass Correlation Coefficients

The ICC coefficients (κ) for the horizontal distances head–head medial and lateral showed very good intra- and interrater reliabilities (κ>0.9). The condylar angle measurement showed only satisfactory intra- [between *ICC* κ 0.552, 95% CI -0.292–0.844 and *ICC* κ 0.866, 95% CI 0.655–0.948)] and good interrater reliability (between *ICC* κ 0.845, 95% CI 0.579–0.942), especially in the preoperative measurements. The postoperative condylar angle measurements again showed good to very good agreement (ICC κ>0.9).

ICC coefficients of all three-dimensional parameters (RMSE, MSD, and HD) consistently showed very good intra- and interrater reliability (ICC κ>0.9) (**Supplementary Tables 1** and **2**).

Conventional and Three-Dimensional Analyses

The detailed results of the conventional pre- and postoperative measurements (horizontal medial and lateral head-head distances and left and right condylar angles) are summarized in **Table 2**.

The three-dimensional alignment analyses of the preoperative and virtually planned neomandibula models (= pre-virt = expected deviation from "*ground truth*" model) were associated with a median RMSE of 1.4 (0.4–7.2), MSD of 0.3 (-0.1–2.9), and HD of 0.7 (0.1–3.1). The three-dimensional alignment analyses of preoperative and postoperative models (= pre-post = postoperative, real deviation from "*ground truth*" model) showed a median RMSE of 2.2 (1.5–11.1), MSD of 0.5 (-0.6–6.1), and HD of 1.5 (1.1–6.5) and the differences were significantly different for RMSE (p < 0.001) and HD (p <

TABLE 1 | Overview of enrolled patients with regard to registered parameters: gender, age, indication for surgery, mandibular defect class according to Brown et al. (17), number of segments.

Parameters	n (%)	
Gender female/male	9/11	
Age median (range)	55.5 (23–79)	
Indication	OSCC	5 (25%)
	Secondary reconstruction	5 (25%)
	ORN	4 (20%)
	Ameloblastoma	2 (10%)
	Osteomyelitis	2 (10%)
	MRONJ	1 (5%)
	Ameloblastic fibrosarcoma	1 (5%)
Mandibular defect class	II	15 (75%)
	IV	5 (25%)
Number of segments	1	1 (5%)
	2	11 (55%)
	3	7 (35%)
	4	1 (5%)

OSCC, oral squamous cell carcinoma; ORN, osteoradionecrosis; MRONJ, medication-related osteonecrosis of the jaw.

0.001). The difference was not significantly different for MSD (p = 0.554).

Three-dimensional alignment analyses of the virtual and postoperative models (= virt-post = postoperative, real deviation from planned situation) had a median RMSE of 2.3 (1.3–10.7), MSD of -0.1 (-1.0–5.6), and HD of 1.7 (0.1–5.9) (**Table 2** and **Figure 3**).

The results for the RMSE, MSD, and HD analyses as a function of number of bone segments or mandibular defect class (II *vs.* IV) are shown in **Figure 4**.

Uni- and Multivariate Linear Regression Analyses

Uni- and multivariate regression analyses were performed to analyze possible confounding factors (gender, age, indication for surgery, dignity, mandibular defect class, and number of segments) on the RMSE, MSD, and HD of the virtual postoperative model alignment. Gender and number of segments did not have a significant influence on RMSE, MSD, or HD and were thus excluded from the multivariate linear regression analyses. Dignity (benign *vs.* malign) showed a significant influence on RMSE and MSD (p = 0.047 95% CI = 0.015–1.987 and p = 0.001 95% CI = 0.461–1.767), but not on HD (p = 0.223 95% CI = -0.210–0.886). The significant influence of the factors age, indication, dignity, and mandibular defect class remained in the multivariate linear regression analyses (**Table 3**).

DISCUSSION

This study is one of the few studies on in-house CAD/CAM solutions that presents a critical contemporary three-dimensional evaluation of virtually planned mandibular reconstructions with FFF. Tarsitano et al. described that the use of CAD/CAM-assisted mandibular reconstruction is economically viable, as the money saved by the reduction of operation duration offsets the associated costs of approximately EUR 3,450 (5). Rommel et al. calculated the increased costs for planning and the use of patient-specific cutting guides offered and manufactured by osteosynthesis manufacturers to be EUR 2,250 per case (3). According to reviews and meta-analyses others reported the cost of virtual surgical planning to range from USD 3,000–8,200 (6, 10). These higher costs can be explained by the fact that the studies included in the reviews/meta-analyses were published between 2013 and 2016, at a time when 3D printing, for example, was even more expensive than it is today, and usually included the production of patient-specific reconstruction plates. Costs resulting from cost-effective in-house design and printing solutions are reported to be significantly lower. Bosc et al. calculated their cost per case for in-house design and printing at EUR 989 (13). In contrast, our reported median costs per case were EUR 14.30 (4.50–25.30).

TABLE 2 | Results of conventional and three-dimensional analyses.

Parameter	Absolut median (range)	Median (range) differences	p-value
Pre head–head med	84.4 (76.3–94.4)	-1.9 (-13–8)	0.131#
Post head–head med	85.8 (76.0–100.3)		
Pre head–head lat	119.7 (105.3–130.1)	-0.4 (-7.9–6.1)	0.183#
Post head–head lat	121.2 (107.2–131.5)		
Pre condyle angle right	23.0 (11.0–37.0)	0.0 (-26–23)	0.142#
Post condyle angle right	23.0 (11.3–43.0)		
Pre condyle angle left	-22.0 [-32.0–(-7.0)]	1.4 (22–34.5)	0.042#
Post condyle angle left	-20.3 [-56.9–(-8.0)]		
Parameter	Median (range)	Parameter	Median (range)
Pre-virt RMSE	1.4 (0.4–7.2)	Pre-post RMSE	2.2 (1.5–11.1)
Pre-virt MSD	0.3 (-0.1–2.9)	Pre-post MSD	0.5 (-0.6–6.1)
Pre-virt HD	0.7 (0.1–3.1)	Pre-post HD	1.5 (1.1–6.5)
Virt-post RMSE	2.3 (1.3–10.7)	Diff RMSE pre-post *vs.* pre-virt	0.7 (-2.7–10.5)
Virt-post MSD	-0.1 (-1.0–5.6)	Diff MSD pre-post *vs.* pre-virt	-0.1 (-1.3–6.0)
Virt-post HD	1.7 (0.1–5.9)	Diff HD pre-post *vs.* pre-virt	0.9 (-0.8–6.4)

Head–head med/lat, medial/lateral horizontal distance between condylar heads; pre-virt, preoperative vs. virtual model; virt-post = virtual vs. postoperative model; pre-post = pre- vs. postoperative model; RMSE, root mean square error; MSD, mean surface distance; HD, Hausdorff distance; Diff, difference.

#Wilcoxon signed-rank test.

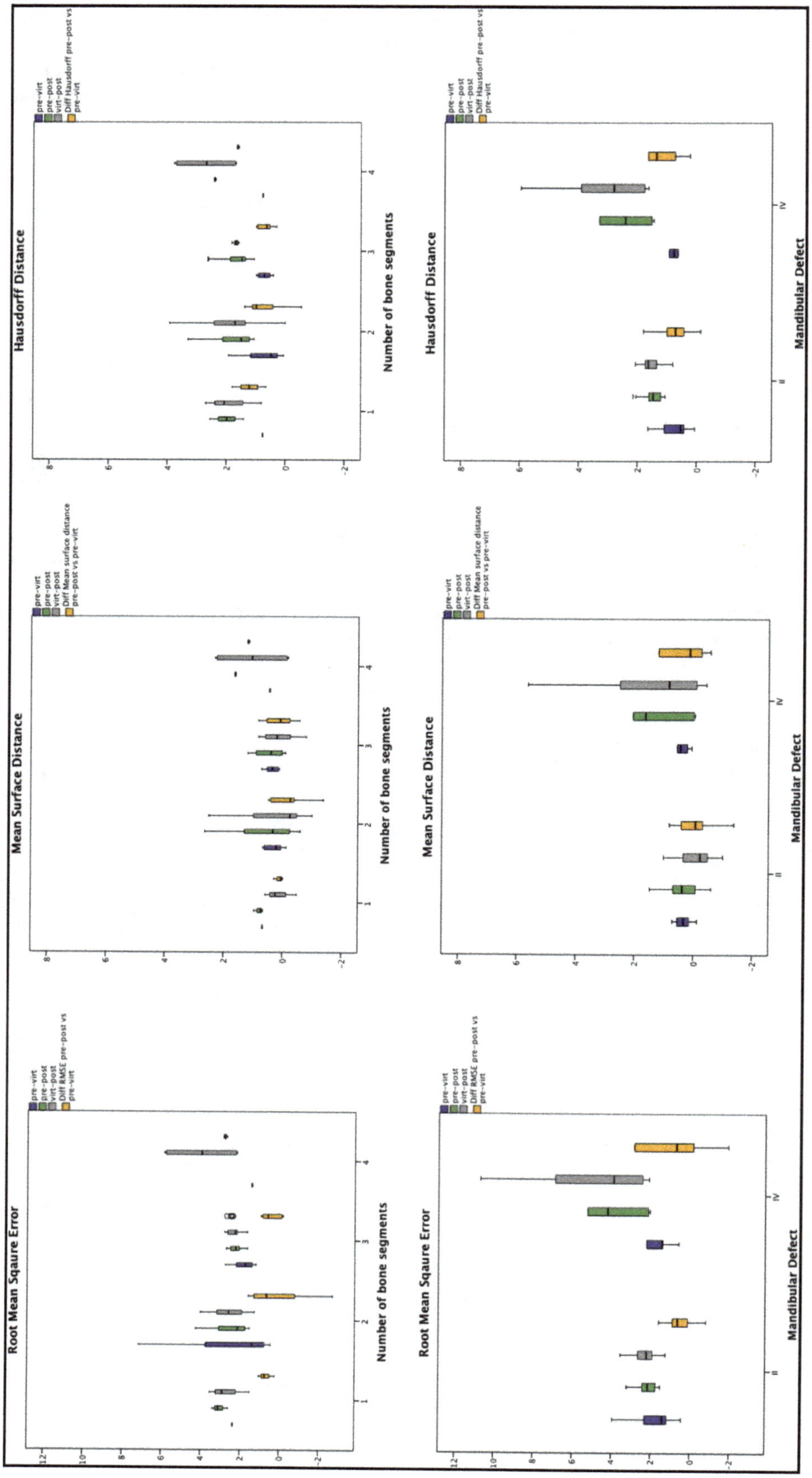

FIGURE 4 | The results for the RMSE, MSD, and HD analyses as a function of number of bone segments (upper row) or mandibular defect class (lower row).

This represents an excellent cost–benefit ratio, We have deliberately omitted recent non-negligible cost items (acquisition and maintenance costs, sterilization time, and planning time of approximately five to six hours, salary, etc.) and did also not calculated overall potential cost savings for simplicity, as have many other authors, and focused exclusively on material costs. More recently, Moe et al. reported their cost per case to be USD 3.87 for in-house design and printing. Dell'Aversana Orabona et al. reported a cost per case of EUR 3 (27). At EUR 14.30, the calculated costs per case are comparable with data from the literature and are completely negligible in relation to the surgical costs. Our slightly higher costs can be explained by two factors: we created and printed repositioning aids for each osteotomy site, and the neomandibula segment was also printed in order to bend the miniplates preoperatively.

The total lead time (planning, designing, printing, post-processing, final preparation with drill sleeves, and sterilization) is two to three days, which agrees very well with the times reported in the literature (13, 14) – and can be expedited further with growing experience and optimization of the processes. Another essential aspect raised by Numajiri et al. is that this form of cost-effective planning is done in the surgeon's time and is not outsourced to the osteosynthesis manufacturers and their clinical engineers as is usually the case (28). Geusens et al. reported that they have employed a full-time clinical engineer, which could be another solution to the altruistic behavior of interested and motivated surgeons (21). According to Tang et al., the economic benefits and limitations associated with the application of virtual surgical planning must be weighed against patient outcomes (4). The introduction of in-house solutions may represent the ideal approach in this respect, as costs can be saved and treatment optimized.

The study design and methodical analyses of the mandibular reconstruction is generally heterogenous among the available studies (4), which makes a direct comparison difficult. In a recent systematic review and meta-analysis on virtual surgical planning in mandibular reconstruction Barr et al. were not able to define a valuable parameter and result for "*accuracy*", even though many authors highlight the introduction of CAD/CAM algorithms as beneficial (6). The reason is again the heterogeneity of parameters. The majority of studies compared the preoperative virtual plan to the postoperative situation by measuring the fibula segment lengths (21, 29–31), point-to-point distances and angles (3, 13, 14), intercondylar distance (32), or intercoronoid distance (21) or by comparing interfragmentary gap distances (33). Numajiri et al. analyzed an algorithm for the production of low-cost cutting guides designed and printed in-house (28). They reported an error deviation of 2.4 mm in 12 studied *in-vitro* model surgeries. For this laboratory setting under ideal conditions, an error deviation of 2.4 mm seems to be quite high. Four years later, Numajiri et al. published a clinical study comparing freehand and in-house-planned CAD/CAM FFF cases (14). Based on a point-to-point analysis, they describe their in-house Blender-based solution as accurate. Interestingly, the results of the more recent study are more precise than the results of their *in vitro* studies, which can probably be attributed to the research group's growing experience with CAD/CAM-based surgical planning and the improvement of the processes. Yu et al. aligned the virtual plan and the postoperative result. But the evaluation was again limited only to distance measurements between corresponding points (8). Bosc et al. analyzed their postoperative results of in-house (Meshmixer or Blender) planned and printed cutting guides after surface alignment using CloudCompare, another potent open-source software solution for this purpose (13). However, the authors only used surface matching to get the maximum points of convergence for better correspondence of analyzed distances and angles. In all studies mentioned, the deviations between planning and operative results were 1–3 mm.

The disadvantage of all "conventional" measurement methods, which essentially involve only the analysis of distances (point-to-point or bone segment lengths) and angles, is that the effect of a small deviation on the entire three-dimensional geometry is neglected. An involuntary deviation from the planned osteotomy angle, fibula segment length, or fibula segment position will result in the derotation of the remaining mandible, and consequently in changes to the condyle angle.

For this reason and unlike most studies that have performed analyses of CAD/CAM-assisted mandibular reconstructions with the FFF, our focus has been on a three-dimensional analysis that encompasses the entire mandibular geometry. For example, Wallner et al. and van Eijnatten et al. applied three-dimensional parameters to compare the accuracy and comparability of open-source software solutions and influence of threshold setting for DICOM data set segmentation (23, 24). This approach seems to be a contemporary and objective way to compare two similar and rather complex objects but has not yet been used routinely in analyses of mandibular reconstructions (11, 12, 27). Each of our examined three-dimensional parameters – RMSE, MSD, and HD – had both excellent intra- and interobserver reliability, making the measured results valid for further analyses and discussion. In contrast, the conventional measurement of condylar angles in particular showed poorer intraobserver reliability for both examiners, which was confirmed by comparable interobserver reliability (**Supplementary Tables 1, 2**). Horizontal distances also revealed very good intra- and interobserver reliabilities. Dell'Aversana Orabona et al. used the open-source software InVesalius for in-house planning in four consecutive cases (27). They reported a distance between three-dimensional pre- and postoperative mesh points of 1.63 mm and a standard deviation of 5.45 mm in a volume overlay analysis. Recently, Moe et al. published results about their in-house workflow and described a mean surface overlay difference of 1.90 mm with an RMSE of 3.72 mm for 29 virtually planned cases, including 24 FFF (12). These results coincide with ours (virt-post MSD -0.1 (-1.0–5.6); virt-post RMSE 2.3 (1.3–10.7)). A novel aspect of our study is the comparison of preoperative situation and virtual model (pre-virt), which reflects the expected deviation from the "ground truth" model. Consequently, the difference between pre-post and pre-virt also reflects the accuracy when the value reaches 0. For this new parameter, we revealed excellent results for RMSE, MSD, and HD (**Table 2**).

TABLE 3 | Uni- and multivariable linear regression model of the virtual-postoperative RMSE, MSD, and HD results and possible confounding factors.

Factor	Root mean square error		Mean surface distance		Hausdorff distance	
	p-value	95% CI	*p*-value	95% CI	*p*-value	95% CI
Univariable linear regression model						
Gender	0.173	-1.561–0.286	0.056	-1.246–0.017	0.148	-0.874–0.135
Age	<0.001	-0.094–(-0.046)	<0.001	-0.054–(-0.018)	<0.001	-0.051–(-0.024)
Indication	<0.001	0.253–0.696	0.026	0.023–0.353	<0.001	0.165–0.402
Dignity	0.047	0.015–1.987	0.001	0.461–1.767	0.223	-0.210–0.886
Mandibular defect type	<0.001	1.092–1.916	<0.001	0.568–1.192	<0.001	0.638–1.075
Number of bone segments	0.416	-1.008–0.421	0.908	-0.526–0.468	0.577	-0.502–0.282
Multivariable linear regression model						
Age	0.01	-0.055–(-0.016)	0.109	-0.029–0.003	0.001	-0.029–(-0.007)
Indication	0.004	0.123–0.602	0.022	0.034–0.426	0.006	0.057–0.331
Dignity	<0.001	1.076–2.654	<0.001	1.056–2.347	/	/
Mandibular defect class	<0.001	0.597–1.391	<0.001	0.298–0.947	<0.001	0.342–0.796

In addition to potential cost savings and increased accuracy, we believe that this in-house planning has a great advantage especially in the training of junior surgeons. Dealing with virtual planning leads to the trainees intensively dealing with the clinical case, and potentially developing a higher demand for the final surgical result. Therefore, in our department, junior surgeons are introduced to virtual in-house fibula planning and learn to independently plan and create resection and repositioning guides. Unlike clinical engineers, they also perform flap elevation and mandibular reconstruction under the guidance of experienced specialists, so they will be involved in all steps of these complex reconstruction cases at an early stage in their careers. But this aspect (e.g. evaluation of junior surgeon´s satisfaction, confidence or virtual planning) was no not evaluated this study.

Limitations, Pitfalls and Solutions

A major drawback of this study was the application of an license-based segmentation software that is associated with an additional acquisition cost (Mimics® 17.0, Materialise; Leuven, Belgium with an one-time acquisition cost in 2014 of EUR 11,700). But, we used Mimics in order to reduce potential software-based pitfalls in our in-house workflow. Nevertheless, there exist reliable and accurate open-source solutions for segmentation like Slicer, as described by Wallner et al. and Egger et al. (23, 34, 35).

Through precise planning the original position of the mandible should be imitated as closely as possible from an esthetic and functional point of view. With regard to occlusion and jaw movement, the correct position of the temporomandibular joint is important, and the course of the neo-alveolar ridge is decisive for subsequent dentoalveolar rehabilitation, while from an esthetic point of view the projection of the chin and jaw angle region is particularly decisive. After a learning period, the planning of complex and heterogenous reconstructive cases with the open-source software Blender was feasible and led to excellent results with regard to the realization of virtual plans (**Figure 5**). But incorrect virtual planning can lead to poor postoperative results even if all surgical steps are basically correct and performed as planned. In the experience of the authors, one key pitfall region is the mandibular ramus. When reconstructing it, the transition of the outer surfaces of the fibula and the remaining cranial ramus portion must blend perfectly. If this is not the case, the application of the osteosynthesis will derotate the ramus portion and consequently change the condyle angle and position. But condylar position changes may occur also later in a longer observational interval than it was in our study (36). But nevertheless, a derotation of the condylar head because of the cranial ramus rotation will be visible immediately. The functional sequalae is uncertain and needs further evaluation (37). A further prerequisite is the optimal design of ramus/collum resection guides. Aspects that should be taken into account here are that the mandibular angle is gripped caudally, so that the correct vertical positioning of the guide is ensured. In addition, the guide must not be too thick cranially to allow sawing; if necessary, an angled micro saw can be used, which is usually not a problem with regard to the general bone thickness in this area.

Lastly, we think that the usage of repositioning guides is an excellent alternative to intraoperative navigation as described by Yu et al. (8) to critically feedback the reconstructive result intraoperatively. Especially the combination of repositioning guides and pre-bent osteosynthesis plates enhance the overall accuracy. This is also reflected by the fact that the number of bone segments had no significant effect on RMSE, MSD, or HD (**Table 3**) and might explain our better results for MSD and RMSE compared to Dell'Aversana Orabona et al. and Moe et al. (12, 27). Regarding the design of the repositioning guides, we recognized that we achieved better fit of the guides when designing multiple, osteotomy-specific guides rather than one large, contiguous guide. The supposed inaccuracy of the large repositioning guides is most likely due to 3D printing itself.

CONCLUSION

After a certain learning period, open-source software facilitates cost-effective and precise in-house virtual planning of mandibular reconstructions with a short lead time and without the need for external companies. Even highly complex reconstructions are thus possible with favorable results. In addition, the open-source

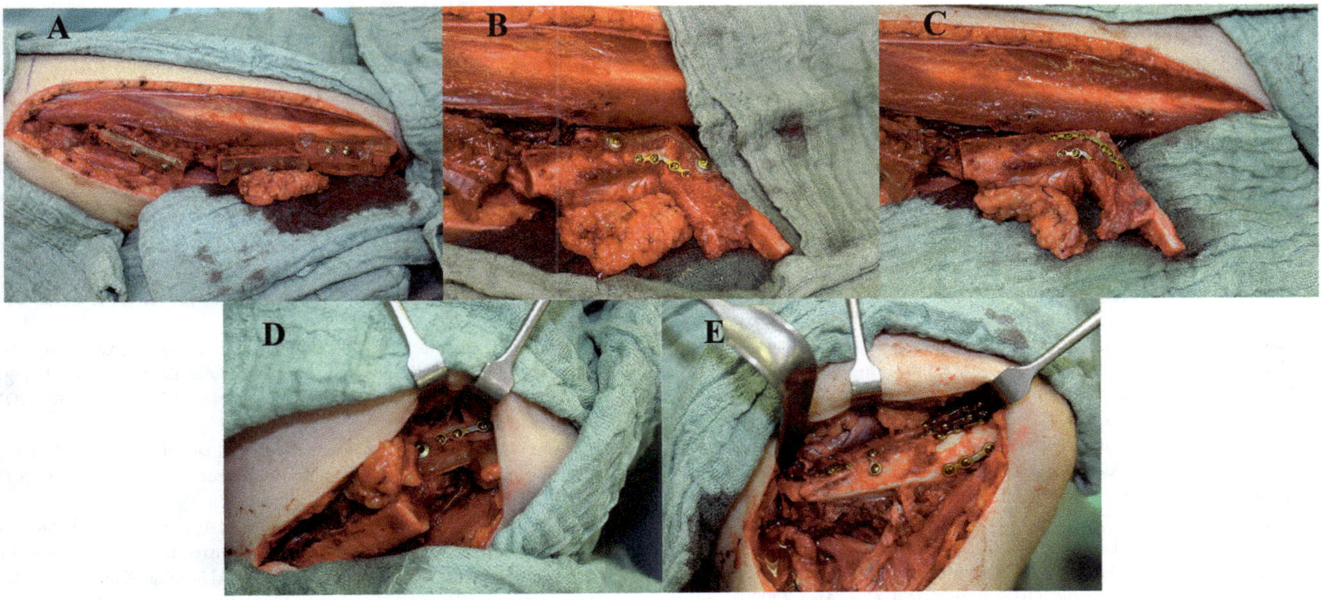

FIGURE 5 | Clinical example with intraoperative images of a case with hemimandibulectomy with exarticulation (Brown IIc) due to chronic osteomyelitis. Reconstruction was performed with a three-segment free fibular flap (FFF), with the corpus section reconstructed with a double-barrel component for better neomandibula contouring and crestal bone position for secondary enossal implant insertion. **(A)** FFF following osteotomies with temporarily applied cutting guides, **(B, C)** reconstruction of the ramus including neo-condylar head and crestal corpus section applying a repositioning aid and pre-bent 2.0 miniplate osteosynthesis, **(D)** positioning of the neomandibula with another repositioning aid, and **(E)** final reconstructive result with the double-barreled caudal FFF section for optimized bony countering.

software offers an excellent possibility to illustrate the surgical procedure. This might enhance the understanding for younger colleagues and increase their likelihood and frequency of an ideal surgical result.

AUTHOR CONTRIBUTIONS

LR: Study design/conduction, operations, data interpretation, and major contribution to manuscript writing and revision. PK: Surface matching and analysis, data acquisition and interpretation, contribution to revision. FG: Surface matching and analysis, data acquisition and interpretation, statistical analysis and contribution to revision. MS: Creation of figures, statistical analysis, contribution to revision. JW: Study design, data interpretation, contribution to revision. MN: Data interpretation, contribution to revision. K-DW: Data interpretation, contribution to revision. AF: Study design/conduction, operations, data interpretation, and major contribution to manuscript writing. All authors contributed to the article and approved the submitted version.

REFERENCES

1. Tarsitano A, Ciocca L, Scotti R, Marchetti C. Morphological Results of Customized Microvascular Mandibular Reconstruction: A Comparative Study. *J Craniomaxillofac Surg* (2016) 44:6. doi: 10.1016/j.jcms.2016.03.007
2. Haddock NT, Monaco C, Weimer KA, Hirsch DL, Levine JP, Saadeh PB. Increasing Bony Contact and Overlap With Computer-Designed Offset Cuts in Free Fibula Mandible Reconstruction. *J Craniofac Surg* (2012) 23:6. doi: 10.1097/SCS.0b013e318257576c
3. Rommel N, Kesting MR, Rohleder NH, Bauer FMJ, Wolff K-D, Weitz J. Mandible Reconstruction With Free Fibula Flaps: Outcome of a Cost-Effective Individual Planning Concept Compared With Virtual Surgical Planning. *J Craniomaxillofac Surg* (2017) 45:8. doi: 10.1016/j.jcms.2017.04.010
4. Tang NSJ, Ahmadi I, Ramakrishnan A. Virtual Surgical Planning in Fibula Free Flap Head and Neck Reconstruction: A Systematic Review and Meta-Analysis. *J Plastic Reconstr Aesthet Surg JPRAS* (2019) 9:1465–77. doi: 10.1016/j.bjps.2019.06.013
5. Tarsitano A, Battaglia S, Crimi S, Ciocca L, Scotti R, Marchetti C. Is a Computer-Assisted Design and Computer-Assisted Manufacturing Method for Mandibular Reconstruction Economically Viable? *J Craniomaxillofac Surg* (2016) 44:7. doi: 10.1016/j.jcms.2016.04.003
6. Barr ML, Haveles CS, Rezzadeh KS, Nolan IT, Castro R, Lee JC, et al. Virtual Surgical Planning for Mandibular Reconstruction With the Fibula Free Flap: A Systematic Review and Meta-Analysis. *Ann Plast Surg* (2020) 84:1. doi: 10.1097/SAP.0000000000002006
7. Ritschl LM, Mücke T, Fichter AM, Roth M, Kaltenhauser C, Pho Duc JM, et al. Axiographic Results of CAD/CAM-Assisted Microvascular, Fibular Free Flap Reconstruction of the Mandible: A Prospective Study of 21 Consecutive Cases. *J Craniomaxillofac Surg* (2017) 45:1. doi: 10.1016/j.jcms.2016.11.001
8. Yu Y, Zhang WB, Liu XJ, Guo CB, Yu GY, Peng X. Three-Dimensional Accuracy of Virtual Planning and Surgical Navigation for Mandibular Reconstruction With Free Fibula Flap. *J Oral Maxillofac Surg* (2016) 74:7. doi: 10.1016/j.joms.2016.02.020
9. Bouchet B, Raoul G, Julieron B, Wojcik T. Functional and Morphologic Outcomes of CAD/CAM-Assisted *Versus* Conventional Microvascular

Fibular Free Flap Reconstruction of the Mandible: A Retrospective Study of 25 Cases. *J Stomatol Oral Maxillofac Surg* (2018) 119:6. doi: 10.1016/j.jormas.2018.07.003

10. Fatima A, Hackman TG, Wood JS. Cost-Effectiveness Analysis of Virtual Surgical Planning in Mandibular Reconstruction. *Plast Reconstr Surg* (2019) 143:4. doi: 10.1097/PRS.0000000000005418
11. Ganry L, Quilichini J, Bandini CM, Leyder P, Hersant B, Meningaud JP. Three-Dimensional Surgical Modelling With an Open-Source Software Protocol: Study of Precision and Reproducibility in Mandibular Reconstruction With the Fibula Free Flap. *Int J Oral Maxillofac Surg* (2017) 46:8. doi: 10.1016/j.ijom.2017.02.1276
12. Moe J, Foss J, Herster R, Powell C, Helman J, Ward BB, et al. An In-House Computer-Aided Design and Computer-Aided Manufacturing Workflow for Maxillofacial Free Flap Reconstruction is Associated With a Low Cost and High Accuracy. *J Oral Maxillofac Surg* (2021) 79:1. doi: 10.1016/j.joms.2020.07.216
13. Bosc R, Hersant B, Carloni R, Niddam J, Bouhassira J, De Kermadec H, et al. Mandibular Reconstruction After Cancer: An in-House Approach to Manufacturing Cutting Guides. *Int J Oral Maxillofac Surg* (2017) 46:1. doi: 10.1016/j.ijom.2016.10.004
14. Numajiri T, Morita D, Yamochi R, Nakamura H, Tsujiko S, Sowa Y, et al. Does an In-House Computer-Aided Design/Computer-Aided Manufacturing Approach Contribute to Accuracy and Time Shortening in Mandibular Reconstruction? *J Craniofac Surg* (2020) 7:317. doi: 10.1097/SCS.0000000000006699
15. Meyer S, Hirsch JM, Leiggener CS, Msallem B, Sigron GR, Kunz C, et al. Fibula Graft Cutting Devices: Are 3d-Printed Cutting Guides More Precise Than a Universal, Reusable Osteotomy Jig? *J Clin Med* (2020) 9:12. doi: 10.3390/jcm9124119
16. Weitz J, Wolff KD, Kesting MR, Nobis CP. Development of a Novel Resection and Cutting Guide for Mandibular Reconstruction Using Free Fibula Flap. *J Craniomaxillofac Surg* (2018) 46:11. doi: 10.1016/j.jcms.2018.09.007
17. Brown JS, Barry C, Ho M, Shaw R. A New Classification for Mandibular Defects After Oncological Resection. *Lancet Oncol* (2016) 17:1. doi: 10.1016/S1470-2045(15)00310-1
18. Wolff KD, Holzle F, Kolk A, Hohlweg-Majert B, Steiner T, Kesting MR. Raising the Osteocutaneous Fibular Flap for Oral Reconstruction With Reduced Tissue Alteration. *J Oral Maxillofac Surg* (2011) 69:6. doi: 10.1016/j.joms.2010.11.040
19. Ritschl LM, Mucke T, Fichter A, Gull FD, Schmid C, Duc JMP, et al. Functional Outcome of CAD/CAM-Assisted *Versus* Conventional Microvascular, Fibular Free Flap Reconstruction of the Mandible: A Retrospective Study of 30 Cases. *J Reconstr Microsurg* (2017) 33:4. doi: 10.1055/s-0036-1597823
20. Mottini M, Seyed Jafari SM, Shafighi M, Schaller B. New Approach for Virtual Surgical Planning and Mandibular Reconstruction Using a Fibula Free Flap. *Oral Oncol* (2016) 59:e6–9. doi: 10.1016/j.oraloncology.2016.06.001
21. Geusens J, Sun Y, Luebbers HT, Bila M, Darche V, Politis C. Accuracy of Computer-Aided Design/Computer-Aided Manufacturing-Assisted Mandibular Reconstruction With a Fibula Free Flap. *J Craniofac Surg* (2019) 30:8. doi: 10.1097/SCS.0000000000005704
22. Ueki K, Yoshizawa K, Moroi A, Iguchi R, Kosaka A, Ikawa H, et al. Changes in Computed Tomography Values of Mandibular Condyle and Temporomandibular Joint Disc Position After Sagittal Split Ramus Osteotomy. *J Craniomaxillofac Surg* (2015) 43:7. doi: 10.1016/j.jcms.2015.05.007
23. Wallner J, Hochegger K, Chen X, Mischak I, Reinbacher K, Pau M, et al. Clinical Evaluation of Semi-Automatic Open-Source Algorithmic Software Segmentation of the Mandibular Bone: Practical Feasibility and Assessment of a New Course of Action. *PloS One* (2018) 13:5. doi: 10.1371/journal.pone.0196378
24. van Eijnatten M, van Dijk R, Dobbe J, Streekstra G, Koivisto J, Wolff J. CT Image Segmentation Methods for Bone Used in Medical Additive Manufacturing. *Med Eng Physics* (2018) 51:6–16. doi: 10.1016/j.medengphy.2017.10.008
25. Ritschl LM, Wolff K-D, Erben P, Grill FD. Simultaneous, Radiation-Free Registration of the Dentoalveolar Position and the Face by Combining 3D Photography With a Portable Scanner and Impression-Taking. *Head Face Med* (2019) 15:1. doi: 10.1186/s13005-019-0212-x
26. Wolff K-D, Grill FD, Ritschl LM. Comparative Photographic, Retrospective Analysis of Nonsyndromic Cleft Noses Treated With or Without NAM. *Plast Reconstr Surg Global Open* (2020) 8:9. doi: 10.1097/GOX.0000000000003045
27. Dell'Aversana Orabona G, Abbate V, Maglitto F, Bonavolonta P, Salzano G, Romano A, et al. Low-Cost, Self-Made CAD/CAM-Guiding System for Mandibular Reconstruction. *Surg Oncol* (2018) 27:2. doi: 10.1016/j.suronc.2018.03.007
28. Numajiri T, Nakamura H, Sowa Y, Nishino K. Low-Cost Design and Manufacturing of Surgical Guides for Mandibular Reconstruction Using a Fibula. *Plast Reconstr Surg Global Open* (2016) 4:7. doi: 10.1097/GOX.0000000000000682
29. Hanasono MM, Skoracki RJ. Computer-Assisted Design and Rapid Prototype Modeling in Microvascular Mandible Reconstruction. *Laryngoscope* (2013) 123:3. doi: 10.1002/lary.23717
30. Succo G, Berrone M, Battiston B, Tos P, Goia F, Appendino P, et al. Step-By-Step Surgical Technique for Mandibular Reconstruction With Fibular Free Flap: Application of Digital Technology in Virtual Surgical Planning. *Eur Arch Otorhinolaryngol* (2015) 272:6. doi: 10.1007/s00405-014-3078-3
31. Schepers RH, Raghoebar GM, Vissink A, Stenekes MW, Kraeima J, Roodenburg JL, et al. Accuracy of Fibula Reconstruction Using Patient-Specific CAD/CAM Reconstruction Plates and Dental Implants: A New Modality for Functional Reconstruction of Mandibular Defects. *J Craniomaxillofac Surg* (2015) 43:5. doi: 10.1016/j.jcms.2015.03.015
32. Metzler P, Geiger EJ, Alcon A, Ma X, Steinbacher DM. Three-Dimensional Virtual Surgery Accuracy for Free Fibula Mandibular Reconstruction: Planned *Versus* Actual Results. *J Oral Maxillofac Surg* (2014) 72:12. doi: 10.1016/j.joms.2014.07.024
33. Stirling Craig E, Yuhasz M, Shah A, Blumberg J, Salomon J, Lowlicht R, et al. Simulated Surgery and Cutting Guides Enhance Spatial Positioning in Free Fibular Mandibular Reconstruction. *Microsurgery* (2015) 35:1. doi: 10.1002/micr.22229
34. Egger J, Pfarrkirchner B, Gsaxner C, Lindner L, Schmalstieg D, Wallner J. Fully Convolutional Mandible Segmentation on a Valid Ground- Truth Dataset. *Conf Proc IEEE Eng Med Biol Soc* (2018) 2018:29–33. doi: 10.1109/EMBC.2018.8512458
35. Wallner J, Schwaiger M, Hochegger K, Gsaxner C, Zemann W, Egger J. A Review on Multiplatform Evaluations of Semi-Automatic Open-Source Based Image Segmentation for Cranio-Maxillofacial Surgery. *Comput Methods Programs Biomed* (2019) 182:105102. doi: 10.1016/j.cmpb.2019.105102
36. Wang W, Shan XF, Liang J, Xie S, Zhang J, Cai ZG. Changes in Condylar Position After Mandibular Reconstruction With Condylar Head Preservation by Computed Tomography. *J Oral Maxillofac Surg* (2019) 77:6. doi: 10.1016/j.joms.2018.12.037
37. Tang Q, Li Y, Yu T, Chen X, Zhou Z, Huang W, et al. Association Between Condylar Position Changes and Functional Outcomes After Condylar Reconstruction by Free Fibular Flap. *Clin Oral Investig* (2021) 25:1. doi: 10.1007/s00784-020-03338-w

18

Navigation-Guided Transnasal Endoscopic Delineation of the Posterior Margin for Maxillary Sinus Cancers: A Preclinical Study

Stefano Taboni[1,2,3,4,5], Marco Ferrari[1,2,3,4,6], Michael J. Daly[3], Harley H. L. Chan[3], Donovan Eu[1,3], Tommaso Gualtieri[1,3,7], Ashok R. Jethwa[1], Axel Sahovaler[1,3,8], Andrew Sewell[1], Wael Hasan[1,3], Ilyes Berania[1], Jimmy Qiu[3], John de Almeida[1], Piero Nicolai[2], Ralph W. Gilbert[1] and Jonathan C. Irish[1,3]*

[1] Department of Otolaryngology—Head and Neck Surgery/Surgical Oncology, Princess Margaret Cancer Centre, University Health Network, Toronto, ON, Canada, [2] Section of Otorhinolaryngology—Head and Neck Surgery, Department of Neurosciences, University of Padua—"Azienda Ospedaliera di Padova", Padua, Italy, [3] Guided Therapeutics (GTx) Program, Techna Institute, University Health Network, Toronto, ON, Canada, [4] University Health Network (UHN) Guided Therapeutics (GTx) Program International Scholar, Toronto, ON, Canada, [5] Artificial Intelligence in Medicine and Innovation in Clinical Research and Methodology (PhD Program), Department of Clinical and Experimental Sciences, University of Brescia, Brescia, Italy, [6] Technology for Health (PhD Program), Department of Information Engineering, University of Brescia, Brescia, Italy, [7] Unit of Otorhinolaryngology—Head and Neck Surgery, Department of Medical and Surgical Specialties, Radiologic Sciences, and Public Health, University of Brescia—"ASST Spedali Civili di Brescia", Brescia, Italy, [8] Head & Neck Surgery, University College London Hospital, London, United Kingdom

***Correspondence:**
Marco Ferrari
marco.ferrari@unipd.it*

Background: The resection of advanced maxillary sinus cancers can be challenging due to the anatomical proximity to surrounding critical anatomical structures. Transnasal endoscopy can effectively aid the delineation of the posterior margin of resection. Implementation with 3D-rendered surgical navigation with virtual endoscopy (3D-SNVE) may represent a step forward. This study aimed to demonstrate and quantify the benefits of this technology.

Material and Method: Four maxillary tumor models with critical posterior extension were created in four artificial skulls (Sawbones®). Images were acquired with cone-beam computed tomography and the tumor and carotid were contoured. Eight head and neck surgeons were recruited for the simulations. Surgeons delineated the posterior margin of resection through a transnasal approach and avoided the carotid while establishing an adequate resection margin with respect to tumor extirpation. Three simulations were performed: 1) unguided: based on a pre-simulation study of cross-sectional imaging; 2) tumor-guided: guided by real-time tool tracking with 3D tumor and carotid rendering; 3) carotid-guided: tumor-guided with a 2-mm alert cloud surrounding the carotid. Distances of the planes from the carotid and tumor were classified as follows and the points of the plane were classified accordingly: "red": through the carotid artery; "orange": <2 mm from the carotid; "yellow": >2 mm from the carotid and within the tumor or <5 mm from the tumor; "green": >2 mm from the carotid and 5–10 mm from the tumor; and "blue": >2 mm from the carotid and >10 mm from the tumor. The three techniques (unguided, tumor-guided, and carotid-guided) were compared.

Results: 3D-SNVE for the transnasal delineation of the posterior margin in maxillary tumor models significantly improved the rate of margin-negative clearance around the tumor and reduced damage to the carotid artery. "Green" cuts occurred in 52.4% in the unguided setting *versus* 62.1% and 64.9% in the tumor- and carotid-guided settings, respectively ($p < 0.0001$). "Red" cuts occurred 6.7% of the time in the unguided setting *versus* 0.9% and 1.0% in the tumor- and carotid-guided settings, respectively ($p < 0.0001$).

Conclusions: This preclinical study has demonstrated that 3D-SNVE provides a substantial improvement of the posterior margin delineation in terms of safety and oncological adequacy. Translation into the clinical setting, with a meticulous assessment of the oncological outcomes, will be the proposed next step.

Keywords: intraoperative navigation (NIV), 3D-virtual endoscopy, surgical margins, maxillary sinus cancers, transnasal endoscopic surgery

INTRODUCTION

Resection of advanced maxillary sinus cancers can be particularly challenging due to the anatomical proximity to surrounding neural and vascular structures. This challenge creates a dilemma for surgical treatment as one is balancing between an adequate margin of resection and potential morbidity. Over the last three decades, the evolution of transnasal endoscopic surgery and improvements in adjuvant treatments have been considerably impacting the management of sinonasal cancer (1–13). Transnasal endoscopy can be considered the standard of treatment for many adequately selected nasoethmoidal malignancies; in addition, it can effectively aid the delineation of critical margins of resection even in the setting of open approaches for advanced sinonasal cancers (i.e., endoscopic-assisted maxillectomy and cranioendoscopic resection) (13, 14). With the era of endoscopic and minimal access surgical ablations, there has been increasing reliance on imaging for patient selection and for prediction of volume of ablation. The ability to increasingly employ intraoperative near real-time on-the-table surgical navigation (SN) to improve margin-negative resection is upon us.

With the advent of new technologies, particularly in the area of intraoperative imaging, the ability to increase the confidence and performance of margin-negative tumor resections while maximizing the preservation of normal anatomical structures is imminent. Specifically, determining the posterior margin (PM) of the resection during maxillectomy surgery is a challenge and has prompted researchers to propose solutions addressing this problem (13, 15–19). Correct delineation of the PM of a maxillectomy requires the surgeon to build a three-dimensional (3D) mental image of the tumor based on preoperative imaging. Even in the hands of experienced surgeons, this process can be difficult, and minor deviations in the position and orientation of the margin can significantly affect the cut trajectory with respect to the tumor and critical anatomical structures.

Since the early 1990s, SN has emerged as a useful aid and evolved parallel to transnasal endoscopic surgery, particularly with the intent to avoiding complications (20). SN in the craniomaxillofacial region has been proven to be useful in the assessment of the adequacy of reconstruction and for the planning of osteotomies during oncologic ablations (21–23). Moreover, SN has provided improved accuracy of craniomaxillofacial osteotomies (24, 25), and proportional improvement of clinical outcomes can be hypothesized based on preliminary experiences (26–29). Implementation of endoscopy with 3D-rendered SN with virtual endoscopy (3D-SNVE) may represent a significant step forward.

The aims of this preclinical study were to test and quantify the benefits provided by 3D-SNVE in terms of adequate delineation of the PM in models of advanced maxillary tumors that would require an open maxillectomy.

MATERIALS AND METHODS

Tumor Model Preparation

Four artificial skulls (Sawbones®, Vashon Island, WA, USA) and a moldable material (Play-Doh®, Hasbro®, Pawtucket, RI, USA) mixed with acrylic glue were employed to build four models (S1–S4) of locally advanced maxillary sinus tumors with varying degrees of posterior tumor extension. The degree of posterior extension in each model is described in terms of the involvement of anatomical spaces/structures and the closest distance from the internal carotid artery (ICA) (tumor–carotid distance, T–C distance), as follows: 1) invasion of the pterygopalatine fossa (PPF) (T–C distance = 14.9 mm, model S1); 2) invasion of the medial pterygoid plate, pterygoid fossa, and base of the pterygoid process (T–C distance = 10.2 mm, model S2); 3) complete invasion of the pterygoid process (T–C distance = 6.2 mm, model S3); and 4) invasion of the anterior foramen lacerum and upper parapharyngeal space (T–C distance = 3.5 mm, model S4) (**Figure 1**). Each tumor model was created based on actual cases of maxillary cancers treated between January 2016 and December 2018 in the Unit of Otorhinolaryngology – Head and Neck Surgery of the University of Brescia (Brescia, Italy). The tumor models were based on preoperative magnetic resonance imaging (MRI) (**Figure 1**). Soft tissues in the models were simulated using

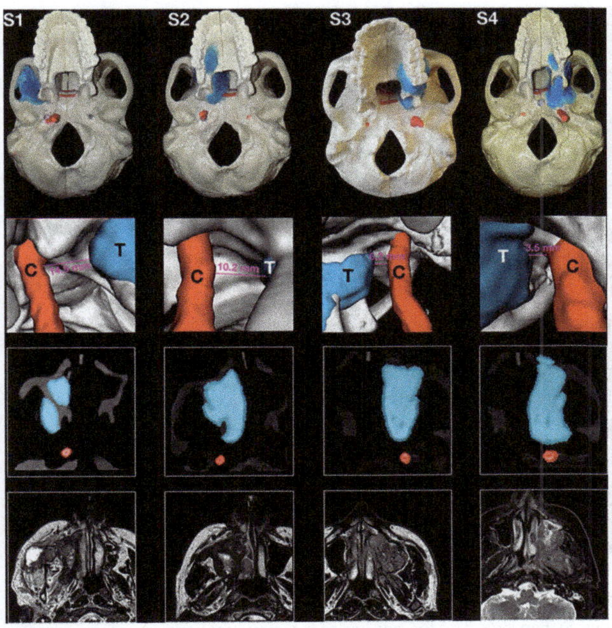

FIGURE 1 | Panel with four phantoms, as seen from an inferior perspective (*superior row*); 3D rendering of the tumor and the carotid alongside the tumor–carotid distance for each model (*second row*); and appearance of tumors at the computed tomography imaging alongside contouring of the tumor and the carotid (*third row*); and preoperative magnetic resonance imaging (MRI) of four actual cases of maxillary cancers (*inferior row*).

medical gauzes to restrict tumor visualization to only the endoscopic and transoral views (i.e., simulating tumors ulcerating into the sinonasal and/or oral cavity). The anterior third of the nasal septum was simulated with a 3-mm slice of silicon, fixed orthotopically to the skull with acrylic glue. As a result of silicon elasticity, the anterior nasal septum could be partially tilted and displaced with the scope and instruments during simulations. The ICAs in the models were created from an angio-CT that was done in a neurological workup for an anonymized patient and were semi-automatically contoured through Mimics® (Materialise, Leuven, Belgium). Firstly, a global threshold was applied to provide a quick gross segmentation, and then manual refinement was used to smooth the segmentation. Respective stereolithography (STL) files were generated and ICAs were 3D printed (3D Printer Dimension 1200es System; Stratasys, Eden Prairie, MN, USA) and painted with red dye mixed with iodine solution for CT contrast (Omnipaque; GE Healthcare, Chicago, IL, USA). A carotid canal was manually created in the base of the artificial skulls, and each ICA was fixed in the anatomical situation. The area for simulation of transnasal PM delineation was marked by horizontal lines in the phantoms and further classified into a superior and an inferior part based on the plane passing through the inferior aspect of the nasopharyngeal vault (**Figure 2C**).

Surgical Pointer Tool Preparation

Custom surgical pointers were designed using Autodesk Fusion 360 software (San Rafael, CA, USA) and 3D printed on a Dimension 1200es System (Stratasys, Eden Prairie, MN, USA).

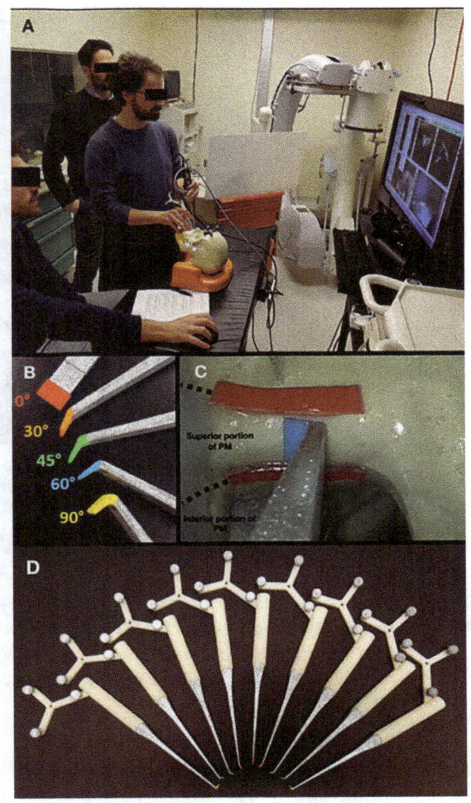

FIGURE 2 | **(A)** Simulation setting. **(B)** Pointers with different types of angled tips. **(C)** Endoscopic view, with *red lines* indicating the superior and inferior potions of the posterior margin (PM); **(D)** Pointers with angled tips with different angles (0°, 30°, 45°, 60°, and 90°) and directions (right or left).

Surgeons participating in the simulations were provided with color-coded pointers with different angulations (0°, 30°, 45°, 60°, and 90°) (**Figures 2A, B, D**). Each pointer was meant to simulate the trajectory of delineation of the PM of resection, so that the surgeon could select which trajectory best represented the way he/she would have set the PM of resection from a transnasal perspective.

Image Acquisition and Tumor Contouring

Three-dimensional images of each skull model were acquired using a prototype cone-beam computed tomography (CBCT) imaging system on a mobile C-arm (30, 31). The mentioned flat-panel imaging system was validated for guidance of head and neck procedures involving significant bone resection and/or complex anatomical reconstruction (32). In this study, 3D volumes (256 × 256 × 192) covered a field of view of 20 × 20 × 15 cm^3 using isotropic 0.8-mm 3D voxels. On CBCT imaging, the tumor and carotid models were clearly distinguishable from the artificial bone, as they showed a much higher X-ray attenuation (**Figures 1** and **3**). Contouring of the tumors and the ICAs was obtained semi-automatically using a two-step process within the NIRFAST-Slicer software (33). Firstly, a global threshold was applied to provide a quick,

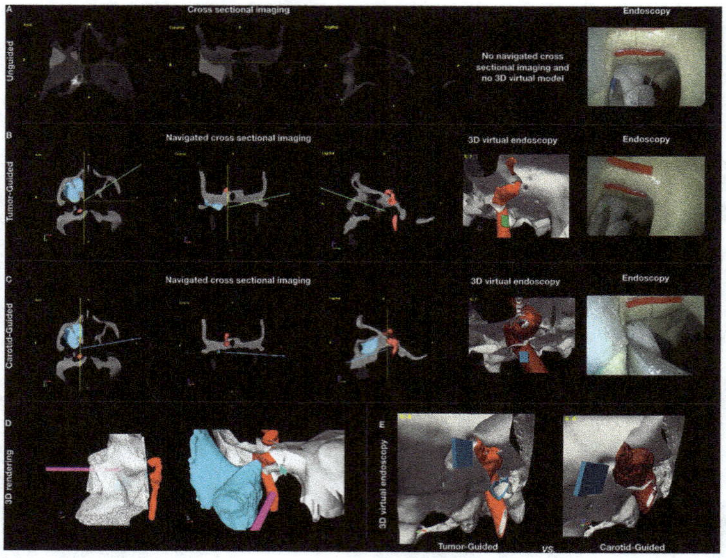

FIGURE 3 | **(A–C)** Panel showing the appearance of the different settings of data acquisition: unguided simulations with cross-sectional imaging pre-simulation analysis **(A)**, tumor-guided **(B)**, and carotid-guided **(C)** simulations with real-time surgical navigation indicating the position of the instrument and the posterior margin delineation. **(D)** Pictures showing the appearance of the 3D rendering of the skull with the positions of the scope and pointer. Virtual margin delineation, simulating the cut of 3D objects (skull, tumor, and carotid). **(E)** Comparison of the 3D virtual endoscopy appearance in the tumor-guided and carotid-guided settings.

coarse segmentation, and then manual refinement was used to smooth the segmentation. To visualize a virtual surgical margin around the ICA (**Figure 3**), a semi-transparent wireframe was generated at 2 mm from the vessel surface using volumetric image dilation processing in MATLAB software (MathWorks, Natick, MA, USA).

Navigation System

CBCT images were displayed within an in-house navigation software package (GTx-Eyes) based on the open-source Image-Guided Surgery Toolkit (34, 35). Tumor and margin segmentations were superimposed on three-planar views and separately as 3D surface renderings. Surgical tool tracking in this study was provided by a stereoscopic infrared camera (Polaris Spectra, NDI, Waterloo, Canada). Image-to-tracker registration was obtained by paired-point matching of predrilled divots by means of a tracked pointer. A small four-sphere reference tool (NDI, Waterloo, Canada) was anchored to the skull throughout the registration and simulations. A registration error of 1 mm or less was considered acceptable for the navigation experiments. A four-sphere reference (Medtronic, Jacksonville, FL, USA) was secured to each 3D printed tool (surgical pointer) and to a Storz® endoscope (Karl Storz Group, Tuttlingen, Germany), which was then calibrated using a custom calibration jig. Angled pointer navigation was implemented using software features for virtual planar tool clipping (e.g., osteotome or saw) and colored accuracy indicators for distance, pitch, and roll developed previously for orthopedic oncology applications (36) and subsequently applied to open head and neck procedures (24, 25, 37). In this study, for transnasal simulations, the 3D rendering of the virtual endoscopic view could be freely rotated and the skull rendering clipped along the virtual cutting plane during the transnasal delineation of the PM (**Figure 3**).

Surgical Simulation

Surgeons from the Department of Otolaryngology - Head and Neck Surgery of the University Health Network (Toronto, ON, Canada) and from the Unit of Otorhinolaryngology - Head and Neck Surgery of the University of Brescia (Brescia, Italy) were recruited for the simulations. Each surgeon received a brief explanation of the steps of the simulation and of the subsequent analysis methods. The surgical task was to choose among pointers with different angulations (0°, 30°, 45°, 60°, and 90°) and position the selected pointer under transnasal endoscopy guidance within the delineated areas (i.e., superior and inferior parts of the PM of resection) to provide a clear margin from the tumor posterior surface while avoiding intersection with the ipsilateral ICA. No physical cuts were performed to allow reuse of the models; rather, the pointer position and orientation were recorded when the surgeon gave vocal confirmation of his/her proposed delineation of the margin, and the analysis was performed on the virtual trajectory. Surgeons were asked to define the superior and posterior parts of the PM with two endoscopes (0° and 45°), first using only the surgical corridor of the ipsilateral nasal cavity and then through either a bilateral (i.e., with the scope through one nostril and pointer through the other) or a contralateral approach (i.e., with both scope and the pointer through the contralateral nostril). Surgeons were required to perform the PM delineation in three settings—1) unguided, 2) tumor-guided, and 3) carotid-guided—as shown in **Figure 3**. In the unguided simulation, the surgeons could only view the cross-sectional images (i.e., axial, sagittal, and coronal) prior to starting transnasal endoscopy, with no access to the real-time navigation system or the 3D tumor/margin renderings. In the tumor-guided simulation, virtual angled pointers were guided using real-time tool tracking and the 3D tumor and carotid segmentation (**Figure 3**). Finally, in the carotid-guided simulation, a 2-mm alert cloud surrounding the carotid was added to the tumor-guided setting; in this setting, a sonic alarm reproducing the arterial flow sound at Doppler examination was sounded when the trajectory of the PM definition was through the proximity alert zone (38), and a beeping sonic alarm was activated when the trajectory of the PM definition was through the ICA (**Figure 3**).

To avoid recall bias, the phantoms were randomized for each surgeon and the sequence of the phantoms was arranged such that the guided and unguided simulations were never performed at close intervals. The rationale for this was based on the belief that guided simulations could have enhanced adequate pointer orientation in a subsequent unguided task. Written informed consent was obtained from the individuals for the publication of any potentially identifiable images or data included in this article.

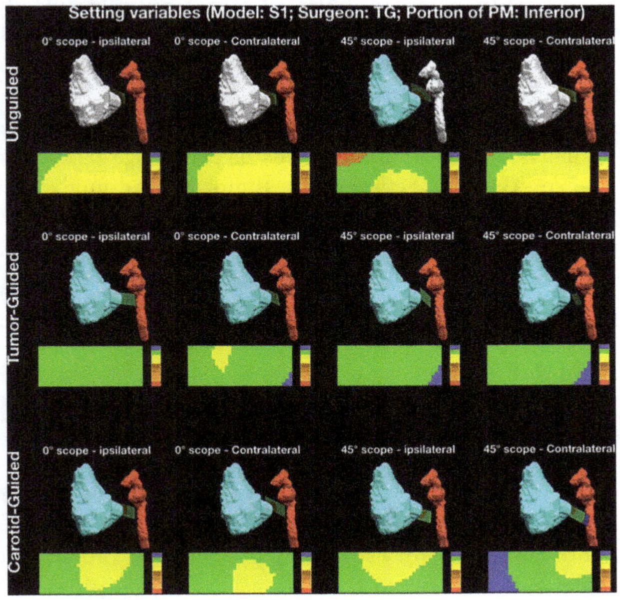

FIGURE 4 | Example of the analysis of posterior margin delineation. Each *point* of the isolated area was classified as follows: "red" (*R*), into the internal carotid artery (ICA); "orange 1" (*O1*), <2 mm from the ICA and into the tumor; "orange 2" (*O2*), <2 mm from the ICA and <5 mm from the tumor; "orange 3" (*O3*), <2 mm from the ICA and 5–10 mm from the tumor; "orange 4" (*O4*), <2 mm from the ICA and >10 mm from the tumor; "yellow 1" (*Y1*), >2 mm from the ICA and into the tumor; "yellow 2" (*Y2*), >2 mm from the ICA and <5 mm from the tumor; "green" (G), >2 mm from the ICA and 5–10 mm from the tumor; and "blue" (*B*), >2 mm from the ICA and >10 mm from the tumor. *PM*, posterior margin.

Virtual Cutting Plane Analysis

Analysis of the cutting planes was performed by means of MATLAB software (MathWorks, Natick, MA, USA). An area of 30-mm length along the longitudinal axis of the cut and 11-mm width (5.5 mm on both sides with respect to the longitudinal axis) was isolated from each plane starting from the pointer tip. The minimal distance with respect to the tumor and ICA surfaces was calculated for each point making up the isolated area and reproduced as a distribution of distances shown as a 30 × 11-mm^2 (length × width) color-scaled image (**Figure 4**). The cutting plane was deemed to be "intratumoral" when the distance from the cutting plane to the tumor was ≤0 mm and "adequate" when it was >0 mm. If the cutting plane was ≤0 mm to the ICA wall, the ICA was considered "damaged", while a 0- to 2-mm margin to the ICA was deemed to be a "danger zone". An "adequate" distance was defined as >2 mm. Each point of the isolated area was classified as follows: "red" (R), into the ICA; "orange 1" (O1), <2 mm from the ICA and into the tumor; "orange 2" (O2), <2 mm from the ICA and <5 mm from the tumor; "orange 3" (O3), <2 mm from the ICA and 5–10 mm from the tumor; "orange 4" (O4), <2 mm from the ICA and >10 mm from the tumor; "yellow 1" (Y1), >2 mm from the ICA and into the tumor; "yellow 2" (Y2), >2 mm from the ICA and <5 mm from the tumor; "green" (G), >2 mm from the ICA and 5–10 mm from the tumor; and "blue" (B), >2 mm from the ICA and >10 mm from the tumor. Each isolated area was described as a distribution among the above-mentioned categories.

Surgeon Questionnaire

At the end of the simulations, each surgeon was asked to complete a validated questionnaire (38) (**Table 1**) in order to quantify opinions about the gain in terms of speed, accuracy, and self-confidence using tool tracking and the proximity alerts alongside the readiness for clinical translation of the technology.

Statistical Analysis

Statistical analysis was run through XLSTAT® (Addinsoft®, Long Island, NY, USA). Simulations were grouped into three

TABLE 1 | Questionnaire answers and surgeons' responses.

Statements for questionnaire (38)	Median (IQR)[a]
I felt faster to perform surgery when aided by the virtual view.	6.0 (6.0–6.8)
The system appeared to be sufficiently accurate for its intended use.	6.0 (6.0–6.0)
The dynamic tool tracking allowed me to quickly assess my proximity to critical structures without significantly interrupting dissection.	6.0 (6.0–6.8)
Proximity alerts increased my confidence during ablation close to critical structures.	6.0 (6.0–6.8)
The current technology is ready for clinical trial without significant changes.	5.5 (4.3–6.0)

IQR, interquartile range.
[a]*Based on a seven-point Likert scale (7 = strongly agree; 1 = strongly disagree).*

categories: unguided, tumor-guided, and carotid-guided. These three groups were compared in terms of the distance distributions through a bilateral Kruskal–Wallis test and the Steel–Dwass–Critchlow–Fligner *post-hoc* test. The rates of intratumoral and intra-ICA virtual cuts among the three groups of simulations were assessed with Fisher's exact test. Intraindividual differences in terms of percentage of adequate distance (G area) between the tumor/carotid-guided and unguided groups of simulations were calculated and considered as the "gain" provided by 3D-SNVE. The level of significance was set at 0.05 for all statistical tests.

RESULTS

Eight head and neck surgeons with heterogeneous experience (ranging from 3 to 13 years of experience) in oncologic endoscopic resections participated in the study. Five surgeons completed head and neck fellowship training, while three were attending a residency training program at the time of simulations. Overall, 612 PM transnasal delineations were simulated, namely, 204 per group (i.e., unguided, tumor-guided, carotid-guided). The registration error was <1 mm in all simulations. Surgeons chose to use the 0°, 30°, 45°, 60°, and 90° pointers in 0 (0%), 61 (11%), 99 (18%), 246 (45%), and 138 (25%) transnasal simulations, respectively. Surgeons indicated that the surgical exposure was not adequate in 68 (11%) of the simulations, of which 61 (90%) were through a transnasal ipsilateral approach, and no plane trajectories were recorded in these cases.

The virtual delineation of the PM of resection in maxillary tumor models transgressed the tumor in 47 (25.4%), 7 (4.0%), and 4 (2.2%) cases in the unguided, tumor-guided, and carotid-guided procedures, respectively ($p < 0.0001$). The virtual margin delineation was more than 2 mm to the ICA in 80 (43.2%), 104 (59.4%), and 111 (60.3%) cases in the unguided, tumor-guided, and carotid-guided procedures, respectively ($p < 0.0001$) and involved the ICA in 79 (42.7%), 30 (17.1%), and 25 (13.6%) cases in the unguided, tumor-guided, and carotid-guided procedures, respectively ($p < 0.0001$).

Simulation tumor model S1 had a significantly lower rate of points falling into the carotid (at least one point into the carotid in 6% of simulations) and in the 2-mm carotid alert zone (at least one point into the alert zone in 7% of simulations) when compared to phantoms S2, S3, and S4 (32%, 30%, and 18% of intra-carotid simulations and 32%, 36%, and 35% of intra-alert zone simulations, respectively; $p < 0.0001$ for both comparisons). The rate of clear margin (i.e., margin not crossing the tumor) was not significantly different among the four phantoms (92%, 86%, 90%, and 87% for S1, S2, S3, and S4, respectively; $p = 0.33$).

The percentage of points falling within the tumor volume was significantly higher in the group of unguided simulations compared to the tumor- and carotid-guided ones ($p < 0.0001$) (**Table 2**). In a bivariate analysis, the guidance proved to be associated with a higher rate of clear margin ($p < 0.0001$) and a lower rate of carotid damage ($p < 0.0001$), independently of the increasing difficulty of the tumor–carotid model.

3D-SNVE significantly improved the rate of identification of an adequate plane of dissection while reducing the risk of carotid damage: the percentage of "red" points was significantly lower in the two guided groups with respect to the unguided group ($p < 0.0001$) (**Table 2**), and the percentage of points with an adequate distance from the carotid and the tumor simultaneously (i.e., "green" points) was significantly higher in the guided groups when compared to the unguided group ($p < 0.0001$) (**Table 2**).

The gain of margin delineation provided by 3D-SNVE (considering both tumor- and carotid-guided settings) was, on average, 24.2% (ranging from 0.0% to 33.3%, when analyzing single-surgeon results) in terms of obtaining clear margins and 25.7% (ranging from 1.8% to 59.6%, when analyzing single-surgeon results) in terms of avoiding carotid damage. The heterogeneity of training and experience resulted in a significant variability of the rates of intratumoral unguided cuts between surgeons (average value = 9.6%, range = 0.0%–16.7%, $p = 0.039$), but the gain in the adequacy of margin delineation provided by 3D-SNVE was statistically independent of the operator ($p = 0.202$).

Surgeon Preference

All surgeons preferred using a bilateral transseptal approach to have better vision and working volume in all models. Surgeons felt more self-confident using the 0° and 45° scopes in 68% and 32% of unguided simulations and in 46% and 54% of guided simulations, respectively. When using 3D-SNVE, surgeons

TABLE 2 | Average percentage of points of the virtual margin delineation in each category of the "color code" according to the guidance setting.

Color code	Description	% of Cutting planes			*p*-value
		Unguided	Tumor-guided	Carotid-guided	
Red	Into the carotid	6.7	0.9	1.0	$p < 0.0001$
Orange 1	<2 mm carotid, into the tumor	0.0	0.0	0.0	NS
Orange 2	<2 mm carotid, <5 mm tumor	0.3	0.2	0.3	NS
Orange 3	<2 mm carotid, 5–10 mm tumor	4.3	2.8	2.1	$p < 0.0001$
Orange 4	<2 mm carotid, >10 mm tumor	1.6	0.2	0.4	$p < 0.0001$
Yellow 1	>2 mm carotid, into the tumor	3.6	0.4	0.2	$p < 0.0001$
Yellow 2	>2 mm carotid, <5 mm tumor	19.1	23.8	23.5	$p = 0.041$
Green	>2 mm carotid, 5–10 mm tumor	52.4	62.1	64.9	$p < 0.0001$
Blue	>2 mm carotid, >10 mm tumor	12.1	9.5	7.5	NS

NS, not significant.

preferred the carotid-guided setting in 61% of the simulations and the tumor-guided in 39%.

Questionnaire Score

The seven-point Likert scale questionnaire statements and median (interquartile range, IQR) responses are shown in **Table 1**. No subject strongly disagreed (scores 1–2) with any of the statements. Only one gave a negative response (score of 3) to question 1. One gave a negative response (score of 3) and two gave a neutral response (score of 4) to question 7. There was universal agreement (scores 5–7) for all other questions, with uniform responses across the subjects.

DISCUSSION

The present preclinical study demonstrates the beneficial role of 3D-SNVE in PM delineation and ICA preservation in ablative surgery for advanced maxillary tumors.

The frequency of "positive" margins decreased from 27% to 3% when the surgeon used navigation during the simulation, and carotid damage decreased from 41% to 15%. Since margin control still represents a challenging goal in the surgical management of such cancers, implementation of 3D-SNVE into surgical practice is a promising strategy for the future. Furthermore, the possibility of adding 3D rendering of the critical structures on virtual views and cross-sectional imaging with associated sound alerts may increase the confidence of the surgeon during the procedure and help avoid life-threatening complications.

While surgery combined with neoadjuvant and adjuvant radiation and chemotherapy has improved the overall outcomes of advanced sinonasal cancers, surgery still remains the principal modality of treatment (39–41). Clear-margin resection has been proven to significantly impact patient prognosis and can be considered the most important surgeon-controllable variable (13, 42–45). Endoscopic surgery has been shown to improve the surgical precision and to reduce the morbidity of certain procedures. The benefits of guiding margin delineation in open maxillectomies through an endoscopic transnasal approach was demonstrated by Deganello et al. (13), who reported this technique as facilitating the detachment of the maxilla from the skull base and allowing for a more precise delineation of the posterior and medial margins of resection. This endoscopic technique was used to treat 79 advanced tumors involving the maxilla with a low rate of microscopic involvement of the PM (3.8%) (13). The authors classified posterior endoscopic resection into three types according to the anatomical structures progressively involved and found that, even in the most complex scenario (i.e., type 3 resection), the rate of free PM was remarkably high (87.5%) (13).

In previous clinical studies by Catanzaro et al. (26) and Tarsitano et al. (29), 3D navigation was helpful in achieving a significantly higher rate of clear deep margin when implemented to the standard procedure for advanced maxillary, oral, or orbital cancers (i.e., ablation followed by mapping of the surgical bed with frozen section biopsies). More recently, in studying maxillectomy surgery, Ricotta et al. (46) confirmed that the rate of overall positive margins was higher in the control group (10 patients) compared to that in a group of 18 patients operated on with SN.

A preclinical study by Ferrari et al. (24) was performed using a previous version of the same in-house navigation system employed here. That study evaluated cutting planes for osteotomies in open surgery of sinonasal advanced cancers and demonstrated a substantial benefit in the delineation of the virtual osteotomies both for novel and experienced surgeons.

The present study adds to this previous work by testing the navigation system in a more complex setting, with critical anatomical structures close to the tumor. In addition to the complexity of the tumor–vessel model, further development of real-time tool tracking with 3D virtual endoscopy for angled endoscopes allowed visual overlay of the structures beyond the confines of the nasal wall and further allowed clipping of the endoscopic 3D rendering along the angled pointer trajectory.

The surgical treatment of maxillary tumors requires accurate delineation of the posterior boundary of the resection in a very complex area with surrounding critical anatomical structures. The surgeon needs to base the ablation planning on a mental representation of the tumor and surrounding structures, relying upon specific anatomical landmarks identified throughout the dissection, and this task becomes particularly challenging at the PM owing to poor visualization and maneuverability. Furthermore, cancers frequently have an irregular shape and have complex patterns of invasion into neighboring structures (47). The use of 3D navigation provides the surgeon with a real-time direct visualization of the tumor and the adjacent critical structures and facilitates positioning and orienting the margin with respect to the tumor and critical structures. The clinical translation of this navigation approach may help in achieving a balance between the adequacy of the oncological resection and preservation of the uninvolved surrounding anatomical structures. This benefit of the navigation has already been demonstrated in the field of pelvic tumor resection (36).

In our preclinical study, a significant improvement in the virtual delineation of maxillectomy PM with high rates of complete and ICA-sparing virtual resection was demonstrated when 3D-SNVE was employed. The benefit of margin delineation guided by SN in terms of oncologic adequacy and critical structure preservation was remarkable (average gain of 24.2% in obtaining clear margins and 25.7% in avoiding carotid damage). Despite the heterogeneity of training and experience, which resulted in a significant variability of the rates of intratumoral unguided cuts (p = 0.039), the gain in the adequacy of margin delineation when relying on 3D-SNVE was statistically independent of the surgeon (p = 0.202). This result suggests that SN could be beneficial both for expert and novice surgeons. The most reasonable explanation is that the 3D visualization of the tumor facilitates margin delineation, thus partially compensating for lack of experience in 3D mental representation of the tumor position and boundaries. In addition, with more extensive use of this technology, a learning curve with further improvements in surgical precision and time required can be expected, as already observed in other studies focusing on SN in the sinonasal area (21).

Margins were not classified into either adequate or close for two main reasons: 1) the definition of a "negative", "close", or a "positive" margin is not clear for sinonasal cancer resections, and 2) a complete resection with a 5-mm or wider margin is hardly ever achievable in sinonasal cancers. In the present study, we created phantoms with tumor models mimicking real cases with a very critical posterior extension, in which the minimal distance between the ICA and the tumor was 8.7 mm, on average (median = 8.2 mm, range = 3.5–14.9 mm).

The preclinical nature of the present study represents its main limitation, as the results could be potentially biased by the "ideal" conditions of the laboratory setting. Therefore, the benefits conferred by 3D-SNVE should be interpreted cautiously. However, the preliminary clinical data published in the literature are in agreement with the conclusion of our experiment (26, 28, 29, 37, 46). Translation of 3D-SNVE into clinical research should be the next step in order to test the potential benefits on patient outcomes with application in live surgery and in the environment of an operating room. Another limitation was that an arbitrary area of 30 × 11 mm was chosen to simulate the endoscopic PM delineation; in real surgery, the margin shape would result more irregular and variably sized.

The authors acknowledge that repeating simulations with the same technology, even if with different guidance modalities, may have caused a "learning effect". Future studies will also investigate the benefits of navigation across a wider range of experience levels, including senior staff.

CONCLUSION

This preclinical study has demonstrated the substantial benefit of 3D-SNVE for PM definition in advanced maxillary tumors. This technology is expected to improve resection margins and potentially reduce critical structure injury, thus optimizing the oncological adequacy and overall safety of the resection simultaneously. Translation into the clinical setting, with a thoughtful analysis of oncological outcomes, is the proposed next step.

AUTHOR CONTRIBUTIONS

ST, MF, MD, JI, RG, and PN contributed to the study concepts. MF, MD, ST, and HC designed the study. ST, MD, MF, TG, DE, AJ, ASa, WH, ASe, IB, and JD helped with data acquisition. All authors analyzed and interpreted the data. ST, MF, and MD performed the statistical analysis. ST, MF, and MD prepared the manuscript. ST, MF, MD, JI, RG, and PN edited the manuscript. All authors contributed to the article and approved the submitted version.

REFERENCES

1. Nicolai P, Castelnuovo P, Bolzoni Villaret A. Endoscopic Resection of Sinonasal Malignancies. *Curr Oncol Rep* (2011) 13(2):138–44. doi: 10.1007/s11912-011-0151-6
2. Hanna E, DeMonte F, Ibrahim S, Roberts D, Levine N, Kupferman M. Endoscopic Resection of Sinonasal Cancers With and Without Craniotomy: Oncologic Results. *Arch Otolaryngol Head Neck Surg* (2009) 135(12):1219–24. doi: 10.1001/archoto.2009.173
3. Lund V, Howard DJ, Wei WI. Endoscopic Resection of Malignant Tumors of the Nose and Sinuses. *Am J Rhinol* (2007) 21(1):89–94. doi: 10.2500/ajr.2007.21.2957
4. Castelnuovo P, Battaglia P, Turri-Zanoni M, Tomei G, Locatelli D, Bignami M, et al. Endoscopic Endonasal Surgery for Malignancies of the Anterior Cranial Base. *World Neurosurg* (2014) 82(6 Suppl):S22–31. doi: 10.1016/j.wneu.2014.07.021
5. Moya-Plana A, Bresson D, Temam S, Kolb F, Janot F, Herman P. Development of Minimally Invasive Surgery for Sinonasal Malignancy. *Eur Ann Otorhinolaryngol Head Neck Dis* (2016) 133(6):405–11. doi: 10.1016/j.anorl.2016.06.001
6. Snyderman CH, Carrau RL, Kassam AB, Zanation A, Prevedello D, Gardner P, et al. Endoscopic Skull Base Surgery: Principles of Endonasal Oncological Surgery. *J Surg Oncol* (2008) 97(8):658–64. doi: 10.1002/jso.21020
7. Lund VJ, Wei WI. Endoscopic Surgery for Malignant Sinonasal Tumours: An Eighteen Year Experience. *Rhinology* (2015) 53(3):204–11. doi: 10.4193/Rhin14.318
8. Nicolai P, Battaglia P, Bignami M, Bolzoni Villaret A, Delù G, Khrais T, et al. Endoscopic Surgery for Malignant Tumors of the Sinonasal Tract and Adjacent Skull Base: A 10-Year Experience. *Am J Rhinol* (2008) 22(3):308–16. doi: 10.2500/ajr.2008.22.3170
9. Villaret AB, Yakirevitch A, Bizzoni A, Bosio R, Bignami M, Pistochini A, et al. Endoscopic Transnasal Craniectomy in the Management of Selected Sinonasal Malignancies. *Am J Rhinol Allergy* (2010) 24(1):60–5. doi: 10.2500/ajra.2010.24.3397
10. Lund VJ, Stammberger H, Nicolai P, Castelnuovo P, Beal T, Beham A, et al. European Position Paper on Endoscopic Management of Tumours of the Nose, Paranasal Sinuses and Skull Base. *Rhinol Suppl* (2010) 22:1–143.
11. Ferrari M, Bossi P, Mattavelli D, Ardighieri L, Nicolai P. Management of Sinonasal Adenocarcinomas With Anterior Skull Base Extension. *J Neurooncol* (2020). doi: 10.1007/s11060-019-03385-8
12. Snyderman CH, Pant H, Carrau RL, Prevedello D, Gardner P, Kassam AB. What are the Limits of Endoscopic Sinus Surgery?: The Expanded Endonasal Approach to the Skull Base. *Keio J Med* (2009) 58(3):152–60. doi: 10.2302/kjm.58.152
13. Deganello A, Ferrari M, Paderno A, Turri-Zanoni M, Schreiber A, Mattavelli D, et al. Endoscopic-Assisted Maxillectomy: Operative Technique and Control of Surgical Margins. *Oral Oncol* (2019) 93:29–38. doi: 10.1016/j.oraloncology.2019.04.002
14. Naunheim MR, Goyal N, Dedmon MM, Chambers KJ, Sedaghat AR, Bleier BS, et al. An Algorithm for Surgical Approach to the Anterior Skull Base. *J Neurol Surg Part B Skull Base* (2016) 77(4):364–70. doi: 10.1055/s-0036-1580598
15. Balm AJM, Smeele LE, Lohuis PJFM. Optimizing Exposure of the Posterolateral Maxillary and Pterygoid Region: The Lower Cheek Flap. *Eur J Surg Oncol EJSO* (2008) 34(6):699–703. doi: 10.1016/j.ejso.2007.08.009
16. Chatni SS, Sharan R, Patel D, Iyer S, Tiwari RM, Kuriakose MA. Transmandibular Approach for Excision of Maxillary Sinus Tumors Extending to Pterygopalatine and Infratemporal Fossae. *Oral Oncol* (2009) 45(8):720–6. doi: 10.1016/j.oraloncology.2008.11.005
17. Kreeft AM, Smeele LE, Rasch CR, Hauptmann M, Rietveld DH, Leemans CR, et al. Preoperative Imaging and Surgical Margins in Maxillectomy Patients. *Head Neck* (2012) 34(11):1652–6. doi: 10.1002/hed.21987
18. Sun J, Shen Y, Weng Y-Q, Li J, Zhang Z-Y. Lateral Lip-Splitting Approach for

Total and Subtotal Maxillectomy. *J Oral Maxillofac Surg* (2009) 67(6):1197–205. doi: 10.1016/j.joms.2008.06.078

19. McMahon JD, Crowther J, Taylor WM, Wong LS, Paterson T, Devine J, et al. Anterolateral Corridor Approach to the Infratemporal Fossa and Central Skull Base in Maxillectomy: Rationale and Technical Aspects. *Br J Oral Maxillofac Surg* (2015) 53(9):814–9. doi: 10.1016/j.bjoms.2015.06.006
20. Citardi MJ, Yao W, Luong A. Next-Generation Surgical Navigation Systems in Sinus and Skull Base Surgery. *Otolaryngol Clin North Am* (2017) 50(3):617–32. doi: 10.1016/j.otc.2017.01.012
21. Azarmehr I, Stokbro K, Bell RB, Thygesen T. Surgical Navigation: A Systematic Review of Indications, Treatments, and Outcomes in Oral and Maxillofacial Surgery. *J Oral Maxillofac Surg Off J Am Assoc Oral Maxillofac Surg* (2017) 75(9):1987–2005. doi: 10.1016/j.joms.2017.01.004
22. Schramm A, Gellrich NC, Gutwald R, Schipper J, Bloss H, Hustedt H, et al. Indications for Computer-Assisted Treatment of Cranio-Maxillofacial Tumors. *Comput Aided Surg Off J Int Soc Comput Aided Surg* (2000) 5 (5):343–52. doi: 10.1002/1097-0150(2000)5:5<343::AID-IGS4>3.0.CO;2-1
23. Schramm A, Suarez-Cunqueiro MM, Barth EL, Essig H, Bormann KH, Kokemueller H, et al. Computer-Assisted Navigation in Craniomaxillofacial Tumors. *J Craniofac Surg* (2008) 19(4):1067–74. doi: 10.1097/SCS.0b013e3181760fc0
24. Ferrari M, Daly MJ, Douglas CM, Chan HHL, Qiu J, Deganello A, et al. Navigation-Guided Osteotomies Improve Margin Delineation in Tumors Involving the Sinonasal Area: A Preclinical Study. *Oral Oncol* (2019) 99:104463. doi: 10.1016/j.oraloncology.2019.104463
25. Bernstein JM, Daly MJ, Chan H, Qiu J, Goldstein D, Muhanna N, et al. Accuracy and Reproducibility of Virtual Cutting Guides and 3D-Navigation for Osteotomies of the Mandible and Maxilla. *PloS One* (2017) 12(3): e0173111. doi: 10.1371/journal.pone.0173111
26. Catanzaro S, Copelli C, Manfuso A, Tewfik K, Pederneschi N, Cassano L, et al. Intraoperative Navigation in Complex Head and Neck Resections: Indications and Limits. *Int J Comput Assist Radiol Surg* (2017) 12(5):881–7. doi: 10.1007/s11548-016-1486-0
27. Guo R, Guo YX, Feng Z, Guo CB. Application of a Computer-Aided Navigation Technique in Surgery for Recurrent Malignant Infratemporal Fossa Tumors. *J Craniofac Surg* (2015) 26(2):e126–32. doi: 10.1097/SCS.0000000000001350
28. Feichtinger M, Pau M, Zemann W, Aigner RM, Kärcher H. Intraoperative Control of Resection Margins in Advanced Head and Neck Cancer Using a 3D-Navigation System Based on PET/CT Image Fusion. *J Cranio-Maxillo-fac Surg Off Publ Eur Assoc Cranio-Maxillo-fac Surg* (2010) 38(8):589–94. doi: 10.1016/j.jcms.2010.02.004
29. Tarsitano A, Ricotta F, Baldino G, Badiali G, Pizzigallo A, Ramieri V, et al. Navigation-Guided Resection of Maxillary Tumours: The Accuracy of Computer-Assisted Surgery in Terms of Control of Resection Margins - A Feasibility Study. *J Cranio-Maxillo-fac Surg Off Publ Eur Assoc Cranio-Maxillo-fac Surg* (2017) 45(12):2109–14. doi: 10.1016/j.jcms.2017.09.023
30. Daly MJ, Siewerdsen JH, Moseley DJ, Jaffray DA, Irish JC. Intraoperative Cone-Beam CT for Guidance of Head and Neck Surgery: Assessment of Dose and Image Quality Using a C-Arm Prototype. *Med Phys* (2006) 33(10):3767–80. doi: 10.1118/1.2349687
31. Siewerdsen JH, Moseley DJ, Burch S, Bisland SK, Bogaards A, Wilson BC, et al. Volume CT With a Flat-Panel Detector on a Mobile, Isocentric C-Arm: Pre-Clinical Investigation in Guidance of Minimally Invasive Surgery. *Med Phys* (2005) 32(1):241–54. doi: 10.1118/1.1836331
32. King E, Daly MJ, Chan H, Bachar G, Dixon BJ, Siewerdsen JH, et al. Intraoperative Cone-Beam CT for Head and Neck Surgery: Feasibility of Clinical Implementation Using a Prototype Mobile C-Arm. *Head Neck* (2013) 35(7):959–67. doi: 10.1002/hed.23060
33. Jermyn M, Ghadyani H, Mastanduno MA, Turner W, Davis SC, Dehghani H, et al. Fast Segmentation and High-Quality Three-Dimensional Volume Mesh Creation From Medical Images for Diffuse Optical Tomography. *J BioMed Opt* (2013) 18(8):86007. doi: 10.1117/1.JBO.18.8.086007
34. Enquobahrie A, Cheng P, Gary K, Ibanez L, Gobbi D, Lindseth F, et al. The Image-Guided Surgery Toolkit IGSTK: An Open Source C++ Software Toolkit. *J Digit Imaging* (2007) 20(Suppl 1):21–33. doi: 10.1007/s10278-007-9054-3
35. Daly MJ, Chan H, Nithiananthan S, Qiu J, Barker E, Bachar G, et al. *Clinical Implementation of Intraoperative Cone-Beam CT in Head and Neck Surgery*, Vol. 796426. KH Wong, DR Holmes III, editors (2011). doi: 10.1117/12.878976
36. Sternheim A, Daly M, Qiu J, Weersink R, Chan H, Jaffray D, et al. Navigated Pelvic Osteotomy and Tumor Resection: A Study Assessing the Accuracy and Reproducibility of Resection Planes in Sawbones and Cadavers. *J Bone Joint Surg Am* (2015) 97(1):40–6. doi: 10.2106/JBJS.N.00276
37. Hasan W, Daly MJ, Chan HHL, Qiu J, Irish JC. Intraoperative Cone-Beam CT-Guided Osteotomy Navigation in Mandible and Maxilla Surgery. *Laryngoscope* (2020) 130(5):1166–72. doi: 10.1002/lary.28082
38. Dixon BJ, Daly MJ, Chan H, Vescan A, Witterick IJ, Irish JC. Augmented Real-Time Navigation With Critical Structure Proximity Alerts for Endoscopic Skull Base Surgery. *Laryngoscope* (2014) 124(4):853–9. doi: 10.1002/lary.24385
39. Castelnuovo P, Turri-Zanoni M, Battaglia P, Antognoni P, Bossi P, Locatelli D. Sinonasal Malignancies of Anterior Skull Base: Histology-Driven Treatment Strategies. *Otolaryngol Clin North Am* (2016) 49(1):183–200. doi: 10.1016/j.otc.2015.09.012
40. Ferrari M, Ioppi A, Schreiber A, Gualtieri T, Mattavelli D, Rampinelli V, et al. Malignant Tumors of the Maxillary Sinus: Prognostic Impact of Neurovascular Invasion in a Series of 138 Patients. *Oral Oncol* (2020) 106:104672. doi: 10.1016/j.oraloncology.2020.104672
41. López F, Lund VJ, Suárez C, Snyderman CH, Saba NF, Robbins KT, et al. The Impact of Histologic Phenotype in the Treatment of Sinonasal Cancer. *Adv Ther* (2017) 34(10):2181–98. doi: 10.1007/s12325-017-0605-9
42. Paulino AC, Marks JE, Bricker P, Melian E, Reddy SP, Emami B. Results of Treatment of Patients With Maxillary Sinus Carcinoma. *Cancer* (1998) 83 (3):457–65. doi: 10.1002/(SICI)1097-0142(19980801)83:3<457::AID-CNCR14>3.0.CO;2-V
43. Nishio N, Fujimoto Y, Fujii M, Saito K, Hiramatsu M, Maruo T, et al. Craniofacial Resection for T4 Maxillary Sinus Carcinoma: Managing Cases With Involvement of the Skull Base. *Otolaryngol Head Neck Surg Off J Am Acad Otolaryngol Head Neck Surg* (2015) 153(2):231–8. doi: 10.1177/0194599815586770
44. Ozsaran Z, Yalman D, Baltalarli B, Anacak Y, Esassolak M, Haydaroğlu A. Radiotherapy in Maxillary Sinus Carcinomas: Evaluation of 79 Cases. *Rhinology* (2003) 41(1):44–8.
45. Bristol IJ, Ahamad A, Garden AS, et al. Postoperative Radiotherapy for Maxillary Sinus Cancer: Long-Term Outcomes and Toxicities of Treatment. *Int J Radiat Oncol Biol Phys* (2007) 68(3):719–30. doi: 10.1016/j.ijrobp.2007.01.032
46. Ricotta F, Cercenelli L, Battaglia S, Bortolani B, Savastio G, Marcelli E, et al. Navigation-Guided Resection of Maxillary Tumors: Can a New Volumetric Virtual Planning Method Improve Outcomes in Terms of Control of Resection Margins? *J Cranio Maxillofac Surg* (2018) 46(12):2240–7. doi: 10.1016/j.jcms.2018.09.034
47. Ferrari M, Montalto N, Nicolai P. Novel Approaches in Surgical Management: How to Assess Surgical Margins. In: JB Vermorken, V Budach, CR Leemans, JP Machiels, P Nicolai, B O'Sullivan, editors. *Critical Issues in Head and Neck Oncology*. Springer, Cham (2021). doi: 10.1007/978-3-030-63234-2_7

19

Augmented Reality to Assist Skin Paddle Harvesting in Osteomyocutaneous Fibular Flap Reconstructive Surgery: A Pilot Evaluation on a 3D-Printed Leg Phantom

Laura Cercenelli[1], Federico Babini[1], Giovanni Badiali[2], Salvatore Battaglia[3], Achille Tarsitano[2], Claudio Marchetti[2] and Emanuela Marcelli[1]*

[1] eDIMES Lab - Laboratory of Bioengineering, Department of Experimental, Diagnostic and Specialty Medicine, University of Bologna, Bologna, Italy, [2] Maxillofacial Surgery Unit, Head and Neck Department, IRCCS Azienda Ospedaliera Universitaria di Bologna, Department of Biomedical and Neuromotor Sciences, Alma Mater Studiorum University of Bologna, Bologna, Italy, [3] Maxillofacial Surgery Unit, Policlinico San Marco University Hospital, University of Catania, Catania, Italy

***Correspondence:**
Laura Cercenelli
laura.cercenelli@unibo.it

Background: Augmented Reality (AR) represents an evolution of navigation-assisted surgery, providing surgeons with a virtual aid contextually merged with the real surgical field. We recently reported a case series of AR-assisted fibular flap harvesting for mandibular reconstruction. However, the registration accuracy between the real and the virtual content needs to be systematically evaluated before widely promoting this tool in clinical practice. In this paper, after description of the AR based protocol implemented for both tablet and HoloLens 2 smart glasses, we evaluated in a first test session the achievable registration accuracy with the two display solutions, and in a second test session the success rate in executing the AR-guided skin paddle incision task on a 3D printed leg phantom.

Methods: From a real computed tomography dataset, 3D virtual models of a human leg, including fibula, arteries and skin with planned paddle profile for harvesting, were obtained. All virtual models were imported into Unity software to develop a marker-less AR application suitable to be used both *via* tablet and *via* HoloLens 2 headset. The registration accuracy for both solutions was verified on a 3D printed leg phantom obtained from the virtual models, by repeatedly applying the tracking function and computing pose deviations between the AR-projected virtual skin paddle profile and the real one transferred to the phantom *via* a CAD/CAM cutting guide. The success rate in completing the AR-guided task of skin paddle harvesting was evaluated using CAD/CAM templates positioned on the phantom model surface.

Results: On average, the marker-less AR protocol showed comparable registration errors (ranging within 1-5 mm) for tablet-based and HoloLens-based solution. Registration accuracy seems to be quite sensitive to ambient light conditions. We found a good success rate in completing the AR-guided task within an error margin of 4 mm (97% and 100% for tablet and HoloLens, respectively). All subjects reported greater usability and ergonomics for HoloLens 2 solution.

Conclusions: Results revealed that the proposed marker-less AR based protocol may guarantee a registration error within 1-5 mm for assisting skin paddle harvesting in the clinical setting. Optimal lightening conditions and further improvement of marker-less tracking technologies have the potential to increase the efficiency and precision of this AR-assisted reconstructive surgery.

Keywords: augmented reality, virtual planning, 3D printing, Head and Neck Cancer, Microsoft HoloLens, registration, reconstructive surgery, 3D modeling

1 INTRODUCTION

Augmented reality (AR) in medicine is a technology that expands on image-guided surgery, allowing intraoperative guidance and navigation. This technique integrates imaging information with the real-world surgical field to give the surgeon a sort of "x-ray vision".

In recent years, AR technology has been proposed and applied in neurosurgery (1, 2), urology (3–5), orthopedics (6, 7) and craniomaxillofacial surgery (8, 9), among others.

A variety of technologies including traditional projectors, mobile devices such as tablets and smartphones, and head mounted displays (HMDs) have been proposed and used to perceive the augmented surgical field (8, 10). Specifically, several commercial optical see-through HMDs, such as Microsoft HoloLens (Microsoft, Redmond, WA) and Google Glass (Google Inc., Mountain View, California, USA), have gained broad availability and are being explored for applications in surgery. However, a small number of AR-based solutions for intraoperative surgical guidance have been successfully demonstrated in humans, e.g. for spine and hip surgery (11–13), while other promising solutions have been described and demonstrated on phantom (14–16).

In craniomaxillofacial surgery, the AR technology can be considered an evolution of the navigation-assisted surgery, and it represents a promising tool in aiding complex surgical procedures, such as mandible reconstruction with fibula flap, with potential to avoid or limit the use of cutting guide technology. The osteomyocutaneous microvascular fibular flap harvesting represents the reconstructive gold standard for complex mandibular defects resulting from tumor resections, trauma or malformations (17). For these cases, the use of 3D technologies and computer-aided design/computer-aided manufacturing (CAD/CAM) is essential to provide an accurate planning and to enhance the quality of the surgical outcomes. While CAD/CAM has become a quite common practice to virtually plan the bony resection and reconstruction, for skin paddle incision the surgeon still relies on measurements made on radiological imaging which are then reported on the patient's skin. Besides computerized tomographic angiography and magnetic resonance tomography, Doppler sonography is an affordable and harmless method commonly used to preoperatively determine arterial supply to the lower extremity. i.e. to identify the cutaneous perforators in fibula osteocutaneous free tissue transfer patients (18–20).

Only few recent experiences reported the use of accurate virtual planning and CAD/CAM technology for skin paddle harvesting and localization of the cutaneous perforator vessels of the fibula vascular anatomy for supplying the free flap (21, 22). In this field, the AR technology may offer an alternative or combined approach to assist intraoperatively the surgeon in skin paddle harvesting.

It would be possible to plan and reproduce the soft tissue resection and reconstruction and not only the bony part of the 3D-aided surgery. In order to achieve this goal, once the planning is carried out either on the resection and on the fibular skin area planned for soft tissue reconstruction, the reconstructed 3D virtual plan may be transferred to AR technology. This will give the surgeon the opportunity to reproduce the planned reconstruction, based on the three-dimensional position and reciprocal position to the bony segments and flap insetting, in restoring the defect.

As great advantage, the AR technology, when deployed on a wearable head mounted display, allows the direct view of the planned resection and reconstruction on the surgical field without the need for the surgeon to alternate viewing between the surgical field and external monitors such as in the case of standard navigation systems, with potential clinical benefits of reducing operative time and improving surgical outcomes. We have recently reported preliminary case series where the feasibility of a proof-of-concept AR based protocol implemented on a tablet for assisting procedures of free fibula bone harvest (23) and of galeo-pericranial flap harvest (24) was demonstrated. In those experiences the AR guidance was based on a marker-less registration, i.e. without the need of invasive placement of fixed fiducial markers on the patients. However, the provided registration accuracy between the real and the virtual content, that will affect the reliability of the virtual planning overlaying the patient anatomy, requires to be systematically evaluated before widely promoting this AR protocol in the clinical practice. Indeed, virtual-to-real scene registration, patient position tracking and projection of the digital content onto the targeted anatomical structures are crucial steps of AR-guided navigation systems (8, 25, 26).

In this paper, we describe the AR based protocol we developed for assisting skin paddle harvesting in osteomyocutaneous fibular flap reconstructive procedure, usable both with a handheld device, such as a tablet, and with a HMD, such as Microsoft HoloLens 2 smart glasses. The study was also designed to evaluate the registration errors associated with the two display solutions, and the achievable success rate when simulating the AR-guided task of skin paddle harvesting on a 3D printed human leg phantom.

2 MATERIALS AND METHODS

The study was designed in order to first implement the AR based protocol on both the tablet and the HoloLens 2 smart glasses. Then, a first testing session to quantify the achievable registration accuracy with the two display solutions, and a second testing session to evaluate the success rate in executing the AR-guided skin paddle incision task on a 3D printed leg phantom were performed.

In the following sections the development and implementation phase, as well as the experimental phase of the study were reported.

2.1 Development Phase

This phase consists of three steps: A) Image segmentation and virtual content preparation; B) Design and manufacturing of the human leg phantom; C) Development of the AR application (**Figure 1**).

2.1.1 Image Segmentation and Virtual Content Preparation

The process started from acquisition of real computed tomography angiography (CTA) datasets of a patient lower leg, which represents the donor-site for osteomyocutaneous fibular flap harvesting procedure. CTA scans were acquired after administering nonionic contrast media intravenously (Xenetix 350 Guerbet) and with a slice thickness of 0.6 mm (Lightspeed VCT LS Advantage 64 slices; General Electric Medical System).

Anatomical areas of interest of the subject's leg were segmented using D2P™ software (3D Systems Inc., Rock Hill, SC, USA): bones (tibia and fibula), arterial vessels (popliteal, fibular, tibial and perforating arteries) and leg skin (distinguishing the skin paddle profile for harvesting, according to the virtual planning for mandibular reconstruction).

Three-dimensional meshes were then generated from all the segmented masks, and saved in STL format.

2.1.2 Design and Manufacturing of Human Leg Phantom

From the virtual models obtained in the previous step, a tangible phantom made of photosensitive resin was produced *via* a stereolithography (SLA) 3D printer (Form 3, Formlabs, Somerville, MA, USA).

To make the virtual leg model compatible with the build volume of Form 3 printer (14.5 × 14.5 × 17.5 cm), CAD processing was carried out using MeshMixer software (Autodesk

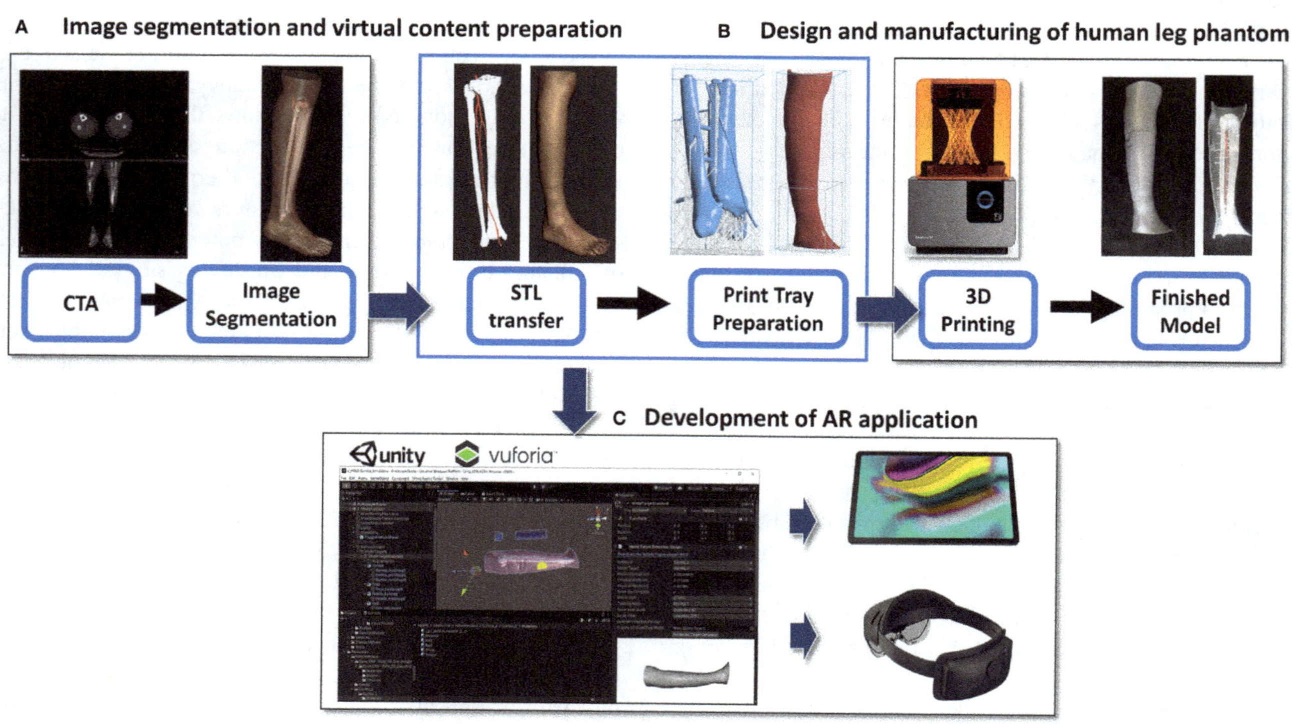

FIGURE 1 | Description of the development work flow. **(A)** Image segmentation and virtual content preparation; **(B)** Design and manufacturing of the human leg phantom; **(C)** Development of the AR application.

Inc., CA, US) in order to create a modular phantom composed of several parts. In detail, for the skin layer and the bones/vessels block, three cross sections were designed, each divided into two symmetrical portions defined by a longitudinal cutting plane, and a set of joints among the various separate parts was created. Each component was printed individually, using a grey resin for the skin (4 mm thick shell) and a clear resin for bone and vessel structures. Then, arteries were colored red to differentiate them from bones, and all pieces were assembled (**Figure 2**).

2.1.3 Development of AR Application

The obtained virtual models of the lower leg, i.e. bone anatomy, arteries and the planned skin paddle profile with the corresponding selected perforator vessel, were imported into Unity 3D software (Unity Technologies, San Francisco, CA, USA) extended with a specific software development kit for creating augmented reality apps (Vuforia Engine package, PTC, Inc., Boston, MA, USA).

The tracking algorithm and registration between the virtual content and the real scene were implemented using the "Model Target" function of Vuforia Engine, which allows the marker-less tracking of a physical object in the real world by recognition of the shape of the 3D object itself observed from a certain perspective. Model Target function enables to recognize and track objects in the real world based on their shape. To make a Model Target for a particular object the 3D model data for the object, such as a 3D CAD model or a 3D scan of the object, is necessary. A Model Target requires that the user holds the AR display device at a particular angle relative to the object, and at a particular distance to initialize the tracking. To aid with this process, the application typically draws an image ("guide view") showing an approximation of the object shape from this distance and viewing angle, so that the user just needs to move the AR display until the object matches this guide view. After that, tracking can begin (**Figure 3**).

In this study, the CAD model of the leg skin was used as Model Target for virtual-to-real scene registration. The created AR application was built both as an Android app for mobile devices then deployed on a Samsung Galaxy TAB S5E (**Figure 4**), and as a UWP (Universal Windows Platform) app deployed on Microsoft HoloLens 2 smart glasses (**Figure 5**).

In both cases, the AR application generates "holographic" overlays, by rendering the bony and vascular anatomy of the simulated patient leg, and also the planned skin paddle profile for harvesting to be used as guiding information during the experimental task performed on leg phantom.

Interactable user interface toggles (check boxes) were added to turn off and on the rendering of each virtual anatomical structure

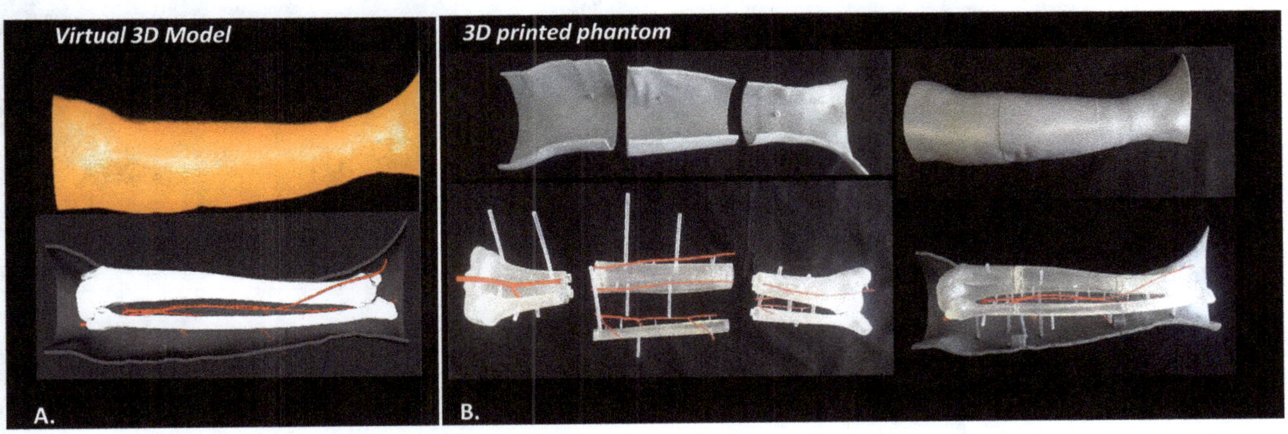

FIGURE 2 | Virtual **(A)** and 3D printed **(B)** model of the designed human leg phantom, used for the experimental phase.

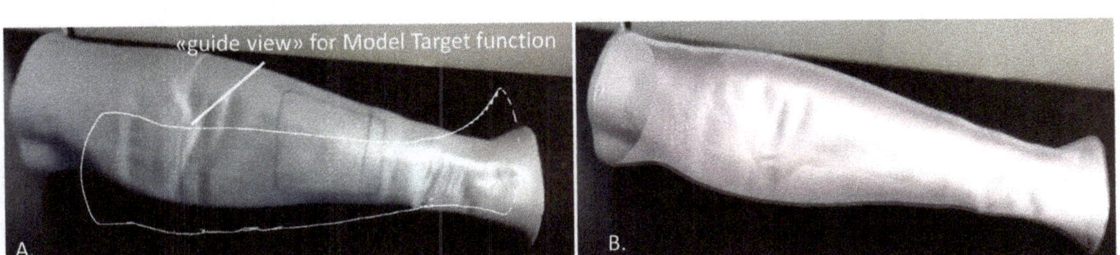

FIGURE 3 | Example of the "guide view" in the Model Target function **(A)**, showing an approximation of the object shape used for tracking the phantom leg and matching to it the virtual content **(B)**.

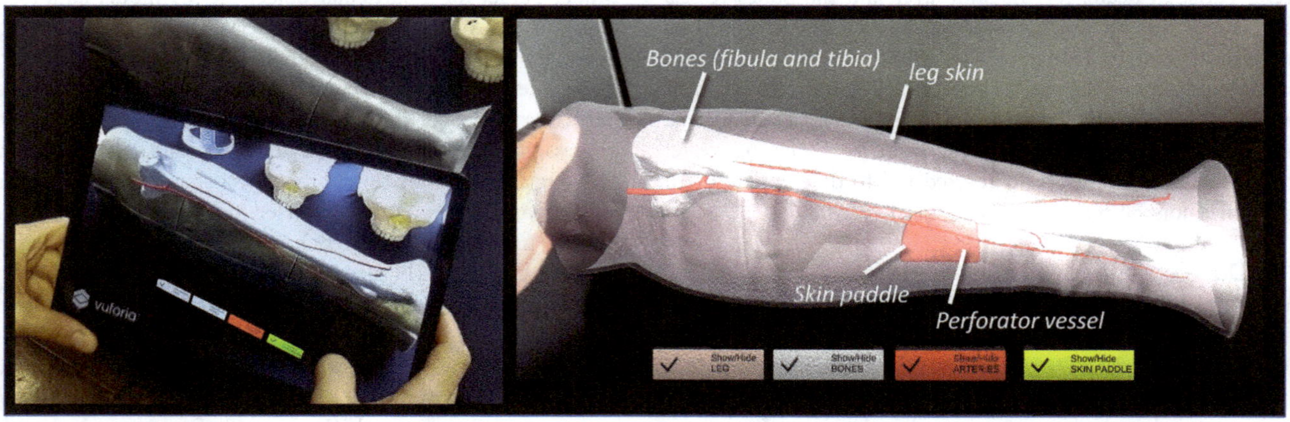

FIGURE 4 | The AR application generating the holographic overlays superimposed on the real phantom anatomy, as displayed to surgeon *via* tablet.

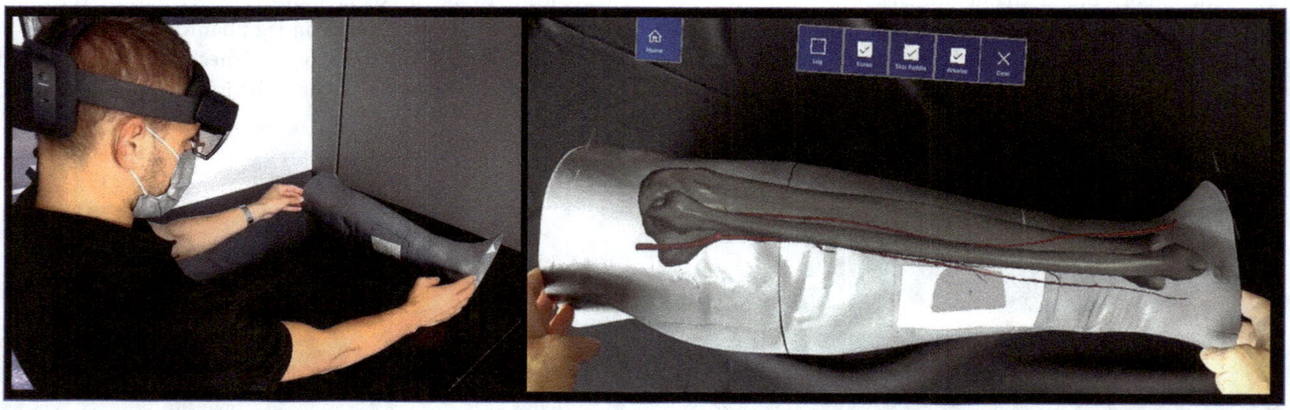

FIGURE 5 | The AR application generating the holographic overlays superimposed on the real phantom anatomy, as displayed to surgeon *via* HoloLens 2 smart glasses.

(skin paddle, bones, vessels) (see **Suppl_Video_1_Tablet_DEMO** and **Suppl_Video_2Holo_DEMO**).

For the HoloLens application, voice commands to show/hide the virtual anatomical structures were also implemented in order to provide a completely hand-free AR guidance system.

A portable high-performance workstation (Intel(R) Core i7-10750H, CPU@ 2.60GHz, 16GB RAM, NVIDIA GeForce RTX 2070) was used for the virtual content preparation and for development of the AR application that was then deployed and run directly in the tablet or HoloLens 2 smart glasses.

2.2 Experimental Phase

Experimental tests on phantom were carried out in the following two phases.

2.2.1 Test Session 1

We evaluated the registration error of the two AR display types (tablet-based and HoloLens-based). For each solution, we tested two lighting conditions: 1) environment illuminated by natural daylight (OFF_lamp); 2) artificial lamp light that points directly on the phantom (ON_lamp).

In order to evaluate the registration error, the "real" skin paddle profile and the virtual one projected in AR were compared. The "real" skin paddle profile was obtained from the planned skin paddle: from patient CT angiography the 3D model of the chosen perforator vessel was also reconstructed, then the skin paddle outline was drawn in order to centre this perforator, as we have already described in a previous work (23). Then, we designed and printed a customized guide (template) based on calf proximal and distal diameters, that includes the planned skin paddle outline centering the perforator, and we used this CAD/CAM template to transfer the planned skin paddle profile to the 3D printed phantom (**Figure 6**).

The real profile was obtained by tracing a line on an adhesive tape applied over the leg phantom while following the groove of the CAD/CAM template (**Figure 6B**). The 3D printed template was also provided with a central hole in the paddle (diameter = 1.5 mm) which was used to trace on the tape the central point of

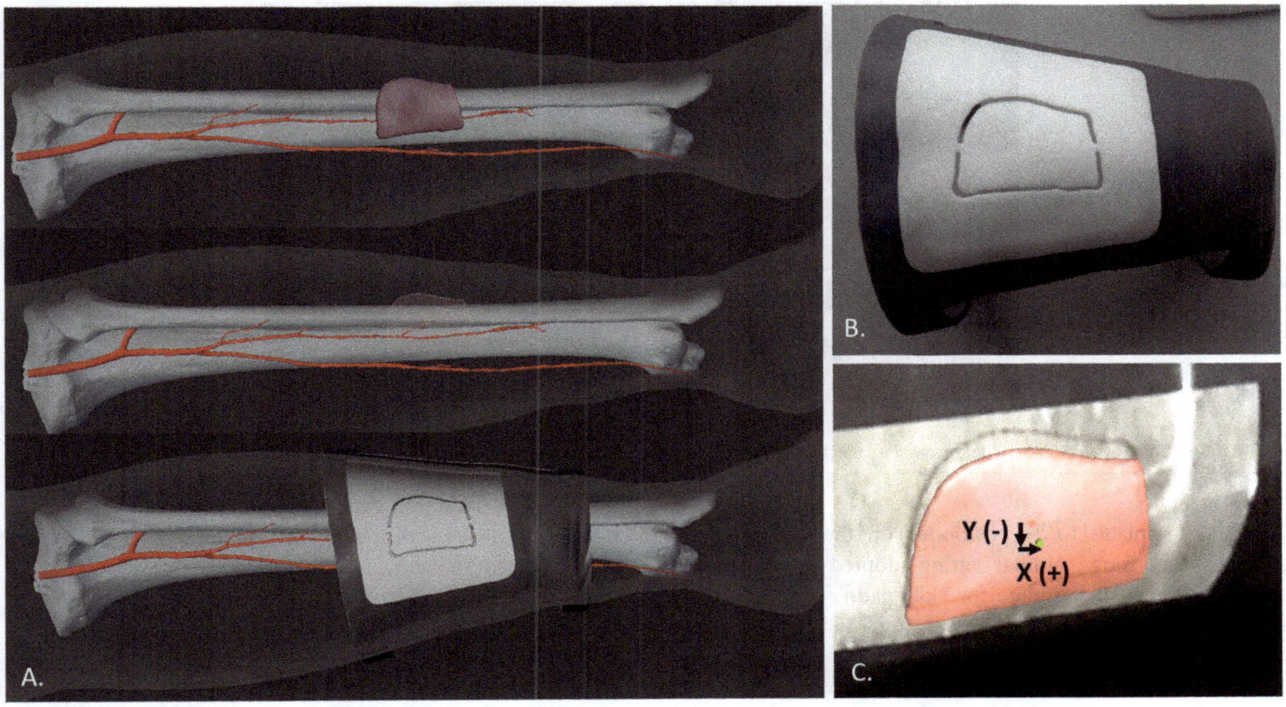

FIGURE 6 | The virtual planning of the skin paddle outline centering the perforator **(A)** and the CAD/CAM template used to transfer this planned skin paddle profile to the 3D printed phantom **(B)**. Comparison between the virtual paddle projected in AR and the real one obtained from the CAD/CAM template applied to the leg phantom **(C)**.

the paddle. The same central point was included in the virtual paddle as a green dot. Registration error was quantified as mean deviations between the central point traced on the tape and the virtual one, both in horizontal (X) and vertical (Y) directions (**Figure 6C**). The X, Y deviations were automatically calculated using a Matlab code applied to screenshots acquired for each test. Each testing condition was repeated 12 times and means values ± SD were calculated.

2.2.2 Test Session 2

As second phase, we quantified the success rate in performing on the leg phantom the AR-guided task of skin paddle profile tracing by a group of 8 subjects (5 females and 3 males, aged between 25 and 50, being students, researchers and engineers at University of Bologna, without specific experience with augmented reality systems). Each subject performed the task using both the tablet-based and the HoloLens-based AR application.

The virtual skin paddle profile was designed and displayed as a dashed line to facilitate the optimal visibility of both the virtual and the real trajectory drawn gradually with the pencil during the execution of the AR-guided task, thus avoiding that the line traced by the user become occluded, to some extent, by holograms (**Figure 7**). Push buttons and voice commands allow to control the appearance and disappearance of the virtual objects, thus facilitating the optimal visibility of relevant elements during the task (e.g. the skin layer used as Model Target for marker-less registration can be removed after having checked the achievement of a good registration).

For tests using tablet, the mobile device was anchored to an articulated arm fixed to the table on which the leg phantom was placed. By means of the articulated arm the tablet can be oriented and locked in the most appropriate position to allow the correct visualization of the holographic overlay, and the user to freely carry out the task.

For tests using HoloLens 2, a preliminary user experience with the mixed reality headset was provided, also including the calibration procedure which is required to ensure the best hologram viewing experience for each subject.

Each subject was instructed that the primary goal of the test was to accurately trace a line following the virtual skin paddle profile displayed in AR (see **Suppl_Video_3_Tablet_TASK**), both through the tablet, and through the HoloLens 2 smart glasses.

For both test sessions, the AR-guided task was performed after the tracking of leg phantom profile has been achieved, and the optimal registration between the holographic virtual content and the real phantom has been visually checked and verified using the cutting guide.

A 0.5 mm pencil was used to draw the perceived profile on an adhesive tape applied over the leg phantom surface. The success rate in tracing the AR-displayed profile was evaluated using

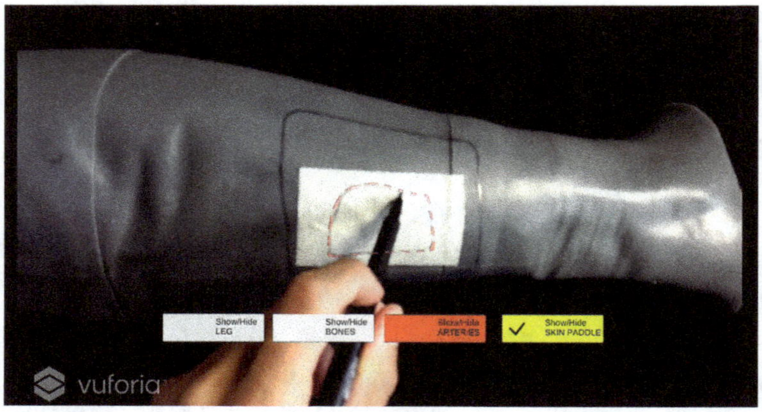

FIGURE 7 | Example of virtual skin paddle profile displayed as a dashed line to avoid occlusion of the real scene by holograms.

CAD/CAM templates to be positioned on the surface of the phantom model using a similar setting adopted in our previous works (14, 16). Each template for skin paddle outline can be uniquely positioned on the leg phantom as it is a customized CAD/CAM design starting from the leg model reconstructed from CT scan. The anatomical fitting of each template on phantom calf is obtained thanks to the shape of the template itself: two customized flanges embrace circumferentially the proximal and distal portions of the leg, allowing to position it univocally in all dimensions (**Figure 8**).

The templates were 3D printed (Form 3, Formlabs) with a groove of different widths (4 mm, 2 mm, 1 mm) in order to evaluate three levels of achievable accuracy: ± 2.0 mm, ± 1.0 mm, and ± 0.5 mm (**Figure 8**). A millimeter adhesive tape was associated to each template and used to measure the cumulative length of the traced skin paddle profile falling within the groove, and then to calculate the percentage of successful traced trajectories ("percentage success rate") (**Figure 8**). We considered as successful competition of the task (100% success rate) those trials in which the traced skin paddle profile fell within the groove of the cutting guide along its entire length (16.5 cm).

2.3 Statistics

All results about the registration errors (Test Session 1) and the percentage of success rate in performing the AR-guided task (Test Session 2) were reported as mean values and standard deviation (SD).

For Test Session 1, T-test for unpaired data was used to compare the mean registration errors, both in X and Y direction, for the tablet-based and HoloLens-based groups, as well as to evaluate for each AR display type the difference of mean values between the "OFF_lamp" and "ON_Lamp" lightening condition.

For Test Session 2, the difference of the mean percentage success rate obtained with the two AR display types was evaluated using T-test for paired samples.

SPSS software (IBM, Armonk, New York, US) was used to perform the statistical analysis, and a p value of <0.05 was considered statistically significant.

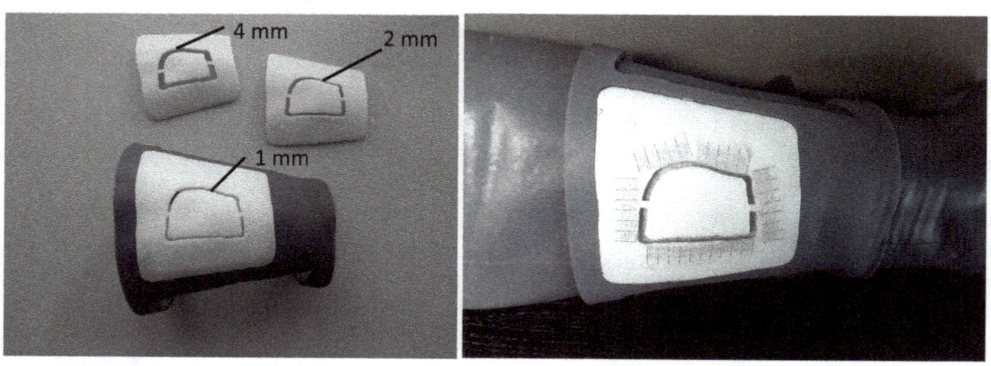

FIGURE 8 | CAD/CAM templates used to evaluate the success rate in performing the AR-guided task, using different levels of accuracy (template "1 mm", template "2 mm", template "4 mm").

3 RESULTS

On average, we found a similar registration errors for tablet-based and HoloLens-based solutions, ranging between 1-5 mm (**Figure 9**). The largest deviations between virtual and real content were in the vertical (Y) direction for "OFF_lamp" lightening condition, while lower registration errors (within 2 mm) resulted in the horizontal (X) direction (blue bars in **Figure 9**).

For tablet-based application, the "ON-Lamp" lightening condition provided a statistically significant reduction of the registration error in the vertical direction if compared with "OFF-lamp" condition (3.6 ± 0.7 mm vs 5.0 ± 0.9 mm, $p < 0.005$), while the registration error in horizontal direction did not significantly change. The "ON-Lamp" lightening condition seems to reduce also the registration error for Hololens-based application, particularly in vertical direction, although this reduction did not result statistically significant (2.7 ± 1.2 mm vs 4.2 ± 2.4 mm, $p = 0.072$).

Results from Test Session 2 are summarized in **Table 1**. With HoloLens 2 all subjects (100%) were able to successfully trace the skin paddle profile with an accuracy level of ±2.0 mm (verified with the "4 mm" template); with tablet, on average, the 97% of the traced trajectories was within ±2.0 mm accuracy level.

For accuracy level ±1 mm and ±0.5 mm, lower success rates resulted for both tablet and HoloLens solutions (53%, 19% and 71%, 41%, respectively), (**Table 1**). We found no statistically significant difference in success rate between tablet-based and HoloLens-based AR application, except for ±0.5 mm accuracy level, where AR guidance with HoloLens 2 showed a success rate higher than the one achievable with tablet ($p<0.05$).

From Test Session 1 we realized that the implemented marker-less registration is quite sensitive to environment lightening conditions, and that holograms can appear to project accurately over the leg phantom only from a certain perspective (i.e. a quite frontal perspective corresponding to the one chosen for Model Target creation in Vuforia Engine), whereas from other perspectives the hologram revealed very inaccurate placement.

In performing Test Session 2, we observed some inherent drawbacks of the marker-less registration based on the recognition of the 3D object profile using Vuforia Engine Model Target function. Especially in tablet-based application we observed that the hologram tends to shift away a little bit from the optimal registration position as soon as the subject approaches the hand to the phantom to start drawing the AR-guided trajectory. This behavior may be due to the fact that the subject places his hand between the camera and the tracked real object, thus interfering with the correct recognition of the skin layer profile of the leg phantom used as Model Target.

In terms of user experience, all subjects reported greater usability and ergonomics of the HoloLens solution, although the brightness of the virtual content was lower than the one displayed on the tablet.

4 DISCUSSION

AR is a promising technology for craniofacial surgeons to obtain a "see-through" effect in the operating room. However, some problems with AR, such as depth perception (27) and registration errors (28), i.e. the difference between virtual content and actual reality resulting in bias for users, still remain.

The present study aims to increase the information regarding the achievable registration accuracy with a marker-less AR

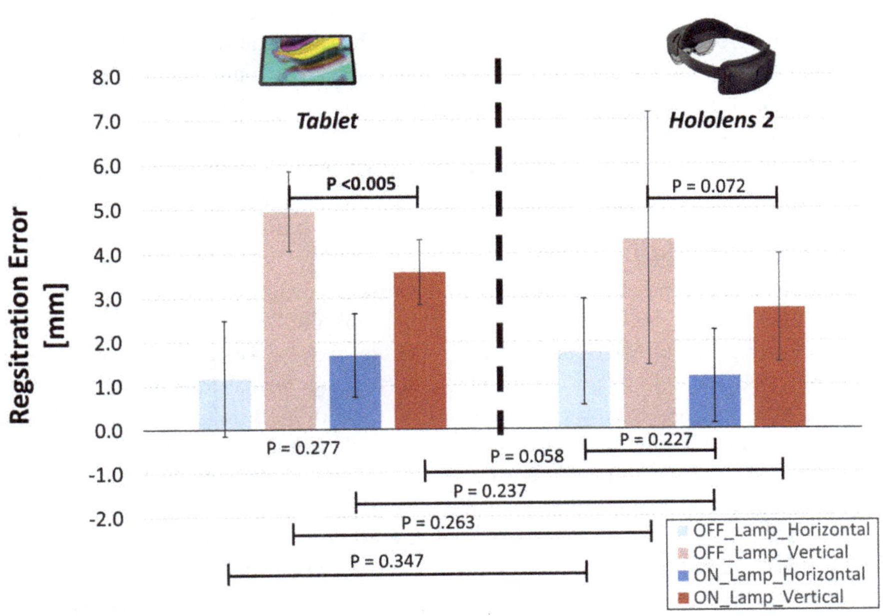

FIGURE 9 | Resulting registration errors calculated as mean horizontal and vertical deviations between the real and virtual content, for two lighting conditions: environment illuminated by natural daylight (OFF_Lamp); artificial lamp light that points directly on the phantom (ON_Lamp).

TABLE 1 | Resulting mean percentage success rate in performing the AR-guided task using both tablet and HoloLens 2, for different accuracy levels ("1 mm", "2 mm", "4 mm" templates).

Subject	Tablet			HoloLens 2		
	Template 1 mm (± 0.5 mm)	Template 2 mm (± 1 mm)	Template 4 mm (± 2 mm)	Template 1 mm (± 0.5 mm)	Template 2 mm (± 1 mm)	Template 4 mm (± 2 mm)
1	30%	48%	100%	33%	94%	100%
2	15%	48%	91%	28%	36%	100%
3	6%	76%	100%	21%	45%	100%
4	24%	45%	100%	45%	91%	100%
5	21%	52%	100%	48%	82%	100%
6	27%	42%	100%	30%	42%	100%
7	3%	30%	82%	76%	97%	100%
8	24%	79%	100%	45%	82%	100%
Mean	**19%**	**53%**	**97%**	**41%**	**71%**	**100%**
SD	10%	17%	7%	17%	25%	0%

Bold values are used to identify/highlight the mean values.

application usable *via* a tablet and a HoloLens 2 headset, that we developed for assisting skin paddle harvesting in osteomyocutaneous fibular flap procedure for mandibular reconstruction. The perspective of clinical application of the proposed AR protocol for head and neck reconstruction is the 3D planning of the soft tissue resection and reconstruction, having the opportunity to reduce the donor site morbidity, improving eventually the three-dimensional reconstructive outcome.

From a technical point of view, the primary challenge that needs to be addressed for AR to become a viable tool for surgery is the accuracy of registration between the displayed virtual content and the real scene. The registration error, mainly caused by registration method and camera performance, results in a "misalignment" effect in the subjective perception for virtual and reality image. The registration error is divided into static registration error and dynamic registration error. The static registration error deals with the error caused by the system when the user's viewpoint is still at rest with the real object, whereas the dynamic registration error refers to the error that occurs when the real object has relative motion in the user's view or environment (29). In our study we quantified the static registration error obtained for both tablet and HoloLens solutions, when using a marker-less tracking method based on the recognition of the 3D object profile.

Most of the current AR approaches are limited to invasive marker fixation to provide virtual-to-patient registration. In craniomaxillofacial surgery, AR solutions based on a marker-less tracking, like the one we propose, may offer the advantage to overcome the inherent drawbacks of standard navigation systems, such as the use of reference marks to be positioned on the patient, and the need for a quite long registration procedure. Therefore, a marker-less tracking approach offers a less intrusive solution and limits the need for manufacturing dedicated CAD/CAM trackers anchored for example to occlusal splints, which may obstruct the operative field.

On the other hand, marker-less solutions, as we observed in our experiments, may suffer from poor robustness, being sensitive to ambient light conditions, to changes in viewpoint, to contrast image and to the integrity of the 3D object profile used as Model Target. Indeed, in our previous experience in real clinical setting (23) we observed evident registration errors due to the posterior leg soft tissue displacing after the skin incision, since this surgical action alters the correct recognition of the leg profile used for registration. In general, while hard tissues can be registered with a high degree of success, the ability to accurately track mobile or deformable anatomy still remains a challenge, since soft tissue deformations during intraoperative maneuver reduce the stability of AR tracking which is based on a static rigid 3D model.

In the present study we found mean registration errors ranging within 1-5 mm, for both tablet-based and HoloLens-based solution, considering two dimensions, i.e. horizontal (X) and vertical (Y) directions. Our findings were quite in line with other studies on HoloLens accuracy for surgical applications that reported visualization errors up around 2 millimeters (30–32) and more than 5 millimeters in one case (33).

We observed largest deviations in the vertical (Y) direction. This may be due to the "Model Target" registration function which is based on recognition of the shape of a 3D object (i.e. the leg) observed from a certain perspective. In horizontal direction (X) there is an excellent fitting between the real and virtual content since the proximal and distal edge of the leg are correctly recognized and matched; however, the virtual-to-real matching with the Model Target function can occur also with a persisting rotational component along the leg long axis; this leads to a more relevant misalignment of the projected skin paddle profile in the vertical direction (Y).

Typically, the skin paddle used for reconstruction is a soft tissue area of average 6x4cm^2 at least, so a sub-millimetric accuracy in virtual-to-real registration is not required and even an error of 5-10 millimeters can be acceptable, since it does not affect the clinical outcome. Therefore, our findings are satisfying in terms of accuracy since the resulting average registration errors are absolutely compatible with the objectives and clinical applications of the proposed AR protocol.

For marker-less tracking we chose the external profile of the leg skin as Model Target to be used in Vuforia Engine package; this means that all the virtual structures of interest to be projected in AR (fibula, arterial vessels, skin paddle profile) are included in the chosen Model Target. This could be a favorable aspect to minimize the registration error, since the farther the augmented virtual object is from the object used for tracking, the greater the registration error.

For the AR-guided task we found a good success rate (around 100%) in completing the task within an error margin of 4 mm for both AR display solutions. These results have to take into account that for each test we started from a condition of optimal registration error (around 2 mm), which was visually checked before the subject started tracing the trajectory under the AR guidance, in order to maximize the achievable success rate.

Regarding AR display types, HMDs are emerging as efficient and promising media to support complex manual surgical tasks typically performed under direct vision (8, 34), since they allow the surgeon to maintain a "surgeon-centered' point of view and to leave his/her hands free to operate on the patient. Nowadays, optical-see-through HMD, like Microsoft HoloLens 2 smart glasses, are the leading wearable AR technology that are being explored also for applications in surgery. Nevertheless, technological and human-factor limitations, such as the small augmentable field of view, the low contrast image, and the still limited registration accuracy for high-precision surgical tasks, still hinder their routine use.

This does not exclude that they can be useful and usable, as in the case of the present study, to assist surgical procedures where there are no stringent accuracy requirements (i.e. submillimetric accuracy). Indeed, the expectation for AR system accuracy should be commensurated with the surgical tasks for which the tool is intended. In our study, all the performed AR-guided tracings on phantom encompassed appropriate skin regions to include the planned perforator vessel for fibular flap harvesting, also in those cases where low percentage of success rate resulted from accuracy verification through CAD/CAM templates.

When surgeons need to accomplish extremely delicate procedures such as precise drilling or cutting in narrow operative areas, AR systems specifically designed for high-precision surgical tasks, i.e. capable of guaranteeing a submillimetric accuracy level, should be preferred (8, 14, 35, 36).

From our experience, comparing the tablet-based and the HoloLens-based solution the following pros and cons emerged. The major advantage of a tablet solution is the good brightness of the virtual rendered anatomy. On the other hand, the advantage of a "surgeon-centered' point of view is lost, and it is necessary to fix the mobile device in a suitable position that allows the AR view for the surgeon and at the same time the possibility to perform manually the AR-guided surgical task.

Regarding HoloLens 2 we received feedbacks from users of a quite comfortable and ergonomics headset, that offers the advantages of optical see-through technology and hands-free operation. However, the provided contrast image is quite low.

The preoperative planning time for the proposed AR protocol is about 3 hours: 2 hours for CT image segmentation and virtual content preparation, if good quality imagining is provided, and 1 hour for AR application development and its deployment on HoloLens smart glasses. This time would not represent a limitation for clinical use. Indeed, the proposed AR protocol for skin paddle incision can be used as an alternative to CAD/CAM approach based on skin paddle outline guides that require a comparable or even longer preoperative planning time (if we consider also the 3D printing time). Moreover, the AR technology, implemented in a mark-less way, has the great potential of being a "streamlined", non-obstructive technology, which can be easily transferred and applied in the surgical setting.

Our study has some limitations. In Test Session 1 we quantified only the static registration error, while dynamic misalignment that occurs when the leg phantom has relative motion in the user's view or environment was not evaluated.

Moreover, in Test Session 2, each subject performed the task consecutively using the two different AR display types, so in the second execution of the same task he/she could have benefited from a little training effect. We tried to limit this bias, inverting the order of execution of the test with tablet and HoloLens between one subject and another.

As future development, we plan to enriched the AR based protocol with additional features that allow the simultaneous tracking of multiple 3D objects, e.g. a target anatomical region and a movable bone segment to be repositioned or displayed relative to the target. This may open the way to exploring new surgical or outpatient applications of augmented reality in the craniomaxillofacial field.

Future perspective will address to transfer the proposed AR protocol in the real clinical field to assist the skin paddle harvesting in osteomyocutaneous fibular flap reconstructive surgery. Surely, the head mounted display such as the HoloLens 2 solution is the most promising and viable option for use in the operating room setting. So, our future efforts will be focused on promoting a clinical study on the use of the AR protocol with HoloLens 2 headset.

5 CONCLUSIONS

In this study we present the development of a marker-less AR based protocol proposed to assist skin paddle harvesting in osteomyocutaneous fibular flap procedure for mandibular reconstruction. The developed AR guidance system was evaluated on a 3D printed leg phantom, thus allowing a systematic comparison of the achievable static registration accuracy and of the success rate in performing the AR-guided skin paddle harvesting task, when using two different AR display solutions, i.e. a tablet and HoloLens 2 headset. Results revealed that the AR based protocol provides a registration error within the range 1-5 mm for assisting skin paddle harvesting in the clinical setting, in both solutions. Greater usability and ergonomics resulted for HoloLens 2. Optimal lightening conditions and further improvement of marker-less tracking technologies have the potential to increase the efficiency and precision of this AR-assisted reconstructive surgery.

AUTHOR CONTRIBUTIONS

LC: study concept and design, manuscript preparation, and dataanalysis. FB: software development, and data collection and analysis. GB, SB, and AT: study design and data interpretation. CM: study supervision. EM: study concept and study supervision. LC, GB, AT, CM, SB, and EM: contributed to the manuscript review. All authors contributed to the article and approved the submitted version.

SUPPLEMENTARY MATERIAL

Video 1 | Use of the AR application on the phantom, via tablet.

Video 2 | Use of the AR application on the phantom, via HoloLens 2 smart glasses.

Video 3 | Execution of the AR-guided task on phantom.

REFERENCES

1. Chidambaram S, Stifano V, Demetres M, Teyssandier M, Palumbo MC, Redaelli A, et al. Applications of Augmented Reality in the Neurosurgical Operating Room: A Systematic Review of the Literature. *J Clin Neurosci* (2021) 91:43–61. doi: 10.1016/j.jocn.2021.06.032
2. Hersh A, Mahapatra S, Weber-Levine C, Awosika T, Theodore JN, Zakaria HM, et al. Augmented Reality in Spine Surgery: A Narrative Review. *HSS J* (2021) 17(3):351–8. doi: 10.1177/15563316211028595
3. Reis G, Yilmaz M, Rambach J, Pagani A, Suarez-Ibarrola R, Miernik A, et al. Mixed Reality Applications in Urology: Requirements and Future Potential. *Ann Med Surg* (2021) 66:102394. doi: 10.1016/j.amsu.2021.102394
4. Schiavina R, Bianchi L, Lodi S, Cercenelli L, Chessa F, Bortolani B, et al. Real-Time Augmented Reality Three-Dimensional Guided Robotic Radical Prostatectomy: Preliminary Experience and Evaluation of the Impact on Surgical Planning. *Eur Urol Focus* (2021) 7(6):1260–7. doi: 10.1016/j.euf.2020.08.004
5. Schiavina R, Bianchi L, Chessa F, Barbaresi U, Cercenelli L, Lodi S, et al. Augmented Reality to Guide Selective Clamping and Tumor Dissection During Robot-Assisted Partial Nephrectomy: A Preliminary Experience. *Clin Genitourin Cancer* (2021) 19(3):e149–55. doi: 10.1016/j.clgc.2020.09.005
6. Verhey JT, Haglin JM, Verhey EM, Hartigan DE. Virtual, Augmented, and Mixed Reality Applications in Orthopedic Surgery. *Int J Med Robot* (2020) 16 (2):1–9. doi: 10.1002/rcs.2067
7. Matthews JH, Shields JS. The Clinical Application of Augmented Reality in Orthopaedics: Where Do We Stand? *Curr Rev Musculoskelet Med* (2021) 14 (5):316–9. doi: 10.1007/s12178-021-09713-8
8. Badiali G, Cercenelli L, Battaglia S, Marcelli E, Marchetti C, Ferrari V, et al. Review on Augmented Reality in Oral and Cranio-Maxillofacial Surgery: Toward “Surgery-Specific” Head-Up Displays. *IEEE Access* (2020) 8:59015–28. doi: 10.1109/ACCESS.2020.2973298
9. Benmahdjoub M, van Walsum T, van Twisk P, Wolvius EB. Augmented Reality in Craniomaxillofacial Surgery: Added Value and Proposed Recommendations Through a Systematic Review of the Literature. *Int J Oral Maxillofac Surg* (2021) 50(7):969–78. doi: 10.1016/j.ijom.2020.11.015
10. Mezger U, Jendrewski C, Bartels M. Navigation in Surgery. *Langenbecks Arch Surg* (2013) 398(4):501–14. doi: 10.1007/s00423-013-1059-4
11. Molina CA, Sciubba DM, Greenberg JK, Khan M, Witham T. Clinical Accuracy, Technical Precision, and Workflow of the First in Human Use of an Augmented-Reality Head-Mounted Display Stereotactic Navigation System for Spine Surgery. *Oper Neurosurg Hagerstown Md* (2021) 20 (3):300–9. doi: 10.1093/ons/opaa398
12. Yahanda AT, Moore E, Ray WZ, Pennicooke B, Jennings JW, Molina CA. First in-Human Report of the Clinical Accuracy of Thoracolumbar Percutaneous Pedicle Screw Placement Using Augmented Reality Guidance. *Neurosurg Focus* (2021) 51(2):E10. doi: 10.3171/2021.5.FOCUS21217
13. Kiarostami P, Dennler C, Roner S, Sutter R, Fürnstahl P, Farshad M, et al. Augmented Reality-Guided Periacetabular Osteotomy-Proof of Concept. *J Orthop Surg* (2020) 15(1):540. doi: 10.1186/s13018-020-02066-x
14. Cercenelli L, Carbone M, Condino S, Cutolo F, Marcelli E, Tarsitano A, et al. The Wearable VOSTARS System for Augmented Reality-Guided Surgery: Preclinical Phantom Evaluation for High-Precision Maxillofacial Tasks. *J Clin Med* (2020) 9(11):E3562. doi: 10.3390/jcm9113562
15. Glas HH, Kraeima J, van Ooijen PMA, Spijkervet FKL, Yu L, Witjes MJH. Augmented Reality Visualization for Image-Guided Surgery: A Validation Study Using a Three-Dimensional Printed Phantom. *J Oral Maxillofac Surg* (2021) 79(9):1943.e1–1943.e10. doi: 10.1016/j.joms.2021.04.001
16. Condino S, Fida B, Carbone M, Cercenelli L, Badiali G, Ferrari V, et al. Wearable Augmented Reality Platform for Aiding Complex 3d Trajectory Tracing. *Sensors* (2020) 20(6):E1612. doi: 10.3390/s20061612
17. Kumar BP, Venkatesh V, Kumar KAJ, Yadav BY, Mohan SR. Mandibular Reconstruction: Overview. *J Maxillofac Oral Surg* (2016) 15(4):425–41. doi: 10.1007/s12663-015-0766-5
18. Futran ND, Stack BC, Zaccardi MJ. Preoperative Color Flow Doppler Imaging for Fibula Free Tissue Transfers. *Ann Vasc Surg* (1998) 12(5):445–50. doi: 10.1007/s100169900182
19. Goetze E, Kämmerer PW, Al-Nawas B, Moergel M. Integration of Perforator Vessels in CAD/CAM Free Fibula Graft Planning: A Clinical Feasibility Study. *J Maxillofac Oral Surg* (2020) 19(1):61–6. doi: 10.1007/s12663-019-01215-y
20. González Martínez J, Torres Pérez A, Gijón Vega M, Nuñez-Villaveiran T. Preoperative Vascular Planning of Free Flaps: Comparative Study of Computed Tomographic Angiography, Color Doppler Ultrasonography, and Hand-Held Doppler. *Plast Reconstr Surg* (2020) 146(2):227–37. doi: 10.1097/PRS.0000000000006966
21. Battaglia S, Maiolo V, Savastio G, Zompatori M, Contedini F, Antoniazzi E, et al. Osteomyocutaneous Fibular Flap Harvesting: Computer-Assisted Planning of Perforator Vessels Using Computed Tomographic Angiography Scan and Cutting Guide. *J Cranio-Maxillo-fac Surg* (2017) 45(10):1681–6. doi: 10.1016/j.jcms.2017.07.017
22. Battaglia S, Ricotta F, Maiolo V, Savastio G, Contedini F, Cipriani R, et al. Computer-Assisted Surgery for Reconstruction of Complex Mandibular Defects Using Osteomyocutaneous Microvascular Fibular Free Flaps: Use of a Skin Paddle-Outlining Guide for Soft-Tissue Reconstruction. A Technical Report. *J Cranio-Maxillo-fac Surg* (2019) 47(2):293–9. doi: 10.1016/j.jcms.2018.11.018
23. Battaglia S, Badiali G, Cercenelli L, Bortolani B, Marcelli E, Cipriani R, et al. Combination of CAD/CAM and Augmented Reality in Free Fibula Bone Harvest. *Plast Reconstr Surg Glob Open* (2019) 7(11):e2510. doi: 10.1097/GOX.0000000000002510
24. Battaglia S, Ratti S, Manzoli L, Marchetti C, Cercenelli L, Marcelli E, et al. Augmented Reality-Assisted Periosteum Pedicled Flap Harvesting for Head and Neck Reconstruction: An Anatomical and Clinical Viability Study of a Galeo-Pericranial Flap. *J Clin Med* (2020) 9(7):E2211. doi: 10.3390/jcm9072211
25. Linte CA, Davenport KP, Cleary K, Peters C, Vosburgh KG, Navab N, et al. On Mixed Reality Environments for Minimally Invasive Therapy Guidance: Systems Architecture, Successes and Challenges in Their Implementation From Laboratory to Clinic. *Comput Med Imaging Graph* (2013) 37(2):83–97. doi: 10.1016/j.compmedimag.2012.12.002
26. Pérez-Pachón L, Poyade M, Lowe T, Gröning F. Image Overlay Surgery Based on Augmented Reality: A Systematic Review. *Adv Exp Med Biol* (2020) 1260:175–95. doi: 10.1007/978-3-030-47483-6_10
27. Bremers AWD, Yöntem AÖ, Li K, Chu D, Meijering V, Janssen CP. Perception of Perspective in Augmented Reality Head-Up Displays. *Int J Hum-Comput Stud* (2021) 155:102693. doi: 10.1016/j.ijhcs.2021.102693
28. Tokunaga DM, Corrêa CG, Bernardo FM, Bernardes J, Ranzini E, Nunes FLS, et al. Registration System Errors Perception in Augmented Reality Based on RGB-D Cameras. In: R Shumaker, S Lackey, editors. *Virtual, Augmented and Mixed Reality.* Cham: Springer International Publishing (2015). p. 119–29. Lecture Notes in Computer Science.
29. Jiang J, Huang Z, Qian W, Zhang Y, Liu Y. Registration Technology of Augmented Reality in Oral Medicine: A Review. *IEEE Access* (2019) 7:53566–84. doi: 10.1109/ACCESS.2019.2912949
30. Moreta-Martinez R, García-Mato D, García-Sevilla M, Pérez-Mañanes R, Calvo-Haro J, Pascau J. Augmented Reality in Computer-Assisted Interventions Based on Patient-Specific 3D Printed Reference. *Healthc Technol Lett* (2018) 5(5):162–6. doi: 10.1049/htl.2018.5072
31. Liu H, Auvinet E, Giles J, Rodriguez Y Baena F. Augmented Reality Based Navigation for Computer Assisted Hip Resurfacing: A Proof of Concept Study. *Ann BioMed Eng* (2018) 46(10):1595–605. doi: 10.1007/s10439-018-2055-1

32. Meulstee JW, Nijsink J, Schreurs R, Verhamme LM, Xi T, Delye HHK, et al. Toward Holographic-Guided Surgery. *Surg Innov* (2019) 26(1):86–94. doi: 10.1177/1553350618799552
33. Condino S, Carbone M, Piazza R, Ferrari M, Ferrari V. Perceptual Limits of Optical See-Through Visors for Augmented Reality Guidance of Manual Tasks. *IEEE Trans BioMed Eng* (2020) 67(2):411–9. doi: 10.1109/TBME.2019.2914517
34. Ferrari V, Carbone M, Condino S, Cutolo F. Are Augmented Reality Headsets in Surgery a Dead End? *Expert Rev Med Devices* (2019) 16(12):999–1001. doi: 10.1080/17434440.2019.1693891
35. Badiali G, Cutolo F, Cercenelli L, Carbone M, D'Amato R, Ferrari V, et al. The Vostars Project: A New Wearable Hybrid Video and Optical See-Through Augmented Reality Surgical System for Maxillofacial Surgery. *Int J Oral Maxillofac Surg* (2019) 48:153. doi: 10.1016/j.ijom.2019.03.472
36. Cutolo F, Freschi C, Mascioli S, Parchi PD, Ferrari M, Ferrari V. Robust and Accurate Algorithm for Wearable Stereoscopic Augmented Reality With Three Indistinguishable Markers. *Electronics* (2016) 5(3):59. doi: 10.3390/electronics5030059

20

Navigational Transmaxillary Endoscopic Approach for Inferomedial Tumors

Cheng-Hsien Wu[1,2], Yi-Yun Ho[1], Tzu-Lun Liu[1], Tzu-Ying Wu[2,3], Han-Chieh Cheng[1,2] and Chieh-Chih Tsai[4,5]*

[1] *Oral and Maxillofacial Surgery, Department of Stomatology, Taipei Veterans General Hospital, Taipei, Taiwan,*
[2] *Department of Dentistry, School of Dentistry, National Yang Ming Chiao Tung University, Taipei, Taiwan,*
[3] *Orthodontic and Pediatric Dentistry, Department of Dentistry, Taipei Veterans General Hospital, Taipei, Taiwan,*
[4] *Department of Ophthalmology, Taipei Veterans General Hospital, Taipei, Taiwan,* [5] *Department of Ophthalmology, School of Medicine, National Yang-Ming Chiao Tung University, Taipei, Taiwan*

Correspondence:
Cheng-Hsien Wu
wu_ch@vghtpe.gov.tw

Orbital tumors encompass a heterogeneous range of histopathology and usually variable in location. Traditionally, transconjunctival medial orbitotomy is used to access the medial orbital wall. However, it creates potential risk of soft tissue sequelae such as scarring, lid contracture, or entropion/ectropion. For the lesions close to the orbital apex, increased risk of optical nerve injury should be cautious during orbitotomy procedure. Transnasal endoscopic approach to the orbital walls has been applied since 1999. Although it provides good surgical visualization and prevents the soft tissue and neural complications, the narrow nasal corridor increases the surgical complexity. Extensive sphenoethmoidectomy is usually required to gaining access. Furthermore, the resultant medical orbital defect is difficult to repair. The maxillary sinus is the largest paranasal sinuses which is located beneath the orbital floor. It provides an ample working space for instrumentation. Meanwhile, repair of the orbital floor defect is feasible and with high degree of accuracy under navigation control. In this report, we propose a novel computer-assisted endoscopic protocol to excise the medial orbital tumors with immediate repair of the wall defect.

Keywords: transmaxillary, endoscope, orbital tumor, navigation, computer assisted, minimally invasive

1 INTRODUCTION

Orbital tumors encompass a heterogeneous range of histopathology, which 64% are benign and 46% are malignant according to a large cohort survey (1). According to its relationship with the extraocular muscle cones, the orbital tumors are classically divided into intraconal and extraconal position (2). Surgical excision is sometimes challenging to achieve balance among the optimal operative visualization, preserving function and minimize morbidities. Several transorbital and extraorbital surgical approaches has been developed for orbital tumor excision (3). However, for deep-seated lesions or those close to the orbital apex, the surgical filed is usually confined and risky to the surrounding neurovascular structures. Traditionally, surgical approaches to the lesions located in the medioposterior orbit are transconjunctival medial orbitotomy, and medial lateral orbitotomy (3–5). Although those approaches are straightforward, however, the soft tissue sequalae secondary to scarring e.g. lid retraction, ectropion/entropion, epiphora may anticipate (6). For large medial orbital lesions or those located close to the orbital apex, increased risk of optic nerve compressive injury during dissection should not be overlooked. Since the rapid progress of sinonasal endoscopic surgery, this technique is gradually applied in the orbital tumor or infectious condition management (7). The paranasal sinuses located at the medial and inferior parts of the orbital cavity provide a natural surgical access to the orbital tumors. The first case of transnasal endoscopic approach (TNEA) excision of the medioposterior orbital cavernous hemangioma was reported in 1999 (8). Although the nasal cavity provides a natural corridor for surgical access to the medial orbital wall, extensive sphenoethmoidectomy is usually required to gain better visualization and surgical freedom (9). In some cases, a second surgeon is needed for additional suction and irrigation procedures to improve visualization. This may require a septoplasty for additional instrumentation and the four-hands technique further increase the complexity of the operation (10). The maxillary sinus is the largest paranasal sinuses and located just beneath the orbital floor. Naturally, it provides a good access to the orbital floor and even to the medial and lateral walls. By using the traditional Caldwell Luc's approach, this wide opening sinus window become the direct portal to the orbital floor. In this report, we demonstrated the algorithm of the computer-assisted transmaxillary endoscopic approach (TMEA). The technical part will be explicated in four orbital tumor cases.

2 MATERIALS AND METHODS

Four cases with tumors located in the inferomedial compartment of orbit were enrolled. Written informed consent was obtained from these patients for the publication of any potentially identifiable images or data included in this article. The demographic data and presenting symptoms/signs were listed in the **Table 1**. The image-guided transmaxillary surgical scheme is proposed in the following sequence: image processing and virtual model creation, virtual surgical simulation and transfer, navigational TMEA, and post-operative evaluation. The step-by-step workflow is listed below:

2.1 Image Processing and Virtual Model Creation

Creation of an ideal virtual model is all the beginning of computer-assisted surgery. To optimize the skeletal image rendering quality, the volumetric CBCT scan with slice thickness of 0.3mm were used (NewTom NT, QR, Verona, Italy). The orbital tumors were best visualized with MRI sequences as the T1W, T1W with contrast and fat suppression technique, and T2W. The digital imaging and communications

TABLE 1 | Clinical characteristics and surgical parameters.

	Patient No. 1	Patient No. 2	Patient No. 3	Patient No. 4	Average
Clinical parameters					
Age (years)	85	64	48	51	62 ± 14.6
Gender	Male	Female	Female	Male	
Localization	Intraconal	Extraconal	Extraconal	Intraconal	
Laterality	Right	Left	Left	Right	
Quadrant of the orbit	Inferomedial	Inferomedial	Inferomedial	Superomedial/inferomedial	
Symptoms & signs	Near complete vision loss, proptosis	Progressive blurred vision and mild proptosis	Painful swelling	Progressive blurred vision and proptosis	
Histopathology	Schwannoma	Cavernous venous malformation	Idiopathic orbital inflammation	Cavernous venous malformation	
Size (cm^3)	13.4 (2.8x2.0x2.4)	1.2 (1.3x1.0x0.9)	2.3 (1.2x0.9x2.1)	7.8 (2.0x2.3x1.7)	6.2 ± 4.9
Hospital stays (days)	4	3	3	5	3.8 ± 0.8
Surgical parameters					
Operation time (min)	155	180	174	300	202.3 ± 57.2
Blood loss (ml)	65	20	30	170	71.3 ± 59.4
Orbital floor reconstruction	Bio-membrane	Bio-membrane with titanium mesh	None	MEDPORE	
Early complication	Paranasal paresthesia (+) for 2 months with complete recovery Nasal congestion (+) 3 weeks	Paranasal paresthesia (+) for 1 month with complete recovery Nasal congestion (-)	Paranasal paresthesia (+) for 1 month with complete recovery Nasal congestion (+) for 1month	Paranasal paresthesia (+) for at least 2 months with progressive recovery Nasal congestion (+) for 1month	
	Diplopia cannot evaluate due to poor vision	Diplopia (+), complete resolve within 2 months	Diplopia (+), complete resolve within 2 months	Diplopia (+) for at least 2 months with progressive recovery	
Late complications	Mild enophthalmos	None	None	Mild enophthalmos	

in medicine (DICOM) data were imported to the iPlan® CMF Version 3.0 software platform (Brainlab AG, Feldkirchen, Germany) for subsequent planning. Automatic image fusion algorithm is ran first to coordinate the image datasets (11). This is a critical step that ensure all the objects created from different image datasets will register in the same spatial cranial position. Segmentation of the craniofacial bones was then done by the preset templates of the software or manual segmentation of the region of interest by bone-specific Hounsfield units (**Figure 1A**, green). The tumor was mapped based on the MRI for better soft tissue and tumor border delineation. If the orbital walls surrounding the tumor are destructed, a mirrored image is created from the healthy orbit and superimposed onto the affected side (**Figure 1A**, orange). Then surgeon could fine-tune the position of the mirrored object and outlines the margins to achieve symmetry. This will facilitate intraoperative guidance by printing out the physical model for pre-contouring the reconstructive material, plus by real-time navigation to ensure the implant position. The trajectories design allows surgeon to design the path of entry to the medial orbit and define the ideal entry point on the sinus roof/orbital floor (**Figure 1B**). The virtual surgical plan is then transferred to the navigator for intraoperative guidance. The according 3D segmented objects are exported in the form of stereolithographic (STL) files to manufacturing the physical models.

2.2 Navigational Transmaxillary Endoscopic Approach

2.2.1 Navigation Coordinate Registration

The VSP done by the iPlan was imported into the infrared-based navigation system (Kick®, Brainlab AG, Feldkirchen, Germany). This stereoscopic infrared camera provides real-time tracking and displaying instrument positions intraoperatively. To ensure the operation is in the same coordinate system of the navigation image datasets, registration is the crucial preliminary step to re-orient the patient in the operating theatre. A "skull reference frame" with reflective marker spheres is fixed onto the patient's skull. Then the registration is completed by using the optical surface matching device (Z touch®, Brainlab AG, Feldkirchen, Germany) plotting the skin points on the T zone of the forehead and nasal region. Optical tracking pointer is used to verify the accuracy of registration. The resulting point-to-point target registration error (TRE) should less than 1mm to optimize the accuracy of registration (12, 13).

2.2.2 Caldwell Luc Approach and Trajectorial-Guided Orbital Floor Entry

The surgeon position stands at the same site of the affected eye facilitate medial dissection of the orbit. The patient's head position is upward extended and turned away from the surgeon side. Upper lip is retracted upward to reveal the buccogingival sulcus. Supravestibular incision to maintain a mucosal cuff is done from the canine to the second molar. The anterior wall of the maxillary sinus is exposed by elevating the subperiosteal flap. The infraorbital neurovascular bundle is identified and preserved. A rectangular bony window is prepared for antrostomy after pre-fixed a miniplate on the bone fragment to facilitate later reposition (**Figure 2**). To optimize the freedom of surgery, the bony window should be designed as large as possible for sufficient surgical corridor. The maxillary sinus is entered and a 0-degree, 4mm endoscope (Karl Storz and Co, Tuttlingen, Germany) is introduced to visualize the surgical field. There are two surgical landmarks identified: the infraorbital canal (IOC) and the maxillary ostium (**Figure 3A**). The IOC presents as linear protuberance running from the junction between the superior and posterior sinus walls to the infraorbital foramen. The IOC separate the orbital floor to a thinner medial part (1.0-2.0mm) and a thicker lateral part (2.5-4.0mm) (14). The maxillary ostium sited at the posterior-superior corner of the medial sinus wall. After identified the medial part of the orbital floor, the navigation pointer is introduced to locate the entry site. The reflective marker spheres can also attach onto the surgical instruments by adapter array for real-time guidance. The length, diameter, and vector of the instruments can be easily calibrated by the

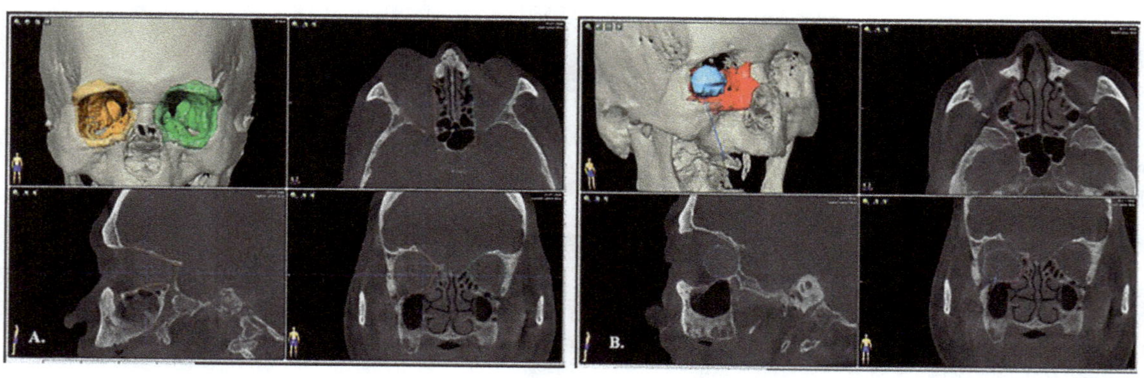

FIGURE 1 | Image segmentation by bone-specific Hounsfield units. **(A)** segmentation of the normal, non-destructive orbital wall (green); the mirrored image from the contralateral normal orbital wall to rebuild the destructed right side medio-inferior orbital walls (orange). **(B)** The orbital tumor was segmented with fusion MRI and CT images to optimize the tumor boundaries (blue). A trajectory through the maxillary sinus that indicated the path of entry to orbital tumor was designed for intraoperative guidance.

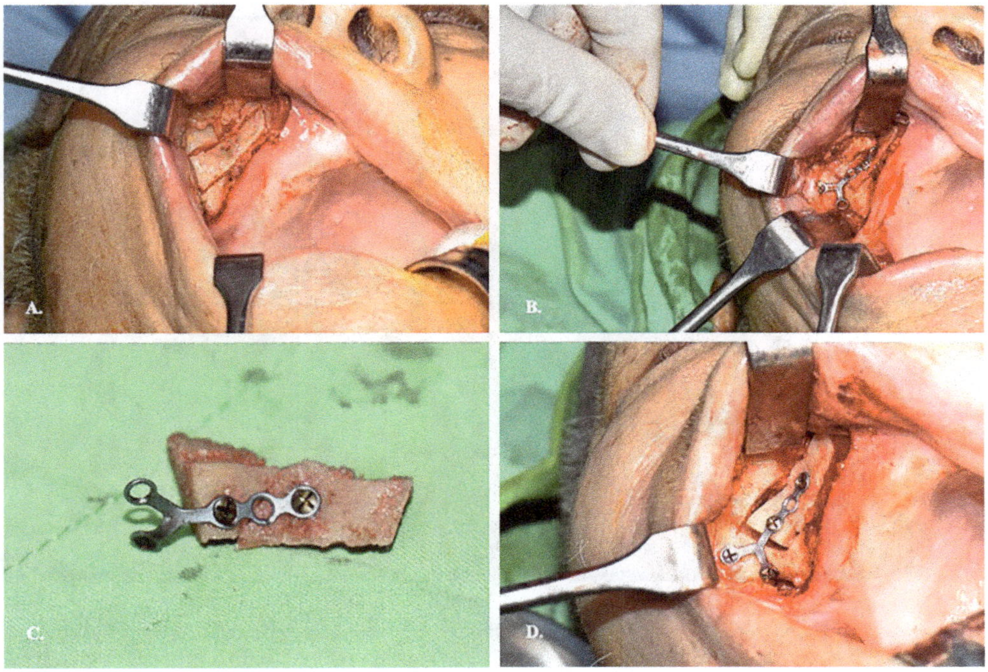

FIGURE 2 | Preparation of the bone window on the anterior wall of maxillary sinus. **(A)** Supravestibular incision to expose sinus anterior wall. **(B)** Prebend the miniplate before osteotomy of the sinus wall. **(C)** Illustration of the miniplate-prefix bony wall. **(D)** Reposition of the bony wall after completion of the orbital surgery.

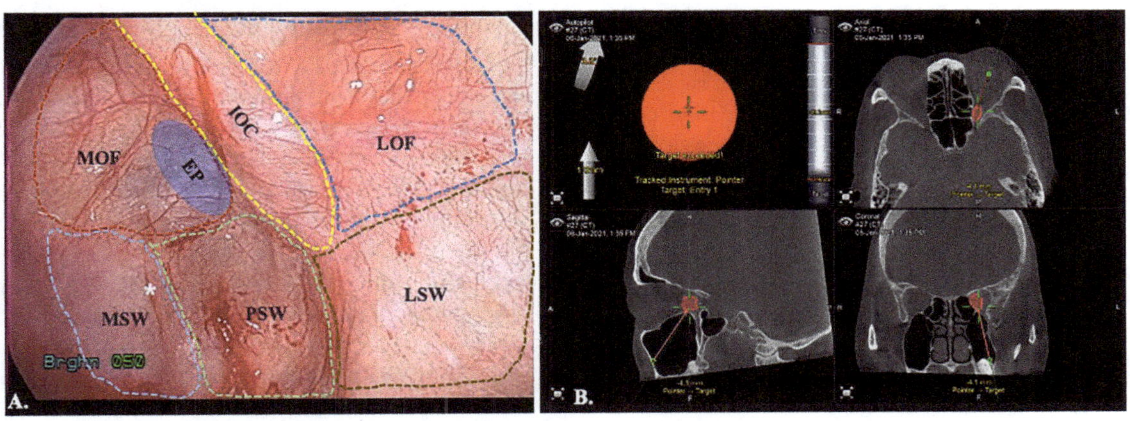

FIGURE 3 | Endoscopic view of transmaxillary approach with the trajectorial-guided entry to the orbit. **(A)**. MOF, medial orbital floor; IOC, infraorbital canal; LOF, lateral orbital floor; MSW, medial sinus wall; PSW, posterior sinus wall; LSW, lateral sinus wall; EP, entry point; *maxillary ostium. **(B)** Trajectorial-guided orbital entry.

instrument calibration matrix. By combining the autopilot function, the trajectorial-guided surgical dissection could be done in accuracy and safe (**Figure 3B**). The periorbita is readily seen after the orbital floor is opened.

2.2.3 Periorbita Dissection and Image-Controlled Tumor Excision

After creation of the orbital floor window, the navigation pointer is used to locate the tumor position (**Figure 4A**). The surrounding bone is carefully removed with rongeur or rotating bur. It should be cautious that adequate protection is necessary to prevent periorbita from accidentally drawn in by the rotating airflow. This could result in catastrophic injury to the extraocular muscles and nerves. The incision is performed longitudinal to the long axis of the orbit. Once the periorbita is opened, the medial and inferior rectus muscles (MR and IR) are seen as dissection landmarks (**Figure 4B**). Extraconal lesions are usually easily identified and less need for dissection after

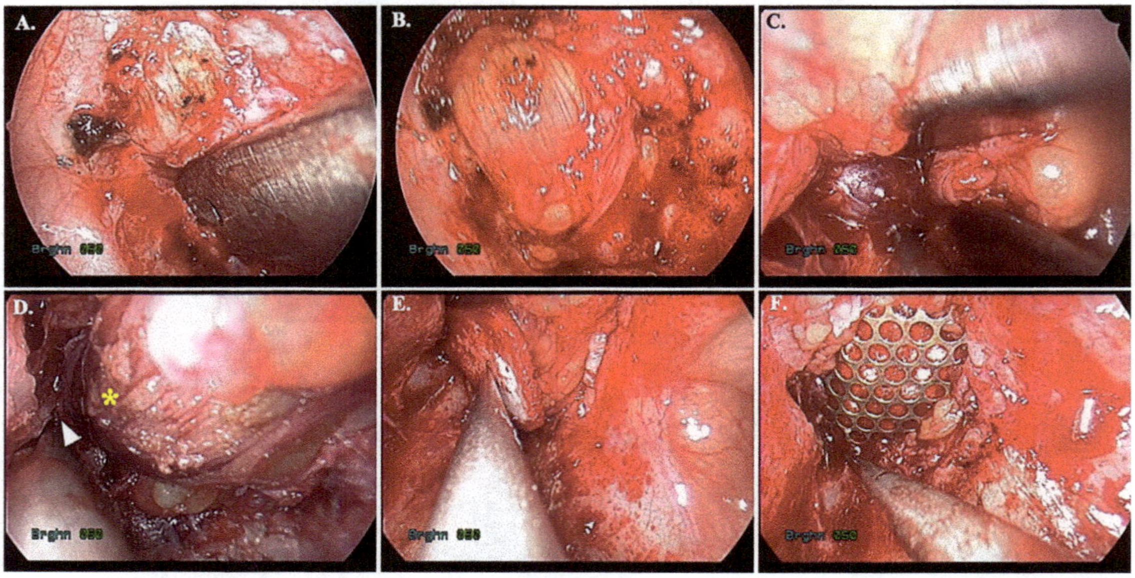

FIGURE 4 | Image-controlled surgical excision of medial orbital tumor with reconstruction. **(A)** entry of the medial orbit; **(B)** periorbita and inferior rectus muscle; **(C)** identify the tumor; **(D)** image after tumor excision, the arrowhead: ethmoid sinus, star: medial rectus muscle; **(E)** bio-collagen membrane repair of the defect; **(F)** Ti-mesh reinforcement of the inferomedial strut.

periorbita incision and navigator identification (**Figures 4C, D**). For intraconal tumors, the MR and IR can mobilize medially/laterally and superiorly. For the lesions sited superomedially, a larger orbital floor surgical defect allows to mobilize the entire orbit inferiorly which provide access to the area (15, 16). With transmaxillary endoscopic approach, the surgical target could safely reach medially to the ethmoid sinus and even superiorly to the sphenoid sinus and optic canal under navigation control. After identifying the tumor, the dissection is proceeded under image controlled and the cryoprobe may assist in cryoextraction of the tumor in some scenario (17).

2.2.4 Imaged-Controlled Medial/Inferior Orbital Walls Repair

The orbital floor (or with the medial wall defect) can be repaired straightforward after removal of the tumor. For small defects that are not involving the inferomedial strut, an alloplastic material, e.g. biocollagen membrane, or porous polyethylene implants is sufficient for endoscopic reconstruction (**Figure 4E**). For larger defects or those involving the inferomedial strut, the titanium mesh could be applied to reinforce the structure and prevent diplopia from orbital malposition (**Figure 4F**). The mesh can easily be pre-bended by the physical model and inserted into the surgical defect under endoscope. Navigation provides the accurate position control (**Figure 5**). Forced duction test should be performed to preclude any soft tissue entrapment by the material.

2.2.5 Reposition the Anterior Maxillary Wall and Wound Closure

After completion of the orbital floor repair, the bony fragment of the maxillary anterior wall is repositioned and fixed with miniplate. The buccogingival incision is primarily close with resorbable sutures.

RESULTS

Four cases with TMEA excision of medial orbital tumor were performed. All patients underwent surgery with radical intent, and a complete resection was obtained. The clinical characteristics were listed in the **Table 1**. Clinically, all patients had various degrees of visual impairment and proptosis. The individual patient presentation on the diagnosis were listed as followed:

Patient 1 was in a status of nearly complete vision loss due to optic nerve compression. Meanwhile, he had limited upward and lateral gaze of the affected orbit. The MRI showed a retrobulbar intraconal well-demarcated ovoid mass about 2.8x2.0x2.4cm. The tumor showed heterogenous appearance on T2W sequences with some internal cystic component, and significant contrast enhancement. The tumor deviated the right optic nerve upward and causing right proptosis (**Figure 6A**).

Patient 2 experienced mild symptoms with progressive blurred vision and proptosis. The CT showed an ovoid, well-defined with contrast-enhanced mass at the medioposterior extraconal space and medial to the apical region of the optic nerve. MRI images showed slight hypointensity in T1W sequences and hyperintensity in T2W sequences. The radiographic feature was favored of cavernous venous malformation (**Figure 6B**).

Patient 3 complained of painful swelling over left side orbit. The images showed a 1.2x0.9x2.1cm enhancing mass at medial side of left intraconal region, which involving the medial rectus muscle (**Figure 6C**). Suspected orbital lymphoma or idiopathic inflammation pseudotumor.

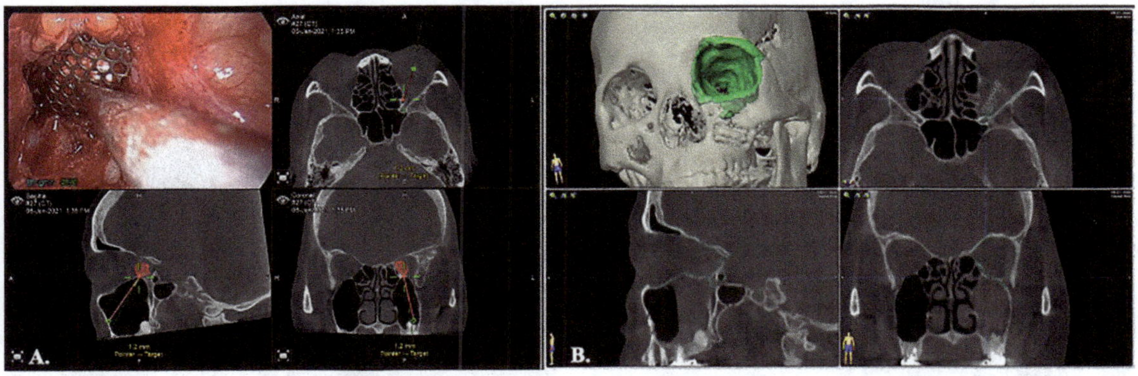

FIGURE 5 | Image-controlled orbital floor reconstruction. **(A)** position control of the Ti-mesh by real time navigation. **(B)** post-op image showed high level of accuracy with orbital floor reconstruction. Green: pre-operative orbital wall.

Patient 4 presented with progressive blurred vision for 2 years. The visual exam demonstrated decreased visual acuity, color sense, limited abduction, and mild exophthalmos of right sided eye. Orbital MRI revealed a heterogeneously enhancing mass lesion at the right intraconal space, medial to the optic nerve, and measuring about 2.0x2.3x1.7cm. With mass effect causing deviation of the right orbital nerve laterally. The lesion showed hyperintense T2 and hypointense T1FS appearance. Suspected cavernous venous malformation (**Figure 6D**).

Four lesions were difficult to approach by traditional transorbital route. We applied TMEA and successfully excised the lesions. For extraconal lesions, the surgical dissection was straightforward with limited periorbital dissection. However, the intraconal lesions need more muscle traction and may need fat extirpation especially close to the orbital apex. The surgical procedure in case 4 was shown in **Figures 7A–H**. The mean operation time were 202.3 ± 57.2minutes including the setup of navigator. The hospital stay was about 3.8 ± 0.8 days. All patients experienced a short duration of paranasal paresthesia, but all recovered within post-op 2 months except for the case 4. He still had numbness of the paranasal region at 2 months followed up. But the degree of numbness decreases over time. Patient 2 and 3 had post-op diplopia due to edematous change of the orbital content. It resolved within 2 months and no residual limitation of extraocular muscles was found. Patient 1 cannot evaluate the post-op diplopia due to near-complete vision loss before operation. However, his light perception immediate recover after operation. The visual acuity showed complete improved in patient 2 and dramatically improved in patient 1 from the initial no light perception state. The case 4 presented with persisted diplopia at upward and downward gaze after 2 months of followed up. However, the degree of diplopia showed progressive recovery. The summary of visual outcomes was listed in **Table 2**. Biocollagen membrane (ABCcolla® Collagen Membrane, ACRO Biomedical Co., Ltd. Kaohsiung, Taiwan) was used for orbital floor reconstruction in case 1 and case 2 (**Figure 4E**). Titanium mesh (MatrixORBITAL ™ DePuySynthes, Oberdorf, Switzerland) was used for structural reinforcement of medial orbital struct in patient 2 (**Figure 4F**). Porous polyethylene implant (Medpor®, Stryker CMF, Kalamazoo, MI 49002, USA) was used in patient 4 (**Figure 7F**). Compared the reconstructive results, the patient 1 showed mild enophthalmos for only using biocollagen membrane reconstruction. In patient 2, 3 the post-operative CT images showed true-to-original reconstructed orbital floor without periorbita or muscular herniation (**Figure 9**). Preoperative and postoperative CT images of case 1,2,4 showed well restored orbital volume (**Figures 8–10**). The patient 4 has mild enophthalmos after operation even the CT images showed well bony reconstruction (**Figure 10**). The enophthalmos is suspected related to fat volume reduction during operation from its intraconal position and size. The clinical photo of case 1 and case 2 were shown in **Figure 11**. The images showed well orbital volume preservation after surgery and no interference on orbital movement.

4. DISCUSSION

Orbital tumor treatment is often challenging for both functional and esthetic considerations. Among them, orbital vascular malformations (OVMs) are the most common orbital masses, which are often misinterpretation as "tumor" in the context of cavernous hemangiomas, lymphangiomas … etc (18). In our cases, two were pathologically diagnosed as capillary venous malformation. In same study, Colletti et al. proposed three subtypes of OVMs, which are relevant to planning corresponding treatment modalities and predict the possible complications. Unlike the type 2 and type 3 OVMs which are connected to the venous system of the orbit (and sometimes intracranially), the type 1 OVM is excluded from the surrounding venous system. This feature allows relatively easiness on surgical dissection, and less bleeding during procedure. In terms of surgical approaches, transnasal endoscopic approach is fitted for the extraconal/intraconal type 1 OVM that situated at the medial quadrants of the orbit (18, 19). In this report, we proposed an alternative route to the medial OVMs from the floor. For the extraconal lesions, the dissection is relative straightforward. Once the lesion is localized under navigation, the periorbita was excised as needed and the dissection could be limited

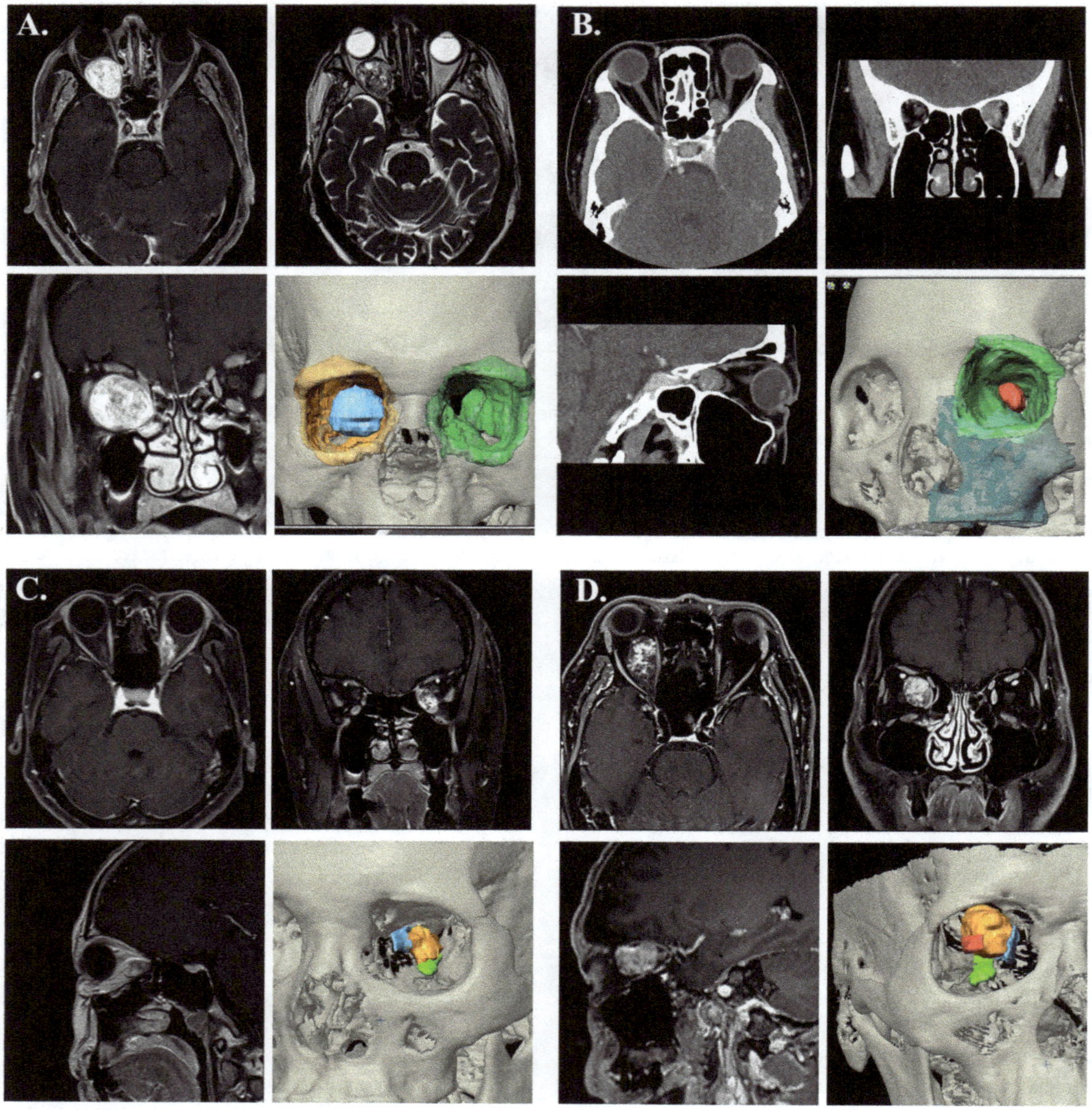

FIGURE 6 | Image characteristics of the cases. **(A)** The contrast-enhanced MRI showed a retrobulbar intraconal well-demarcated ovoid mass of right orbit. The tumor showed heterogenous appearance on T2W sequences with some internal cystic component, and significant contrast enhancement. The tumor deviated the right optic nerve upward and causing right proptosis. 3D image rendering tumor lesion was demonstrated (blue). **(B)** The CT showed an ovoid, well-defined with contrast-enhanced mass at the medioposterior extraconal space and medial to the apical region of the optic nerve. 3D image rendering tumor lesion was demonstrated (red). **(C)** The MRI demonstrated an enhancing mass at medial side of left intraconal space (orange), which involving the medial rectus muscle (blue) and superior to inferior rectus muscle (green). **(D)** The MRI revealed a heterogeneously enhancing mass lesion at the right intraconal space (orange), medial to the optic nerve (red) that displaced laterally. (Blue: medial rectus muscle; Green: inferior rectus muscle)

with endoscopic assistance. For the case 2 and 3, the patients experienced limited diplopia but fully recovered within 2 months is possibly related to post-operative tissue edematous change. For the intraconal lesions, dissection between inferior and medical rectus muscles is usually necessary. During procedure, the prolonged and excessive muscle traction will cause swelling and even ischemic change of the muscle that may cause diplopia after surgery (20–22). Especially when the lesion is close to the orbital apex, the surgical corridor is limited by the convergence of muscle cones which further increase the incidence of muscle injury. In our cases, although all the patients experienced diplopia immediate after operation. However, the diplopia is transient and all resolve in 2 months except the case 4. He still presented with limitation on upward and downward gaze after 2 months followed up but with progressive improvement. The position of this intraconal lesion was close to the orbital apex make surgical dissection more complicated. The postoperative images showed swelling of the inferior and medial rectus muscle reflect the intense inflammatory reaction

TABLE 2 | Preoperative and postoperative ophthalmic evaluation.

	Patient 1			Patient 2		
	Pre-op	**Post-op 1wk**	**Post-op 2M**	**Pre-op**	**Post-op 1 wk**	**Post-op 2M**
Visual acuity	NLP*	20/200	20/50	20/30	20/25	20/20
Hertel Exophthalmometer (mm)	14	9	9	16	Not perform	14
EOM	Restriction in all directions except abduction	No change	Mild to moderate improvement	Full and free	Mild restriction in supraaduction	Full and free
		Patient 3			**Patient 4**	
Visual acuity	20/20	20/20	20/20	20/40	20/20	20/20
Hertel Exophthalmometer (mm)	14/14	14/14	14/13	21	Not perform	16
EOM	Full and free	Mild infraduction and lateroduction limitation	Full and free	Full and free	Infraduction and supraduction	Progressive improve

**NLP, no light perception.*

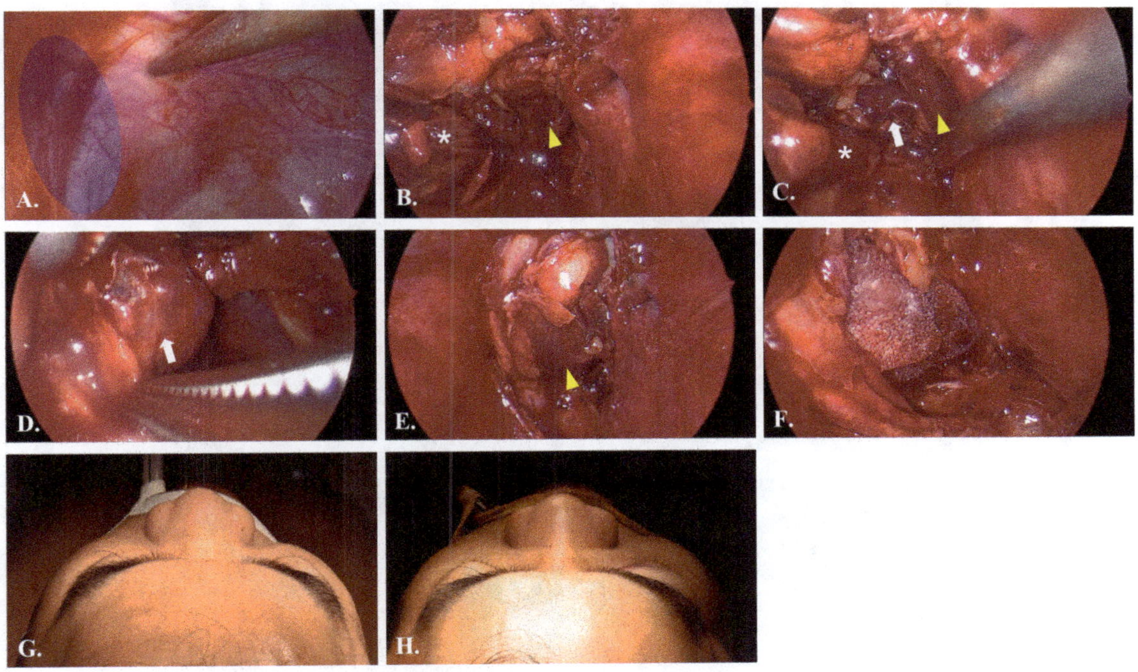

FIGURE 7 | Intraoperative views of Case 4. **(A)** Endoscopic view of case 4. The pointer indicated the location of infraorbital nerve. The blue area is the entry point. **(B)** After incision of the periorbita, the inferior rectus muscle (yellow arrowhead) and medial rectus muscle (white star) were identified. **(C)** Dissection between inferior rectus and medial rectus muscle to identify the lesion (white arrow). **(D)** Dissection of the lesion from peripheral orbital tissue. **(E)** Return of inferior rectus muscle to original position after removal of the lesion. **(F)** The orbital floor was repaired with porous polyethylene mesh (MEDPOR). **(G)** Preoperative view showed mild proptosis of right eye. **(H)** Postoperative view showed symmetry orbital position.

and muscle dysfunction (**Figure 10**). This phenomenon is not seen in case 1. Although the lesion was also in intraconal position, it could be easily dissection off between medial and inferior rectus muscles from its more anterior location that made it away from the narrow apical region.

The traditional transorbital route has limited access to the posterior orbital tumors especially in the inferomedial and apical region (23). The operation on this tight, crowding space that packing with numerous critical neurovascular structures is just like "The devil's touch". Combination of extensive fronto-temporo-orbital-zygomatic dysjunction is sometimes indicated for complete excision, however, the potential neural complications, such as subdural hematoma, brain edema, CSF leakage, vision loss, postoperative seizure should be cautious (24) not mentioned to the complexity of the operation. Recently, the TNEA is gaining popularity for orbital tumor excision especially

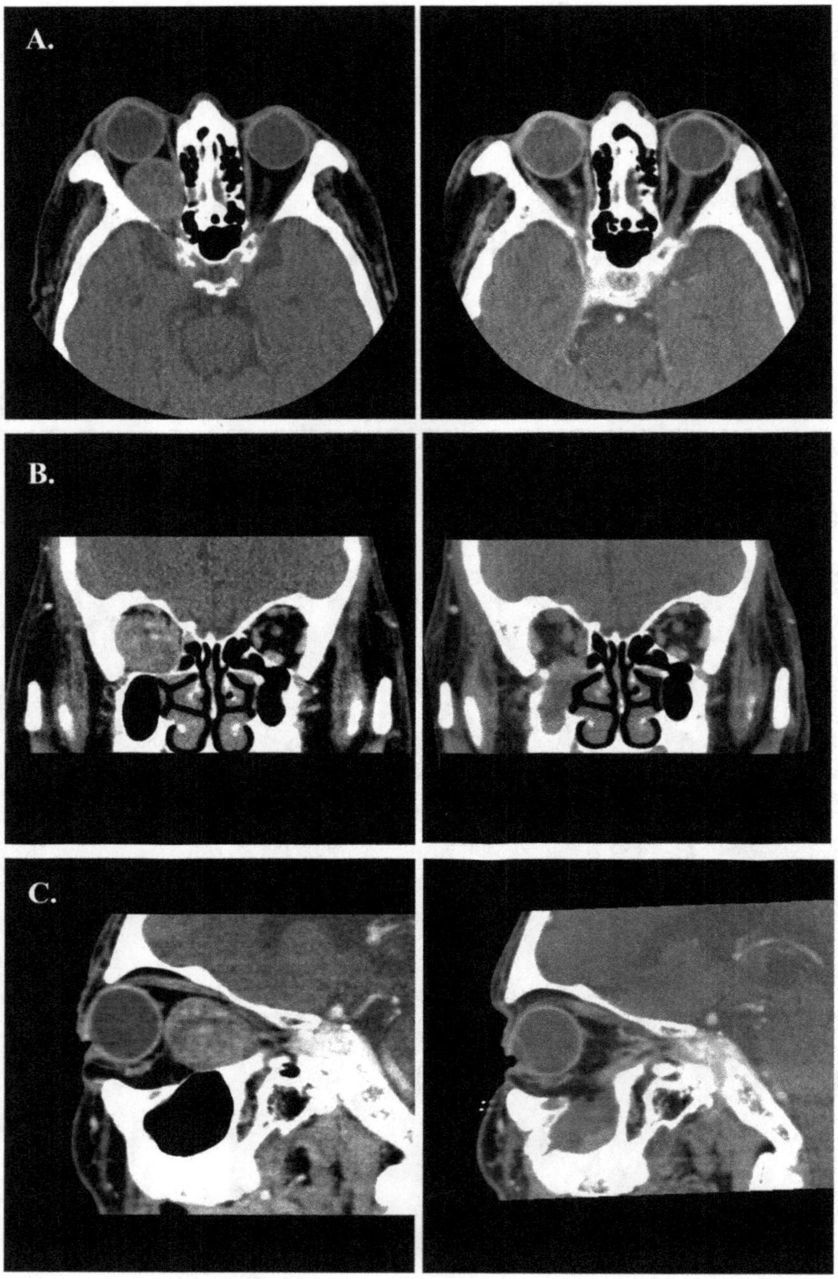

FIGURE 8 | (A–C) Preoperative and postoperative images of Case 1. The left-side axial, coronal and sagittal images were the preoperative CT scans. The right-side postoperative CT images showed normal extraocular muscles position and well restored orbital volume.

for intraconal lesions located inferiorly and medially to the optic nerve and the extraconal lesions adjacent to the paranasal sinuses (8, 19, 25, 26). Anatomically, the lamina papyracea is the only thin barrier between medial orbit and the ethmoid sinus. The transnasal route provides the shortcut to the orbit thus avoids plethoric muscle detachment and potential neurovascular compression from transorbital approach. The outcome of the purely TNEA excision of orbital tumors has been well elaborate in the systemic review (20). In this review, it demonstrated that TNEA can effectively excise a diverse array of intraconal/extraconal orbital lesions. However, almost one-third of cases had postoperative sequalae, which diplopia was the most frequent reported followed by enophthalmos. Although 76.2% of complications were transient, the overall complication rate was slightly higher than the reported rate from traditional orbitotomy procedures (21). Techniquewise, the TNEA usually begin with sphenoethmoidectomy to reach the lamina papyracea and then enter to the medial orbit after removing this thin bony

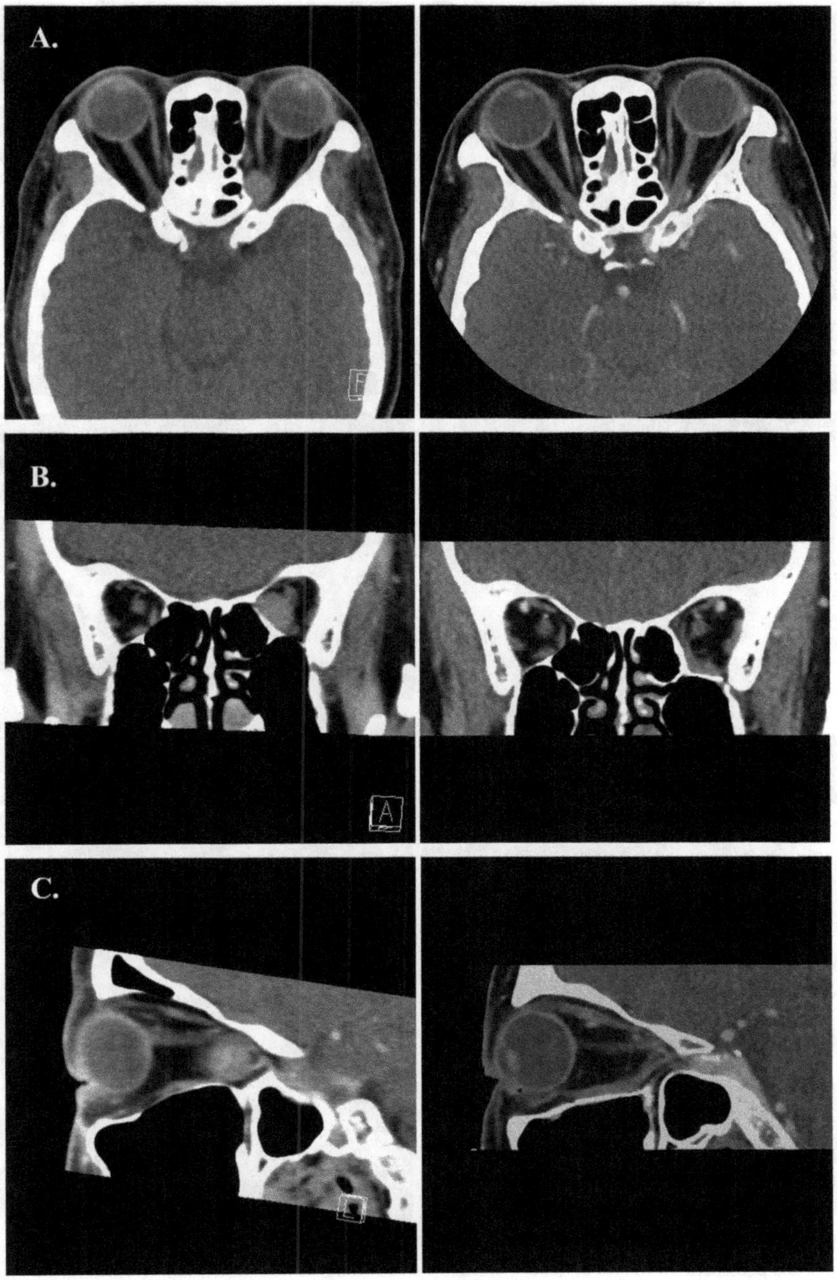

FIGURE 9 | (A–C) Preoperative and postoperative images of Case 2. The left-side axial, coronal and sagittal images were the preoperative CT scans. The right-side postoperative CT images showed normal extraocular muscles position and well restored orbital volume with Titanium mesh.

barrier. The "sword fighting effect" that from narrow surgical corridor may limited the working channel for the intraconal lesions or those close to the orbital apex. To improve the maneuverability, the four-handed binostril procedure, extensive medial antrostomy, posterior septectomy may employ (27, 28). However, these maneuvers may increase the nasal complication rate and crusting (29). The TMEA provides an excellent operative window for instrumentation. According to the recent anatomical study from Donofrio CA et al. (30), the mean operative window for TMEA was 278.9 ± 43.8 mm^2, which was significantly larger than the TNEA (240.8 ± 21.5mm^2). The larger operative window improves the maneuverability of instruments. Furthermore, the surgical path of TMEA is a direct line of sight which is more intuitive for surgeons. The ample space from maxillary sinus tolerates different surgical instruments in the same channel. By creating a large antrum window, we could deploy the endoscope and dissecting instruments in a direct and single surgical port. The dissection

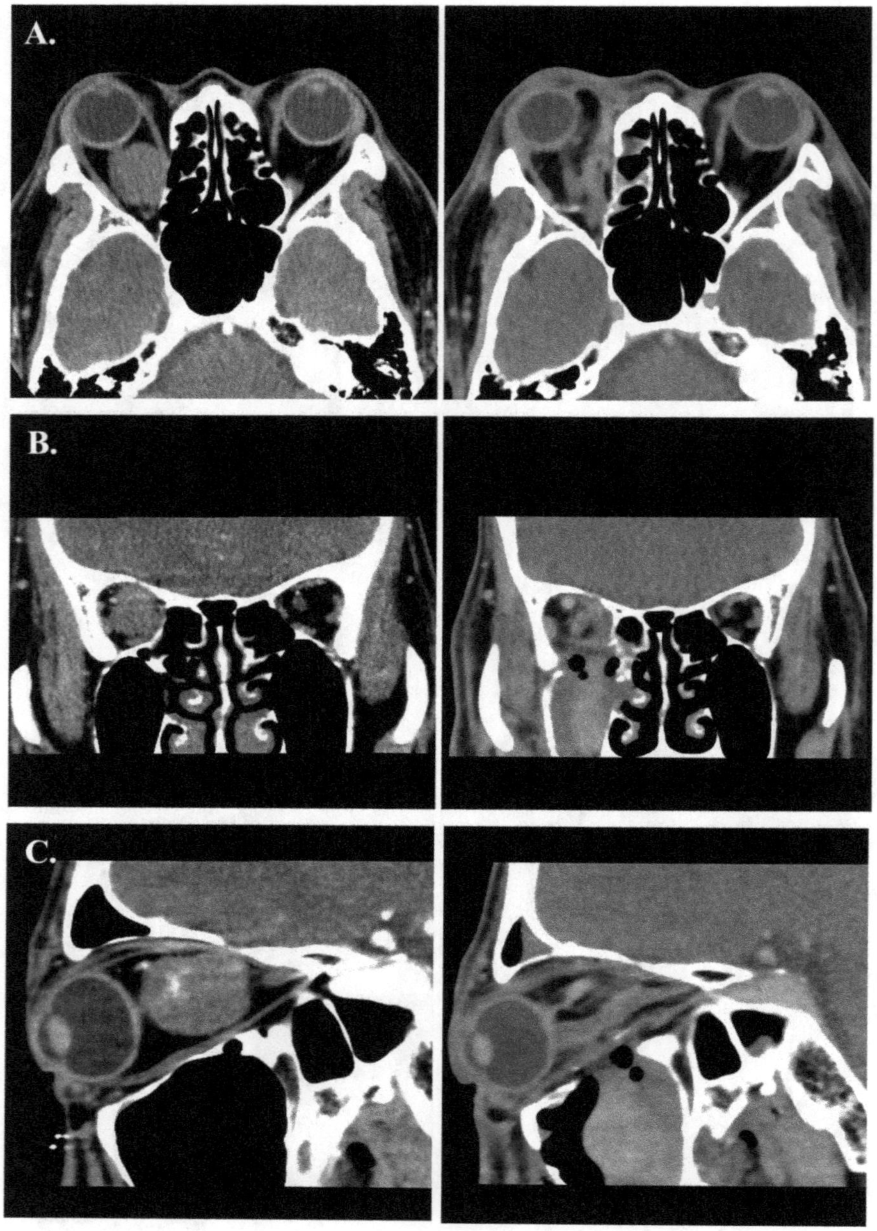

FIGURE 10 | **(A–C)** Preoperative and postoperative images of Case 4. The left side axial, coronal and sagittal images were the preoperative CT scans. The right-side immediate postoperative CT images showed swelling of the medial rectus and mild distortion of medial rectus muscle.

was done straightforward, and the operation time could be controlled within 3 hours including the setup of navigation and orbital wall reconstruction. The distance of pivotal point of the instruments to the orbital floor is greater in TMEA, which produces a larger angle of attack than TNEA (45°-65° vs. 20°-30°, respectively) (30). Meaning that TMEA could cover the entire orbital floor as surgical field. In our experience, the TMEA could easily target posteriorly to the medial orbital apex and superiorly to the lateral wall of the sphenoid sinus after removing the orbital floor. According to the comparative study of different endoscopic approach to the anterolateral skull base, TMEA offers better surgical freedom and head-on approach than TNEA (31). This superior surgical flexibility is well demonstrated in our case 2. The lesion was located at the inferomedial aspect of the orbital apex and lateral to the sphenoid sinus. With the three-dimensional image rendering, virtual surgical trajectory was planned preoperatively. The orbital floor osteotomy and surgical dissection was accurately executed by real-time navigation control. The surgical freedom of TMEA is primarily limited by the size of antrum window. For patients with atrophic maxillary sinus, with mixed dentition stage, incomplete pneumatization are not indicated for this approach (32). We

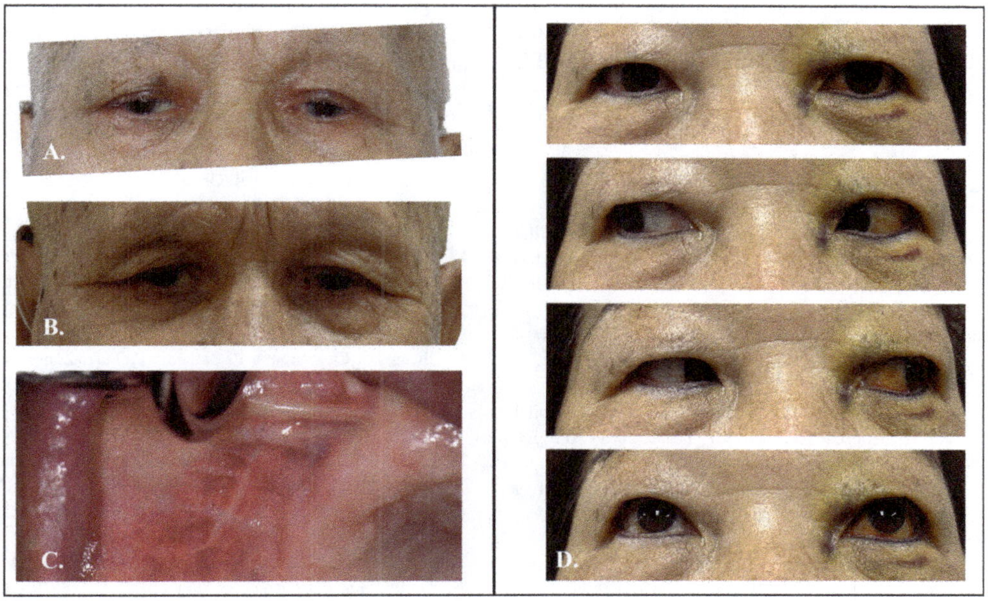

FIGURE 11 | Preoperative and postoperative clinical photo of Case 1 and 2. **(A)** Preoperative photo of case 1 showed mild proptosis over right-side eye. **(B)** Symmetry of eye position after TMEA excision of orbital tumor. **(C)** Postoperative oral wound healed well. **(D)** Two weeks postoperative photo of case 2 showed well functional orbital movement.

recommend creating the antrum window as large as possible, even including the entire anterior maxillary wall but the infraorbital foramen to avoid nerve injury. By using piezo osteotomy, the bone cutting is precise and atraumatic which facilitate later reposition of the bone fragment with miniplates. This temporary antrum window protocol preserves the integrity of the maxillary sinus, which reduces the soft tissue contracture on the surgical site and formation of oro-antral fistula. Although transient facial numbness may develop from traction injury to the infraorbital nerve, all our patients completely recovered within 2 months. The reported rhinological morbidities in TNEA such as epistaxis, nasal synechiae, nasal crusting, nasolacrimal duct injuries are free from TMEA (28, 33).

The other advantage from the ample surgical field provided by TMEA is the possibility of reconstruction of the orbital wall. The orbital floor osteotomy created for surgical access could be repaired under endoscope by alloplastic materials, such as collagen membrane, porous polyethylene implants, or titanium plates depending on the defect size and the strength need. The implant is easily inserted through the antrum window and placed between the periorbita and the bony orbit. Navigation is then used to ensure the position is true to original. This procedure prevents the herniation of the periorbita into the sinus, which avoid post-operative enophthalmos and long-term diplopia. In the literature, the risk of developing post-operative enophthalmos is 5.9% for TNEA, which is mainly due to fail to restore the orbital volume (34). Currently, there is no consensus on the best reconstruction option for TNEA, although the bone fragments, pedicle naso-septal flap, or allograft had been used (35). The limited surgical corridor in TNEA makes the medial or inferior orbital walls reconstruction difficult and most of the surgeons choose not to repair it. However, there were several excellent results of medical wall reconstruction by porous polyethylene mesh after traumatic injury and tumor excision from TNEA by Colletti et al. (36–40). With experienced hands, the medial wall defects could be repaired *via* TNEA and further prevent post-operative enophthalmos. The TMEA creates defects at the orbital floor, either biocollagen membrane or porous polyethylene mesh is suitable material for reconstruction. However, if the defects across the orbital supporting construct, more rigid material, e.g. Titanium mesh is the material of choice. With the experience on endoscopic orbital floor reconstruction in blow out fracture patients, orbital wall repair with Titanium mesh *via* TMEA is feasible and has more controllable outcome with the assistance of endoscope and navigation (41, 42).

5. CONCLUSION

Endoscopic surgery opens an eye for minimal invasive orbital tumor excision. The TMEA provides a versatile surgical corridor to the inferior and medial orbit and even to the orbital apex region. It provides an intuitive dissection corridor and an alternative surgical view to TNEA. In this computer-assisted workflow, we implement virtual surgical planning, intraoperative navigation, and true-to-original orbital wall reconstruction that is beneficial for patients by shorten surgical time, hospital stays, and minimal complications. We believe the application could be expanded to most of the orbital tumor surgery.

AUTHOR CONTRIBUTIONS

C-HW: protocol design, manuscript preparation, data collection, analysis, and final approval of the manuscript. Y-YH, T-LL, T-YW, H-CC, and C-CT: data collection and analysis. T-YW: image processing and virtual surgical planning. All authors are responsible for the manuscript. All authors contributed to the article and approved the submitted version.

REFERENCES

1. Shields JA, Shields CL, Scartozzi R. Survey of 1264 Patients With Orbital Tumors and Simulating Lesions: The 2002 Montgomery Lecture, Part 1. *Ophthalmology* (2004) 111(5):997–1008. doi: 10.1016/j.ophtha. 2003.01.002
2. Darsaut TE, Lanzino G, Lopes MB, Newman S. An Introductory Overview of Orbital Tumors. *Neurosurg Focus* (2001) 10(5):E1. doi: 10.3171/ foc.2001.10.5.2
3. Cockerham KP, Bejjani GK, Kennerdell JS, Maroon JC. Surgery for Orbital Tumors. Part II: Transorbital Approaches. *Neurosurg Focus* (2001) 10(5):E3. doi: 10.3171/foc.2001.10.5.4
4. Bejjani GK, Cockerham KP, Kennerdel JS, Maroon JC. A Reappraisal of Surgery for Orbital Tumors. Part I: Extraorbital Approaches. *Neurosurg Focus* (2001) 10(5):E2. doi: 10.3171/foc.2001.10.5.3
5. Maroon JC, Kennerdell JS. Surgical Approaches to the Orbit. Indications and Techniques. *J Neurosurg* (1984) 60(6):1226–35. doi: 10.3171/jns.1984. 60.6.1226
6. Mullins JB, Holds JB, Branham GH, Thomas JR. Complications of the Transconjunctival Approach. A Review of 400 Cases. *Arch Otolaryngol Head Neck Surg* (1997) 123(4):385–8. doi: 10.1001/archoto.123.4.385
7. Raponi I, Giovannetti F, Buracchi M, Priore P, Battisti A, Scagnet M, et al. Management of Orbital and Brain Complications of Sinusitis: A Practical Algorithm. *J Craniomaxillofac Surg* (2021) 49(12):1124–9. doi: 10.1016/ j.jcms.2021.09.005
8. Herman P, Lot G, Silhouette B, Marianowski R, Portier F, Wassef M, et al. Transnasal Endoscopic Removal of an Orbital Cavernoma. *Ann Otol Rhinol Laryngol* (1999) 108(2):147–50. doi: 10.1177/000348949910800208
9. Felippu A, Mora R, Guastini L, Peretti G. Transnasal Approach to the Orbital Apex and Cavernous Sinus. *Ann Otol Rhinol Laryngol* (2013) 122(4):254–62. doi: 10.1177/000348941312200407
10. Castelnuovo P, Pistochini A, Locatelli D. Different Surgical Approaches to the Sellar Region: Focusing on the "Two Nostrils Four Hands Technique". *Rhinology* (2006) 44(1):2–7.
11. Essig H, Rana M, Meyer A, Eckardt AM, Kokemueller H, von See C, et al. Virtual 3D Tumor Marking-Exact Intraoperative Coordinate Mapping Improve Post-Operative Radiotherapy. *Radiat Oncol* (2011) 6:159. doi: 10.1186/1748-717X-6-159
12. Rana M, Essig H, Eckardt AM, Tavassol F, Ruecker M, Schramm A, et al. Advances and Innovations in Computer-Assisted Head and Neck Oncologic Surgery. *J Craniofac Surg* (2012) 23(1):272–8. doi: 10.1097/SCS.0b013e 318241bac7
13. Tarsitano A, Ricotta F, Baldino G, Badiali G, Pizzigallo A, Ramieri V, et al. Navigation-Guided Resection of Maxillary Tumours: The Accuracy of Computer-Assisted Surgery in Terms of Control of Resection Margins - A Feasibility Study. *J Craniomaxillofac Surg* (2017) 45(12):2109–14. doi: 10.1016/j.jcms.2017.09.023
14. Gonul E, Erdogan E, Duz B, Timurkaynak E. Transmaxillary Approach to the Orbit: An Anatomic Study. *Neurosurgery* (2003) 53(4):935–41. doi: 10.1227/ 01.neu.0000084164.22028.10
15. Paluzzi A, Gardner PA, Fernandez-Miranda JC, Tormenti MJ, Stefko ST, Snyderman CH, et al. "Round-The-Clock" Surgical Access to the Orbit. *J Neurol Surg B Skull Base* (2015) 76(1):12–24. doi: 10.1055/s-0033-1360580
16. Donofrio CA, Capitanio JF, Riccio L, Herur-Raman A, Caputy AJ, Mortini P. Mini Fronto-Orbital Approach: "Window Opening" Towards the Superomedial Orbit - A Virtual Reality-Planned Anatomic Study. *Oper Neurosurg (Hagerstown)* (2020) 19(3):330–40. doi: 10.1093/ons/opz420
17. Castelnuovo P, Arosio AD, Volpi L, De Maria F, Ravasio A, Donati S, et al. Endoscopic Transnasal Cryo-Assisted Removal of Orbital Cavernous Hemangiomas: Case Report and Technical Hints. *World Neurosurg* (2019) 126:66–71. doi: 10.1016/j.wneu.2019.01.235
18. Colletti G, Biglioli F, Poli T, Dessy M, Cucurullo M, Petrillo M, et al. Vascular Malformations of the Orbit (Lymphatic, Venous, Arteriovenous): Diagnosis, Management and Results. *J Craniomaxillofac Surg* (2019) 47(5):726–40. doi: 10.1016/j.jcms.2018.09.009
19. Bleier BS, Castelnuovo P, Battaglia P, Turri-Zanoni M, Dallan I, Metson R, et al. Endoscopic Endonasal Orbital Cavernous Hemangioma Resection: Global Experience in Techniques and Outcomes. *Int Forum Allergy Rhinol* (2016) 6(2):156–61. doi: 10.1002/alr.21645
20. Dubal PM, Svider PF, Denis D, Folbe AJ, Eloy JA. Short-Term Outcomes of Purely Endoscopic Endonasal Resection of Orbital Tumors: A Systematic Review. *Int Forum Allergy Rhinol* (2014) 4(12):1008–15. doi: 10.1002/ alr.21402
21. Purgason PA, Hornblass A. Complications of Surgery for Orbital Tumors. *Ophthalmic Plast Reconstr Surg* (1992) 8(2):88–93. doi: 10.1097/00002341- 199206000-00002
22. Dallan I, Seccia V, Lenzi R, Castelnuovo P, Bignami M, Battaglia P, et al. Transnasal Approach to the Medial Intraconal Space: Anatomic Study and Clinical Considerations. *Minim Invasive Neurosurg* (2010) 53(4):164–8. doi: 10.1055/s-0030-1263106
23. Leone CRJr., Wissinger JP. Surgical Approaches to Diseases of the Orbital Apex. *Ophthalmology* (1988) 95(3):391–7. doi: 10.1016/s0161-6420(88)33174-x
24. Rose GE. The "Devil's Touch"; Visual Loss and Orbital Surgery. A Synopsis of the Mustarde Lecture, 2006. *Orbit* (2007) 26(3):147–58. doi: 10.1080/ 01676830701539331
25. Almond MC, Cheng AG, Schiedler V, Sires BS, Most SP, Jian-Amadi A. Decompression of the Orbital Apex: An Alternate Approach to Surgical Excision for Radiographically Benign Orbital Apex Tumors. *Arch Otolaryngol Head Neck Surg* (2009) 135(10):1015–8. doi: 10.1001/archoto.2009.147
26. Mir-Salim PA, Berghaus A. [Endonasal, Microsurgical Approach to the Retrobulbar Region Exemplified by Intraconal Hemangioma]. *HNO* (1999) 47(3):192–5. doi: 10.1007/s001060050381
27. Abuzayed B, Tanriover N, Gazioglu N, Eraslan BS, Akar Z. Endoscopic Endonasal Approach to the Orbital Apex and Medial Orbital Wall: Anatomic Study and Clinical Applications. *J Craniofac Surg* (2009) 20 (5):1594–600. doi: 10.1097/SCS.0b013e3181b0dc23
28. Castelnuovo P, Turri-Zanoni M, Battaglia P, Locatelli D, Dallan I. Endoscopic Endonasal Management of Orbital Pathologies. *Neurosurg Clin N Am* (2015) 26(3):463–72. doi: 10.1016/j.nec.2015.03.001
29. Healy DYJr., Lee NG, Freitag SK, Bleier BS. Endoscopic Bimanual Approach to an Intraconal Cavernous Hemangioma of the Orbital Apex With Vascularized Flap Reconstruction. *Ophthalmic Plast Reconstr Surg* (2014) 30 (4):e104–6. doi: 10.1097/IOP.0b013e3182a22ed1
30. Donofrio CA, Riccio L, Pathmanaban ON, Fioravanti A, Caputy AJ, Mortini P. Endoscopic Sublabial Transmaxillary Approach to the Inferior Orbit: Pearls and Pitfalls-A Comparative Anatomical Study. *Neurosurg Rev* (2021) 44 (6):3297-307. doi: 10.1007/s10143-021-01494-5
31. Wilson DA, Williamson RW, Preul MC, Little AS. Comparative Analysis of Surgical Freedom and Angle of Attack of Two Minimal-Access Endoscopic Transmaxillary Approaches to the Anterolateral Skull Base. *World Neurosurg* (2014) 82(3-4):E487–E93. doi: 10.1016/j.wneu.2013.02.003
32. Schultheiss S, Petridis AK, El Habony R, Maurer P, Scholz M. The Transmaxillary Endoscopic Approach to the Orbit. *Acta Neurochir* (2013) 155(1):87–97. doi: 10.1007/s00701-012-1525-8
33. McKinney KA, Snyderman CH, Carrau RL, Germanwala AV, Prevedello DM, Stefko ST, et al. Seeing the Light: Endoscopic Endonasal Intraconal Orbital

Tumor Surgery. *Otolaryng Head Neck* (2010) 143(5):699–701. doi: 10.1016/j.otohns.2010.07.010

34. Zoli M, Sollini G, Milanese L, La Corte E, Rustici A, Guaraldi F, et al. Endoscopic Approaches to Orbital Lesions: Case Series and Systematic Literature Review. *J Neurosurgery* (2021) 134(2):608–20. doi: 10.3171/2019.10.Jns192138
35. Lenzi R, Bleier BS, Felisati G, Muscatello L. Purely Endoscopic Trans-Nasal Management of Orbital Intraconal Cavernous Haemangiomas: A Systematic Review of the Literature. *Eur Arch Otorhinolaryngol* (2016) 273(9):2319–22. doi: 10.1007/s00405-015-3733-3
36. Colletti G, Saibene AM, Pessina F, Duvina M, Allevi F, Felisati G, et al. A Shift in the Orbit: Immediate Endoscopic Reconstruction After Transnasal Orbital Tumors Resection. *J Craniofac Surg* (2017) 28(8):2027–9. doi: 10.1097/SCS.0000000000003879
37. Colletti G, Pipolo C, Lozza P, Felisati G, Allevi F, Biglioli F, et al. Orbital Medial Wall Fractures: Purely Endoscopic Endonasal Repair With Polyethylene Implants. *Clin Otolaryngol* (2018) 43(1):396–8. doi: 10.1111/coa.12675
38. Colletti G, Saibene AM, Giannini L, Dessy M, Deganello A, Pipolo C, et al. Endoscopic Endonasal Repair With Polyethylene Implants in Medial Orbital Wall Fractures: A Prospective Study on 25 Cases. *J Craniomaxillofac Surg* (2018) 46(2):274–82. doi: 10.1016/j.jcms.2017.11.017
39. Colletti G. The Reconstruction of the Medial Wall of the Orbit: A Change in Philosophy. *J Invest Surg* (2020) 33(7):653–4. doi: 10.1080/08941939.2018.1554017
40. Pagnoni M, Giovannetti F, Amodeo G, Priore P, Iannetti G. Endoscopic Endonasal Versus Transfacial Approach for Blowout Fractures of the Medial Orbital Wall. *J Craniofac Surg* (2015) 26(3):e247–9. doi: 10.1097/SCS.0000000000001660
41. Yang JR, Liao HT. Functional and Aesthetic Outcome of Extensive Orbital Floor and Medial Wall Fracture *via* Navigation and Endoscope-Assisted Reconstruction. *Ann Plas Surg* (2019) 82:S77–85. doi: 10.1097/Sap.0000000000001700
42. Said M, Gill AS, Strong EB. Utility of Endoscope-Assisted Orbital Fracture Repair for Atraumatic Reduction of Entrapped Muscle Tissue and Surgical Education. *J Oral Maxil Surg* (2019) 77(11):2298–301. doi: 10.1016/j.joms.2019.04.032

21

Advances in the Resection and Reconstruction of Midfacial Tumors through Computer Assisted Surgery

Max Wilkat, Norbert Kübler and Majeed Rana*

Department for Oral & Maxillofacial Surgery, University Hospital Düsseldorf, Düsseldorf, Germany

***Correspondence:**
Max Wilkat
Max.Wilkat@med.uni-duesseldorf.de

Curatively intended oncologic surgery is based on a residual-free tumor excision. Since decades, the surgeon's goal of R0-resection has led to radical resections in the anatomical region of the midface because of the three-dimensionally complex anatomy where aesthetically and functionally crucial structures are in close relation. In some cases, this implied aggressive overtreatment with loss of the eye globe. In contrast, undertreatment followed by repeated re-resections can also not be an option. Therefore, the evaluation of the true three-dimensional tumor extent and the intraoperative availability of this information seem critical for a precise, yet substance-sparing tumor removal. Computer assisted surgery (CAS) can provide the framework in this context. The present study evaluated the beneficial use of CAS in the treatment of midfacial tumors with special regard to tumor resection and reconstruction. Therefore, 60 patients diagnosed with a malignancy of the upper jaw has been treated, 31 with the use of CAS and 29 conventionally. Comparison of the two groups showed a higher rate of residual-free resections in cases of CAS application. Furthermore, we demonstrate the use of navigated specimen taking called tumor mapping. This procedure enables the transparent, yet precise documentation of three-dimensional tumor borders which paves the way to a more feasible interdisciplinary exchange leading e.g. to a much more focused radiation therapy. Moreover, we evaluated the possibilities of primary midface reconstructions seizing CAS, especially in cases of infiltrated orbital floors. These cases needed reduction of intra-orbital volume due to the tissue loss after resection which could be precisely achieved by CAS. These benefits of CAS in midface reconstruction found expression in positive changes in quality of life. The present work was able to demonstrate that the area of oncological surgery of the midface is a prime example of interface optimization based on the sensible use of computer assistance. The fact that the system makes the patient transparent for the surgeon and the procedure controllable facilitates a more precise and safer treatment oriented to a better outcome.

Keywords: midfacial tumors, computer assisted surgery, navigated resection, computer assisted reconstruction, orbital volume measurement

INTRODUCTION

Progress in the planning and implementation of computer assisted surgery (CAS) with the aid of 3D images for the area of the jaw and facial tumors has been recorded over the past two decades, particularly in order to optimize the interface-supporting procedure in tumor surgery (1, 2). Especially during staging, computer-assisted planning and multi-planar as well as -modal evaluation and analysis of data (CT, MRT) have become indispensable and represent an essential pillar of tumor surgery and tumor management.

The complex 3D structures of the face and head require a lot of experience and skill on the part of the surgeon. Without computer-assisted planning and navigation, therapy is only possible with difficulty (3–5). Tumor resection is often associated with the loss of essential, functional structures of the face (6). To reconstruct the affected areas of the face, patient-specific autogenic or alloplastic solutions are used. Computer-assisted systems are increasingly used today to determine the optimal anatomical position and for navigation (7). These systems make use of the possibility of visualizing tumors and their boundaries in CT data as well as planning the reconstruction on virtual three-dimensional models, which delivers very good results in individual planning. However, the planning effort and the costs of previous systems are still high and additional tools and engineering know-how are required to perform the segmentation in the various data sets (MRT, CT, CBCT) manually and in a complex manner. In addition to multimodal image analysis, modern image analysis platforms allow the automatic segmentation of tumors (8, 9), the extension of this segmentation by a defined safety distance, the simulation of the bony reconstruction, the import of preformed three-dimensional reconstructions such as titanium grid structures, as well as the image fusion of the planning with the postoperative result (1, 10). It is suitable for preoperative analysis as well as intraoperative, interactive image information exploitation (navigation, intraoperative CT/CBCT) as well as for connection to other interfaces, such as postoperative tumor staging or radiation planning.

In our study we focused on application possibilities of CAS for oncologic surgery of the midface. These anatomically complex tumors require a highly sophisticated treatment planning in terms of resection and reconstruction. This is enabled through the usage of CAS. Moreover, CAS might contribute to a better interdisciplinary networking and an improved quality of life for the patient.

The task of the present work was therefore to evaluate to what extent oncological surgery of the midface can benefit from the use of CAS and in which areas it is superior to conventional therapy.

MATERIALS AND METHODS

Study Design

This prospective clinical study was approved by the local ethics committee at the Hannover Medical School, Germany. The patient collective considered in this work was treated within the period from 2011 to 2019 in the Department for oral and maxillofacial surgery at the Hannover Medical School and at the University Hospital Düsseldorf.

31 patients with tumors of the upper jaw were treated through computer-assisted tumor resection including tumor mapping and primary reconstruction. A retrospectively analyzed patient sample of 29 cases which were treated through conventional methods without the use of computer assisted surgery served as a control group. The patients of the control group were selected with regard to tumor sizes and tumor locations that were comparable with the random sample of 31 patients that had been treated using CAS.The two groups were compared with regard to descriptive data, resection results and quality of life.

Due to the tumor extent, 15 of the above mentioned 31 patients had defects involving the orbit which needed primary orbit reconstruction. These 15 cases of primary reconstruction of the midface involving the orbit were evaluated for the pre- and postoperative volume of the orbit.

Conventional Tumor Resection

For conventional tumor resection the surgeon evaluated the tumor extent on basis of the clinical findings involving inspection and palpation and the contemplation of the preoperative standard imaging procedure. The resection border was chosen to include a safety margin of 1 centimeter. Afterwards, the resection was performed followed by taking of circular resection-bed driven specimen of the mucosal resection margin and the deep resection margin for frozen section control. The mucosal resection margin was removed with a minimum of two specimen, while the deep resection margin was removed with a minimum of 1 specimen. In cases of extraoral skin resection, the skin resection margin was collected with a minimum of 2 specimen. The anatomical orientation of these taken resection margins were marked by indicating sutures whose orientation was written into the accompanying pathology request document. In case of positive frozen sections further resection was performed in the area indicated by the pathologist. The final resection status which also involved the bony margins was described in the definitive pathology report.

Computer Assisted Surgery - Digital Workflow

The whole workflow of data acquisition, preoperative planning, tumor resection and mapping using intraoperative real-time navigation as well as reconstruction of midfacial defects involving the orbit after ablative surgery using CAD/CAM is demonstrated (see **Figure 1**).

Data Acquisition and Preoperative Planning

The process of digital planning was carried out using the planning software iPlan® (version 3.0.5, Brainlab, Feldkirchen, Germany). With regard to intraoperative navigation-supported tumor mapping and tumor resection, imaging was acquired first (see **Figure 2**).

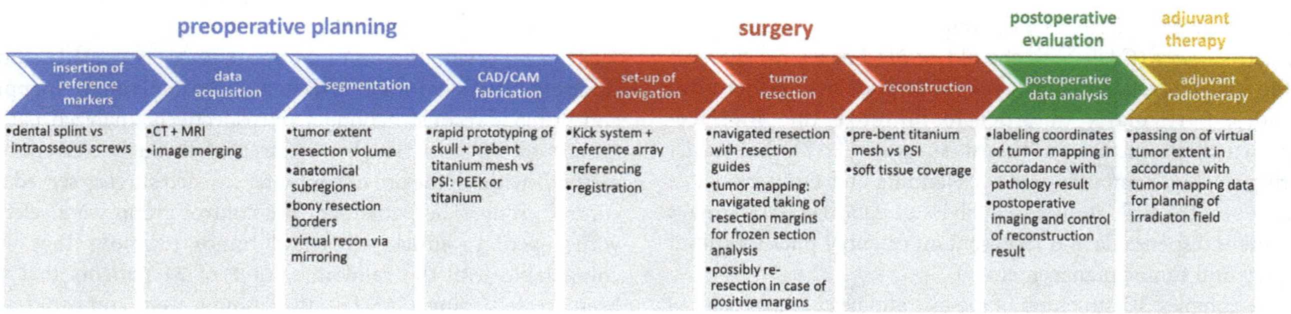

FIGURE 1 | Complete workflow of computer-assisted surgery. Computer-assisted surgery involving preoperative planning with data acquisition and processing including segmentation and virtual resection and reconstruction as shown in blue, surgery with real-time navigation, resection with tumor mapping and reconstruction as shown in red, postoperative evaluation as shown in green. Except for adjuvant radiotherapy as shown in yellow, the illustrated workflow has been used as clinical routine for treatment of midface tumors.

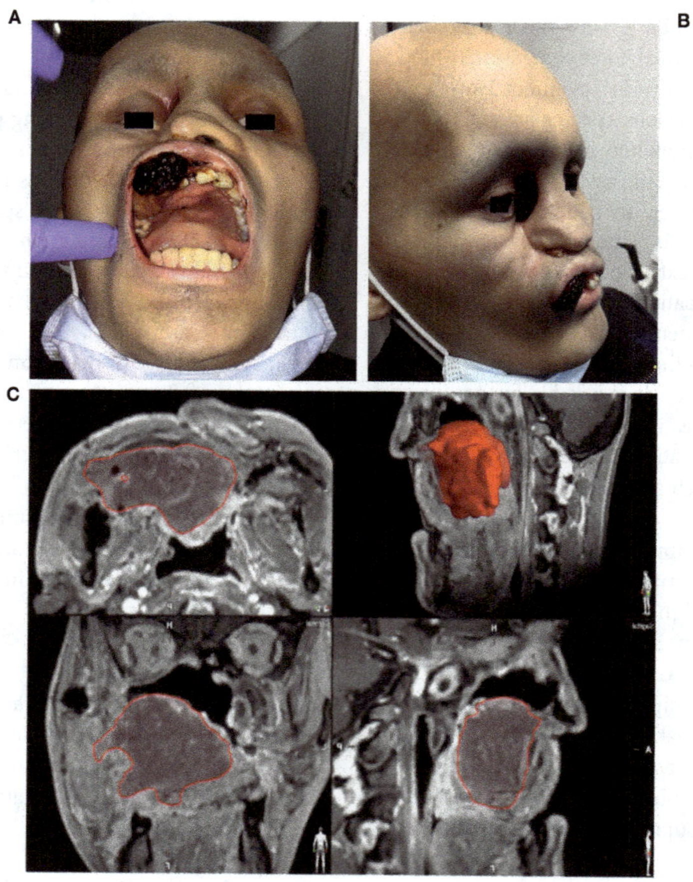

FIGURE 2 | Clinical findings and virtual data in a case of Ewing's sarcoma of the midface. **(A)** Frontal/intraoral and **(B)** side view of a 19-year-old patient with an Ewing's sarcoma of the midface presenting with an ulcerating neoplasm in the area of the hard palate, the maxillary vestibule and the right medial nasal slope which has lead to a sinking of the right eyeball. **(C)** Segmented tumor extent (red) in the multi-planar view of the MRI images.

Imaging data was collected following a standard procedure for all cases. CT data was acquired during arteriovenous phase using contrast medium (field of view 20 cm, pitch 1.0, slice thickness 1.0 mm, 140-160 mA, pixel density 512 × 512). MRI imaging was additionally collected (T1- and T2-weighted images, 1.5T (1T = 800 kA/m), slice thickness 2 mm, pixel density 512 × 512) and merged *via* iPlan® software (version 3.0.5, Brainlab, Feldkirchen, Germany) using the automatic 'best fit' algorithm.

After automated fusion the result was manually checked in a multi-planar view considering the axial, coronal and sagittal planes. Conformation of best fit was indicated by manually accepting the result.

As soon as the image data were available in the required format, segmentation followed (see **Figure 3**). Segmentation was performed by the same senior surgeon as investigator for all 31 cases. In particular, the extent of the primary tumor was segmented, and the area of resection was defined by adding a three-dimensional safety margin in a freely selectable distance. Safety margin was set at 1 centimeter. On the basis of the segmented resection volume the bony resection margins were defined and used for designing resection guides. Moreover, anatomical subunits were segmented such as the bony orbit and the alveolar process of the upper jaw which both could be mirrored from the unaffected site for reconstruction purposes if applicable (see **Figures 3, 4**).

Set Up of Intraoperative Navigation

During the acquisition of the CT data set, either an individual dental splint with 4 additional titanium mini screws or in cases of a reduced or loosened set of teeth or planned resection which involved more than half of the dental arch in the upper jaw four surgically inserted 2.0 cross-drive titanium mini screws (DePuy Synthes®) have been used as reference markers during the individual registration of the patient.

Before the operation, the patient was placed in a headrest. The reference star was fixed on the skull *via* the "Skull Reference-Array" plus osteosynthesis (see **Figure 5A**). The reference star was identified by the infrared camera of the navigation system Kick® (Brainlab, Feldkirchen, Germany). identifying the exact position of the patient during operation. As mentioned above the previously inserted reference markers (a dental splint with additional titanium mini screws or titanium mini screws inserted to the skull) were navigated to in order to match their position to the coordinates of the reference markers previously saved in the data record. Additionally, a landmark test was carried out in order to compare the patient on the operating table with the virtual image in the data set and ensure that referencing has been successful.

The time for intraoperative navigation set-up has been measured to evaluate the mean surgery prolongation.

Navigation-Guided Tumor Resection and Tumor Mapping

The treatment of midfacial tumor patients involving the tumor resection and the reconstruction was performed by only one team with the same senior surgeon being in charge during all CAS operations. Using the navigation probe, the extent of the virtually planned resection could be transferred to the intraoperative situation. Moreover, resection guides indicated the virtually planned resection margins concerning the bony margin (see **Figure 6A**). After navigated resection of the tumor (see **Figures 6B, C**), the resection-bed driven margins for frozen section analysis were collected with the aid of navigation by setting intraoperative landmarks with the help of the iPlan software (Version 3.0.5). At least 12 specimens were taken from the mucosal resection margin following the clockwork technique accompanied by at least four specimens from the deep resection margin. In cases of extraoral skin resection further specimen were taken following the clockwork technique. Coordinates of every three-dimensional position of a taken specimen were saved in the software. All these coordinates were thereby integrated into the virtual data to determine the exact three-dimensional position of the taken specimen of the resection margin. Moreover, screenshots of every coordinate

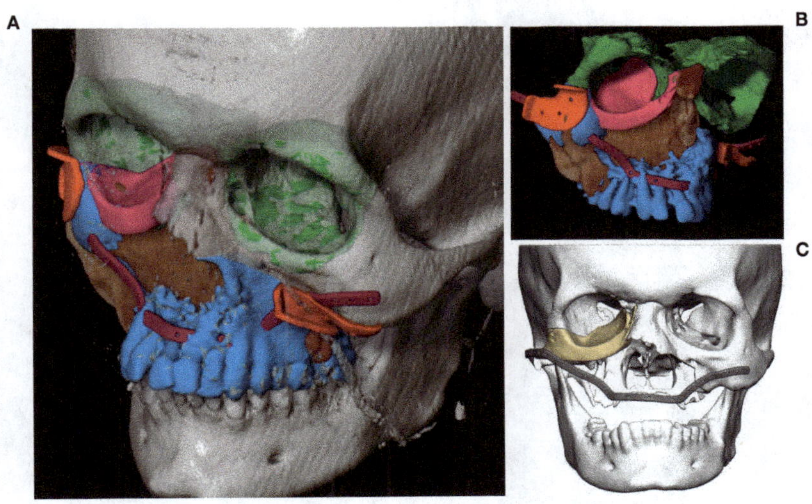

FIGURE 3 | Virtual segmentation and planning of the functional defect reconstruction in a case of Ewing's sarcoma of the midface. **(A, B)** Segmentation of the tumor extent (brown) and the planned bony resection (blue) with the resection border indicated by the cutting guides (red). The anatomical subunit of the left orbit has been mirrored to reconstruct the right orbit (both green) as a planning template for the right orbital floor reconstruction with a patient specific PEEK implant (pink). The outer contour of the maxilla is reconstructed with a patient specific titanium reconstruction plate (purple). **(C)** Both PSIs are displayed.

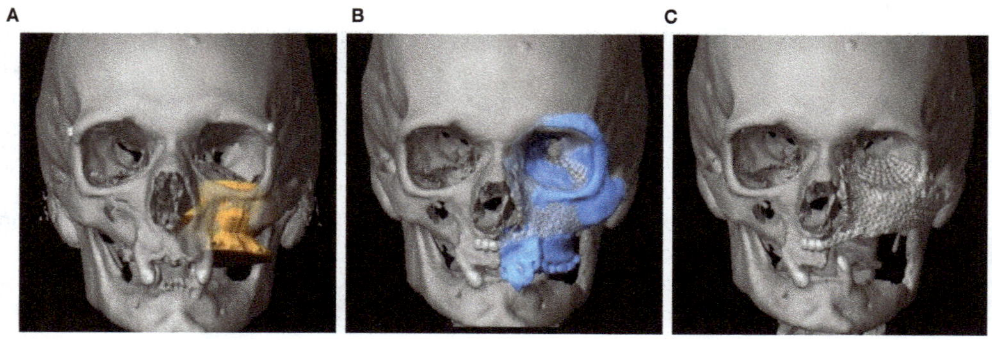

FIGURE 4 | Virtual reconstruction planning using the principle of mirroring. **(A)** Segmented tumor of the left maxillary sinus with infiltration into the left floor of the orbit (yellow). **(B)** Template of the healthy right midface mirrored to the left (blue). **(C)** Postoperative CT shows the reconstruction of the orbit and the midface using two PSIs.

were acquired, printed out and send to the pathologist accompanied by the specimen and the pathology request document to pass on the three-dimensional localization of the taken specimen. The information of specimen position has been linked to the pathology result of the corresponding specimen later on by color-coding: red meaning the specimen was positive for tumor residual, green meaning the specimen was tumor-free (see **Figure 5**).

In order to evaluate whether the method of intraoperative navigation-assisted tumor resection and mapping was successful in the sense that more complete resections could be carried out, tumor resection of the upper jaw with CAS were compared with the control group. Resection status was defined by the final report of the pathologist. This report considered the main tumor resection specimen - including the bony margins which needed more time for processing compared to soft tissue margins due to the necessary decalcification - as well as the taken resection margin specimen for frozen section analysis. It was differentiated between complete resection (R0), microscopically residual tumor mass (R1) and macroscopically residual tumor mass (R2).

Primary Reconstruction After Ablative Surgery

The analysis of the tumor and resection margins showed the extent to which the reconstruction was restricted. Midface reconstruction true to original using titanium mesh structures

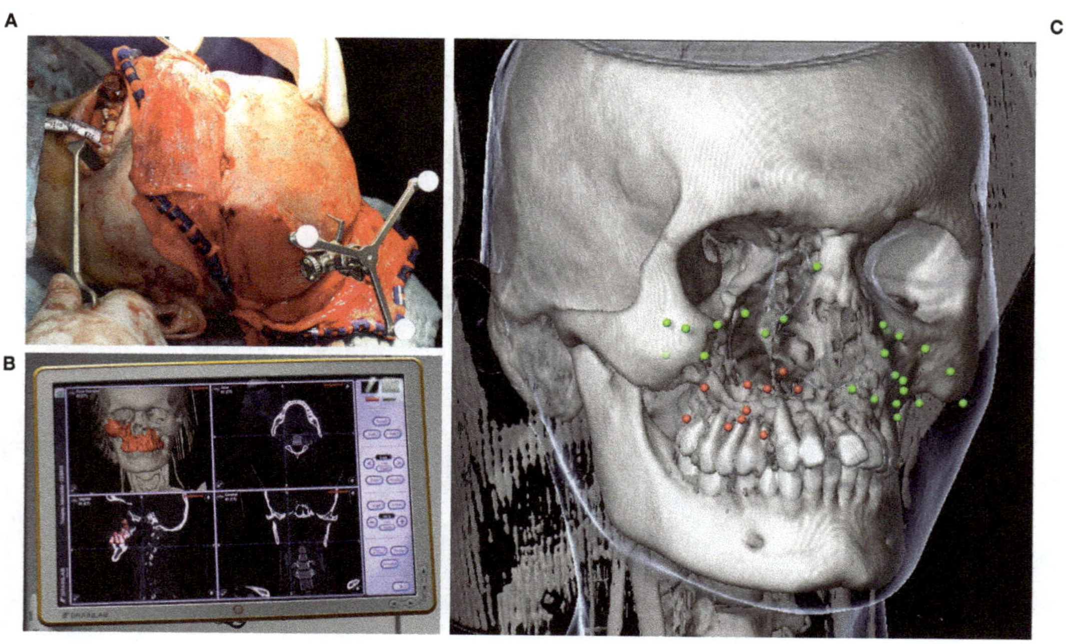

FIGURE 5 | Intraoperative navigation during midfacial tumor ablation in a case of Ewing's sarcoma of the midface. **(A)** Skull reference array attached for intraoperative navigation after coronal approach. **(B)** Real time navigation monitor showing the planned bony resection segmented in red color. **(C)** Data post-processing of the landmarks set intraoperatively after receipt of the histopathological report (green = tumor-free, red = tumor residual).

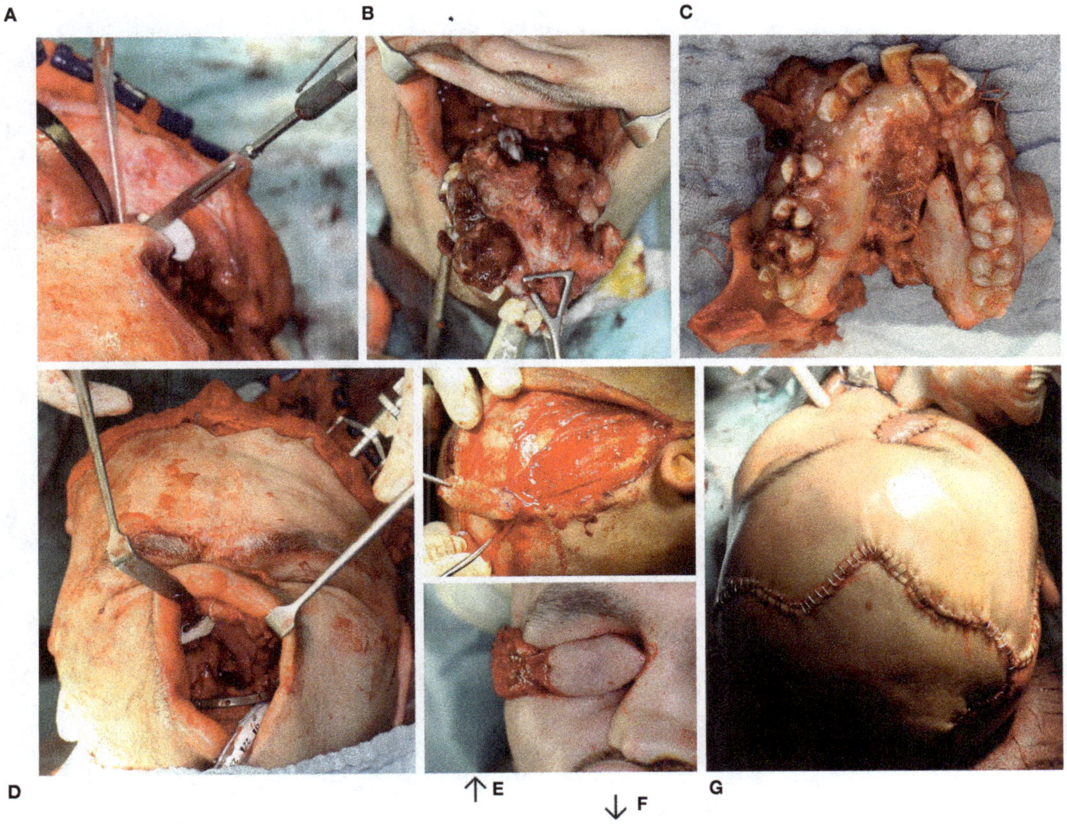

FIGURE 6 | Resection of Ewing's sarcoma of the midface with primarily functional reconstruction. **(A)** Bone resection using a cutting guide. **(B, C)** Tumor resection en bloc preserving the eyeball. **(D)** Primarily functional reconstruction reconstruction of the zygomatic bone and orbit floor using two patient specific implants (combined SLM titanium and PEEK (KLS Martin®, Tuttlingen) using the virtually mirrored left orbit as a template) both visible intraorally. **(E, F)** Dissection of the temporal muscle flap. **(G)** Wound closure with temporal muscle flap sewn in.

or PEEK implants with soft tissue transplants was the aim (see **Figures 6D–G**). With unilateral tumor growth the virtual mirroring of the opposite healthy side served as a reference point for the reconstruction of the shape and the volume of the orbit true to the original so that not only the functional but also the aesthetic restoration was achieved (see **Figure 4**). The virtual reconstruction planning was exported as a stereolithography file (STL format) and printed out three-dimensionally or milled *via* "rapid prototyping" to create a bio-model made of cheap composite materials, which could also be autoclaved. On the basis of the virtual model a patient-specific 3D implant was pre-formed by cold forming titanium mesh. Alternatively, a PEEK implant or a titanium implant was manufactured *via* additive CAD/CAM procedure by KLS Martin (Tuttlingen, Germany) (see **Figure 3**). During the intraoperative navigation, the reference probe was used to check whether the implant has been inserted anatomically correctly, since the data set acted as a virtual template. For pre-bent titanium meshes the thickness of the mesh itself had to be considered. Therefore an offset according to the used mesh thickness has been used during navigational reconstruction control. In cases of CAD/CAM processed implants the STL-file of the implant itself was integrated into the data set for navigation control.

The software iPlan 4.0 beta was used to measure the intra-orbital volume. It is able to virtually subtract a pre-formed cuboid with a defined volume from the segmented bony boundaries so that the volume can be calculated. This algorithm is integrated in the currently available software and enables the surgeon to calculate the volume by simply clicking on the "Orbital cavity" button (see **Figure 7**).

Patient specific implants were covered by autologous soft tissue transplants (see **Figure 8**). Transplants were selected according to the resulting soft tissue deficiency to ensure a sufficient soft tissue coverage of the implant to prevent implant exposure.

Determination and Definition of the Irradiation Field

The use case of integration of the data of tumor mapping into the irradiation protocol has not yet been established as a clinical routine during the time of the treatment of the 31 CAS patients. However, in 3 cases the information of tumor mapping collected intraoperatively was post-processed and forwarded to the radiation therapist. The data was stored in the preoperative data set in XBrain format. After receipt of the histological findings the virtual points were marked in color depending on

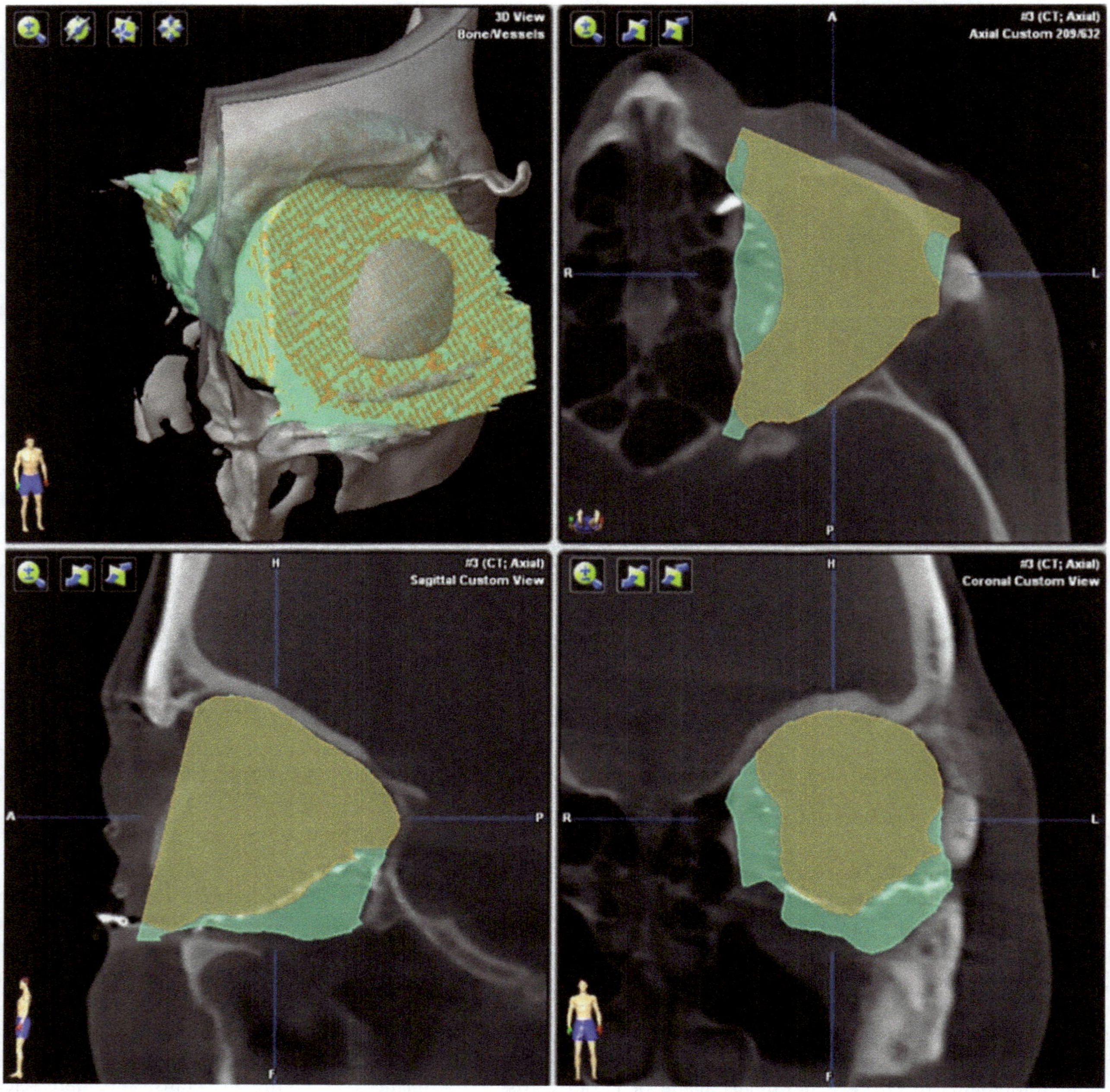

FIGURE 7 | Calculation of orbit volume. Orbital cavity algorithm calculates the orbit volume not only within the bony boundaries (green), but also on the adjacent orbit 3D mesh (yellow). The volume calculation works automatically.

the resection status result. The virtual points that were not within the calculated safety distance were also marked in color accordingly. Thus, the radiation therapist could recognize in the data set which points indicated the supposed residual tumor, which points marked an excessively small safety distance and which points were free of tumor tissue.

After the operative reconstruction of the bony midface, the reconstruction result was checked with the help of a postoperative CBCT by default. The XBrain data was merged with the postoperative CBCT data set. Thus, the preoperative data set, the intraoperative tumor marking, the postoperative data set and the tumor mapping, which had been post-processed depending on the histological findings were available to the radiation therapist as an entire DICOM data set for his irradiation field planning. Moreover, the radiation therapist had the option of merging the data made available by the surgeon with a planning CT for irradiation.

Quality of Life

The quality of life of patients was measured using the University of Washington Quality of Life Questionnaire (UW-QOL v4)

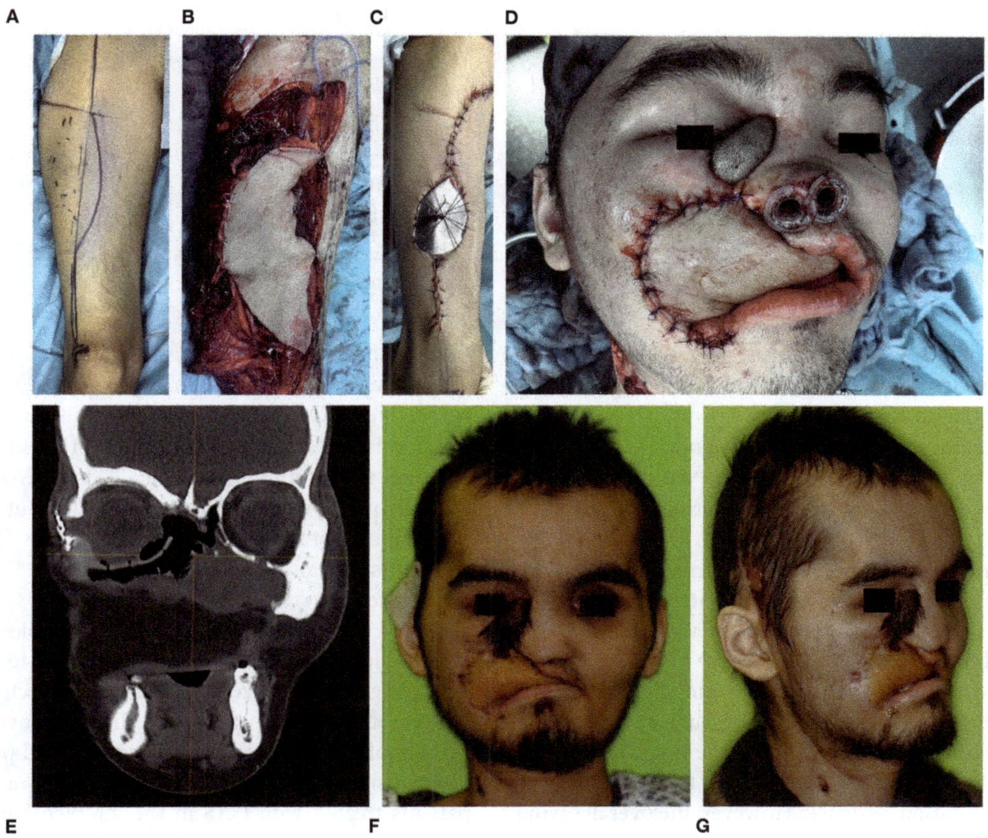

FIGURE 8 | Early secondary soft tissue reconstruction of the upper lip and jaw using an anterolateral thigh flap in a case of Ewing's sarcoma of the midface. **(A–C)** Skin marking, flap harvest and wound closure of the anterolateral thigh flap of the right lower extremity. **(D)** Anterolateral thigh flap sewed in. **(E)** Postoperative CT scan in coronal plane shows the patient specific implant *in situ* reconstructing the right orbital floor while the symmetrical position of the eyeball has been restored. **(F)** Frontal and **(G)** half site view of the patient two months after tumor resection and two stage reconstruction (primary orbital floor and early secondary soft tissue of the upper lip and jaw).

(11), a short multifactorial questionnaire that contains specific questions about head and neck tumors. It consists of twelve domains (appearance, activity, recovery, mood, fear, pain, swallowing, chewing, speech, shoulder, taste, saliva). Each of these domains relates to the last seven days and should be rated on a scale that ranges from symptom-free to severe impairment. In addition, the patients should indicate which of these areas was most important to them in the past week. Finally, three global questions were asked about the current state of mind, health-related quality of life and overall quality of life, which were to be answered on a five-point Likert scale. The questionnaire has a high level of validity and is particularly suitable for the questions at hand, as it addresses the specific problems of the patient collective (12, 13).

Statistical Evaluation

The statistical analyzes were calculated with SPSS for MAC OS X version 22.0 (SPSS Inc., Chicago, IL, USA). The socio-demographic data were analyzed using descriptive statistics. The mean values and standard deviations are given for interval-scaled data and the frequencies are given for ordinal-scaled data. In the case of interval-scaled data, t-tests were calculated for independent samples to compare the mean values. The chi-square test was calculated for the ordinal scaled data. A p-value less than 0.05 was considered significant for all tests.

RESULTS

Time for Set-Up of Intraoperative Navigation

Table 1 gives an overview of the intraoperative navigation times. The registration process in the form of comparing the instruments with the markers took an average of 3.7 minutes with a standard deviation of 1.1 minutes. The duration of the registration depended on the landmarks used. In 22 cases dental splints were used for referencing. Preoperatively intraosseous inserted, screws were used in 9 cases. There was no significant difference in the duration of the registration process comparing dental splints with intraosseous screws, as the screw heads were not covered by skin after preoperative insertion, which abolished the need for exposure. The registration accuracy was measured in

TABLE 1 | Time and accuracy of intraoperative navigation.

	M (min)	SD (min)
time of		
-referencing	3,2	0,3
-registration	3,7	1,1
-intraoperative navigating	8,8	1,3
-export of data	3,9	0,9
total time of intraoperative navigation	**19,6**	**2,8**
	M (mm)	**SD (mm)**
accuracy of registration	**1,2**	**0,4**

Bold values are the main results.

millimeters and in the case of the present patient collective was 1.2 mm with a standard deviation of 0.4 mm. The registrations carried out from time to time during the operation to compare the registration accuracy did not show any significant deviations from the original registration accuracy. There was no significant difference in the registration accuracy comparing dental splints with intraosseously inserted screws.

The intra-operative navigation took 8.8 minutes (SD = 1.3 min.), The data transfer to the navigation system including the co-registration with the planning data was carried out automatically and took 3.9 minutes (SD = 0.9 min.).

While set-up of navigation requires a certain amount of time, navigation itself helps to save time during surgery due to the following aspects: improved orientation in the imaging data set, improved selection of the biopsy position and faster surgery due to the real-time navigation feedback. However, the overall saving of time cannot be quantified due to the lack of a comparison of the highly individual cases. Besides assumably shortened operating time CAS offers also advantages concerning quality control due to instant merging of pre- and intraoperative data sets, high consistency between pre-, intra- and postoperative data sets and automatic data saving for postoperative quality control.

Intraoperative Tumor Marking and Resection

Table 2 shows the distribution of the descriptive characteristics of the patients with a tumor of the upper jaw treated with CAS as the intervention group compared to those patients treated conventionally without CAS as the control group. The two groups mostly match in their composition. There is no statistically significant difference between the means of the two groups: neither in age calculated by t-test, nor in gender, TNM classification, adjuvant therapy (radiotherapy and chemotherapy), mode of reconstruction or diagnosis checked for by chi-square tests.

In the CAS group, 19 (61.3%) patients suffered from squamous cell carcinoma, 4 patients (12.9%) had an adenocystic carcinoma and two patients (6.6%) had an ossifying fibroma. One person each (3.2%) suffered from a keratocyst, a sinunasal carcinoma, a mucoepidemoid carcinoma, a B-cell non-hodgkin lymphoma, an Ewing's sarcoma or an osteosarcoma as displayed in **Table 2**.

With a number of 16 (51.6%) most patients of the intervention group treated with CAS were reconstructed with a latissimus dorsi flap, three patients (9.7%) were reconstructed with a radial forearm flap and for another four patients (12.9%) a local primary wound closure was sufficient. A serratus anterior muscle flap and an upper arm flap were used in 2 patients (6.5%), respectively. One patient (3.2%) was reconstructed with a temporal muscle flap, one patient (3.2%) with a pedicled palatinal flap and one patient (3,2%) received an anterolateral thigh flap. One of the patients (3.2%) was not reconstructed but received an obturator prosthesis. 8 patients (25.8%) received a chemotherapy after the surgical procedure, 23 patients (74.2%) a radiotherapy.

In the CAS group, frozen sections samples were collected in higher numbers and smaller sizes compared to the control group. An average of 15.3 frozen sections were collected per CAS patient with an average size of 8.7 mm. In the conventional group an average of 5.3 frozen sections were collected per patient with an average size of 23.2 mm. More R0 resections were achieved in patients treated with CAS in the intervention group compared with the control group as displayed in **Figure 9**. In the CAS group, an R0 resection could be performed in 22 patients (71.0%), while in the control group there were 16 patients (55.2%). An R1 resection was performed in 8 patients (25.8%) in the CAS group compared to 12 patients (41.4%) in the control group. In both groups one patient showed an R2 resection (CAS = 3.2%; control group = 3.4%), which was performed because the tumor had infiltrated the internal carotid artery as a vital structure. However, the differences are not significant (df = 58; t = -1.112; p = 0.271).

Reconstruction After Ablative Surgery

Resection defects after the loss of hard and soft tissue due to ablative surgery of the midface result in considerable functional and aesthetic deficits. These changes are even more dramatic if the orbit is affected by the resection. Once the orbital bony boundaries and/or the intra-orbital soft tissues are impaired, the resulting imbalance between the eyeball and the supporting structures lead to symptoms such as enophthalmus, double vision and facial asymmetry. This particularly applies for orbital prosthesis in cases of anophthalmic patients. Reconstruction of these cases involves a repositioning of the eye globe/prosthesis which might need a reduction of the intra-orbital volume due to intra-orbital soft tissue loss achieved by a reforming of the boundaries of the orbital cavity. Due to the intricate three-dimensional anatomy and the wish for a better prediction of the result, it is advisable to use modern principles of CAS in these cases. CAS allows a backwards planning, which enables the virtual planning of the desired

TABLE 2 | Test characteristics of patients with tumors of the upper jaw treated with the help of CAS in the intervention group compared to the control group treated conventionally without CAS.

	CAS	no CAS (conservatively)	p
age (M ± SD)	63 ± 17,7	65 ± 10,7	.350
gender (m/f)	22/9	15/14	.126
pT			.688
2	0	0	
3	9	7	
4	22	22	
pN			.397
0	23	23	
1	4	5	
2	4	1	
pM			
0	0	0	
R			.431
0	22	16	
1	8	12	
2	1	1	
radiotherapy (yes/no)	26/5	19/10	.100
chemotherapy (yes/no)	8/23	2/27	.080
	CAS	**no CAS (conservatively)**	**p**
mode of reconstruction			.462
obturator prosthesis = no surgical reconstruction	1	2	
Latissimus dorsi flap	16	15	
Serratus anterior muscle flap	2	1	
local primary closure	4	2	
upper arm flap	2	2	
radial forearm flap	3	2	
local flap	0	4	
gingiva flap	0	1	
Anterolateral thigh flap	1	0	
M. temporalis flap	1	0	
pedicled palatinal flap	1	0	
	CAS	**no CAS (conservatively)**	**p**
diagnosis			.491
squamous cell carcinoma	19	25	
adenocystic carcinoma	4	2	
mucoepidermoid carcinoma	1	1	
osteosarcoma	1	1	
ossifying fibroma	2	0	
keratocyst	1	0	
sinunasal carcinoma	1	0	
B-cell non-hodgkin lymphoma	1	0	
Ewing's sarcoma	1	0	

position of the eyeball/eye prosthesis first followed by the calculation of the necessary intra-orbital volume reduction and thus the needed recontouring of the orbital boundaries. This recontouring is achieved *via* rapid prototyping and prebenting of titanium meshes. The anatomically correct positioning is monitored *via* intraoperative navigation. The extra-orbital soft tissue defect can be replaced *via* autologous tissue transfer.

Here we present data of 15 primary cases in need of midfacial reconstruction after ablative tumor surgery involving the orbit. Pre-operative planning took 25 min for the surgeon and 60 min for the technical staff on average, while manufacturing of the model and the implant took 2 working days. **Table 3** compares the pre- and postoperative volumes of these patients after ablative surgery using CAS. In all cases the intra-orbital volume was reduced, which led to a more symmetrical positioning of and improved support for the eye globe/ prosthesis and thereby for the accompanying structures like the eye lids.The mean preoperative volume for primary reconstructions was 30.97 cm^3 (SD = 3.25 cm^3) and the postoperative volume was 28.23 cm^3 (SD = 3.70 cm^3). A t-test for independent samples showed that the mean difference between the pre- and postoperative volumes was significant (df = 28; t = 2.085; p = 0.046) (see **Figure 10**).

Optimization of the Interface Between Surgery and Radiation Therapy Using CAPP and CAS

So far, only the treatment results of three patients could be evaluated, because although the data could be passed on from the surgeon to the radiation therapist, the radiation therapists do

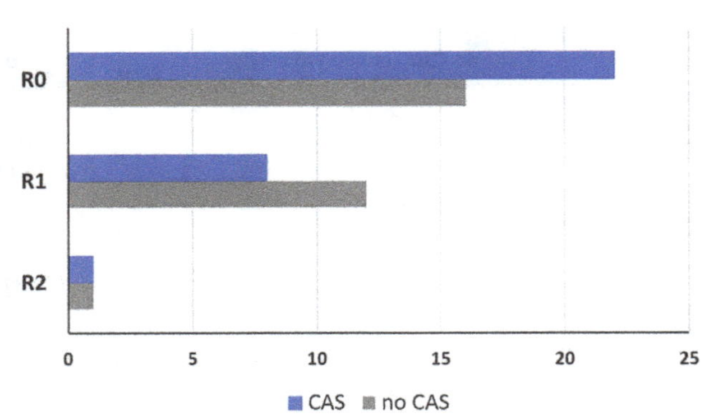

FIGURE 9 | Resection result of the group that was treated using the CAS, compared to the control group. R0: No tumor detectable in the organism R1: Microscopic residual tumor at the resection border R2: Macroscopically tumor or metastases remaining in the patient. Dark blue = intervention group treated with CAS, grey = control group treated without CAS.

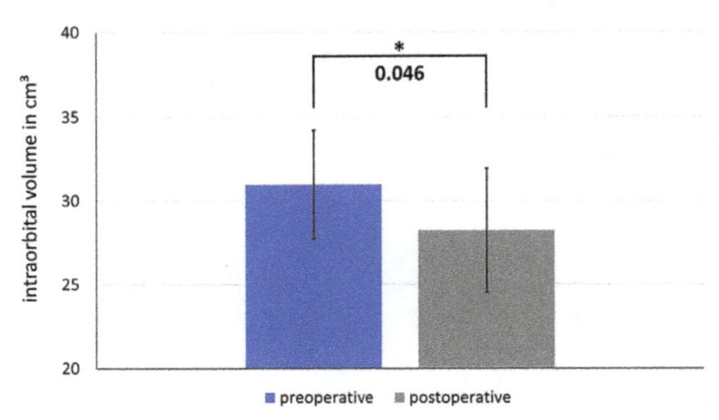

FIGURE 10 | Comparison of the pre- and postoperative intraorbital volumes after ablative surgery and primary reconstruction using CAS. The difference between the preoperative and postoperative volume is significant. * shows significance with a p-value < 0.05

not yet routinely include this information, but rather use their planning CTs as a basis for their therapy. However, since the first results are very promising, our efforts are aimed at routinely providing the protocols, which were mainly prepared with the help of the CAS, to the radiotherapists in order to use these protocols as a basis for their therapy. We assume that this procedure will gain a foothold in routine clinical practice. Since this method is still new, the post-processing of the data for passing on to the radiation therapist currently still takes some time. According to previous experiences, this takes about 10 minutes.

Case Study of Selective Irradiation After Virtual Tumor Marking With the Help of CAS

With the help of this case study, the advantages of intraoperative data collection and transfer to the radiation therapists are explained. A 67-year-old patient with a primary SCC of the left maxilla invading the orbital floor (cT4) was operated on using CAS. Intraoperative, navigation-assisted tumor mapping and tumor resection were used. The histopathological findings near the base of the skull still showed parts of a residual tumor in two localizations of the tumor map, there were no close margin areas. This information was highlighted in color in the intra-operative tumor map.

Due to the location of the residual and the reduced general health condition of the patient a further resection could not be performed. Therefore, the files were passed on to the radiation therapist in DICOM format. The iPlan 4.0 beta software was used. Only those coordinates (voxels) that represented a positive histology or a close-margin resection were marked with the Houndsfield unit of 3500 H. This value has been chosen well above the usual maximum limit of 3100 H to ensure that the original DICOM data record could not be manipulated any further.

TABLE 3 | Pre- and postoperative volumes of the patients with a primary reconstruction of the orbit using the CAS.

patient number	affected site	preoperative volume (cm^3)	postoperative volume (cm^3)
primary reconstruction			
1	r	30.900	23.642
2	r	27.777	24.128
3	l	29.826	27.174
4	l	32.193	30.987
5	r	30.038	24.878
6	l	28.396	25.656
7	r	31.971	28.624
8	l	30.378	28.375
9	l	39.378	36.895
10	r	31.407	29.343
11	r	34.535	32.535
12	r	25.073	23.488
13	l	33.258	32.360
14	l	27.517	25.912
15	l	31.960	29.423
mean	***p = 0.046***	**30.97**	**28.23**
standard deviation		**3.25**	**3.70**

Bold values are the main results.

This provided another advantage as the marked points could be quickly found again using the threshold algorithm. This improved data set was exported as "enhanced DICOM format" (enDICOM) and could be imported into common irradiation devices.

In this case, the enDICOM data set was imported in the Oncentra MasterPlan System (version 3.3, Nucletron, Netherlands/USA) and co-registered with the postoperative radiation therapy planning CT scan. With this additional information, a more selective irradiation of the midface resulting in smaller volumes of high dose irradiation could be guaranteed.

Quality of Life

For the calculation, the responses of the intervention group that were treated using CAS for tumors of the upper jaw were compared to the responses from the control group which were treated conventionally without CAS. A mean value comparison was calculated using the t-test for independent samples. Out of the included 60 patients a total of 42 patients fully completed and returned the QoL-questionnaire and thereby were included in the calculation. The group that was treated using CAS had a response rate of 68% and the control group a response rate of 72% which results in 21 patients of each group.

Figure 11 shows the distribution of the score rating with regard to the global question about health-related quality of life and overall quality of life. For both, the CAS group tends to have a better scoring (health-related quality of life: M = 3.70; SD = 0.66, overall quality of life: M = 3.60; SD = 0.75) than the control group (health-related quality of life: M = 3.35; SD = 0.90, overall quality of life: M = 3.20; SD = 1.01). However, the differences do not become significant neither in terms of health-related quality of life (df = 38; t = 1.872; p = 0.069) nor for the overall quality of life (df = 38; t = 1.424; p = 0.163).

When looking at the question of how the patients are doing compared to the months prior to diagnosis, the group treated with CAS (M = 2.80; SD = 1.19) tended to have better scores than the control group (M = 2.65; SD = 1.23) without the difference becoming significant (df = 38; t = -0.392; p = 0.698).

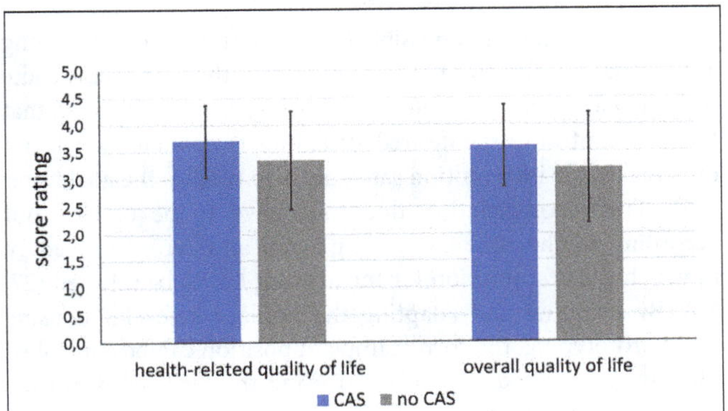

FIGURE 11 | Comparison of health-related and overall quality of life of the patients of the intervention group treated using CAS compared to the control group treated conventionally without CAS.

With regard to the domains, it was found that there tended to be differences in the areas of mood and appearance. In the control group, more patients stated that they were bothered by their appearance and that their mood was impaired. There were no differences between the groups with regard to the other domains. **Figure 12** compares the results of both groups with regard to the variables appearance and mood. For the sake of clarity, the items have been combined into two or three statements.

DISCUSSION

The routine use of CAPP and CAS in the treatment of upper and lower jaw tumors in the maxillofacial surgery was often prevented by the high costs and poor user friendliness due to the high technical complexity and the demanding operation of the systems. Regarding the costs we have the beneficial situation in Germany that the total use of computer-assisted surgery and orbital reconstruction is being reimbursed because of many publications and the clear consensus in the indication having the benefit of precise reconstruction, excellent surgical results and saving time in terms of operation hours.However, there is a need for a comprehensive system with which the entire procedure, from planning to implementation and result control, can be carried out efficiently and easily in order to optimize patient treatment and reduce overall costs. In the present work such a method for the therapy optimization of tumors of the upper jaw and midface area with the necessary treatment steps was presented and evaluated based on the analysis of 31 patients with a tumor of the midface and their surgical treatment with the help of CAS. The preoperative planning, intraoperative navigation with navigated tumor resection and tumor mapping, the reconstruction after ablative surgery and optimization of the interface between surgery and radiation therapy were examined in detail. The CAPP and CAS introduce a new level of quality control and quality assurance and thus promote the professionalization of surgery, because the success of the treatment can now be quantified. From a medico-legal perspective, the surgeon can protect himself externally with the CAPP and CAS, since the documentation of the individual operative sub-steps makes all therapeutic measures transparent, traceable and verifiable at all times. At the same time, the demands on one's own performance increase because the intervention is no longer carried out intuitively or on the basis of experience. Due to the technical possibilities, the aim is to plan and implement the intervention down to the millimeter.

Advantages of these procedures has been presented before (14–18). The current study provides data of a prospective clinical study including 31 patients with midfacial tumors treated with CAS in comparison with 29 patients treated conventionally.

Intraoperative Navigation

The steps associated with intraoperative navigation such as referencing, registration, intraoperative navigation and data transfer took an average of 19.6 minutes (SD = 2.8 minutes).

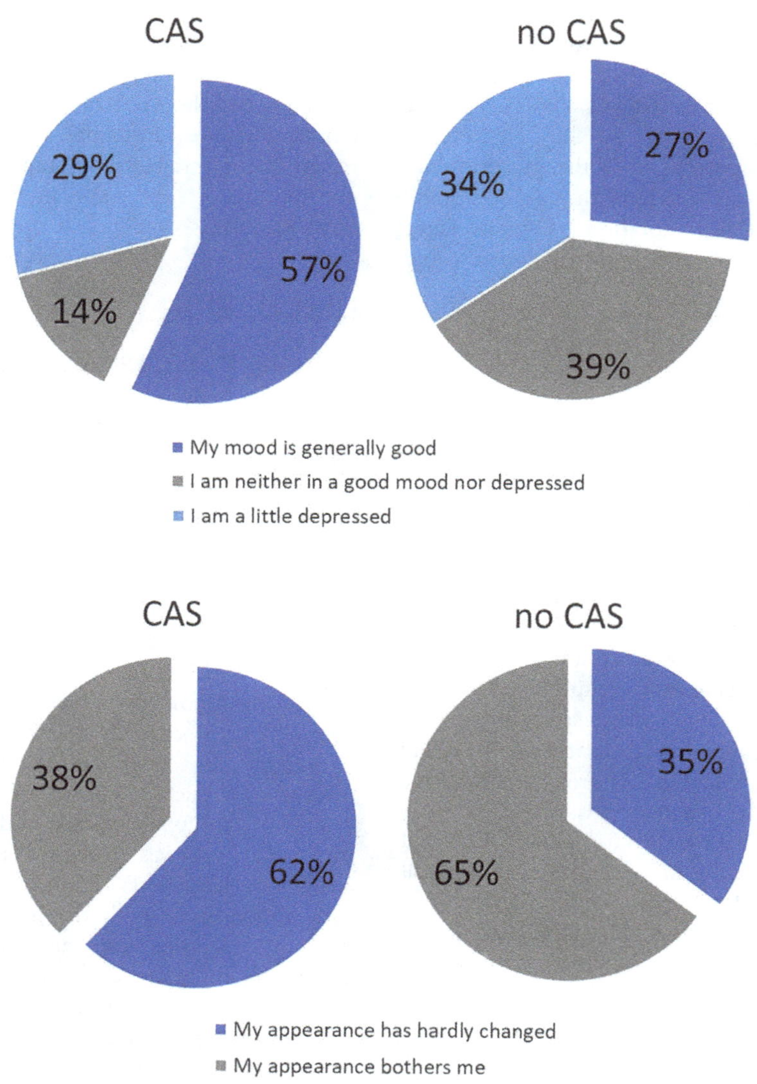

FIGURE 12 | Distribution of answers of the intervention group treated with CAS compared to the control group treated without CAS. In the upper part distribution of answers regarding the question of the mood in recent weeks are displayed while in the lower part distribution of answers regarding the question of 'how you feel about your own external appearance in recent weeks' are shown.

In order to be able to decide whether this additional effort pays off in terms of a cost-benefit ratio, the additional time effort must be compared with indicators of the benefit. Initial studies show that the additional time invested of around 30 minutes predominates (19, 20) and that the more experienced the user is with the method of navigation, the quicker the intra-operative set-up of navigation devices (21). First of all, the operating time itself is important, but it is difficult to quantify objectively, as the operating time depends on the patient's individual clinical situation. However, there are already studies that have shown a shortening of the operating time (22, 23). In addition to the time saved, the qualitative benefit for the patient should also be taken into account (24). With regard to the time savings, it should be remembered that the detailed preparation for the operation means that all structures are known and that better orientation in the image data set is possible (25). Due to the prior planning and virtual simulation of the access routes, the best access route including alternatives is determined before the operation, so that targeted control of the desired structures is possible, which not only makes the intervention safer, but also reaches the goal faster (26). The reconstruction does not have to be carried out according to the time-consuming "trial and error" procedure in which the best position for the implant has to be selected (27, 28). By planning and adapting the implant beforehand using rapid prototyping, the correct implant position can be controlled directly and immediately adapted using the feedback from the intraoperative navigation (29). It is also positive that the patient is not exposed to further radiation during surgery due to the x-rayless navigation system. A high degree of consistency between the pre-, intra- and postoperative data evaluated through the merging of the data sets allows a statement to be made about the success of the intervention and thus makes the procedure more transparent for all involved (30–32). By storing all the data sets, the patient has the benefit of a complete treatment plan, since the radiation therapist can also benefit from the data and can plan his therapy precisely tailored to the patient (33).

Navigation-Assisted Tumor Resection and Tumor Mapping

A considerable problem of conventional tumor resection without navigation is that the anatomical three-dimensional position of the specimen is described in words written down in the surgery report and in the pathology request document by the operating surgeon. The achieved accuracy can hardly be compared to the method of navigated tumor resection and tumor mapping. This method links the specimen to a coordinate in the three-dimensional anatomy of the patient. Technically this coordinate represents one precise point in space which refers to a sphere-shaped volume with a radius of 1.2 mm due to the measured registration accuracy during navigation. With a mean specimen size of the taken resection margins of 8.7 mm the virtual coordinate does not congruently match in full size. However, by taking at least 12 specimen the outline of the resection margin is adequately captured. Together with the histopathological result, this serves as an objective virtual marking of the true tumor extent. This higher number of taken specimen seems only applicable with the help of CAS since differentiation during relocation cannot be achieved with conventional location- and orientation-labeling by simple word description. The orientation-labeling and achieved accuracy of relocation with intraoperative navigation method adequately serves the technical achievable accuracy especially in cases of re-resection and should lie above the accuracy of the previous used conventional method. Even in view of soft tissue shifting presenting a well-known problem with intraoperative navigation (24, 34, 35), the presented method of mapping of midfacial tumors seems still applicable because in the anatomical region of the midface there are many bony structures giving stability to the adjacent soft tissue and thereby limiting the bias of soft tissue shifting.

In combination with the preoperative virtual planning of the resection extent which relies on merging of different imaging modalities combining the different information of these modalities (36), this method of navigated tumor resection and tumor mapping harbors promising results. In our study, we showed that with this method there were more R0 resection possible within tumors of the upper jaw compared to the conventional tumor resection. However, the difference between the two groups was not significant probably due to the sample size. It seems debatable that the observed increase in R0 resections in the CAS group may be achieved by the higher number of frozen sections rather than the use of navigation and CAS. However, in our opinion this high number of frozen sections cannot be adequately labeled with conventional methods allowing precise relocation in case of re-resection. Therefore, a technically applicable sampling of a high number of frozen sections is only reasonably achievable through CAS as already stated above. The comparison of the groups with regard to age, gender, radiation, diagnosis and reconstruction method shows that the groups did not differ in any respect. The CAS is therefore not only indicated for certain patients but can be used in all cases in everyday clinical practice. It has been proven to be particularly advantageous in the case of T4-tumors, since here, a successful operation without the use of CAS in terms of free resection margins is less likely (37, 38).

Even though no clear statements can be made about the long-term success of the CAS compared to previous methods, it should be noted that the CAS makes it easier to maintain the safety margin (37–39). Longitudinal studies will show whether the recurrence rate can be reduced in the long term, as this is already the case in other disciplines (40–42).

Another advantage of the CAS is that all information about the patient's anatomy is available preoperatively. This means that it is known how far the safety distance can be maintained before the intervention. If, for example, the safety margin touches the base of the skull, bony structures can be removed or preserved with greater certainty, since the distance to intracranial perforation is known. Our experience has shown that CAS has proven itself particularly well in the midface area, since most tumors are closely related to bony structures. This is precisely why the CAS is particularly suitable for T3 and T4 tumors.

Reconstruction After Ablative Surgery

The loss of hard and soft tissue after tumor resection is associated with substantial functional and aesthetic deficits (43). CAS in the form of computer-assisted design and models (CAD/CAM) has by far improved the possibilities of reconstructive surgery, especially in the planning of symmetrical aspects of the bony contour (28, 44–47). With regard to the primary reconstruction of the midface, the focus of the functional and aesthetic rehabilitation is, in addition to the chewing function, on the reconstruction of the orbital region. Since the secondary reconstruction can be expected to show poorer functional and aesthetic results due to various challenges, the focus should be on the primary reconstruction, in which the implants are inserted directly after the tumor resection. In doing so, not only the resection but also the implant insertion is carried out with the help of a template, since the position of the implant can be planned preoperatively according to the prosthetic situation. With the rapid prototyping or computer-assisted design/modeling (CAD/CAM) process, it is possible to create a virtual template for unilateral defects using simple processes such as mirroring the unaffected side onto the affected side, through which the midface can be restored (3). If there are bilateral defects, there is also the option of importing the midface from the atlas segmentation and adapting it to the remaining bony structures (elastic and rigid deformation) (48). This is used, for example, for complex tumors of the midface. Once the tumor has been resected, the periorbital region is reconstructed with alloplastic materials and autologous bone grafts. Various CAS procedures can be used here.

These procedures have opened up new possibilities and also a new claim for reconstructive surgery of the facial skull since it is now possible to achieve better aesthetic results through the symmetrical and thus faithful restoration of the removed structures. While prior to the introduction of these methods it was primarily a matter of repositioning the vascular or avascular bone in such a way that functionality was restored, the steps necessary to completely restore the face can now be planned preoperatively, taking into account the aesthetic subtleties (44, 45).

Our data showed that when the orbit is reconstructed after tumor surgery using CAS, the postoperative volume decreases. The postoperative reduction in volume is needed in cases of intra-orbital soft tissue deficiencies. Moreover, potential soft tissue atrophy and scaring may occur after surgery in this area which can cause enophthalmus. Therefore, we preferred a slight undercorrection rather than an overcorrection But even if the intra-orbital soft tissue was not touched, the postoperative volume was decreased. On the one hand, this is due to the fact, that a new implant is inserted which has its own volume, which must be taken into account. The segmented orbit mesh has an average volume of about 1.3 cm^3. If this number was added to the postoperative orbital volume, the difference between the pre- and postoperative volumes would no longer be significant. Deviations are also more likely with regard to the orbit compared to midface reconstruction since the structures are more filigree and complex and manual adjustments are therefore often necessary. On the other hand, the orbit mesh is bent manually using the STL models, so that minor errors can occur.

Successful Irradiation With Computer-Assisted Surgery

According to Boehm et al. only a few technical solutions for structured data storage and processing of all patient-related data are scientifically described (49). As already described above, after an operation it is necessary to transmit the data to the radiation therapist so that he can optimally plan the therapy. Without the CAS, the radiation therapist has insufficient information available in the form of histological findings, surgical reports and CT data sets, according to which he must plan a strategy. With the help of the CAS, screenshots in form of jpeg files and even enhanced DICOM data sets can be transmitted to the pathologist after the surgical procedure, so that the information can be passed on in a language-independent and unambiguous manner. The 3D volume rendering enables the pathologist to identify the location of the tumor in the image. Based on the histological results, positive boundaries can then be marked in the data set or drawn in in color. As part of further oncological treatment, this data can be saved and transmitted in DICOM format to oncologists, radiologists and pathologists so that they can receive specific tumor information such as the invasion of adjacent structures. Therefore, CAS can serve to enhance the interdisciplinary collaboration and improve patients' outcome. This is especially relevant for the treatment planning of adjuvant radiation therapy. While radiation therapy has been shown to reduce loco-regional recurrence rates (50), it harbors significant side effects such as xerostomia. These side effects occur due to the damaging of healthy tissue surrounding the tumor tissue. The planning of dose distribution during radiation relies on post-operative imaging (51). However, it can be challenging to differentiate on the basis of the imaging data between tissue aberrations due to remaining tumor or due to postoperative changes. The described procedure of tumor mapping can link the pathological information to a definitive three-dimensional coordinate and thereby helps reduce any doubt during interpretation of the imaging data. This allows a more precise dose distribution. However, if this procedure leads to a further reduced loco-regional recurrence rate or to lesser side effects during radiation therapy remains to be seen in further studies focusing on statistically representative patient groups which underwent adjuvant radiation therapy relying on CAS.

Quality of Life

It is difficult to quantify patients' quality of life in terms of CAS due to various problems. On the one hand, due to the lack of a comparison option, the patient is often not even aware that the CAS, for example, was able to remove the tumor more effectively or that vital structures could be better preserved. In addition due to the fact that patients are suffering from cancer and have to undergo an operation, the level of suffering among patients is so high that the quality of life is impaired for all patients, whether they were operated with or without the use of CAS (52–54). Large numbers of cases would be necessary to calculate significant differences between the groups. However, our data showed that those patients who were operated on using CAS had higher scores, especially in the areas of mood and appearance. These factors in turn correlate with one another.

When asked about the worst event since the operation, patients with oral cancer above all mentioned the realization of facial distortions, even if these seemed minor to third parties (55, 56). This shows that the patient's appearance is particularly important, which is understandable in terms of social integration after treatment. Appearance is also related to mood. While in the past the patient's survival was in the foreground and the operation was therefore extremely radical, CAS offers far more options here. By setting a safety distance in advance as part of the preoperative planning, it becomes evident which structures need to be removed, so that the reconstruction of the face can be planned in detail in advance and patient-specific implants can be made. Therefore, there was a tendency towards a higher health-related and overall quality of life, on which the factors appearance and mood exert a decisive influence. In particular for health-related quality of life, our results became almost significant, which suggests that a larger sample might show significant results.

CONCLUSION

The CAS offers great advantages over the previously established therapy methods in ablative tumor surgery, which are primarily reflected in the precision, safety and success of the treatment. Thanks to sophisticated systems for merging data sets from different imaging processes and the resulting possibilities for precise preoperative planning, in which the treatment goal can be determined in advance, taking into account all the necessary information, the operation can be less invasive while still maintaining a successful and more predictable result. Moreover, the possibility of computer-assisted implementation and documentation enables interdisciplinary, language-independent and thus unambiguous communication due to the broad database. Given these advantages of CAS, it is surprising that CAS is not yet routinely used in clinics. Due to the costs and the time required for the implementation and familiarization with the systems it becomes understandable that some surgeons have not yet been convinced of the use of the CAS.

In this study, we showed distinct advantages of CAS in the complex oncologic surgery of the midface. The operation and the planned expected results of the operation can be simulated preoperatively on the computer, afterwards an intraoperative implementation of the simulation is possible with the help of the navigation. The postoperative control through image fusion of the preoperative plan with a postoperative data set enables an evaluation of the reconstruction result with millimeter precision, as it is desired for complex reconstructions.

Another great advantage of this system is that all steps in the diagnosis and therapy of the patient are traceable at any time. If surgical obstacles arise intraoperatively, an alternative procedure with this system can be carried out with a minimum of effort and the complete tumor resection can still be ensured. Thus, the goal of improving the success of the treatment, optimization of interdisciplinary collaboration and the patient's quality of life through complete tumor resection and adequate reconstruction is retained.

AUTHOR CONTRIBUTIONS

MR conceived of the work and participated in its design and coordination. MW and MR made substantial contributions to data acquisition and conception of manuscript. MW drafted and designed the manuscript. MR has been involved in drafting and revising the manuscript. All authors contributed to the article and approved the submitted version.

REFERENCES

1. Schramm A, Suarez-Cunqueiro MM, Barth EL, Essig H, Bormann K-H, Kokemueller H, et al. Computer-Assisted Navigation in Craniomaxillofacial Tumors. *J Craniofac Surg* (2008) 19:1067–74. doi: 10.1097/SCS.0b013e3181760fc0
2. Strauss G, Winkler D, Trantakis C, Schulz T, Meixensberger J. Post-Processing of Radiological Data for Preoperative Planning in Skull Base Surgery. *Laryngo- Rhino- Otologie* (2004) 83:157–63. doi: 10.1055/s-2004-814271
3. Gellrich N-C, Schramm A, Hammer B, Rojas S, Cufi D, Lagrèze W, et al. Computer-Assisted Secondary Reconstruction of Unilateral Posttraumatic Orbital Deformity. *Plast Reconstruct Surg* (2002) 110:1417–29. doi: 10.1097/01.PRS.0000029807.35391.E5
4. Eckardt A, Swennen GRJ. Virtual Planning of Composite Mandibular Reconstruction With Free Fibula Bone Graft. *J Craniofac Surg* (2005) 16:1137–40. doi: 10.1097/01.scs.0000186306.32042.96
5. Wong ME, Kau CH, Melville JC, Patel T, Spagnoli DB. Bone Reconstruction Planning Using Computer Technology for Surgical Management of Severe Maxillomandibular Atrophy. *Oral Maxillofac Surg Clinics North America* (2019) 31:457–72. doi: 10.1016/j.coms.2019.03.008
6. Bell RB. Computer Planning and Intraoperative Navigation in Cranio-Maxillofacial Surgery. *Oral Maxillofac Surg Clinics North Am* (2010) 22:135–56. doi: 10.1016/j.coms.2009.10.010
7. Rana M, Essig H, Eckardt AM, Tavassol F, Ruecker M, Schramm A, et al. Advances and Innovations in Computer-Assisted Head and Neck Oncologic Surgery. *J Craniofac Surg* (2012) 23:272–8. doi: 10.1097/scs.0b013e318241bac7
8. Wilkat M, Singh DD, Lutz I, Möllmann H, Gellrich N-C, Rana M. Use and Evaluation of a Computer-Assisted Examination Method for the Diagnosis and Analysis of Medication-Related Osteonecrosis of the Jaw. *Craniomaxillofac Trauma Reconstruct* (2020) 14:36–42. doi: 10.1177/1943387520922767
9. Rana M, Modrow D, Keuchel J, Chui C, Rana M, Wagner M, et al. Development and Evaluation of an Automatic Tumor Segmentation Tool: A Comparison Between Automatic, Semi-Automatic and Manual Segmentation of Mandibular Odontogenic Cysts and Tumors. *J Cranio-Maxillofac Surg* (2015) 43:355–9. doi: 10.1016/j.jcms.2014.12.005
10. Gellrich N-C, Schramm A, Böckmann R, Kugler J. Follow-Up in Patients With Oral Cancer. *J Oral Maxillofac Surg* (2002) 60:380–6; discussion 387–8. doi: 10.1053/joms.2002.31224. discussion 387-8.
11. Rogers SN, Lowe D. The University of Washington Quality of Life Scale. In: VR Preedy, RR Watson, editors. *Handbook of Disease Burdens and Quality of Life Measures.* New York, NY: Springer New York. (2010) p. 101–28. doi: 10.1007/978-0-387-78665-0_6
12. Chen AM, Daly ME, Farwell DG, Vazquez E, Courquin J, Lau DH, et al. Quality of Life Among Long-Term Survivors of Head and Neck Cancer Treated by Intensity-Modulated Radiotherapy. *JAMA Otolaryngol- Head Neck Surg* (2014) 140:129–33. doi: 10.1001/jamaoto.2013.5988
13. D'Antonio LL, Zimmerman GJ, Cella DF, Long SA. Quality of Life and Functional Status Measures in Patients With Head and Neck Cancer. *Arch Otolaryngol–head Neck Surg* (1996) 122:482–7. doi: 10.1001/archotol.1996.01890170018005
14. Rana M, Chui CHK, Wagner M, Zimmerer R, Rana M, Gellrich N-C. Increasing the Accuracy of Orbital Reconstruction With Selective Laser-Melted Patient-Specific Implants Combined With Intraoperative Navigation. *J Oral Maxillofac Surg* (2015) 73:1113–8. doi: 10.1016/j.joms.2015.02.014
15. Zimmerer RM, Ellis E, Aniceto GS, Schramm A, Wagner MEH, Grant MP, et al. A Prospective Multicenter Study to Compare the Precision of Posttraumatic Internal Orbital Reconstruction With Standard Preformed and Individualized Orbital Implants. *J Cranio-Maxillofac Surg* (2016) 44 (9):1485–97. doi: 10.1016/j.jcms.2016.07.014
16. Schramm A, Suarez-Cunqueiro MM, Rücker M, Kokemueller H, Bormann K-H, Metzger MC, et al. Computer-Assisted Therapy in Orbital and Mid-Facial Reconstructions. *Int J Med Robotics + Comput Assist Surg: MRCAS* (2009) 5 (2):111–24. doi: 10.1002/rcs.245
17. Metzger MC, Hohlweg-Majert B, Schön R, Teschner M, Gellrich N-C, Schmelzeisen R, et al. Verification of Clinical Precision After Computer-Aided Reconstruction in Craniomaxillofacial Surgery. *Oral Surg Oral Med Oral Pathol Oral Radiol Endodontics* (2007) 104(4):e1–10. doi: 10.1016/j.tripleo.2007.04.015
18. Essig H, Rana M, Meyer A, Eckardt AM, Kokemueller H, von See C, et al. Virtual 3D Tumor Marking-Exact Intraoperative Coordinate Mapping Improve Post-Operative Radiotherapy. *Radiat Oncol (London England)* (2011) 6:159. doi: 10.1186/1748-717X-6-159
19. Aponte-Tinao L, Ritacco LE, Ayerza MA, Luis Muscolo D, Albergo JI, Farfall GL. Does Intraoperative Navigation Assistance Improve Bone Tumor Resection and Allograft Reconstruction Results? *Clin Orthopaed Related Res* (2015) 473:796–804. doi: 10.1007/s11999-014-3604-z
20. Barsa P, Fröhlich R, Sebek F, Suchomel P. Intraoperative CT-Based Spinal Navigation: The Initial 295 Implants Experience. *Rozhledy v Chirurgii* (2014) 93:16–20. doi: 10.1007/s00701-014-2184-8
21. Farfalli GL, Albergo JI, Ritacco LE, Ayerza MA, Milano FE, Aponte-Tinao LA. What Is the Expected Learning Curve in Computer-Assisted Navigation for Bone Tumor Resection? *Clin Orthopaed Related Res* (2017) 475:668–75. doi: 10.1007/s11999-016-4761-z
22. Tan X, Hu M, Tao Y, Luo J, Xu J, Liu S. Application of Computer-Aided

Surgery in Fibrous Dysplasia of Cranio-Maxillofacial Bone. *Shanghai Kou Qiang Yi Xue = Shanghai J Stomatol* (2014) 23:62–5.

23. Sießegger M, Mischkowski RA, Schneider BT, Krug B, Klesper B, Zöller JE. Image Guided Surgical Navigation for Removal of Foreign Bodies in the Head and Neck. *J Cranio-Maxillofac Surg* (2001) 29:321–5. doi: 10.1054/jcms.2001.0254
24. Anand M, Panwar S. Role of Navigation in Oral and Maxillofacial Surgery: A Surgeon's Perspectives. *Clin Cosmetic Investigational Dentist* (2021) 13:127–39. doi: 10.2147/CCIDE.S299249
25. Choudhri O, Mindea SA, Feroze A, Soudry E, Chang SD, Nayak JV. Experience With Intraoperative Navigation and Imaging During Endoscopic Transnasal Spinal Approaches to the Foramen Magnum and Odontoid. *Neurosurg Focus* (2014) 36(3):E4. doi: 10.3171/2014.1.FOCUS13533
26. Marmulla R, Niederdellmann H. Precision Control of the Position of the Bone Segments During Surgical Navigation. *Rev Stomatol Chirurgie Maxillo-faciale* (1998) 99:184–7. doi: 10.1016/S1010-5182(98)80067-X
27. Zhang L, Sun H, Yu H, Yuan H, Shen G, Wang X. Computer-Assisted Orthognathic Surgery Combined With Fibular Osteomyocutaneous Flap Reconstruction to Correct Facial Asymmetry and Maxillary Defects Secondary to Maxillectomy in Childhood. *J Craniofac Surg* (2013) 24:886–9. doi: 10.1097/SCS.0b013e31827ff370
28. Zhang WB, Wang Y, Liu XJ, Mao C, Guo CB, Yu GY, et al. Reconstruction of Maxillary Defects With Free Fibula Flap Assisted by Computer Techniques. *J Cranio-Maxillo-Facial Surg* (2015) 43:630–6. doi: 10.1016/j.jcms.2015.03.007
29. Levine JP, Patel A, Saadeh PB, Hirsch DL. Computer-Aided Design and Manufacturing in Craniomaxillofacial Surgery: The New State of the Art. *J Craniofac Surg* (2012) 23:288–93. doi: 10.1097/SCS.0b013e318241ba92
30. Guevara-Rojas G, Figl M, Schicho K, Seemann R, Traxler H, Vacariu A, et al. Patient-Specific Polyetheretherketone Facial Implants in a Computer-Aided Planning Workflow. *J Oral Maxillofac Surg* (2014) 72:1801–12. doi: 10.1016/j.joms.2014.02.013
31. Sun Y, Luebbers HT, Agbaje JO, Schepers S, Vrielinck L, Lambrichts I, et al. Accuracy of Upper Jaw Positioning With Intermediate Splint Fabrication After Virtual Planning in Bimaxillary Orthognathic Surgery. *J Craniofac Surg* (2013) 24:1871–6. doi: 10.1097/SCS.0b013e31829a80d9
32. Ritacco LE, Milano FE, Farfalli GL, Ayerza MA, Muscolo DL, Aponte-Tinao LA. Accuracy of 3-D Planning and Navigation in Bone Tumor Resection. *Orthopedics* (2013) 36(7):e942–50. doi: 10.3928/01477447-20130624-27
33. Guijarro-Martínez R, Gellrich NC, Witte J, Tapioles D, Von Briel C, Kolotas C, et al. Optimization of the Interface Between Radiology, Surgery, Radiotherapy, and Pathology in Head and Neck Tumor Surgery: A Navigation-Assisted Multidisciplinary Network. *Int J Oral Maxillofac Surg* (2014) 43:156–62. doi: 10.1016/j.ijom.2013.09.005
34. Sukegawa S, Kanno T, Furuki Y. Application of Computer-Assisted Navigation Systems in Oral and Maxillofacial Surgery. *Jpn Dental Sci Rev* (2018) 54:139–49. doi: 10.1016/j.jdsr.2018.03.005
35. Lan L, He Y, An J, Zhang Y. Application of Computer-Aided Navigation Technology in the Extraction of Foreign Body From the Face. *J Craniofac Surg* (2020) 31:e166–9. doi: 10.1097/SCS.0000000000006126
36. Sun H, Li B, Shen S, Yang T, Zhang L, Shen SGF, et al. Image-Guided Endoscopic Navigation for the Precise Resection of a Mandibular Condylar Osteochondroma. *J Craniofac Surg* (2013) 24(6):e573–9. doi: 10.1097/SCS.0b013e31829ad374
37. Ricotta F, Cercenelli L, Battaglia S, Bortolani B, Savastio G, Marcelli E, et al. Navigation-Guided Resection of Maxillary Tumors: Can a New Volumetric Virtual Planning Method Improve Outcomes in Terms of Control of Resection Margins? *J Cranio-Maxillofac Surg* (2018) 46:2240–7. doi: 10.1016/j.jcms.2018.09.034
38. Tarsitano A, Ricotta F, Baldino G, Badiali G, Pizzigallo A, Ramieri V, et al. Navigation-Guided Resection of Maxillary Tumours: The Accuracy of Computer-Assisted Surgery in Terms of Control of Resection Margins – A Feasibility Study. *J Cranio-Maxillofac Surg* (2017) 45:2109–14. doi: 10.1016/j.jcms.2017.09.023
39. Sternheim A, Rotman D, Nayak P, Arkhangorodsky M, Daly MJ, Irish JC, et al. Computer-Assisted Surgical Planning of Complex Bone Tumor Resections Improves Negative Margin Outcomes in a Sawbones Model. *Int J Comput Assist Radiol Surg* (2021) 16:695–701. doi: 10.1007/s11548-021-02337-w
40. Li F-Y, Chen X-L, Sai X-Y, Zhang J-S, Hu S, Li J-J, et al. Application of Intraoperative Magnetic Resonance Imaging and Multimodal Navigation in Surgical Resection of Glioblastoma. *Zhonghua Wai Ke Za Zhi [Chinese J Surgery]* (2013) 51(6):542–6.
41. Nandra R, Matharu G, Stevenson J, Parry M, Grimer R, Jeys L. Long-Term Outcomes After an Initial Experience of Computer-Navigated Resection of Primary Pelvic and Sacral Bone Tumours: Soft-Tissue Margins Must be Adequate to Reduce Local Recurrences. *Bone Joint J* (2019) 101-B:484–90. doi: 10.1302/0301-620X.101B4.BJJ-2018-0981.R1
42. Laitinen MK, Parry MC, Albergo JI, Grimer RJ, Jeys LM. Is Computer Navigation When Used in the Surgery of Iliosacral Pelvic Bone Tumours Safer for the Patient? *Bone Joint J* (2017) 99-B:261–6. doi: 10.1302/0301-620X.99B2.BJJ-2016-0149.R2
43. Kokemueller H, Tavassol F, Ruecker M, Gellrich NC. Complex Midfacial Reconstruction: A Combined Technique of Computer-Assisted Surgery and Microvascular Tissue Transfer. *J Oral Maxillofac Surg* (2008) 66:2398–406. doi: 10.1016/j.joms.2007.12.030
44. Terzic A, Scolozzi P. Image Guided Surgical Navigation Integrating "Mirroring" Computational Planning Based on Intra-Operative Cone-Beam CT Imaging: A Promising New Approach for Management of Primary Bilateral Midfacial Fractures. *Comput Aided Surg* (2011) 16:170–80. doi: 10.3109/10929088.2011.581901
45. Hanasono MM, Jacob RF, Bidaut L, Robb GL, Skoracki RJ. Midfacial Reconstruction Using Virtual Planning, Rapid Prototype Modeling, and Stereotactic Navigation. *Plast Reconstruct Surg* (2010) 126:2002–6. doi: 10.1097/PRS.0b013e3181f447e1
46. Palines PA, Ferrer JR, Yoo A, St Hilaire H, Stalder MW. Simplifying Bony Midface Reconstruction With Patient-Specific Titanium Plates. *Plast Reconstruct Surg Global Open* (2021) 9:e3555. doi: 10.1097/GOX.0000000000003555
47. Schramm A, Wilde F. Die Computergestützte Gesichtsschädelrekonstruktion. *HNO* (2011) 59:800–6. doi: 10.1007/s00106-011-2351-7
48. Essig H, Dressel L, Rana M, Rana M, Kokemueller H, Ruecker M, et al. Precision of Posttraumatic Primary Orbital Reconstruction Using Individually Bent Titanium Mesh With and Without Navigation: A Retrospective Study. *Head Face Med* (2013) 9:1–7. doi: 10.1186/1746-160X-9-18
49. Boehm A, Müller S, Pankau T, Straub G, Bohn S, Fuchs M, et al. Computer Assistance to Improve Therapy Planning for Head Neck Oncology. *Laryngo-Rhino- Otologie* (2011) 90:732–8. doi: 10.1055/s-0031-1295410
50. Schiff BA, Roberts DB, El-Naggar A, Garden AS, Myers JN. Selective vs Modified Radical Neck Dissection and Postoperative Radiotherapy vs Observation in the Treatment of Squamous Cell Carcinoma of the Oral Tongue. *Arch Otolaryngol–Head Neck Surg* (2005) 131(10):874–8. doi: 10.1001/archotol.131.10.874
51. Kessel IL, Blanco A. Update in Radiation Therapy for Oral and Maxillofacial Tumors and Dose Mapping. *Oral Maxillofac Surg Clinics North Am* (2014) 26 (2):223–9. doi: 10.1016/j.coms.2014.01.008
52. Rhoten BA, Murphy BA, Dietrich MS, Ridner SH. Depressive Symptoms, Social Anxiety, and Perceived Neck Function in Patients With Head and Neck Cancer. *Head Neck* (2018) 40:1443–52. doi: 10.1002/hed.25129
53. Pandey M, Devi N, Ramdas K, Krishnan R, Kumar V. Higher Distress Relates to Poor Quality of Life in Patients With Head and Neck Cancer. *Int J Oral Maxillofac Surg* (2009) 38:955–9. doi: 10.1016/j.ijom.2009.04.004
54. Rabbels J, Wyzisk M, Siessegger M, Klesper B, Reuther T, Kübler AC. Quality of Life of Patients With Squamous Cell Carcinoma of the Oral Cavity. *Mund- Kiefer- und Gesichtschirurgie: MKG* (2005) 9:300–5. doi: 10.1007/s10006-005-0628-2
55. Chaturvedi SK, Shenoy A, Prasad KMR, Senthilnathan SM, Premlatha BS. Concerns, Coping and Quality of Life in Head and Neck Cancer Patients. *Support Care Cancer* (1996) 4:186–90. doi: 10.1007/BF01682338
56. Duffy SA, Ronis DL, Valenstein M, Fowler KE, Lambert MT, Bishop C, et al. Depressive Symptoms, Smoking, Drinking, and Quality of Life Among Head and Neck Cancer Patients. *Psychosomatics* (2007) 48:142–8. doi: 10.1176/appi.psy.48.2.142

22

Reconstruction of a Large Maxillary Defect with an Engineered, Vascularized, Prefabricated Bone Graft

Tarek Ismail[1,2†], Alexander Haumer[1,2†], Alexander Lunger[1], Rik Osinga[1,3], Alexandre Kaempfen[1,2], Franziska Saxer[4], Anke Wixmerten[2], Sylvie Miot[2], Florian Thieringer[5], Joerg Beinemann[5], Christoph Kunz[5], Claude Jaquiéry[5], Thomas Weikert[6], Felix Kaul[6], Arnaud Scherberich[1,2], Dirk J. Schaefer[1,3] and Ivan Martin[2]*

[1] Department of Plastic, Reconstructive, Aesthetic and Hand Surgery, University Hospital Basel, Basel, Switzerland, [2] Department of Biomedicine, University Hospital Basel, University of Basel, Basel, Switzerland, [3] Center for Musculoskeletal Infections, University Hospital Basel, Basel, Switzerland, [4] Department of Orthopedic Surgery, University Hospital Basel, Basel, Switzerland, [5] Clinic for Craniomaxillofacial and Oral Surgery, University Hospital Basel, Basel, Switzerland, [6] Department of Radiology, University Hospital Basel, Basel, Switzerland

***Correspondence:**
Ivan Martin
ivan.martin@usb.ch

[†]These authors have contributed equally to this work and share first authorship

The reconstruction of complex midface defects is a challenging clinical scenario considering the high anatomical, functional, and aesthetic requirements. In this study, we proposed a surgical treatment to achieve improved oral rehabilitation and anatomical and functional reconstruction of a complex defect of the maxilla with a vascularized, engineered composite graft. The patient was a 39-year-old female, postoperative after left hemimaxillectomy for ameloblastic carcinoma in 2010 and tumor-free at the 5-year oncological follow-up. The left hemimaxillary defect was restored in a two-step approach. First, a composite graft was ectopically engineered using autologous stromal vascular fraction (SVF) cells seeded on an allogenic devitalized bone matrix. The resulting construct was further loaded with bone morphogenic protein-2 (BMP-2), wrapped within the latissimus dorsi muscle, and pedicled with an arteriovenous (AV) bundle. Subsequently, the prefabricated graft was orthotopically transferred into the defect site and revascularized through microvascular surgical techniques. The prefabricated graft contained vascularized bone tissue embedded within muscular tissue. Despite unexpected resorption, its orthotopic transfer enabled restoration of the orbital floor, separation of the oral and nasal cavities, and midface symmetry and allowed the patient to return to normal diet as well as to restore normal speech and swallowing function. These results remained stable for the entire follow-up period of 2 years. This clinical case demonstrates the safety and the feasibility of composite graft engineering for the treatment of complex maxillary defects. As compared to the current gold standard of autologous tissue transfer, this patient's benefits included decreased donor site morbidity and improved oral rehabilitation. Bone resorption of the construct at the ectopic prefabrication site still needs to be further addressed to preserve the designed graft size and shape.

Keywords: complex 3D bone defect, vascularized composite graft, bone–soft tissue interface, regenerative surgery, graft prefabrication

INTRODUCTION

Reconstruction of large bone defects in the maxillofacial region, typically relying on autologous vascularized bone grafts or synthetic biocompatible materials, remains a clinical challenge. Apart from reconstructing the hard and soft tissues, the masticatory rehabilitation of the patient by conventional (removable) or implant-supported prostheses needs to be addressed. Autologous bone grafting is associated with limited availability, significant donor site morbidity, and restrained or even impossible oral rehabilitation. Synthetic materials represent only a temporary solution, not only because of frequency of infections but also due to limited integration and thus inadequate separation of oral and nasal cavities (1–3).

The potential for *de novo* bone formation of cells from the stromal vascular fraction (SVF) of adipose tissue, even if not cultured or primed *in vitro*, has been shown in preclinical and clinical models, if implanted orthotopically (4) or exposed to low doses of bone morphogenetic protein (BMP)-2 (5, 6). Moreover, efficient vascularization of critically sized, SVF-based bone grafts was achieved in a rodent model by the insertion of arteriovenous (AV) bundles (7, 8) by analogy with typical microsurgical techniques (9, 10).

Here we describe the pioneering clinical implementation of an ectopically prefabricated (i.e., including a vascular pedicle for transfer) and prelaminated (i.e., multilayer composite including a soft tissue interface) (11) flap as osteogenic and vasculogenic graft for hemimaxillary reconstruction in a patient with Cordeiro type IIIa maxillectomy. The implant was first constructed in a latissimus dorsi muscle flap by combining a custom-shaped scaffold with autologous SVF cells, BMP-2, and an AV bundle. The resulting prevascularized composite graft was then transferred to the maxilla defect with the ultimate goal to durably restore midface symmetry, separate naso- and oropharyngeal spaces, allow physiological swallowing, and establish airway function.

MATERIALS AND METHODS

In this study, we report the case of a 39-year-old female patient diagnosed with an ameloblastic carcinoma of the left maxilla in September 2010. She underwent subsequent hemimaxillectomy in October 2010, which resulted in a Cordeiro type IIIa (total maxillectomy defect sparing the orbital contents) (12, 13), Okay Type II (14), Brown Type 3 (15) maxillectomy defect. The defect was replaced with a palatal obturator prosthesis (**Figures 1A–C**), which gave an unsatisfactory functional result. The orbital floor has been reconstructed with a titanium mesh (Synthes) during primary ameloblastoma resection. The patient suffered from recurrent infections and had problems drinking water due to insufficient separation of the oral and nasal cavity. After a 5-year cancer-free follow-up, the patient needed adequate and long-term surgical reconstruction of the left maxilla. The complexity of the patient's three-dimensional composite defect, in combination with her young age and her desire to bypass morbidity and limited effectiveness of a free vascularized autologous bone graft (e.g., fibula, scapula or the iliac crest), prompted for the implementation of an innovative strategy. The patient had no other relevant comorbidities. This case study conforms with the Declaration of Helsinki. It was approved by the national competent authority, Swissmedic, under exceptional permission (SBH 16-0172) and by the competent ethical committee (EKNZ), with the patient's written informed consent.

The patient's treatment consisted of a two-step reconstructive plan, namely, an ectopic implant prefabrication (**Figure 1D**), followed by its orthotopic transfer (**Figure 1E**). A three-dimensional scaffold was manufactured, based on the patient's computed tomography (CT) data of the defect site and contralateral side by computer-aided design and computer-aided manufacturing (CAD-CAM) techniques. As scaffolding material, allogenic and decellularized cancellous bone (Tutoplast®, Tutogen Medical, Neunkirchen, Germany) with a porosity of approximately 60% was used. The scaffold, with a total volume of 27.6 cm^3, was designed as a set of four pieces, which could be intraoperatively assembled and fixed with preheated absorbable pins, leaving space for a central tunnel to allow for the intraoperative insertion of an AV bundle (**Figure 1E, Figure 2B**).

All surgeries were performed under general anesthesia. To collect stromal vascular fraction (SVF) cells, a hand-assisted abdominal liposuction was performed and a final volume of 320 ml of sedimented fat was harvested. SVF cells were intraoperatively isolated with an automated device (Celution 800/CRS System, Cytori Therapeutics Inc., UK) and counted with a NucleoCounter NC-200™ (ChemoMetec, Denmark), leading to a total number of 106 × 10^6 cells with a viability of 76.8 +/- 3.2%. After assembling the four Tutoplast pieces with pins, the scaffold was cellularized by gentle loading of 105 × 10^6 SVF cells, resuspended in 8.5 ml of fibrin gel (Tisseel®, Baxter, AT) in the presence of 60 μg/ml recombinant human bone morphogenetic protein-2 (BMP-2, Infuse®, Medtronic, CH) (**Figure 2A**). Following SVF cell seeding, a distally ligated arteriovenous (AV) bundle (serratus branch of the

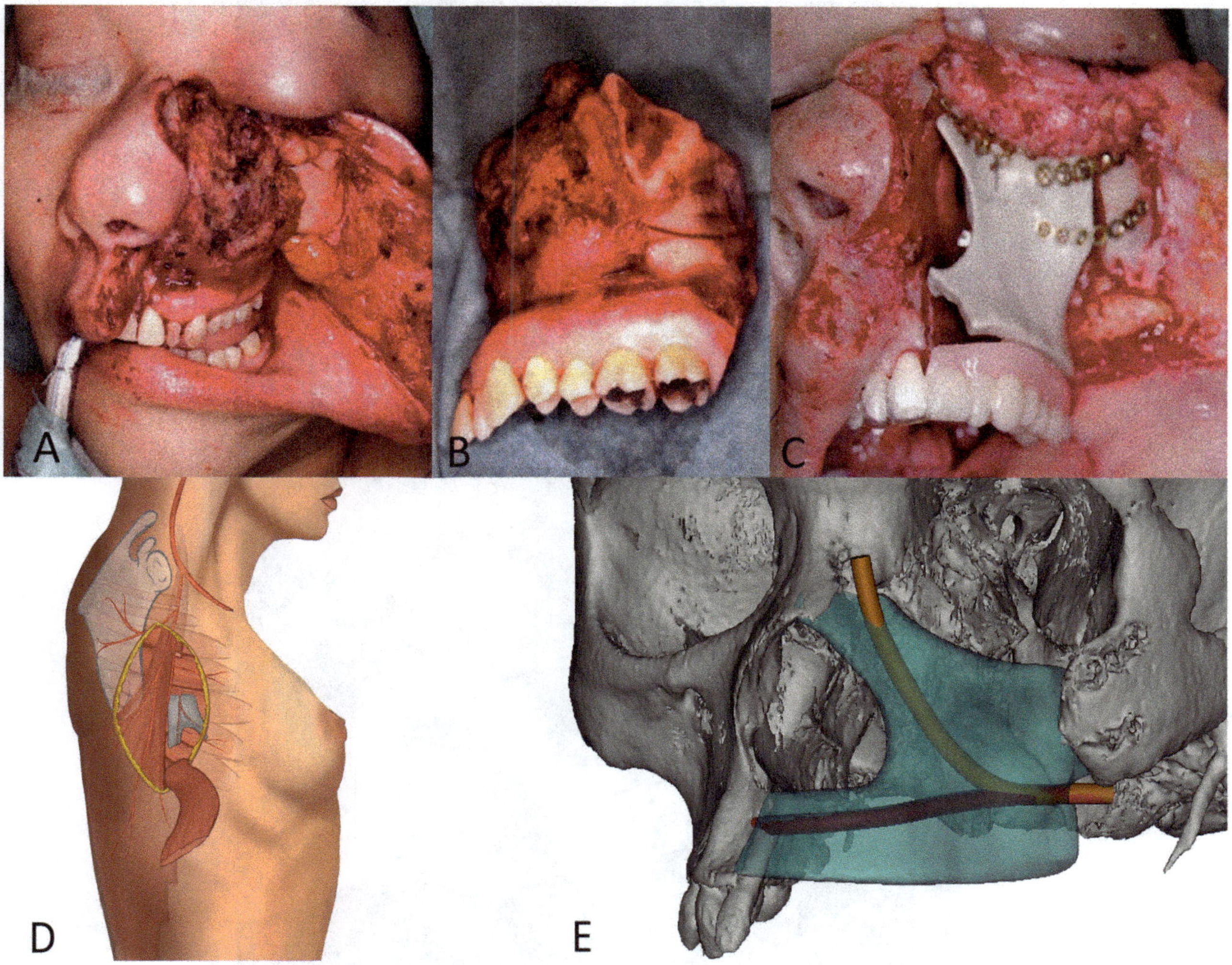

FIGURE 1 | Midface defect, immediate temporary reconstruction, and two-step patient specific planning. **(A)** Intraoperative aspect of exposed ameloblastic carcinoma of the left hemimaxilla prior to resection. **(B)** Left hemimaxillectomy specimen with preservation of midface soft tissue and missing inner nasal lining (mucosa). **(C)** Intraoperative situation after PEEK implantation with obturator prosthesis. **(D)** Ectopic prevascularization by surgical insertion of an arteriovenous (AV) bundle (serratus branch of the thoracodorsal vessel) and wrapping of the construct into a split latissimus muscle. **(E)** CAD-CAM reconstruction on the patients CT scan showing the customized Tutoplast® scaffold with the tunnel planned for the serratus AV bundle and its branching after implantation.

thoracodorsal vessels) was surgically inserted in the central scaffold tunnel for axial prevascularization (**Figure 2B**). The whole construct was wrapped in a split latissimus dorsi muscle flap and placed under the patient's left breast (**Figures 2C, D**). Total surgery time was 6 h and 30 min, while flap raise including vessel dissection and ectopic construct preparation (fixation of the scaffold parts, SVF isolation, seeding of the scaffold) was performed simultaneously.

Vascularization of the construct was analyzed by perfusion magnetic resonance imaging (MRI) after 1 and 6 weeks. Bone metabolism inside the construct was assessed with single-photon emission computed tomography (SPECT) after 6 weeks.

After 8 months and proven neovascularization with manifest bone metabolism as seen on the SPECT scan, the composite graft was harvested and positioned into the recipient site, while a punch biopsy (4 × 5 mm) was taken from the central volume for histological analysis. The thoracodorsal vessels were dissected free, cut, and anastomosed in an end-to-end fashion to the left facial artery and vein. Graft vascularization after transfer was intraoperatively assessed by fluorescent indo cyanine green (ICG) visualization (VisionSense, Philadelphia). The donor site was then settled by primary closure. Postoperative monitoring at the intensive care unit (ICU) was uneventful. Total surgery time was 8 h 18 min. The patient was hospitalized for 7 days. Suction drains at the donor site were removed on the third postoperative day. Antibiotic therapy with amoxicillin/clavulanic acid for a total of 5 days was administered perioperatively.

Regular follow-up appointments were scheduled at 2 and 6 weeks as well as 3, 6, and 12 months post-reconstruction. Final imaging by CT scan and logopedic evaluation to assess speech and swallowing function were conducted 24 months after orthotopic transfer.

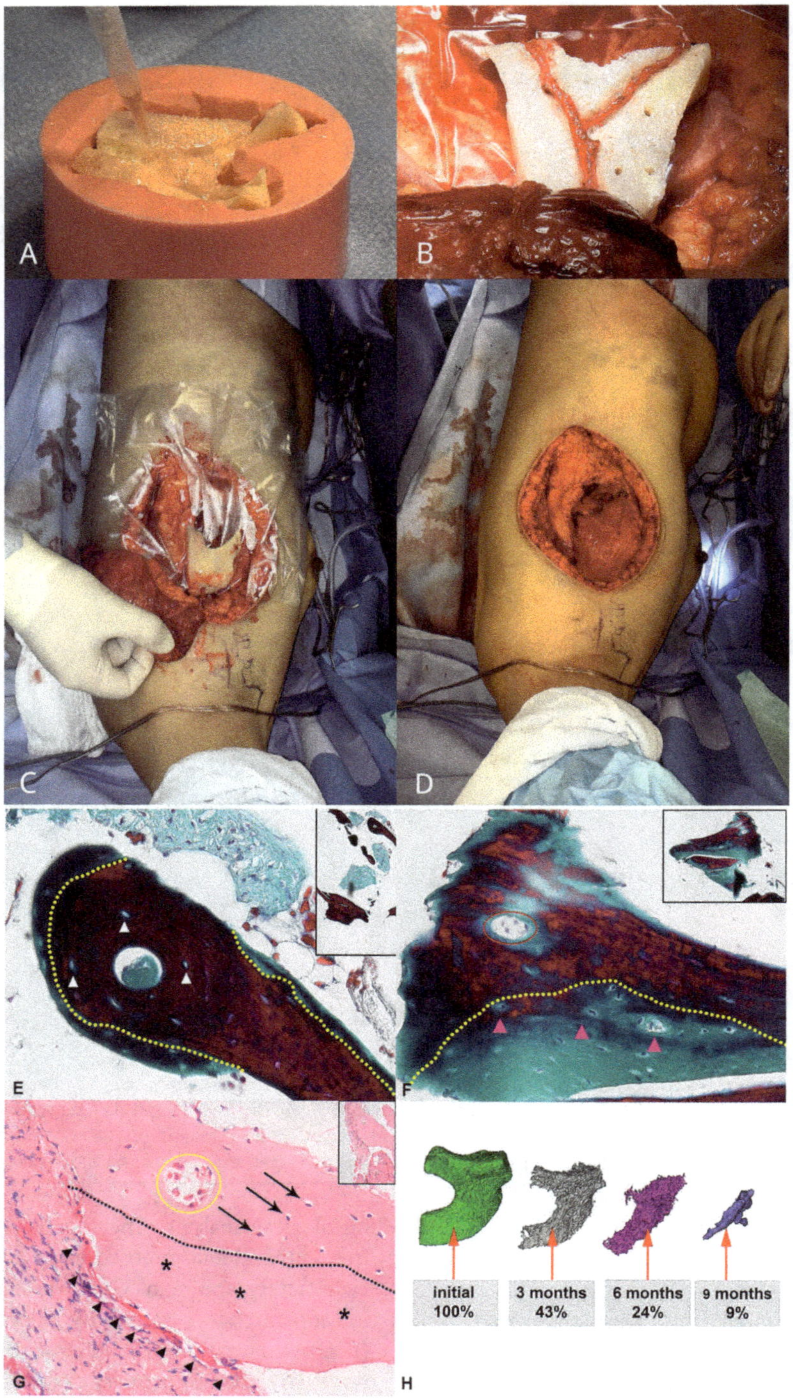

FIGURE 2 | Graft prefabrication and histological analysis (bone biopsy at moment of transfer at week 32) and volume assessment over time. **(A)** 3D scaffold of devitalized bone manufactured to match the patient's defect size and shape and seeded with SVF cells and BMP-2. **(B)** Ectopic implantation with serratus AV bundle. **(C, D)** Construct with vascular pedicle before and after being wrapped in split latissimus muscle. **(E, F)** High magnification of representative figures of bone biopsy after staining with Masson Trichrome. The Tutoplast® scaffold is characterized by purple staining, representing mature bone and cellular lacunae (white arrowheads), showing devitalized bone tissue. Newly formed bone tissue, represented by light green color, is deposited on the Tutoplast® scaffold and contains nuclei (pink arrowheads). The yellow dashed line delineates the original scaffold material and apposition of newly formed bone. A vessel (red circle) demonstrates that the scaffold is vascularized. **(G)** Overview figure shows appositional bone growth on the Tutoplast® scaffold (asterisk). Osteocytes (arrows) are visible in the newly formed bone. The proportion of scaffold vs. new bone formation is close to 50:50. A blood vessel is present within the newly formed bone (yellow circle). Osteoclasts (full arrowheads) fringe the Tutoplast® scaffold (asterisks), which shows clear signs of degradation at site of interaction. There is no major osteoclast infiltration at the level of the newly formed apposed bone and no sign of degradation visible. **(H)** CT-reconstruction and volume calculation show volume decrease over time.

RESULTS

Ectopic Implant Prefabrication

The patient had an uneventful course after ectopic graft placement in December 2016, without intraoperative complications such as major bleeding or pedicle damage. The patient did not report any implant-related discomfort, and neither hematoma nor infection was noted.

Vascularization of the construct was assessed during ectopic graft development after 1 week (**Figure 3A**) and 6 weeks (**Figure 3B**) by dynamic contrast-enhanced MR perfusion imaging. The AV bundle proved to be patent, providing intrinsic perfusion to the construct. The latissimus dorsi muscle wrap was viable, with a perfusion pattern comparable or superior to the subscapularis muscle, chosen as a reference for physiological perfusion in this anatomic region. At both time

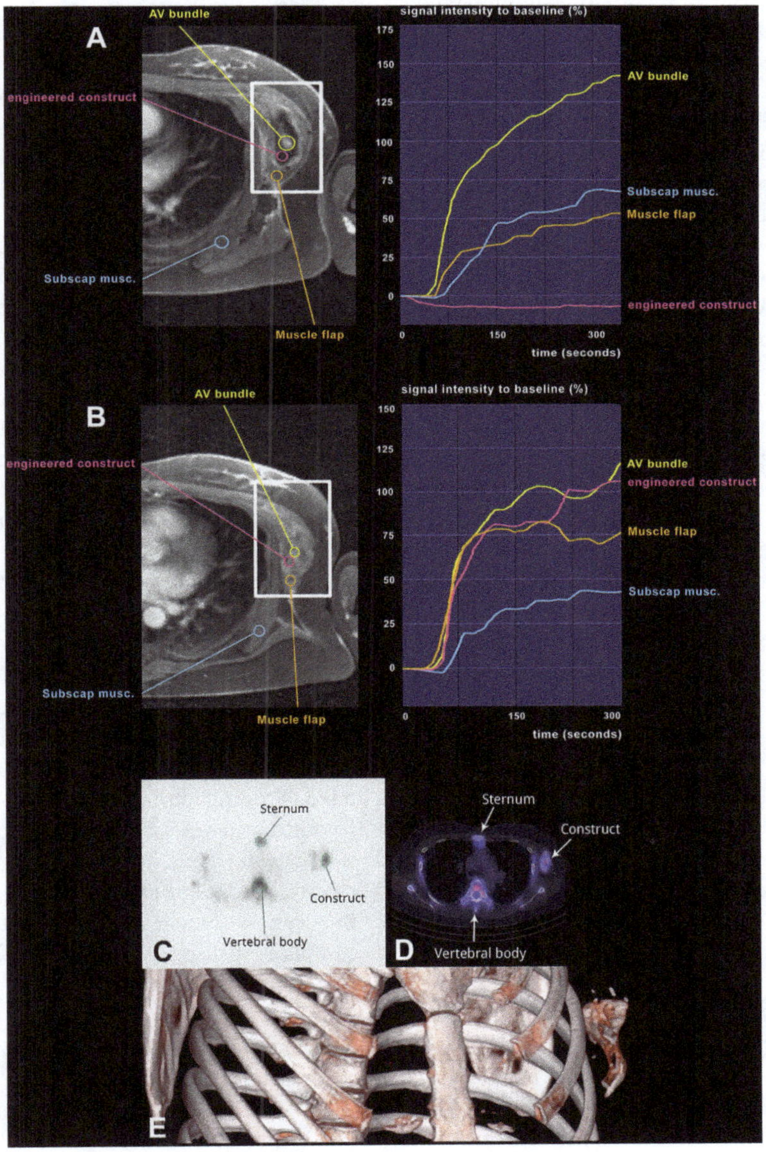

FIGURE 3 | Longitudinal assessment of vascularization and bone formation. Transversal images of a golden-angle radial sparse parallel (GRASP) MRI showing the perfusion of the engineered construct adjacent to the left ribcage over time as well as corresponding signal-time curves at 1 week **(A)** and at 6 weeks **(B)**. The Maxilla construct is highlighted by white rectangles. Signal intensity in relation to t = 0 (injection of contrast agent) on the Y-axis, time in seconds on the X-axis. Violet region of interest (ROI) located in the construct, blue ROI located in the left M. subscapularis *in situ* and yellow ROI encompassing the AV bundle. Orange ROI indicates M. latissimus dorsi flap covering the construct. M. subscapularis was used as a reference for physiological vascularization in this area. Planar images **(C)** and SPECT and SPECT/CT images **(D)** after 6 weeks of the bone scintigraphy, showing strong DPD uptake in the construct, indicating bone turnover and vitality of the construct. In a region-of-interest (ROI) analysis of the maxilla construct at its largest diameter in comparison to the sternum (as a bone with similar structure/size). **(E)** VRT (volume rendering technique) from the SPECT illustrates the location of the prefabricated construct.

points, the subscapularis muscle, the latissimus muscle, and the AV bundle showed a normal, steadily increasing perfusion over time. When focusing on the engineered construct, no signal increase after injection of the contrast agent was observed after 1 week, whereas a steep increase in signal intensity was visible after 6 weeks, demonstrating functional internal vascularization.

Bone metabolism of the construct was assessed after 6 weeks by SPECT/CT (**Figures 3C–E**). Active 3,3-diphosphono-1,2-propanodicarboxylic acid (DPD) uptake in the construct revealed traits of viable bone tissue (maximum counts: 112), in the range between the sternal bone (maximum counts: 95) and the highly compact thoracic vertebral body (maximum counts: 154), used as reference structures of similar size and position (**Figures 3C, D**). Bone biopsy at the phase of construct transfer, 32 weeks after ectopic implantation, morphologically confirmed *de novo* bone formation (**Figures 2E–G**). Masson Trichrome staining showed a clear distinction between the Tutoplast® scaffold material, consisting of devitalized bone, and newly deposited bone matrix. The latter was less dense and less mature, as shown by the green color and reduced lamellar structure. The deposited bone contained stained cell nuclei as sign of living tissue, clearly distinguishable from the devitalized bone of the scaffold, where cells were visible as empty lacunae. Vascularization of the construct was histologically verified by piercing vessels in the scaffold material (**Figures 2F, G**). Osteoclasts were found around the Tutoplast® scaffold, which displayed morphological signs of active resorption. Within the newly formed, apposed bone, there was no major osteoclast infiltration and no signs of degradation. Quantitative histomorphometry of the biopsy specimen indicated an average of 30.2% (SD = 10.3) of newly formed bone over the total bone area.

Mineralized tissue volume in the construct was assessed by CT scan at 3, 6, and 9 months postoperatively (**Figure 2H**). Progressive resorption of the mineralized mass was observed, down to 43%, 24%, and 9% of the initial scaffold volume.

Orthotopic Transplantation

After 32 weeks, despite advanced resorption, the ectopically engineered composite graft was transferred into the maxillary defect. It was anastomosed to the facial artery and external jugular vein as a free tissue transfer (**Figures 4A, B**). The graft was augmented with calvarial bone struts from the patient's left parietal region in order to compensate for the loss of bone volume from the initial design. The postoperative course was uneventful. After one night in the ICU, the patient was transferred to the general ward and dismissed after 7 days. Wound healing and flap integration were satisfactory.

After additional 24 months, oral rehabilitation was evaluated with a clinical assessment of the swallowing and speech function as well as a palatogram and myometric measurement of the lips, tongue, masseter muscle, and mentalis muscle by a speech therapist. The patient yielded a near-to-normal oropharyngeal function with normal speech. She was able to eat an unrestricted diet, presented no ectropion, enophthalmos, or diplopia corresponding to normal globe position and function. No microstomy was observed, and oral competence was restored including normal tongue movement, mouth opening, and oral and lip sensation (**Table 1**). Although the patient reported increased trapezius and suboccipital muscle tonicity and slight drooling on the left side, facial symmetry was achieved with aesthetic satisfaction, based on self- and clinical assessment. The CT scan 24 months after orthotropic transfer showed a resorption of the construct with a remaining bone core (**Figures 4C–H**).

Symmetry and subjective aesthetic outcome were assessed after reconstruction (**Figure 5**).

DISCUSSION

This case describes the unique combination of bone tissue engineering, ectopic prefabrication, and microvascular free-flap strategies for the reconstruction of a highly complex defect of the left hemimaxilla in a young female patient. With this concept, we were able to create a prefabricated, composite maxilla substitute providing both bone and a soft tissue interface, thus avoiding the use of a non-autologous structural support material, such as a titanium cage, and the morbidity associated with autologous vascularized bone tissue transfer.

It is known that midface defects, especially of the maxilla, can have a substantial functional impact. Conventional reconstructive options, including freely transferred or local tissue flaps, typically fail to provide a sufficient anatomical and functional coverage for defects involving the hard and soft palate, as well as the orbital floor (19, 20). This leads to inadequate mastication, food processing, and lack of separation between the oral and nasal cavities. Traditionally, combinations of non-vascularized bone grafts with myocutaneous free flaps as well as free osteomyocutaneous flaps have been used for the coverage of these defects, all of them with specific advantages and disadvantages. Several chimeric free flaps have been described from the fibula or scapula with skin island. Extensive defects involving the palate and orbital floor, as in the patient described, have a better functional outcome and quality of life if reconstructed with free flaps, compared to prostheses. Still, this is a valuable option in mild to moderate-sized palatal defects or in elderly, multimorbid patients (21, 22). Free flaps in general inherently cause a donor site defect and associated complications. In free fibula bone flaps, which are often used in maxillofacial reconstruction, perioperative donor site complications occur in about one-third of cases and long-term morbidities of 17% have been described, including leg weakness, ankle instability, hallux contracture, and decreased ankle mobility (23). Other osteocutaneous flaps, such as the iliac crest flap, can lead to a sensory deficit (up to 27%), chronic pain (8%-26%) (24, 25), or impaired gait and reduced range of hip motion (25%) (26). For the radial forearm osteocutaneous flap, wound breakdown with tendon exposure is known to occur in 5%-46% (27, 28), whereas fracture of the residual radius occurs in 0%-18% (28–30) and chronic pain in 16.7% (31).

To avoid harvesting large amounts of autologous bone tissue, we decided to combine strategies of tissue engineering with approaches of plastic and reconstructive surgery, implementing

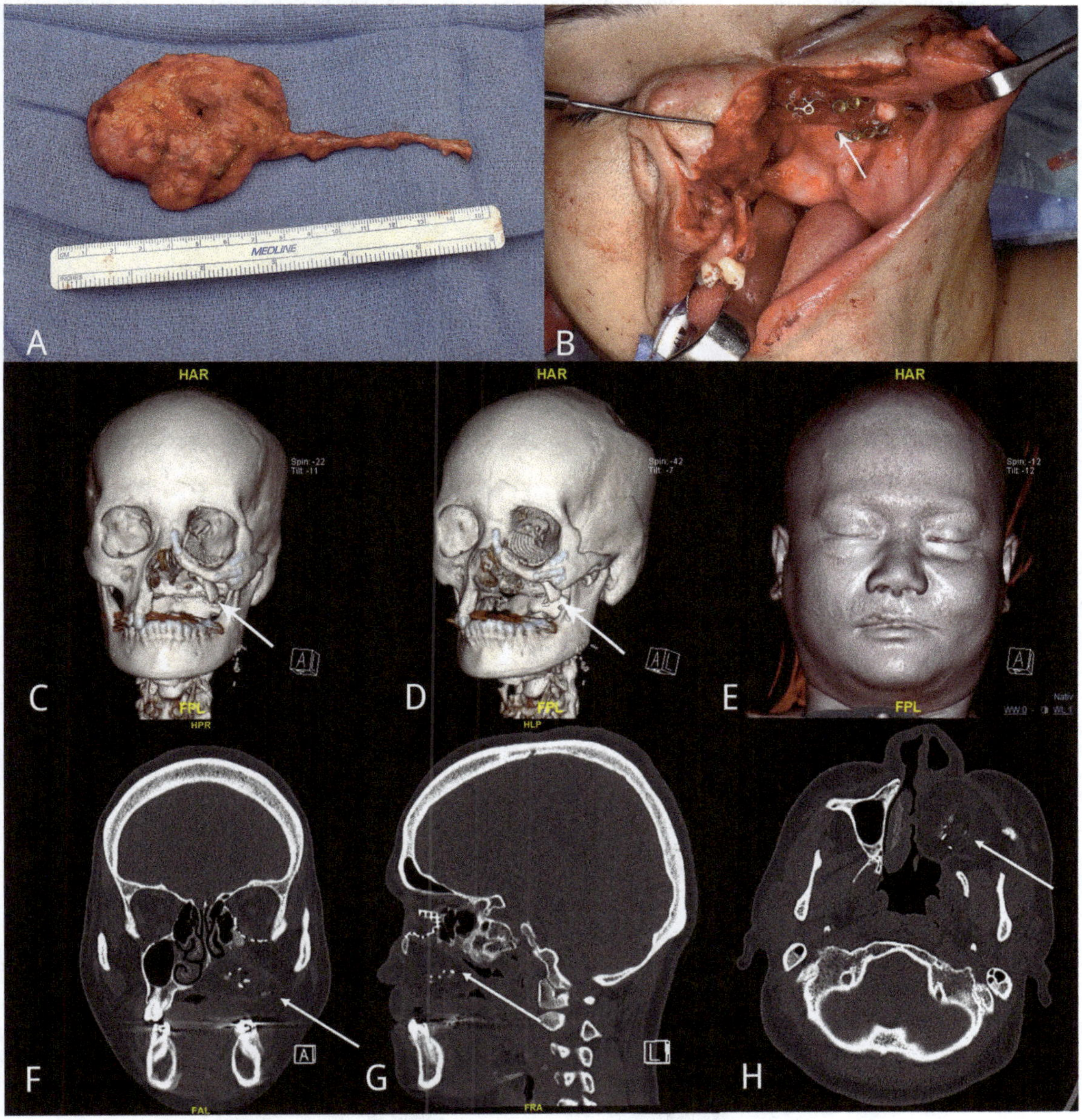

FIGURE 4 | Orthotopic graft transfer and follow-up imaging. Free tissue transfer of the engineered bone-soft tissue composite was performed 9 months after the first step of prefabrication. **(A)** Harvesting of the composite graft, consisting of wrapped latissimus dorsi muscle and the engineered vital bone germ and the AV-bundle. **(B)** Transfacial incision. Exposure of the defect after removal of PEEK implant. **(C, D)** Tabula externa (white arrows) struts served as a substitute for missing bone parts in order to reconstruct the infraorbital rim. **(E)** 3D rendering with symmetric soft tissue coverage. Follow-up CT-imaging 24 months after the orthotopic transfer of the graft from **(F)** coronary, **(G)** sagittal, and **(H)** transverse views. The arrows point to the reconstructed bone tissue present after 24 months.

a "regenerative surgery" paradigm (32). The bone-forming capacity of the engineered graft was based on three traditional osteogenic principles (33), namely, (i) osteoconduction, provided by the allogenic, devitalized scaffolding material, (ii) osteogenesis, through the patient's own osteoprogenitor cells derived from the intraoperatively gained adipose stromal vascular fraction (SVF), and (iii) osteoinduction, through the delivery of BMP-2. The intraoperative tissue engineering approach was substantiated by previous preclinical and clinical studies (4, 5) and bypassed complex, time-consuming and costly *in vitro* cell culture. The engineered graft, ectopically prefabricated with an associated AV bundle, achieved efficient vascularization and bone formation within a confined space. Moreover, its composite nature, including an interface with soft tissues, enabled to restore the patient's anatomical and functional deficit, to provide support to the eye globe, to obliterate the communication between the orbit and the nasopharynx, and to reconstruct the palatal surface.

Table 1 shows in detail the clinical advantages of the developed technique as compared to the expected outcome

TABLE 1 | Comparison of the functional outcome between standard of care with autologous tissue transfer and experimental procedure.

Outcome measures	Experimental procedure (described case)	Standard procedure (%) [Cordeiro PG (16)]	Standard procedure (%) [Moreno MA (17)]	Standard procedure (%) [Sweeny AR (18)]
Speech				
Normal	✓	50	47.5	
Nearly normal	x	34.1	40	
Intelligible	x	13.6	7.5	
Unintelligible	x	2.3	5	
Diet				
Unrestricted	✓	52	55	
Soft	x	42	35	
Liquids	x	6	5	
Feeding tube	x	2	5	
Globe Position and function				
Normal	✓	23.8		
Dystopia	x	4.8		
Diplopia	x	19		8
Enophthalmos	x	4.8		
Ectropion	x	47.6		50
Epiphora	x			29
Exposure keratopathy	x			25
Lagopthalmos	x			16
Fistula	x			8
Midface deformity	x			4
Oral competence				
Yes	✓	91.7		
No	x	8.3		
Drooling	✓			
Microstomia				
Yes	x	25		
No	✓	75		
Aesthetic results				
Excellent	✓	58.6		
Good	x	35.7		
Fair	x	5.7		
Poor	x	0		

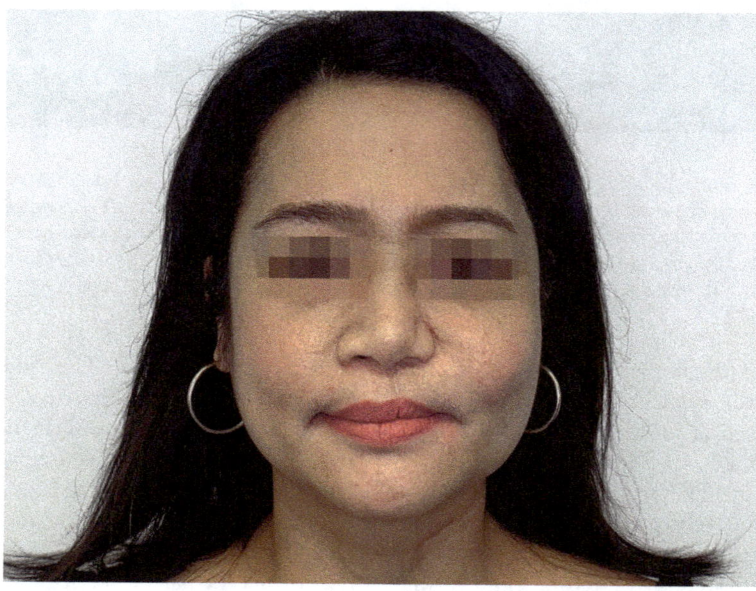

FIGURE 5 | Photographic documentation after reconstruction shows symmetrical and aesthetically pleasing result.

following the standard of care described by Moreno (17), Cordeiro (16), or Sweeney (18). Moreover, in contrast to previously described cases of tissue engineering-based mandibular defect reconstructions, we were able to avoid foreign material (titanium cage), as used by Warnke et al. and Wiltfang et al. (34, 35). By doing so, we avoided not only the postoperative risk of developing an implant-associated infection which, for titanium implants, is reported to be around 7% but also the life-long risk of later hematogenous infection of the implant (36) and the so-called foreign body reactions, where the implant is encapsulated and cannot be integrated with the surrounding tissue (37).

In contrast to previous studies, we used SVF cells from adipose tissue instead of bone-marrow mesenchymal stromal cells (BM-MSC). Adipose stromal cells have recently emerged as a viable source for clinical applications, because of their abundance and easy access. When compared to BM-MSC, SVF cells do require an osteogenic priming, here offered by the BMP2 delivery, but display higher resistance to hypoxia-induced apoptosis and oxidative stress-induced senescence and have more potent proangiogenic activity (38–41).

The main limitation of the developed procedure was a significant resorption of the original scaffold material during the construct prefabrication, so that a sufficient bone stock could not be maintained for dental implants, representing the ultimate solution for mastication and phonation. One possible explanation for the observed resorption might be due to an effect of the supplied BMP-2. Besides their osteoinductive properties, BMPs are known to invoke a seemingly dose-dependent allograft resorption mediated by osteoclasts. Pradhan et al. reported that BMP-2 treatment of a bone graft might cause a higher non-union rate compared with non-treatment, which was attributed to an aggressive bone-resorptive phase prior to osteoinduction (42). Similarly, Vaidya et al. showed that BMP-2-treated bone grafts for spinal fusion lost their original height and structure, likely due to activated bone resorption (43). In addition, Seeherman et al. recently reported that treatment with BMP-2 in a primate bone defect model increased the size of the defect and the number of osteoclasts, so that the expected bone formation was preceded by bone resorption (44). These clinical studies are consistent with experimental evidences that BMP-2 and BMP-7 may reduce bone size by directly or indirectly activating osteoclasts (45). Other possible explanations for the bone resorption observed in the present case could be related to the missing mechanical load during the ectopic prefabrication phase (46) or to the biological influence of the muscle tissue in direct contact with the construct. In fact, it was reported that in calcium sulfate/apatite bone substitutes with direct contact to muscle, the calcium sulfate phase was resorbed after 6 weeks and the hydroxyapatite content decreased significantly over time (47).

Further studies are therefore required to identify the underlying cause of bone resorption and to possibly counteract it. For example, combined anti-resorptive therapies, such as bisphosphonates, have been preclinically validated in a variety of bone repair models, especially to reduce BMP catabolic effects (48–51), and may be considered in future developments. More bone mass would allow the patient to receive tooth implants after the primary procedure and without need of additional bone transfer to the defect site.

Despite this limitation, the engineered graft and its surgical implementation achieved a separation between the oral and nasal cavities in the setting of a critical maxilla defect and provided structural support to the orbital floor. This was of substantial benefit to the patient, without drawbacks of free vascularized autologous bone grafting procedures or foreign body implantation. The clinical case thus represents a proof of principle for a "regenerative surgery"-based prefabrication concept and warrants consideration for reconstruction of complex composite defects in functionally and aesthetically highly demanding areas.

AUTHOR CONTRIBUTIONS

TI and AH were responsible for the conception and design, acquisition of data, analysis and interpretation of data, and writing and revision of the manuscript. TI, AH, DS, AL, AK, FT, CK, and CJ performed the surgery. AL, RO, AK, FT, and FS contributed to the analysis and interpretation of data and revision of the manuscript. JB conceived and designed the analysis, collected the data, and contributed data or analysis tools. TW and FK contributed to the conception and design, acquisition of data, and analysis and interpretation of data. AS, DS, and IM provided senior advice, counseling, writing support, and revision of the manuscript. AW and SM provided conception and design and regulatory aspects. All authors contributed to the article and approved the submitted version.

REFERENCES

1. Järvinen S, Suojanen J, Kormi E, Wilkman T, Kiukkonen A, Leikola J, et al. The Use of Patient Specific Polyetheretherketone Implants for Reconstruction of Maxillofacial Deformities. *J Cranio-Maxillofac Surg* (2019) 47:1072–6. doi: 10.1016/j.jcms.2019.03.018
2. Alonso-Rodriguez E, Cebriàn JL, Nieto MJ, Del Castillo JL, Hernàndez-Godoy J, Burgueño M. Polyetheretherketone Custom-Made Implants for Craniofacial Defects: Report of 14 Cases and Review of the Literature. *J Cranio-Maxillofac Surg* (2015) 43:1232–8. doi: 10.1016/j.jcms.2015.04.028
3. Jonkergouw J, van de Vijfeijken SECM, Nout E, Theys T, Van de Casteele E, Folkersma H, et al. Outcome in Patient-Specific PEEK Cranioplasty: A Two-Center Cohort Study of 40 Implants. *J Cranio-Maxillofac Surg* (2016) 44:1266–72. doi: 10.1016/j.jcms.2016.07.005
4. Saxer F, Scherberich A, Todorov A, Studer P, Miot S, Schreiner S, et al. Implantation of Stromal Vascular Fraction Progenitors at Bone Fracture Sites: From a Rat Model to a First-In-Man Study. *Stem Cells* (2016) 34:2956–66. doi: 10.1002/stem.2478
5. Mehrkens A, Saxer F, Güven S, Hoffmann W, Müller AM, Jakob M, et al. Intraoperative Engineering of Osteogenic Grafts Combining Freshly Harvested, Human Adipose-Derived Cells and Physiological Doses of Bone Morphogenetic Protein-2. *Eur Cells Mater* (2012) 24:308–19. doi: 10.22203/eCM.v024a22

6. Jeon O, Song SJ, Kang SW, Putnam AJ, Kim BS. Enhancement of Ectopic Bone Formation by Bone Morphogenetic Protein-2 Released From a Heparin-Conjugated Poly(L-Lactic-Co-Glycolic Acid) Scaffold. *Biomaterials* (2007) 28:2763–71. doi: 10.1016/j.biomaterials.2007.02.023
7. Ismail T, Osinga R, Todorov AJ, Haumer A, Tchang LA, Epple C, et al. Engineered, Axially-Vascularized Osteogenic Grafts From Human Adipose-Derived Cells to Treat Avascular Necrosis of Bone in a Rat Model. *Acta Biomater* (2017) 63:236–45. doi: 10.1016/j.actbio.2017.09.003
8. Epple C, Haumer A, Ismail T, Lunger A, Scherberich A, Schaefer DJ, et al. Prefabrication of a Large Pedicled Bone Graft by Engineering the Germ for *De Novo* Vascularization and Osteoinduction. *Biomaterials* (2019) 192:118–27. doi: 10.1016/j.biomaterials.2018.11.008
9. Tanaka Y, Sung K-C, Tsutsumi A, Ohba S, Ueda K, Morrison W. Tissue Engineering Skin Flaps: Which Vascular Carrier, Arteriovenous Shunt Loop or Arteriovenous Bundle, has More Potential for Angiogenesis and Tissue Generation? *Plast Reconstr Surg* (2003) 112:1636–44. doi: 10.1097/01.PRS.0000086140.49022.AB
10. Erol OO, Sira M. New Capillary Bed Formation With a Surgically Constructed Arteriovenous Fistula. *Plast Reconstr Surg* (1980) 66:109–15. doi: 10.1097/00006534-198007000-00021
11. Pribaz JJ, Fine NA. Prefabricated and Prelaminated Flaps for Head and Neck Reconstruction. *Clin Plast Surg* (2001) 28:261–+. doi: 10.1016/S0094-1298(20)32362-2
12. Halvorson EG, Cordeiro PG, Disa JJ, Wallin EF, Mehrara BJ. Superficial Temporal Recipient Vessels in Microvascular Orbit and Scalp Reconstruction of Oncologic Defects. *J Reconstr Microsurg* (2009) 25:383–7. doi: 10.1055/s-0029-1220859
13. Disa JJ, Cordeiro PG. Mandible Reconstruction With Microvascular Surgery. *Semin Surg Oncol Vol* (2000) 19:226–34. doi: 10.1002/1098-2388(200010/11)19:3<226::AID-SSU4>3.0.CO;2-N
14. Okay DJ, Genden E, Buchbinder D, Urken M. Prosthodontic Guidelines for Surgical Reconstruction of the Maxilla. *J Prosthet Dent* (2001) 86:352–63. doi: 10.1067/mpr.2001.119524
15. Brown JS, Rogers SN, McNally DN, Boyle M. A Modified Classification for the Maxillectomy Defect. *Head Neck* (2000) 22:17–26. doi: 10.1002/(SICI)1097-0347(200001)22:1<17::AID-HED4>3.0.CO;2-2
16. Cordeiro PG, Chen CM. A 15-Year Review of Midface Reconstruction After Total and Subtotal Maxillectomy: Part I. Algorithm and Outcomes. *Plast Reconstruct Surg* (2012). doi: 10.1097/PRS.0b013e318221dca4
17. Moreno MA, Skoracki RJ, Hanna EY, Hanasono MM. Microvascular Free Flap Reconstruction Versus Palatal Obturation for Maxillectomy Defects. *Head Neck* (2010). doi: 10.1002/hed.21264
18. Sweeney AR, Walker B, Bhrany AD, Chang SH, Jian-Amadi A. Ophthalmic Changes Following Maxillectomy With or Without Postoperative Radiation Therapy. *J Craniofac Surg* (2019). doi: 10.1097/SCS.0000000000005437
19. Andrades P, Militsakh O, Hanasono MM, Rieger J, Rosenthal EL. Current Strategies in Reconstruction of Maxillectomy Defects. *Arch Otolaryngol - Head Neck Surg* (2011) 137:806–12. doi: 10.1001/archoto.2011.132
20. Spiro RH, Strong EW, Shah JP. Maxillectomy and its Classification. *Head Neck* (1997) 19:309–14. doi: 10.1002/(SICI)1097-0347(199707)19:4<309::AID-HED9>3.0.CO;2-4
21. Genden EM, Rinaldo A, Suárez C, Wei WI, Bradley PJ, Ferlito A. Complications of Free Flap Transfers for Head and Neck Reconstruction Following Cancer Resection. *Oral Oncol Vol* (2004) 40:979–84. doi: 10.1016/j.oraloncology.2004.01.012
22. Muñoz-Guerra MF, Naval-Gías L, Capote-Moreno A. Le Fort I Osteotomy, Bilateral Sinus Lift, and Inlay Bone-Grafting for Reconstruction in the Severely Atrophic Maxilla: A New Vision of the Sandwich Technique, Using Bone Scrapers and Piezosurgery. *J Oral Maxillofac Surg* (2009) 67:613–8. doi: 10.1016/j.joms.2008.09.004
23. Momoh AO, Yu P, Skoracki RJ, Liu S, Feng L, Hanasono MM. A Prospective Cohort Study of Fibula Free Flap Donor-Site Morbidity in 157 Consecutive Patients. *Plast Reconstr Surg* (2011) 128:714–20. doi: 10.1097/PRS.0b013e318221dc2a
24. Shpitzer T, Neligan PC, Gullane PJ, Boyd BJ, Gur E, Rotstein LE, et al. The Free Iliac Crest and Fibula Flaps in Vascularized Oromandibular Reconstruction: Comparison and Long-Term Evaluation. *Head Neck* (1999) 21:639–47. doi: 10.1002/(SICI)1097-0347(199910)21:7<639::AID-HED8>3.0.CO;2-T
25. Valentini V, Cassoni A, Marianetti TM, Terenzi V, Fadda MT, Iannetti G. Craniomaxillofacial Fibrous Dysplasia: Conservative Treatment or Radical Surgery? A Retrospective Study on 68 Patients. *Plast Reconstr Surg* (2009) 123:653–60. doi: 10.1097/PRS.0b013e318196bbbe
26. Ling XF, Peng X, Samman N. Donor-Site Morbidity of Free Fibula and DCIA Flaps. *J Oral Maxillofac Surg* (2013) 71:1604–12. doi: 10.1016/j.joms.2013.03.006
27. Arganbright JM, Tsue TT, Girod DA, Militsakh ON, Sykes KJ, Markey J, et al. Outcomes of the Osteocutaneous Radial Forearm Free Flap for Mandibular Reconstruction. *JAMA Otolaryngol - Head Neck Surg* (2013) 139:168–72. doi: 10.1001/jamaoto.2013.1615
28. Werle AH, Tsue TT, Toby EB, Girod DA. Osteocutaneous Radial Forearm Free Flap: Its Use Without Significant Donor Site Morbidity. *Otolaryngol - Head Neck Surg* (2000) 123:711–7. doi: 10.1067/mhn.2000.110865
29. Shnayder Y, Tsue TT, Toby EB, Werle AH, Girod DA. Safe Osteocutaneous Radial Forearm Flap Harvest With Prophylactic Internal Fixation. *Craniomaxillofac Trauma Reconstr* (2011) 4:129–36. doi: 10.1055/s-0031-1279675
30. Zenn MR, Hidalgo DA, Cordeiro PG, Shah JP, Strong EW, Kraus DH. Current Role of the Radial Forearm Free Flap in Mandibular Reconstruction. *Plast Reconstr Surg* (1997) 99:1012–7. doi: 10.1097/00006534-199704000-00014
31. Sinclair CF, Gleysteen JP, Zimmermann TM, Wax MK, Givi B, Schneider D. Assessment of Donor Site Morbidity for Free Radial Forearm Osteocutaneous Flaps. *Microsurgery* (2012) 32:255–60. doi: 10.1002/micr.21950
32. Martin I, Jakob M, Schaefer DJ. From Tissue Engineering to Regenerative Surgery. *EBioMed Vol* (2018) 28:11–2. doi: 10.1016/j.ebiom.2018.01.029
33. Hanna I, Tran H, Swope J, Peleg M. Tissue Engineering Techniques for the Reconstruction of the Atrophic and Local Maxillary Defect. In: *Regenerative Strategies for Maxillary and Mandibular Reconstruction*. Cham: Springer (2019). p. 87–108. doi: 10.1007/978-3-319-93668-0_8
34. Warnke P, Springer I, Wiltfang PJ, Acil PY, Eufinger PH, Wehmöller M, et al. Growth and Transplantation of a Custom Vascularised Bone Graft in a Man. *Lancet* (2004) 364:766–70. doi: 10.1016/S0140-6736(04)16935-3
35. Wiltfang J, Rohnen M, Egberts JH, Lützen U, Wieker H, Açil Y, et al. Man as a Living Bioreactor: Prefabrication of a Custom Vascularized Bone Graft in the Gastrocolic Omentum. *Tissue Eng - Part C Methods* (2016) 22:740–6. doi: 10.1089/ten.tec.2015.0501
36. DeCesare G, Deleyiannis F, Losee J. Reconstruction of Osteomyelitis Defects of the Craniofacial Skeleton. *Semin Plast Surg* (2009) 23:119–31. doi: 10.1055/s-0029-1214164
37. Anderson JM, Rodriguez A, Chang DT. Foreign Body Reaction to Biomaterials. *Semin Immunol Vol* (2008) 20:86–100. doi: 10.1016/j.smim.2007.11.004
38. Ariane Christie S, Kornblith LZ, Howard BM, Conroy AS, Kunitake RC, Nelson MF, et al. Characterization of Distinct Coagulopathic Phenotypes in Injury: Pathway-Specific Drivers and Implications for Individualized Treatment. *J Trauma Acute Care Surg* (2017) 82:1055–62. doi: 10.1097/TA.0000000000001423
39. Yoshimura K, Suga H, Eto H. Adipose-Derived Stem/Progenitor Cells: Roles in Adipose Tissue Remodeling and Potential Use for Soft Tissue Augmentation. *Regen Med* (2009) 4:265–73. doi: 10.2217/17460751.4.2.265
40. Eto H, Suga H, Matsumoto D, Inoue K, Aoi N, Kato H, et al. Characterization of Structure and Cellular Components of Aspirated and Excised Adipose Tissue. *Plast Reconstr Surg* (2009) 124:1087–97. doi: 10.1097/PRS.0b013e3181b5a3f1
41. Fraser JK, Wulur I, Alfonso Z, Hedrick MH. Fat Tissue: An Underappreciated Source of Stem Cells for Biotechnology. *Trends Biotechnol* (2006) 24:150–4. doi: 10.1016/j.tibtech.2006.01.010
42. Pradhan BB, Bae HW, Dawson EG, Patel VV, Delamarter RB. Graft Resorption With the Use of Bone Morphogenetic Protein: Lessons From Anterior Lumbar Interbody Fusion Using Femoral Ring Allografts and Recombinant Human Bone Morphogenetic Protein-2. *Spine (Phila Pa 1976)* (2006) 31:277_84. doi: 10.1097/01.brs.0000216442.12092.01

43. Vaidya R, Weir R, Sethi A, Meisterling S, Hakeos W, Wybo CD. Interbody Fusion With Allograft and rhBMP-2 Leads to Consistent Fusion But Early Subsidence. *J Bone Jt Surg - Ser B* (2007) 89:342–5. doi: 10.1302/0301-620X.89B3.18270
44. Seeherman HJ, Berasi SP, Brown CT, Martinez RX, Sean Juo Z, Jelinsky S, et al. A BMP/activin A Chimera Is Superior to Native BMPs and Induces Bone Repair in Nonhuman Primates When Delivered in a Composite Matrix. *Sci Transl Med* (2019) 11. doi: 10.1126/scitranslmed.aar4953
45. Kamiya N, Ye L, Kobayashi T, Mochida Y, Yamauchi M, Kronenberg HM, et al. BMP Signaling Negatively Regulates Bone Mass Through Sclerostin by Inhibiting the Canonical Wnt Pathway. *Development* (2008) 135:3801–11. doi: 10.1242/dev.025825
46. Huiskes R, Rulmerman R, Van Lenthe GH, Janssen JD. Effects of Mechanical Forces on Maintenance and Adaptation of Form in Trabecular Bone. *Nature* (2000) 405:704–6. doi: 10.1038/35015116
47. Wang J-S, Tagil M, Isaksson H, Bostrom M, Lidgren L. Tissue Reaction and Material Biodegradation of a Calcium Sulfate/Apatite Biphasic Bone Substitute in Rat Muscle. *J Orthop Transl* (2016) 6:10–7. doi: 10.1016/j.jot.2015.11.002
48. Little DG, McDonald M, Bransford R, Godfrey CB, Amanat N. Manipulation of the Anabolic and Catabolic Responses With OP-1 and Zoledronic Acid in a Rat Critical Defect Model. *J Bone Miner Res* (2005) 20:2044–52. doi: 10.1359/JBMR.050712
49. Harding AK, W-Dahl A, Geijer M, Toksvig-Larsen S, Tgil M. A Single Bisphosphonate Infusion Does Not Accelerate Fracture Healing in High Tibial Osteotomies. *Acta Orthop* (2011) 82:465–70. doi: 10.3109/17453674.2011.594231
50. Chen R, Schlossman A, Breuer E, Häagele G, Tillmann C, Van Gelder JM, et al. Long-Chain Functional Bisphosphonates: Synthesis, Anticalcification, and Antiresorption Activity. *Heteroat Chem* (2000) 11:470–9. doi: 10.1002/1098-1071(2000)11:7<470::AID-HC5>3.0.CO;2-P
51. Kamiya N. The Role of BMPs in Bone Anabolism and Their Potential Targets SOST and DKK1. *Curr Mol Pharmacol* (2012) 5:153–63. doi: 10.2174/1874467211205020153

Permissions

All chapters in this book were first published by Frontiers; hereby published with permission under the Creative Commons Attribution License or equivalent. Every chapter published in this book has been scrutinized by our experts. Their significance has been extensively debated. The topics covered herein carry significant findings which will fuel the growth of the discipline. They may even be implemented as practical applications or may be referred to as a beginning point for another development.

The contributors of this book come from diverse backgrounds, making this book a truly international effort. This book will bring forth new frontiers with its revolutionizing research information and detailed analysis of the nascent developments around the world.

We would like to thank all the contributing authors for lending their expertise to make the book truly unique. They have played a crucial role in the development of this book. Without their invaluable contributions this book wouldn't have been possible. They have made vital efforts to compile up to date information on the varied aspects of this subject to make this book a valuable addition to the collection of many professionals and students.

This book was conceptualized with the vision of imparting up-to-date information and advanced data in this field. To ensure the same, a matchless editorial board was set up. Every individual on the board went through rigorous rounds of assessment to prove their worth. After which they invested a large part of their time researching and compiling the most relevant data for our readers.

The editorial board has been involved in producing this book since its inception. They have spent rigorous hours researching and exploring the diverse topics which have resulted in the successful publishing of this book. They have passed on their knowledge of decades through this book. To expedite this challenging task, the publisher supported the team at every step. A small team of assistant editors was also appointed to further simplify the editing procedure and attain best results for the readers.

Apart from the editorial board, the designing team has also invested a significant amount of their time in understanding the subject and creating the most relevant covers. They scrutinized every image to scout for the most suitable representation of the subject and create an appropriate cover for the book.

The publishing team has been an ardent support to the editorial, designing and production team. Their endless efforts to recruit the best for this project, has resulted in the accomplishment of this book. They are a veteran in the field of academics and their pool of knowledge is as vast as their experience in printing. Their expertise and guidance has proved useful at every step. Their uncompromising quality standards have made this book an exceptional effort. Their encouragement from time to time has been an inspiration for everyone.

The publisher and the editorial board hope that this book will prove to be a valuable piece of knowledge for researchers, students, practitioners and scholars across the globe.

List of Contributors

Yang Wang, Xingzhou Qu, Junjian Jiang, Jian Sun, Chenping Zhan and Yue He
Department of Oral & Maxillofacial-Head & Neck Oncology, Shanghai Ninth People's Hospital, Shanghai Jiaotong University School of Medicine, Shanghai, China
National Clinical Research Center for Oral Diseases, Shanghai Key Laboratory of Stomatology & Shanghai Research Institute of Stomatology, Shanghai, China
Shanghai Key Laboratory of Stomatology, Shanghai Research Institute of Stomatology, Shanghai, China

Axel Sahovaler
Department of Otolaryngology-Head and Neck Surgery/Surgical Oncology, Princess Margaret Cancer Centre/University Health Network, Toronto, ON, Canada,
Guided Therapeutics (GTx) Program, Techna Institute, University Health Network, Toronto, ON, Canada

Harley H. L. Chan
Guided Therapeutics (GTx) Program, Techna Institute, University Health Network, Toronto, ON, Canada

Tommaso Gualtieri
Department of Otolaryngology-Head and Neck Surgery/Surgical Oncology, Princess Margaret Cancer Centre/University Health Network, Toronto, ON, Canada
Guided Therapeutics (GTx) Program, Techna Institute, University Health Network, Toronto, ON, Canada
Unit of Otorhinolaryngology-Head and Neck Surgery, University of Brescia-ASST "Spedali Civili diBrescia, Brescia, Italy

Michael Daly
Guided Therapeutics (GTx) Program, Techna Institute, University Health Network, Toronto, ON, Canada

Marco Ferrari
Department of Otolaryngology-Head and Neck Surgery/Surgical Oncology, Princess Margaret Cancer Centre/University Health Network, Toronto, ON, Canada
Guided Therapeutics (GTx) Program, Techna Institute, University Health Network,

Toronto, ON, Canada
Unit of Otorhinolaryngology-Head and Neck Surgery, University of Brescia-ASST "Spedali Civili di

Brescia, Brescia, Italy
Section of Otorhinolaryngology-Head and Neck Surgery, University of Padua-Azienda Ospedaliera di Padova, Padua, Italy

Claire Vannelli
Guided Therapeutics (GTx) Program, Techna Institute, University Health Network Toronto, ON, Canada

Donovan Eu
Department of Otolaryngology-Head and Neck Surgery/Surgical Oncology, Princess Margaret Cancer Centre/University Health Network, Toronto, ON, Canada
Guided Therapeutics (GTx) Program, Techna Institute, University Health Network, Toronto, ON, Canada

Mirko Manojlovic-Kolarski, Susannah Orzell, John R. de Almeida and David P. Goldstein
Department of Otolaryngology-Head and Neck Surgery/Surgical Oncology, Princess Margaret Cancer Centre/University Health Network, Toronto, ON, Canada

Alberto Deganello
Unit of Otorhinolaryngology-Head and Neck Surgery, University of Brescia-ASST "Spedali Civili di Brescia, Brescia, Italy

Piero Nicolai
Section of Otorhinolaryngology-Head and Neck Surgery, University of Padua-Azienda Ospedaliera di Padova, Padua, Italy

Ralph W. Gilbert
Department of Otolaryngology-Head and Neck Surgery/Surgical Oncology, Princess Margaret Cancer Centre/University Health Network, Toronto, ON, Canada

Jonathan C. Irish
Department of Otolaryngology-Head and Neck Surgery/Surgical Oncology, Princess Margaret Cancer Centre/University Health Network, Toronto, ON, Canada
Guided Therapeutics (GTx) Program, Techna Institute, University Health Network,Toronto, ON, Canada

Mónica García-Sevilla, Rafael Moreta-Martinez and David García Mato
Departamento de Bioingeñierıa e Ingeñierıa Aeroespacial, Universidad Carlos III de Madrid, Madrid, Spain
Instituto de Investigación Sanitaria Gregorio Marañón, Madrid, Spain

Gema Arenas de Frutos, Santiago Ochandiano and Carlos Navarro-Cuéllar
Instituto de Investigacio´n Sanitaria Gregorio Maraño´ n, Madrid, Spain
Servicio de Cirug´ıa Oral y Maxilofacial, Hospital General Universitario Gregorio Maraño´ n, Madrid, Spain

Guillermo Sanjuán de Moreta
Instituto de Investigacio´ n Sanitaria Gregorio Maraño ´ n, Madrid, Spain
Servicio de Otorrinolaringolog´ıa, Hospital General Universitario Gregorio Maraño´ n, Madrid, Spain

Javier Pascau
Departamento de Bioingenier´ıa e Ingenier´ıa Aeroespacial, Universidad Carlos III de Madrid, Madrid, Spain
Instituto de Investigacio´ n Sanitaria Gregorio Maraño´ n, Madrid, Spain

Santiago Ochandiano
Servicio de Cirug´ıa Oral y Maxilofacial, Hospital General Universitario Gregorio Maraño´ n, Madrid, Spain
Instituto de Investigacio´ n Sanitaria Gregorio Maraño´ n, Madrid, Spain

David García-Mato, Alba Gonzalez-Alvarez, Javier Pascau and Rafael Moreta-Martinez
Departamento de Bioingenier´ıa e Ingenier´ıa Aeroespacial, Universidad Carlos III de Madrid, Madrid, Spain
Instituto de Investigacio´ n Sanitaria Gregorio Maraño´ n, Madrid, Spain

Hongyang Ma, Sohaib Shujaat, Jeroen Van Dessel, Yi Sun, Constantinus Politis and Michel Bila
OMFS IMPATH Research Group, Department of Imaging & Pathology, Faculty of Medicine, KU Leuven, Leuven, Belgium
Department of Oral and Maxillofacial Surgery, University Hospitals Leuven, Leuven, Belgium

Jan Vranckx
Department of Plastic, Reconstructive, and Aesthetic Surgery, University Hospitals Leuven, Leuven, Belgium

Reinhilde Jacobs
OMFS IMPATH Research Group, Department of Imaging & Pathology, Faculty of Medicine, KU Leuven, Leuven, Belgium
Department of Oral and Maxillofacial Surgery, University Hospitals Leuven, Leuven, Belgium
Department of Dental Medicine, Karolinska Institutet, Stockholm, Sweden

Caterina Giannitto
Department of Diagnostic Radiology, Humanitas Clinical and Research Center Istituti di Ricovero e Cura a Carattere Scientifico (IRCCS), Milan, Italy

Giuseppe Mercante
Otorhinolaryngology Unit, Humanitas Clinical and Research Centre Istituti di Ricovero e Cura a Carattere Scientifico (IRCCS), Milan, Italy
Department of Biomedical Sciences, Humanitas University, Milan, Italy

Luca Disconzi
Department of Diagnostic Radiology, Humanitas Clinical and Research Center Istituti di Ricovero e Cura a Carattere Scientifico (IRCCS), Milan, Italy
Department of Biomedical Sciences, Humanitas University, Milan, Italy

Riccardo Boroni
Department of Supply Chain, Humanitas Clinical and Research Center Istituti di Ricovero e Cura a Carattere Scientifico (IRCCS), Rozzano, Milan, Italy

Elena Casiraghi
Department of Computer Science (DI), Università degli Studi di Milano, Milan, Italy

Federica Canzano, Michele Cerasuolo and Francesca Gaino
Otorhinolaryngology Unit, Humanitas Clinical and Research Centre Istituti di Ricovero e Cura a Carattere Scientifico (IRCCS), Milan, Italy

Paolo Oliva
Department of Supply Chain, Humanitas Clinical and Research Center Istituti di Ricovero e Cura a Carattere Scientifico (IRCCS), Rozzano, Milan, Italy

Flavio Ronzoni
Department of Biomedical Sciences, Humanitas University, Milan, Italy

Luigi Terracciano
Department of Biomedical Sciences, Humanitas University, Milan, Italy
Department of Pathology, Humanitas Clinical and Research Center Istituti di Ricovero e Cura a Carattere Scientifico (IRCCS), Milan, Italy

Giuseppe Spriano
Otorhinolaryngology Unit, Humanitas Clinical and Research Centre Istituti di Ricovero e Cura a Carattere Scientifico (IRCCS), Milan, Italy
Department of Biomedical Sciences, Humanitas University, Milan, Italy

Luca Balzarini
Department of Diagnostic Radiology, Humanitas Clinical and Research Center Istituti di Ricovero e Cura a Carattere Scientifico (IRCCS), Milan, Italy

Konstantin S. Yashin, Anton Yu,. Ermolaev and Mikhail V. Ostapyuk
Department of Oncology and Neurosurgery, Institute of Traumatology and Orthopedics, Privolzhsky Research Medical University, Nizhny Novgorod, Russia

Marina V. Rasteryaeva
Department of Radiation Diagnostics, Institute of Traumatology and Orthopedics, Privolzhsky Research Medical University, Nizhny Novgorod, Russia

Sergey G. Mlyavykh
Institute of Traumatology and Orthopedics, PrivolzhskyResearch Medical University, Nizhny Novgorod, Russia

Marina A. Kutlaeva
Department of Radiation Diagnostics, Institute of Traumatology and Orthopedics, Privolzhsky Research Medical University, Nizhny Novgorod, Russia

Sergey G. Mlyavykh
Institute of Traumatology and Orthopedics, Privolzhsky Research Medical University, Nizhny Novgorod, Russia

Igor A. Medyanik
Department of Oncology and Neurosurgery, Institute of Traumatology and Orthopedics, Privolzhsky Research Medical University, Nizhny Novgorod, Russia

Rong Yang, Chenyao Li and Tong Ji
Shanghai Key Laboratory of Stomatology/Shanghai Institute of Stomatology, Department of Oral and Maxillofacial Head and Neck Oncology, National Clinical Research Center for Oral Diseases, School of Medicine, The Ninth People's Hospital, Shanghai Jiao Tong University, Shanghai, China

Puxun Tu and Xiaojun Chen
School of Mechanical and Engineering, Shanghai Jiaotong University, Shanghai, China

Abdelrehem Ahmed
Department of Craniomaxillofacial and Plastic Surgery, Faculty of Dentistry, Alexandria University, Alexandria, Egypt

Thanh Tu Ha and Dominik Cordier
Department of Neurosurgery, University Hospital Basel, Basel, Switzerland

Florian M. Thieringe
Department of Oral and Cranio-Maxillofacial Surgery, University Hospital Basel, Basel, Switzerland Medical Additive Manufacturing Research Group, Department of Biomedical Engineering, University of Basel, Allschwil, Switzerland

Martin Bammerlin
Advanced Osteotomy Tools AG, Basel, Switzerland

Henriette L. Möllmann, Laura Apeltrath, Nadia Karnatz, Max Wilkat, Erik Riedel, Daman Deep Singh and Majeed Rana
Department of Oral and Maxillofacial Surgery, University Hospital Duesseldorf, Duesseldorf, Germany

Wang-yong Zhu, Wing Shan Choi, May Chun Mei Wong, Jingya Jane Pu, Wei-fa Yang and Yu-xiong Su
Division of Oral and Maxillofacial Surgery, Faculty of Dentistry, The University of Hong Kong, Hong Kong, SAR China

Jane J. Pu, Wing Shan Choi, Wei-fa Yang, Wang-yong Zhu and Yu-xiong Su
Division of Oral and Maxillofacial Surgery, Faculty of Dentistry, The University of Hong Kong, Hong Kong, Hong Kong SAR, China

Philippe Korn, Nils-Claudius Gellrich, Philipp Jehn, Simon Spalthoff and Björn Rahlf
Department of Oral and Maxillofacial Surgery, Hannover Medical School, Hannover, Germany

Raúl Antúnez-Conde, José Ignacio Salmerón, Alberto Díez Montiel, Marc Agea, Dafne Gascón, Ángela Sada, Ignacio Navarro Cuéllar, Manuel Tousidonis, Santiago Ochandiano, Gema Arenas and Carlos Navarro Cuéllar
Maxillofacial Surgery Department, Hospital General Universitario Gregorio Marañoˊ n, Madrid, Spain

Michael Knitschke, Anna Katrin Baumgart Christina Bäcker, Daniel Schmermund, Sebastian Böttger, Philipp Streckbein, Hans-Peter Howaldt and Sameh Attia
Department of Oral and Maxillofacial Surgery, Justus-Liebig-University, Giessen, Germany

Christian Adelung and Fritz Roller
Department of Diagnostic and Interventional Radiology and Pediatric Radiology, Justus-Liebig-University, Giessen, Germany

Jie Chen Ruipu Zhang, Ye Liang, Yujie Ma, Saiwen Song and Canhua Jiang
Department of Oral and Maxillofacial Surgery, Center of Stomatology, Xiangya Hospital, Central South University, Changsha, China
Research Center of Oral and Maxillofacial Tumor, Xiangya Hospital, Central South University, Changsha, China
Institute of Oral Cancer and Precancerous Lesions, Central South University, Changsha, China

Lucas M. Ritschl, Paul Kilbertus, Florian D. Grill, Matthias Schwarz, Markus Nieberler, Klaus-Dietrich Wolff and Andreas M. Fichter
Department of Oral and Maxillofacial Surgery, School of Medicine, Technical University of Munich, Klinikum rechts der Isar, Munich, Germany

Jochen Weitz
Department of Oral and Maxillofacial Surgery, School of Medicine, Technical University of Munich, Klinikum rechts der Isar, Munich, Germany
Department of Oral and Maxillofacial Surgery, Josefinum, Augsburg and Private Practice Oral and Maxillofacial Surgery im Pferseepark, Augsburg, Germany

Stefano Taboni
Department of Otolaryngology—Head and Neck Surgery/Surgical Oncology, Princess Margaret Cancer Centre, University Health Network, Toronto, ON, Canada
Section of Otorhinolaryngology—Head and Neck Surgery, Department of Neurosciences, University of Padua—"Azienda Ospedaliera di Padova", Padua, Italy
Guided Therapeutics (GTx) Program, Techna Institute, University Health Network, Toronto, ON, Canada University Health Network (UHN) Guided Therapeutics (GTx) Program International Scholar, Toronto, ON, Canada
Artificial Intelligence in Medicine and Innovation in Clinical Research and Methodology (PhD Program), Department of Clinical and Experimental Sciences, University of Brescia, Brescia, Italy

Marco Ferrari
Department of Otolaryngology—Head and Neck Surgery/Surgical Oncology, Princess Margaret Cancer Centre, University Health Network, Toronto, ON, Canada
Section of Otorhinolaryngology—Head and Neck Surgery, Department of Neurosciences, University of Padua—"Azienda Ospedaliera di Padova", Padua, Italy
Guided Therapeutics (GTx) Program, Techna Institute, University Health Network, Toronto, ON, Canada
University Health Network (UHN) Guided Therapeutics (GTx) Program International Scholar, Toronto, ON, Canada
Technology for Health (PhD Program), Department of Information Engineering, University of Brescia, Brescia, Italy

Michael J. Daly and Harley H. L. Chan
Guided Therapeutics (GTx) Program, Techna Institute, University Health Network, Toronto, ON, Canada

Donovan Eu
Department of Otolaryngology—Head and Neck Surgery/Surgical Oncology, Princess Margaret Cancer Centre, University Health Network, Toronto, ON, Canada

Tommaso Gualtieri
Department of Otolaryngology—Head and Neck Surgery/Surgical Oncology, Princess Margaret Cancer Centre, University Health Network, Toronto, ON, Canada
Guided Therapeutics (GTx) Program, Techna Institute, University Health Network, Toronto, ON, Canada
Unit of Otorhinolaryngology—Head and Neck Surgery, Department of Medical and Surgical Specialties, Radiologic Sciences, and Public Health, University of Brescia—"ASST Spedali Civili di Brescia", Brescia, Italy

Ashok R. Jethwa, John de Almeida and Ralph W. Gilbert
Department of Otolaryngology—Head and Neck Surgery/Surgical Oncology, Princess Margaret Cancer Centre, University Health Network, Toronto, ON, Canada

Axel Sahovaler
Department of Otolaryngology—Head and Neck Surgery/Surgical Oncology, Princess Margaret Cancer Centre, University Health Network, Toronto, ON, Canada
Guided Therapeutics (GTx) Program, Techna Institute, University Health Network, Toronto, ON, Canada
Head & Neck Surgery, University College London Hospital, London, United Kingdom

Andrew Sewell Jonathan C. Irish and John de Almeida
Department of Otolaryngology—Head and Neck Surgery/Surgical Oncology, Princess Margaret Cancer Centre, University Health Network, Toronto, ON, Canada

Wael Hasan and Jonathan C. Irish
Department of Otolaryngology—Head and Neck Surgery/Surgical Oncology, Princess Margaret Cancer Centre, University Health Network, Toronto, ON, Canada
Guided Therapeutics (GTx) Program, Techna Institute, University Health Network, Toronto, ON, Canada

Jimmy Qiu
Guided Therapeutics (GTx) Program, Techna Institute, University Health Network, Toronto, ON, Canada

Laura Cercenelli, Federico Babini and Emanuela Marcelli
eDIMES Lab - Laboratory of Bioengineering, Department of Experimental, Diagnostic and Specialty Medicine, University of Bologna, Bologna, Italy

Giovanni Badiali and Claudio Marchetti
Maxillofacial Surgery Unit, Head and Neck Department, IRCCS Azienda Ospedaliera Universitaria di Bologna, Department of Biomedical and Neuromotor Sciences, Alma Mater Studiorum University of Bologna, Bologna, Italy

Salvatore Battaglia
Maxillofacial Surgery Unit, Policlinico San Marco University Hospital, University of Catania, Catania, Italy

Cheng-Hsien Wu and Han-Chieh Cheng
Oral and Maxillofacial Surgery, Department of Stomatology, Taipei Veterans General Hospital, Taipei, Taiwan
Department of Dentistry, School of Dentistry, National Yang Ming Chiao Tung University, Taipei, Taiwan

Yi-Yun Ho and Tzu-Lun Liu
Oral and Maxillofacial Surgery, Department of Stomatology, Taipei Veterans General Hospital, Taipei, Taiwan

Tzu-Ying Wu
Department of Dentistry, School of Dentistry, National Yang Ming Chiao Tung University, Taipei, Taiwan
Orthodontic and Pediatric Dentistry, Department of Dentistry, Taipei Veterans General Hospital, Taipei, Taiwan

Chieh-Chih Tsai
Department of Ophthalmology, Taipei Veterans General Hospital, Taipei, Taiwan
Department of Ophthalmology School of Medicine, National Yang-Ming Chiao Tung University, Taipei, Taiwan

Max Wilkat, Norbert Kübler and Majeed Rana
Department for Oral & Maxillofacial Surgery, University Hospital Düsseldorf, Düsseldorf, Germany

Tarek Ismail, Alexander Haumer Alexandre Kaempfen and Arnaud Scherberich
Department of Plastic, Reconstructive, Aesthetic and Hand Surgery, University Hospital Basel, Basel, Switzerland
Department of Biomedicine, University Hospital Basel, University of Basel, Basel, Switzerland

Alexander Lunger
Department of Plastic, Reconstructive, Aesthetic and Hand Surgery, University Hospital Basel, Basel, Switzerland

Rik Osinga and Dirk J. Schaefer
Department of Plastic, Reconstructive, Aesthetic and Hand Surgery, University Hospital Basel, Basel, Switzerland
Center for Musculoskeletal Infections, University Hospital Basel, Basel, Switzerland

Franziska Saxer
Department of Orthopedic Surgery, University Hospital Basel, Basel, Switzerland

Anke Wixmerten, Ivan Martin and Sylvie Miot
Department of Biomedicine, University Hospital Basel, University of Basel, Basel, Switzerland

Florian Thieringer, Joerg Beinemann, Christoph Kunz and Claude Jaquiéry
Clinic for Craniomaxillofacial and Oral Surgery, University Hospital Basel, Basel, Switzerland

Thomas Weikert and Felix Kaul
Department of Radiology, University Hospital Basel, Basel, Switzerland

Index